ANTIGEN AND CLONE-SPECIFIC IMMUNOREGULATION

ANNALS OF THE NEW YORK ACADEMY OF SCIENCES
Volume 636

ANTIGEN AND CLONE-SPECIFIC IMMUNOREGULATION

Edited by Richard L. Edelson

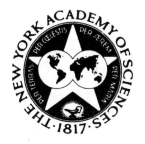

The New York Academy of Sciences
New York, New York
1991

Library of Congress Cataloging-in-Publication Data

Antigen and clone-specific immunoregulation / editor, Richard L. Edelson.
    p. cm. — (Annals of the New York Academy of Sciences; v. 636)
  Includes bibliographical references and index.
  ISBN 0-89766-687-9. — ISBN 0-89766-688-7 (pbk.)
  1. T cells—Congresses. 2. Immune response—Regulation—Congresses. I. Edelson, Richard L. II. Series.
Q11.N5 vol. 636
[QR185.8.T2]
500 s—dc20
[616.07'9]
                                            91-22950
                                                  CIP

Bi-Comp/PCP
Printed in the United States of America
ISBN 0-89766-687-9 (cloth)
ISBN 0-89766-688-7 (paper)
ISSN 0077-8923

ANNALS OF THE NEW YORK ACADEMY OF SCIENCES

Volume 636
December 30, 1991

ANTIGEN AND CLONE-SPECIFIC IMMUNOREGULATION[a]

Editor
RICHARD L. EDELSON

Conference Chairs
RICHARD L. EDELSON AND JONATHAN D. ASHWELL

CONTENTS

---

[a] The papers in this volume were presented at a conference entitled Antigen and Clone-Specific Immunoregulation, which was held by the New York Academy of Sciences in New York City on October 22–24, 1990.

Financial assistance was received from:

Major funders
- THERAKOS
- YALE UNIVERSITY

Supporters
- NATIONAL INSTITUTE OF ALLERGY AND INFECTIOUS DISEASES
- NATIONAL INSTITUTE OF DIABETES AND DIGESTIVE AND KIDNEY DISEASES

Contributors
- AMERICAN CYANAMID COMPANY
- FISONS PHARMACEUTICALS
- GENENTECH, INC.
- MERCK SHARP & DOHME RESEARCH LABORATORIES
- MONSANTO COMPANY
- NATIONAL CANCER INSTITUTE
- PFIZER INC.
- THE R. W. JOHNSON PHARMACEUTICAL RESEARCH INSTITUTE
- SEARLE RESEARCH AND DEVELOPMENT
- STERLING DRUG INC.

Preface

This publication is a compilation of papers delivered at the New York Academy of Sciences Conference on Antigen and Clone-Specific Immunoregulation, held in New York City from October 22 to 24, 1990. The meeting generated substantial interest because of the timeliness and originality of the subject matter, the quality of the internationally recognized speakers, and the interfacing of basic and clinical scientists.

The principal goal of the conference was to place into perspective recent findings which suggest that it may be possible to reduce to clinical practice advances in our understanding of mechanisms of control of aberrant T cells. Normally, the body regulates with great precision the activity of its several million distinct clones of T lymphocytes. This regulation is accomplished on a clone by clone level, with up- and downregulatory signals determining which clones will proliferate, become activated, secrete cytokines and then be appropriately suppressed when no longer needed. This continual fine tuning of the normal immune system is particularly astonishing when one considers that the enormously complex circuitry of the immune system involves, in contrast to that of the nervous system, exceptionally mobile elements capable of great proliferation with which systemic communication must be constantly maintained.

A comparison between the efficiency with which the normal immune system regulates itself and the crudeness of the therapeutic tools with which we deal with diseases caused by undesirably activated T cells is quite sobering. Instead of clone by clone control of these pathogenic T cells, we use such blunt instruments as corticosteroids and antimetabolites, which leads to generalized immunosuppression. Recently, our clinical arsenal has been significantly enhanced by the availability of cyclosporine A, monoclonal anti-T cell subset antibodies, and industrial levels of cytokines. Yet, none of these approaches approximates the precision with which the body regulates its own immune system, and each is associated with major adverse side effects.

Following an introductory session in which we surveyed the means by which the immune system regulates itself, the conference covered three broad topics. Efforts to develop methods to use peptide derivatives of clone-specific T cell receptors to immunize recipients against these clones were discussed in depth. Some success was reported in experimental systems with this approach to the induction of T cells capable of selectively suppressing the activity of the pathogenic T cell clone(s). Whereas this approach is conceptually attractive, it was noted that effective application to the human system remains problematic, since we do not yet know either how many distinct T cell clones are involved in autoimmune diseases or how to identify them, prerequisites for the isolation and purification of the relevant T cell receptor peptides. Nevertheless, the success of this approach in highly defined, artificially produced models of autoimmune disease offers promise with humans.

Methods of producing tolerance to antigens which might be targets of autoreactive immunologic attack were presented. These approaches ranged from experimental shaping of the T cell repertoire to direct induction of tolerance to the antigens themselves. The latter was reported to be successful in certain experimental systems. Applicability to treatment of preexisting human autoimmune disease will require full recognition of the antigens involved.

Provocative clinical responses were described in a malignant proliferation of T cells and in several disorders of T cell immunoregulation by therapies which may involve application of some of the principles investigated in the experimental models. Whereas the mechanisms underlying those clinical responses are not fully established, evidence was presented from several centers that control of individual pathogenic clones of T cells may indeed be possible in the clinical setting with limited side effects.

The interaction between the basic and clinical immunologists was particularly dynamic and productive of a better understanding by both groups of the broad context in which they work. Hopefully, this meeting will encourage the collaboration of these very capable groups as they work towards the common goal of developing precise tools to control disease-causing T cell clones. Optimism is warranted by the progress already made.

RICHARD L. EDELSON

Immunoregulatory Role of γδ T Cells

KEVAN ROBERTS AND ETHAN M. SHEVACH

Laboratory of Immunology
National Institute of Allergy and Infectious Diseases
National Institutes of Health
Building 10, Room 11N315
Bethesda, Maryland 20892

INTRODUCTION

The development of gene cloning technologies such as subtractive hybridization facilitated the isolation in 1984[1,2] of cDNA clones encoding the β-subunit of the T cell receptor (TCR). The same technique was used shortly thereafter to clone a candidate α-chain cDNA clone.[3] Although the deduced amino acid sequence of this latter cDNA had clear similarities to immunoglobulin and the TCR β-chain in structure and sequence, it rapidly became apparent that this cDNA could not encode the TCR α-chain because biochemical studies had demonstrated that α-chains were glycosylated,[4] while the protein deduced from the cDNA contained no consensus sites for asparagine-linked glycosylation. Following the cloning of the authentic TCR α-chain gene in 1985,[5,6] the first α-chain gene was renamed the γ-chain. Expression studies demonstrated that the γ-chain was present at high levels in CD4−, CD8− (double negative, DN) thymocytes.[7] Following the identification in mid-1986 of a T cell subset that expressed a second heterodimeric TCR,[8,9] evidence was quickly obtained that the second chain of this new TCR was not the α- or β-chain. In the summer of 1987, studies of novel genes which were rearranged just upstream of the Jα gene revealed the gene which encoded the TCR δ-chain.[10]

The availability of monoclonal antibodies (mAb) to the γδ TCR of several species has facilitated their isolation and characterization. In man,[11] about 5–10% of peripheral blood T cells express the γδ TCR, while in the mouse about 2–3% of spleen and lymph node cells express this receptor.[12] The γδ T cells are predominantly of the DN phenotype although γδ cells can occasionally be CD8+ and rarely CD4+. Curiously, in the chicken[13] and in the sheep,[14] the proportion of T cells which express the γδ TCR is much higher and can approach 30–40% of total T cells.

One of the most interesting findings with regard to the proposed functional role of γδ T cells is that they appear to be the predominant T cell population in certain localized anatomic sites such as the skin,[15] the intestinal tract,[16] and the vaginal and uterine mucosa.[17] Furthermore, studies of the diversity of the γδ TCR and of the utilization of specific γ and δ gene segments have shown that γδ cells can be subdivided into two populations based on the type of TCR utilized. One population is composed of γδ T cells associated with the skin[18] and with the epithelia of vagina, uterus, and tongue and expresses distinct, but homogenous TCRs.[17] The second population is composed of γδ T cells which localize to peripheral lymphoid tissues and the gut, is generated later in ontogeny, and expresses more diverse TCRs.[19]

1

What is the Function of the γδ TCR?

Although a great deal of information has been accumulated with regard to the molecular and biochemical structure of the γδ TCR, very few conclusions can be drawn at present concerning the role of this unique subpopulation of T cells in immunoregulation. A number of reports have demonstrated that γδ T cells can be alloreactive and can recognize both classical major histocompatibility complex (MHC) class I and class II antigens[20-22] as well as nonclassical MHC antigens such as the products of the TL-region in the mouse[23,34] or the CD1 antigens in man.[25] Although a few reports have shown that γδ T cells can recognize protein or peptide antigens,[26,27] with rare exception the nature of the molecule, if any, which presents the peptide antigen (the restriction element) to the γδ TCR has been very difficult to define. In addition, very little information is available on the possible role of accessory molecules in either the antigen recognition process or in the activation process of γδ T cells. As most γδ cells are DN cells, it remains possible that an as yet undefined cell surface antigen may substitute for CD4/CD8 as an accessory molecule in the process of antigen recognition.

We have been involved for several years in a functional characterization of the γδ T cells which express a dendritic morphology and are found in murine skin

TABLE 1. Effect of Anti-TCR mAbs on IL-4 Production by a Cγ4, Vδ6 T Cell Hybridoma[a]

Culture Conditions	IL-4 Production (CPM × 10⁻³)
Media	70
Anti-CD3 (soluble)	8
Anti-CD3 (plate-bound)	77
Anti-clonotype (soluble)	10

[a] T hybridoma cells (1×10^5) were cultured in media containing FCS in the presence or absence of the indicated anti-TCR mAb in soluble (20 μg/ml) or plate-bound form. Supernatants were collected after 24 hours and assayed for IL-4 content. Results are expressed as CPM and represent ^{3}H-TdR incorporation by the IL-4 dependent CT.4S cells.

(dendritic epidermal T cells, DETC). Although the great majority of murine DETC express the Vγ3Cγ1, Vδ1 TCR,[15,18] we have also isolated a number of T cell lines/clones from the murine epidermis which express the Vγ1.1, Cγ4, Vδ6 TCR.[28] We have attempted to evaluate the activation requirements and growth properties of these cell lines. During the course of studies designed to determine which types of lymphokines are produced by these lines, we made the fortuitous observation[29] that all DETC lines which express the Cγ4, Vδ6 TCR, but not the more common Vγ3, Vδ1 TCR, produced cytokines (IL-4, GM-CSF) spontaneously in culture in the absence of stimulation by an exogenous ligand. Since this observation suggested that a correlation existed between the expression of a particular γδ TCR and spontaneous lymphokine production, we examined the effects of both anti-CD3 and an anti-clonotypic mAb to the TCR expressed by one of these lines and a hybridoma derived from it on IL-4 production (TABLE 1). In the absence of the anti-TCR mAb, high levels of IL-4 were produced; however, in the presence of soluble, but not plate-bound anti-TCR, a marked inhibition of IL-4 production was observed.

The simplest interpretation of these studies was that the soluble anti-TCR mAbs were inhibiting T cell activation by blocking the recognition of antigen present in the culture medium or expressed on the cell surface of the T cells

FIGURE 1. Induction of IL-4 production by FCS. IL-4 produced by the γδ hybridoma which had been adapted for growth in serum-free media was evaluated by incubating the cells for 18 hours in the presence of increasing amounts of FCS. IL-4 content of supernatant was determined by bioassay on IL-4 dependent CT.4S cells. Cells incubated in serum-free media alone produced 2.2 U/ml of IL-4.

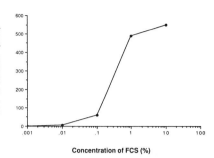

Concentration of FCS (%)

themselves. It is unlikely that mere engagement of the TCR results in inhibition of IL-4 production because plate-bound mAbs did not exert an inhibitory effect. The γδ T cell hybridoma was therefore adapted to serum-free medium in order to assess the possible involvement of antigens present in fetal calf serum (FCS). Supernatants from cells grown in serum-free medium contained no detectable amounts of IL-4, while supplementation of the medium with FCS resulted in dose-dependent IL-4 production (FIG. 1).

The Role of the Vitronectin Receptor (VNR) as an Accessory Molecule for γδ T Cell Activation

Although the studies described above implied that an "antigen" was present in the FCS and that this antigen might be recognized by the γδ TCR, detailed analyses of the components in serum responsible for IL-4 production suggested a number of alternative explanations for the data. One of the major differences between the cells grown serum-free and the cells grown in serum was that the former grew in suspension culture, while the latter grew firmly adherent to the culture vessel. As these observations raised the issue of whether cell adherence was in some way related to cytokine production, we cultured the γδ cell line that had been adapted to serum-free medium on plates coated with a number of extracellular matrix (ECM) proteins (TABLE 2). Surprisingly, culture of the hybridoma on plates coated with FCS, fibronectin, vitronectin, and fibrinogen, but not collagen or bovine serum albumin resulted in the generation of large amounts of IL-4. These findings were not consistent with the hypothesis that the specificity of induction of IL-4 production was mediated by the γδ TCR as these proteins have very little sequence homology, but were in agreement with the specificity of the

TABLE 2. Induction of IL-4 Production by Serum and ECM-Proteins[a]

Coated Plate	IL-4 Production (U/ml)
FCS	1,250
Fibronectin	1,250
Vitronectin	870
Collagen	0
BSA	0

[a] T hybridoma cells which had been adapted to grow in serum-free medium were incubated for 18 hours on plates precoated with FCS or the ECM-proteins indicated. Supernatants were then assayed for IL-4 content on CT.4S cells.

TABLE 3. Properties of the Murine Vitronectin Receptor (VNR)

1. Defined by mAbs H9.2B8 and 8.18E12.
2. Heterodimer consisting of a 140 kD α-chain (reduced 120 kD and 23 kD fragments) noncovalently associated with a 95 kD β-chain. Reactive with antisera to human VNRα and $\beta3$ integrin.
3. Mediated binding to fibronectin, fibrinogen, and vitronectin. Binding inhibited by RGDS, but not RGES. Both mAbs H9.2B8 and 8.18E12 required to inhibit binding.
4. Not expressed on normal thymocytes, LN cells, or spleen cells. Low level expression on 60% of bone marrow cells. Expressed on a high percentage of $\gamma\delta$ and $\alpha\beta$ T cell lines and hybridomas which grow adherent in culture. Inducible on $\alpha\beta$ T cells by chronic (>7 days) activation *in vitro*.

adhesion of this cell line to ECM-proteins mediated by an integrin[30] which has many properties in common with the VNR (TABLE 3). Indeed, the addition of the synthetic peptide RGDS, but not RGES, to plates coated with fibronectin completely inhibited IL-4 production (TABLE 4) in a manner similar to that previously described for inhibition of adherence of this line to the same ECM-protein.[30] The induction of IL-4 production could also be completely inhibited by one of the previously characterized mAbs to this integrin.

Although the ability of RGD-containing ECM-proteins to activate the $\gamma\delta$ hybridoma was mediated by the VNR, engagement of the VNR was not sufficient to induce IL-4 production, as TCR loss mutants of the hybridoma failed to produce IL-4 when stimulated with FCS or ECM-proteins, yet could be induced to produce IL-4 by nonspecific stimulation with ionomycin and phorbol ester (data not shown). This result together with the ability of anti-CD3 to inhibit the response (TABLE 2) strongly suggest that the TCR plays an important role in the induction of IL-4 production.

We have considered three possible explanations for the role of the TCR for VNR-mediated activation of the $\gamma\delta$ hybridoma (FIG. 2, top). One possibility was that the integrin recognizes the RGD sequence in the ECM-protein, while the $\gamma\delta$ TCR recognizes an alternative site in these large molecules. However, this explanation is unlikely because the stimulatory ECM-proteins have very little sequence homology other than RGD and maximal IL-4 production could be induced with a synthetic peptide (Pep Tite 200) which contains only the RGDS cell attachment

TABLE 4. Inhibition of IL-4 Production by Peptides[a]

Culture Conditions	Inhibitor	IL-4 Production (U/ml)
FCS	0	190
	RGDS	0
	RGES	189
	anti-VNR	0
Fibronectin	0	327
	RGDS	0
	RGES	317
	anti-VNR	0

[a] T hybridoma cells grown in serum-free media were cultured for 18 hours in the presence of FCS (10%) or on fibronectin-coated plates. The peptides or the anti-VNR mAb were added to the media at culture initiation. Supernatants were assayed for IL-4 content on CT.4S cells.

sequence and a highly charged sequence of amino acids which facilitate its binding to plastic (data not shown). A second possibility is that activation via the VNR depends on coexpression of the γδ TCR, but that engagement of the TCR by its ligand is not required (FIG. 2, middle). A similar role for the TCR has been postulated for activation of T cells via mAbs to non-TCR cell surface antigens such as Thy-1 and Ly-6.[31] However, this explanation is also unlikely because the

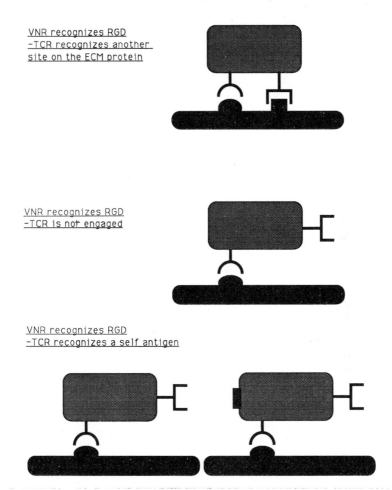

VNR recognizes RGD
-TCR recognizes another
site on the ECM protein

VNR recognizes RGD
-TCR is not engaged

VNR recognizes RGD
-TCR recognizes a self antigen

FIGURE 2. Models for the roles of the γδ TCR and the VNR in the response of the T cell hybridoma to ECM-proteins.

VNR is expressed by many γδ T cell hybridomas and cell lines,[30] yet only those which express the Cγ4, Vδ6 TCR produce cytokines spontaneously.

The hypothesis which is most compatible with our data is that, not only is coexpression of the VNR and TCR required for the induction of IL-4 production, but the TCR must also be engaged by its ligand, most likely a cell surface antigen expressed by the hybridoma itself (FIG. 2, bottom).

Speculations Concerning the Role of Autoreactive γδ T Cells In Vivo

The data presented above strongly favor the view that the combination of Cγ4, and Vδ6 TCR chains results in the expression of a receptor which is likely to recognize an autoantigen. However, the failure of the hybridoma to produce IL-4 in serum-free medium suggests that the reactivity of this TCR for the autoantigen is of the low affinity type and requires the VNR to function as an accessory molecule to produce a high affinity interaction. These results on Cγ4, Vδ6 cells which have been isolated from murine skin confirm and extend the observations of O'Brien et al.[32] who have demonstrated that Cγ4, Vδ6 hybridomas generated from newborn thymocytes are also autoreactive. The nature of the autoantigen recognized by T cells which express the Cγ4, Vδ6 has not been defined.

We are at present considering two distinct, but by no means mutually exclusive, models which will explain the role of this subpopulation of T cells in immunoregulation and which include the possible unique contribution of accessory molecules such as the VNR in their function. First, the studies of O'Brien et al.[32] and Born et al.[33] have convincingly demonstrated that certain hybridomas which bear the Cγ4, Vδ6 TCR in addition to demonstrating a low level of autoreactivity can also be induced to produce IL-2 when stimulated with purified protein derivative (PPD) of *Mycobacterium tuberculosis* and with the mycobacterial heat shock protein, Hsp65. Furthermore, responses have also been obtained with small synthetic peptides derived from mycobacterial Hsp65 and with peptides which contained the homologous (murine) Hsp65 sequence. These results are consistent with the possibility that the true physiologic ligand of these T cells is the bacterial antigen; the reactivity with self Hsp peptides would then represent a crossreaction. The VNR may play a unique role as an accessory molecule for the recognition of bacterial antigens as a number of bacteria have been shown to interact with ECM-proteins.[34] The combined use of certain γδ receptors together with the VNR or other members of the integrin family of ECM-protein receptors may thus be an important mechanism for the generation of host resistance to bacterial antigens. The VNR may prove to play a prominent role in this process as it is a promiscuous integrin which is capable of interacting with one of several ECM proteins.

An alternative view is that the Cγ4, Vδ6 population of T cells is specific for processed peptides of autologous stress proteins and that the reactivity with the mycobacterial peptides represents a crossreaction. In fact, autoreactivity may be the normal function, not only of the Cγ4, Vδ6 subset, but of other γδ cells as Ito et al.[35] have shown that a γδ T cell hybridoma derived from adult thymus recognizes a novel TL-region gene product which has been termed 27[b]. Although the 27[b] molecule may be recognized alone, it may also function as an antigen presenting molecule and present an autoantigen. If other nonclassical MHC antigens function as restriction elements, they may be similarly involved in the presentation of self-peptides. Thus, γδ T cells may play a major role in immunosurveillance and would be particularly important in the recognition of cells modified by tissue damage/injury, carcinogenesis, and chronic infection.

What role would accessory molecules such as the VNR play in this process? Implicit in the hypothesis that γδ T cells are primarily autoreactive is a requirement that the autoreactivity be regulated and at times subverted so as to prevent the induction of autoimmune disease. Regulation of γδ T cell autoreactivity could be most easily accomplished if activation of this T cell subset required the participation of an accessory molecule whose expression or function was finely regulated. The regulation of expression of the VNR, which is only induced after prolonged T cell activation, would serve as an effective means to control the potentially harmful autoreactive T cell. Thus, the resting $\gamma\delta$ cell would be unable to interact with its target ligand because of the low affinity of its TCR; in sites of chronic inflammation or tissue damage, an environment in which the VNR will be induced, the same $\gamma\delta$ T cell would be allowed to interact with self or altered self antigens and mediate its effector functions.

SUMMARY

While the major population of T lymphocytes express T cell receptor (TCR) $\alpha\beta$-chains and recognize peptide antigens in association with either Major Histocompatibility Complex class I or class II molecules, a consensus view does not exist concerning either the nature of the antigen recognized or the nature of the restriction element utilized by the minor population of T cells which express TCR $\gamma\delta$-chains. We have identified a unique subpopulation of $\gamma\delta$ T cells which uniformly express the Cγ4, Vδ6 TCR and which produce a number of cytokines in the absence of exogenous stimulation. Adaption of these cell lines to serum-free culture conditions resulted in a cessation of cytokine production which could then be induced by the addition of extracellular matrix (ECM)-proteins to the culture. The response to the ECM-proteins could be completely inhibited by an antibody to the murine vitronectin receptor (VNR). However, engagement of the VNR by its ligand was not sufficient for the induction of cytokine production as anti-TCR antibodies inhibited the response to ECM-proteins and $\gamma\delta$ TCR loss mutants failed to respond. Collectively, these data demonstrate that not only is coexpression of the VNR and the $\gamma\delta$ TCR required for the induction of cytokine production by this subpopulation of T cells, but that the TCR must also be engaged by its ligand, most likely a cell surface autoantigen expressed by the T cells themselves.

REFERENCES

1. HEDRICK, S. M., D. I. COHEN, E. A. NIELSEN & M. M. DAVIS. 1984. Nature 308: 149–153.
2. YANAGI, Y., Y. YOSHIKAI, K. LEGGETT, S. P. CLARK, I. ALEXANDER & T. W. MAK. 1984. Nature 308: 145–149.
3. SAITO, H., D. M. KRANZ, Y. TAKAGAKI, A. C. HAYDAY & H. N. EISEN. 1984. Nature 309: 757–762.
4. ALLISON, J. P. & L. L. LANIER. 1987. Ann. Rev. Immunol. 5: 503–540.
5. CHIEN, Y. H., D. M. BECKER, T. LINDSTEN, M. OKAMURA, D. I. COHEN & M. M. DAVIS. 1984. Nature 312: 31–35.
6. SAITO, H., D. M. KRANZ, Y. TAKAGAKI, A. C. HAYDAY, H. N. EISEN & S. TONEGAWA. 1984. Nature 312: 36–40.
7. RAULET, D. H., R. D. GARMAN, H. SAITO & S. TONEGAWA. 1985. Nature 314: 103–107.
8. BRENNER, M. B., J. McCLEAN, D. DIALYNAS, J. STROMINGER, J. A. SMITH, F. L. OWEN, J. SEIDMAN, S. IP, F. ROSEN & M. KRANGEL. 1986. Nature 322: 145–149.
9. BANK, I., R. A. DEPINHO, M. B. BRENNER, J. CASSIMERIS, F. W. ALT & L. CHESS. 1986. Nature 322: 179–181.
10. CHIEN, Y., M. IWASHIMA, K. B. KAPLAN, J. F. ELLIOT & M. M. DAVIS. 1987. Nature 327: 677–682.
11. LANIER, L. L., N. A. FEDERSPIEL, J. J. RUITENBERG, J. H. PHILLIPS, J. P. ALLISON, D. LITTMAN & A. WEISS. J. Exp. Med. 165: 1076–1094.
12. CRON, R., F. KONING, W. MALOY, D. PARDOLL, J. COLIGAN & J. BLUESTONE. 1988. J. Immunol. 141: 1074–1082.

13. CHEN, C. H., J. CIHAK, U. LOSCH & M. D. COOPER. 1988. Eur. J. Immunol. **18:** 539–543.
14. MACKAY, C. R., M. F. BEYA & P. MATZINGER. 1989. Eur. J. Immunol. **19:** 1335–1338.
15. KONING, F., G. STINGL, W. M. YOKOYAMA, H. YAMADA, W. L. MALOY, E. TSCHACHLER, E. M. SHEVACH & J. COLIGAN. 1987. Science **236:** 834–837.
16. GOODMAN, T. & L. LEFRANCOIS. 1988. Nature **333:** 855–858.
17. ITOHARA, S., A. G. FARR, J. J. LAFAILLE, M. BONNEVILLE, Y. TAKAGAKI, W. HAAS & S. TONEGAWA. 1990. Nature **343:** 754–757.
18. ASARNOW, D. M., W. A. KUZIEL, M. BONYHADI, R. E. TIGELAAR, P. W. TUCKER & J. P. ALLISON. 1988. Cell **55:** 837–847.
19. RAULET, D. H. 1989. Ann. Rev. Immunol. **7:** 175–207.
20. BLUESTONE, J. A., R. Q. CRON, B. A. COTTERMAN, B. A. HOULDEN & L. A. MATIS. 1988. J. Exp. Med. **168:** 1899–1916.
21. RIVAS, A., J. KOIDE, M. L. CLEARY & E. ENGLEMAN. 1989. J. Immunol. **142:** 1840–1846.
22. MATIS, L. A., A. M. FRY, R. Q. CRON, M. M. COTTERMAN, R. F. DICK & J. A. BLUESTONE. 1989. Science **245:** 746–749.
23. MATIS, L. A., R. CRON & J. A. BLUESTONE. 1987. Nature **330:** 262–264.
24. BONNEVILLE, M., K. ITO, E. G. KRECKO, S. ITOHARA, D. KAPPES, I. ISHIDA, O. KANAGAWA, C. A. JANEWAY, D. B. MURPHY & S. TONEGAWA. 1989. Proc. Natl. Acad. Sci. USA **86:** 5928–5932.
25. PORCELLI, S., M. B. BRENNER, J. L. GREENSTEIN, S. P. BALK, C. TERHORST & P. BLEICHER. 1989. Nature **341:** 447–450.
26. KOZBOR, D., G. TRINCHIERI, D. S. MONOS, M. ISOBE, G. RUSSO, J. HANEY, C. ZMIJEWSKI & C. M. CROCE. 1989. J. Exp. Med. **169:** 1847–1851.
27. VIDOVIC, D., M. ROGLIC, K. MCKUNE, S. GUERDER, C. MACKAY & Z. DEMBIC. 1989. Nature **340:** 646–650.
28. KONING, F., W. M. YOKOYAMA, W. L. MALOY, G. STINGL, T. J. MCCONNELL, D. I. COHEN, E. M. SHEVACH & J. E. COLIGAN. 1988. J. Immunol. **141:** 2057–2062.
29. ROBERTS, K., W. M. YOKOYAMA, P. J. KEHN & E. M. SHEVACH. 1991. J. Exp. Med. **173:** 231–240.
30. MAXFIELD, S. R., K. MOULDER, F. KONING, A. ELBE, G. STINGL, J. E. COLIGAN, E. M. SHEVACH & W. M. YOKOYAMA. 1989. J. Exp. Med. **169:** 2173–2190.
31. SUSSMAN, J. J., T. SAITO, E. M. SHEVACH, R. N. GERMAIN & J. D. ASHWELL. 1988. J. Immunol. **140:** 2520–2526.
32. O'BRIEN, R. L., M. P. HAPP, A. DALLAS, E. PALMER, R. KUBO & W. BORN. Cell **57:** 667–674.
33. BORN, W., L. HALL, A. DALLAS, J. BOYMEL, T. SHINNICK, D. YOUNG, P. BRENNAN & R. O'BRIEN. 1990. Science **249:** 67–69.
34. MOSHER, D. F. & R. A. PROCTOR. 1980. Science **209:** 927–929.
35. ITO, K., L. VAN KAER, M. BONNEVILLE, S. HSU, D. B. MURPHY & S. TONEGAWA. 1990. Cell **62:** 549–561.

T Cell V-Gene Usage in Man in Some Normal and Abnormal Situations[a]

H. WIGZELL,[b] J. GRUNEWALD,[b] M. TEHRANI,[b] S. ESIN,[b]
H. MELLSTEDT,[c] A. ÖSTERBORG,[c] H. DERSIMONIAN,[d]
M. BRENNER,[d] R. ÅHLBERG,[e] A. K. LEFVERT,[e] M. ÖRN,[f]
A. EKLUND,[f] AND C. H. JANSON[b]

[b]Department of Immunology
Karolinska Institute
Box 60 400
S-104 01 Stockholm, Sweden

[c]Department of Oncology
Karolinska Hospital
S-104 01 Stockholm, Sweden

[d]Dana-Farber Cancer Institute
Harvard Medical School
Boston, Massachusetts

[e]Department of Medicine
Karolinska Hospital

[f]Thorax Clinic
Karolinska Hospital

INTRODUCTION

T lymphocytes hold a central position in the regulation and initiation of specific immune responses. They act as effector cells as well as major regulators of other cell types within the immune system, including other T cells. Drawing from an inherent pool of minigene families T lymphocytes generate receptors for antigen allowing a subsequent selection of a population of T cells tailor-made for function in the very same individual. This selection serves as a safeguard against unwanted autoimmune diseases but is not fail proof. The present article will discuss some results and views on how T lymphocytes are selected for specificity, in normal development as well as in certain sets of diseases. Based on these results and experiments obtained in animal systems future prospects for attempted therapy in diseases involving damaging T lymphocytes in man will be elaborated.

Selection of Specific T Cells

The normal generation of T lymphocytes with regard to specificity to a major extent takes place in the thymus. In animal systems it has been clearly shown that

[a] This work was supported by the Swedish Cancer Society, the Swedish Medical Research Council, and by National Institutes of Health Grant AR 39582.

9

elimination of cells with potentially aggressive behavior against self-antigens as well as positive selection for cells with specific reactivity to other self-antigens occurs within the thymus. This is particularly clear for more readily defined effector functions such as helper or killer T cell activities, whereas the selection principles for T cells with specific suppressive consequences for other T cells are largely unsolved. The actual physiological mechanisms underlining the different consequences of having a reaction between the antigen-binding receptor, TcR, on the developing T lymphocyte and specific antigen are as yet speculative. However, an increasing number of observations indicate that a reaction occurring in the absence of additional physiological signals (involving additional adjunct surface molecules and growth factors) may lead to death via apoptosis.[1,2] It would accordingly seem clear that the state of maturation and activation of the T lymphocytes and the actual conditions surrounding the events of antigen-presentation may all have profound consequences whether the signal will be of a positive or negative kind for the individual lymphocyte.

After leaving the thymus the mature T cells now act as thymus-independent cells. This can be exemplified by the fact that administration of low numbers of mature T lymphocytes into thymus-lacking animals will result in the expansion of such T cells into comparatively normal T cell numbers.[3] The maintenance or expansion of normal T cells in the periphery would seem to require accessibility to the corresponding MHC molecules, that is, class II for the CD4 T cells and class I for the CD8 T lymphoctyes.[4,5]

Select Alteration in Adult Animals of T Cell Specificity

Several situations exist in the clinic where a select elimination of a subset of T cells with a particular TcR composition would be advantageous. The most obvious is a condition where malignancy has resulted in T cell leukemia or lymphoma. Here, the TcR molecules on the malignant cells would constitute a "tumor-unique" marker antigen allowing a select attack. The stability of the rearranged TcR genes would here be of significant advantage compared to the corresponding situation in B cells, in particular the failure to display somatic mutations in the variable regions of the TcR genes.[6] Likewise, TcR molecules have a much lower tendency to become soluble compared to Ig molecules. A second condition would be autoimmune diseases with T cell involvement where the corresponding lymphocytes could be identified via a restricted usage of variability conferring genes for their TcRs. A third desire would be to eliminate in a recipient of an organ graft (or a donor of a bone marrow graft) those T lymphocytes having TcRs making them aggressive against the MHC molecules of the other individual.

The first studies attempting to achieve the above principles were initiated in the 70s, that is, before TcRs had been defined at the genetic or structural level.[8] Here, advantage was taken of the use of inbred rats or mice differing at the MHC locus. The initial studies employed F1-hybrids between such strains assuming them to be selectively devoid of T cells with TcRs reactive aggressively against the respective parental MHC molecules.[7] Accordingly, it should be possible to immunize an (AxB)F animal against AxA T cells with TcRs against B strain MHC molecules. The principle was found valid and in occasional animals antibodies were produced having the capacity for selective wipe of A T cells from reacting against B but not a third strain, C, MHC molecules as determined by GvH, MLR or CTL reactions. The studies were subsequently expanded to involve "vaccination" of AxA animals against autologous T blasts previously expanded *in vitro* with specificity for B MHC antigens.[8,9] These latter experiments were extremely demanding requiring large expansions of T blasts *in vitro* coupled with a low frequency of success in initiating the select autoimmune TcR reactivity in the vaccinated animals. However, in the few successful animals the reduced immune response was selective and could be expressed at both antibody and T cell level. Once induced, it behaved like a lifelong select immunosuppression. TABLE 1 provides a summary of conclusions drawn on our earlier data in these systems. Several other groups have since performed similar studies, mostly in autoimmune systems with, in principle, the same kind of results (see reports in this volume).

With the new knowledge of TcR genetics and structure it has now become possible to approach the possibility of elimination of certain TcR-positive T cells in a much more succinct from than was possible using as immuno-gen T lymphocytes or blasts. As this is covered in more detail later in this section, we shall only briefly comment on some animal studies done so far. We are aware of one successful attempt to eliminate animal T cell-tumors via an attack on the TcRs they express.[10] In autoimmune systems there are a few excellent reports where knowledge on TcR usage has been useful in the elimination of a capacity to develop a defined autoimmune disease.[11,12] In mice and rats V-beta 8 is predominant in the T

TABLE 1. Early Studies on Specific T Cell Regulation Using Immune Reactions Directed against TCR Epitopes

System
Reduction in specific MHC reactivity in rodents (Andersson, Binz, Häyry, Lindenmann, Wigzell)
Features
Low frequency of success
Physical elimination of idiotypic T cells
Actively induced: life-long suppression
Passively induced: Recovery with time
No side effects

cells involved in allergic encephalomyelitis. In mice, this made it possible to eliminate the capacity of V-beta 8-antibody treated animals to develop this disease.[11] In rats, the usage of a V-beta 8-specific 21 aminoacid long peptide such as immunogen allowed the induction of an autoimmune process eliminating the ability of such animals to subsequently develop the disease upon immunization with brain antigen.[12] In transplantation systems a similar elegant study has been carried out in a particular rat strain combination where a majority of the T cells involved used a singular V-beta gene component.[13] Also here immunization against this V-beta gene product largely eliminated in a select manner the capacity of T cells from such rats to induce GvH-disease in F1-hybrids between these two strains.

In all, the above studies do allow certain statements: a) It is biologically possible to eliminate T cells with a given TcR type via active or passive immunity. This would also indicate that no complete tolerance could be demonstrated against variability-conferring gene products present in autologous TcRs, although some tolerance may exist. b) No significant side effects have so far been noted. In the earlier experiments[7-9] the autoimmunized and selectively immunosuppressed A-anti(A-anti-B) rats were followed for up to one year without any evidence of immune complex disease or susceptibility to other diseases. Still, this question has to be followed in a most careful manner in the future in both human and animal studies, especially as at least the actively induced immunity against subsets of autologous TcR gene products may be lifelong.

Studies on Human TCR-V-Genes Using Monoclonal Antibodies. The "Normal" Distribution of V-Alpha or -Beta Genes

We have for the last few years been involved in the production of monoclonal antibodies against human TcR V-genes and subsequent usage of such antibodies in normal and diseased conditions. Through our work and via collaboration with other scientists and research groups we have at present available B monoclonal antibodies against discrete V-alpha or -beta gene products.[14] They cover altogether around 25% of the total CD3 positive T cell population. In TABLE 2 are shown seven of these antibodies, their presumed reactivity (they may X-react with additional V-gene family members) and reactivity pattern with PBL T cells from a cohort of normal blood donors subdivided into CD3, CD4 and CD8 + T cells.[15] Two findings are worth commenting on: a) There is a skewed distribution amongst some V-genes as to their expression in relation to CD4 or CD8 T cells[15] and b) The range of frequency scatter amongst CD8 cells is much broader than that on CD4 T cells.

V-beta 5.1 can be chosen as displaying clearcut skewing towards CD4 versus CD8 T cell expression. PBL samples from 24 individual blood donors all had V-beta 5.1 at a higher frequency in the CD4 than in the CD8 population. Such a skewed distribution could be due to events in the periphery, that is, selection amongst mature T lymphocytes in relation to exogenous antigens like superantigens of the staphylococcal enterotoxin type.[16] Alternatively, it may represent the consequences of a profound intrathymic selection during normal T cell differentiation. If so, this would represent a phenomenon linked to CD4/CD8 phenotype at the single positive cell and be unlinked to polymorphic MHC determinants as all individuals had a similar degree of biased distribution. The skewed distribution is most unlikely unrelated to exogenous antigens as the same bias is apparent in PBLs from umbilical cord blood and is in fact present already at the level of the thymus (FIG. 1). By analogy with studies in the mouse we would thus deem it likely that this skewed distribution is due to a positive selection of the corresponding subset of maturing T cells in the thymus which is maintained in the periphery.

TABLE 2. TCR MAb Reactivity with CD4$^+$ and CD8$^+$ PBL Lymphocytes in 24 Blood Donors

MAb	% CD4^{+a}	% CD8^{+a}	P	CD4 > CD8^b
β V 5.1	4.8 (1.8–6.1)	1.5 (0.3–3.8)	<0.001	24
β V 5.2 + 5.3	2.2 (1.6–3.5)	2.6 (1.1–15.1)	0.13	11
β V 5.3	0.8 (0.4–1.6)	0.8 (0.2–13.2)	0.76	12
β V 6	4.4 (0.3–8.8)	1.2 (0.0–12.3)	<0.001	21
β V 8	4.7 (3.1–15.7)	3.1 (1.4–9.3)	<0.001	20
β V 12	1.9 (0.2–2.4)	1.2 (0.5–2.1)	<0.001	20
α V 2.3	3.5 (2.3–5.5)	3.1 (0.6–10.1)	0.31	12

[a] Numbers represent median values. Minimum and maximum values are shown within parentheses.

[b] Figures represent number of individuals (total = 24) with higher reactivity of anti-TCR% MAb within the CD4$^+$ compared to the CD8$^+$ subpopulation.

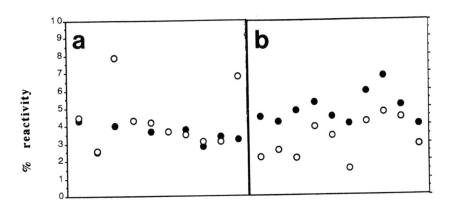

Paired individual observations

FIGURE 1. Reactivity of α V 2.3 **(a)** and β V 5.1 **(b)** in CD4+ CD8− (●) and CD4− CD8+ (○) thymocytes.

With other V-genes showing a biased expression in PBLs of adults the same bias was found at the level of umbilical cord and thymus (data not shown). Likewise, V-genes that in PBL failed to show any biased expression as to CD4/CD8 subsets also failed to show skewed distribution in umbilical cord or thymus T cells.

The second observation, the relatively wider range scatter of CD8 T cells expanding in particular into the higher ranges, would suggest that it is normal for CD8 T cells to undergo more dramatic expansions (and retractions) than CD4 T cells at the "clonal" level in healthy individuals.

TCR V-Gene Distribution in Certain Diseases

An abnormal distribution of human TcR-V genes in T cell populations can be demonstrated by other techniques than monoclonal antibodies such as quantitative PcR.[16] However, monoclonal antibodies have the advantage that they may also serve as tools for enrichment or depletion of select V-gene TcR-types within a T cell population. We have concentrated our studies on three types of diseases in man: a) T cell malignancies; b) B cell malignancies and c) Autoimmune diseases or diseases with T cell involvement but unknown etiology. Our approach would by necessity be better in discovering positively selected cells (expanded "clones") than the opposite, deleted T cells.

Usage of FCR-V-Gene-Specific Antibodies in T Cell Tumor Therapy?

Our primary aim when starting to produce TcR-specific monoclonal antibodies was to use them for the treatment of T cell leukemias.[17] So far, we have only been able to begin to treat a single T cell leukemia patient with a TcR-specific monoclonal antibody.[18] Despite the failure to be able to finish that treatment schedule (the patient had an unrelated heart condition and developed a coronary infarction

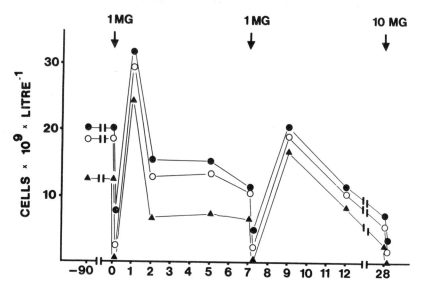

FIGURE 2. Consequences of administration of a monoclonal antibody directed against human v-alpha 2.3 to a patient with a T cell alpha 2.3 positive leukemia. X-axis = time in days. ○ = total white blood cells; ● = total lymphocyte counts; ▲ = alpha-2.3 positive leukemia cells. The monoclonal antibody was administered i.v. in doses indicated. (Data from Janson et al.[18])

between the 2nd and 3rd treatment with antibody) the results are very encouraging. The results of this treatment are summarized in FIG. 2. It can be seen that administration of a total of 2 × 1 mg of monoclonal antibodies (IgG2a) spaced over a 2-week period resulted in a specific elimination of the T cell leukemia cells amounting to close to 80% of the leukemia cells in PBL 4 weeks after initiation of therapy. A major conclusion to be drawn is that the efficiency of antibodies against V-gene products on malignant T cells is much higher than previously found when attempting to treat human B cell malignancies.[19] An additional finding worth commenting upon is the fact that the T cell leukemia numbers continued to fall after any evidence of residual monoclonal antibody could be demonstrated. This suggests the possibility that antibody treatment may have induced an active immune response against the patient's leukemia cells although we have no proof for such an assumption.

The lymphoid system is known to contain an intricate set of networks between the various lymphocyte subsets. In B cell malignancies in man there have been reports on a parallel appearance of oligoclonal T cells in some myeloma patients as determined by RNA/DNA technology.[20,21] Our data[14] confirm and expand these data to show that a) probably all myeloma patients have oligo- or mono-clonal T cells and b) that in PBLs from individual patients dramatic expansions of single TcR V-gene expressions could be demonstrated at the CD4 or CD8 T cell level as shown in TABLE 3. Such T cell "clonality" could also be shown to exist at supposed premalignant B cell conditions such as MGUS (Monoclonal Gammopathy of Unknown Significance). The reason for the positive selection of these "clonal" T cells most likely resides at the level of specific reactions via their TcRs. It is not clear, however, whether their presence is good or bad for the patient. The fact that they can be found in MGUS individuals may, for instance, be used as an argument that they may constitute very early events in the clonal expansion of B cells with an idiotypic match to the specificity of the T cells. Alternatively, the clonal T cell expansion may be secondary to the appearance of a large clone of B cells. Here, such T cells could, *i.e.,* inhibit the outgrowth of those B cells, be functionally neutral or even provide growth signals for the B cells supporting the latter in their multistep progression toward malignancy. It is obvious that this disease may lend itself extremely well to further analysis not only of the specificity of such "clonal" T cells but also of their functional relevance in relation to this type of disease. The monoclonal antibodies would here be most useful tools for T cell enrichment as well as for depletion strategies.

TCR-V-Gene Usage in Certain Autoimmune Diseases

Using our battery against TcR-V-genes of alpha or beta type we have begun to test T lymphocytes from several autoimmune diseases or, alternatively, conditions in the clinic where T cell involvement would seem to be a predominant feature. So far, we have come across three distinct diseases where dramatic expansion and/or biased usage of TcR-V gene expression has been identified.

The first disease is myastenia gravis, MG, a disease where antibodies against the acetylcholine receptor are known to play a decisive part in the disease but where thymus involvement frequently has been implicated. Our findings[22] are summarized in TABLE 4. Using the same argument as before (our battery of monoclonal antibodies detect only around 25% of all T cells) we can deduce that probably all MG patients have dramatically expanded "clones" of alpha/beta T cells in the circulation. Note that in occasional patients close to half of all T cells in a CD4 or CD8 subset may have one V-gene of alpha or beta type, that is, they are oligo- or monoclonal. Another group has likewise indications that MG patients may have a restricted TcR usage.[23] Like the myeloma/MGUS patients we have no evidence of any particular V-alpha or -beta gene being associated with clonal expansion in MG, nor was there any obvious tendency for clonality to be limited to CD4 or DC8 T subsets. The findings of dramatically expanded "clones" of T cells in MG is unlikely to mean that such T cells are of beneficial value to the

TABLE 3. Percent of CD4 and CD8 Positive Peripheral Blood Lymphocytes Reactive with TCR mAbs in MM or MGUS Patients

Pat. No. Out of 16	Diagnosis	Clin. Stage	TCR Monoclonal Antibodies[a]							
			F1	6D6	LC4	1C1	W112	OT145	16G8	S51
CD4										
7	MM	II	**12.4**	1.8	5.1	3.0	1.1	3.1	4.1	2.3
10	MM	II	(2.0)	1.4	2.4	2.9	0.6	1.9	**39.7**	1.1
13	MM	III	3.7	1.6	4.6	2.8	0.9	5.2	4.9	**5.1**
14	MM	III	(2.2)	1.6	(1.6)	(1.4)	0.7	**28.5**	(2.4)	0.9
CD8										
3	MGUS		1.1	**47.0**	2.3	1.7	0.4	3.3	2.3	(0.1)
4	MM	I	0.9	6.4	1.4	1.9	0.9	**34.0**	1.6	0.9
6	MM	I	(0.4)	1.7	(0.2)	(0.3)	(0.1)	0.3	(0.9)	**6.8**
14	MM	III	9.5	11.7	**22.4**	2.1	0.6	1.4	1.8	0.9

[a] Bold numbers indicate a value ≥ twice the normal upper range.

TABLE 4. Percent of CD4 and CD8 Positive Peripheral Blood Lymphocytes Reactive with TCR Monoclonal Antibodies in Patients with Myastenia Gravis

Pat. No. Out of 15	TCR Monoclonal Antibodies[a]							
	α V (F1)	α V12	β V5.1	β V5a	β5b	β V6	β V8	β V12
CD4								
5	(1.4)	2.1	2.7	2.1	0.7	3.5	5.6	**13.7**
7	4.3	0.8	3.9	(1.1)	0.5	**34.2**	4.0	1.1
CD8								
1	0.8	**43.0**	0.4	(0.4)	0.3	0.1	1.8	(0.2)
7	(0.3)	8.2	0.5	(0.5)	0.2	1.1	1.5	**12.4**
15	1.2	2.2	3.0	2.6	1.4	0.8	3.7	**18.0**

[a] Bold figures are > twice the normal range values of the reference population.

patient. The antibodies made against the acetylcholine receptor are predominantly of IgG type and of high affinity with tendencies to clonality.[24] All findings in line with their production being driven by helper T lymphocytes in a somewhat restricted manner. It would thus be logical to expect that a deletion of such restricted, expanded T cell subsets, if anything, would have a beneficial impact on the disease.

Mb Behcet is yet another disease of unknown etiology but with clearcut features of immune dysfunction. We have studied relatively few patients suffering from this disease, which may take a very serious clinical course. Our studies so far involve only PBLs and not local lesions. In this preliminary study we have found a tendency toward abnormal expansions of TcR-restricted subsets of T cells. In one individual, for example, we could identify the two respective V-gene partners, being in the order of 25% of the CD8 T cells. Although studies on the local lesions and their predominant composition of CD8 T cells would be needed to further document the situation, the seriousness of this disease may make it an early prime candidate for attempted therapy against clonally expanded T cells.

Sarcoidosis represents the third disease with T cell involvement for unknown reasons where we have been able to describe an unusual TcR restriction on T cells presumed to be involved in the pathogenic reactions. Sarcoidosis is a granulomatous disease with predominant involvement of the lungs. In our studies we have analyzed both T cells in PBL and in bronchial lavage fluid, BAL, from such patients. As shown in TABLE 5 sarcoidosis patients have a highly abnormal restriction in TcR usage in BAL T cells but not in PBLs, that is, in the actual site of disease. Like for the other diseases the data suggest that probably all sarcoidosis patients have such pathologically expanded TcR-restricted T cells. The "clonal-

TABLE 5. Percent of Anti-TCR MAb Reactivity within CD4+ BAL Lymphocytes/PBL in Patients with Sarcoidosis

Patient No. Out of 11	TCR Monoclonal Antibodies							
	α V 2	α V12	β V5.1	β V 5a	β V 5b	β V 6	β V 8	β V 12+
1	9.0/2.8	0.9/4.4	4.0/4.4	3.4/2.3	1.3/0.8	5.6/9.8	6.7/3.6	1.7/1.1
6	21.7/6.8	1.5/2.2	4.6/5.6	5.3/2.9	2.0/1.3	8.2/5.5	3.3/2.9	3.0/1.9
7	19.6/4.5	1.6/2.3	4.4/4.9	2.1/2.5	0.8/0.9	6.5/3.8	2.8/4.2	0.7/1.1
10	31.9/3.8	0.8/2.8	5.7/6.3	4.0/2.1	2.2/1.0	6.8/6.7	5.8/4.3	1.9/2.1

ity" is very pronounced in BAL CD4 T cells. A highly significant restriction in V-gene usage was noted as 4/11 patients displayed a select expansion in the CD4 BAL T cells of V-alfa 2.3 + T cells. This is particularly remarkable as there was no indication of HLA sharing between these patients, suggesting the possibility that an entity behaving more like a "superantigen" may be linked to the granulomatous tissue damage associated with sarcoidosis. Sarcoidosis is normally a disease with self-limited course and dramatic therapeutic interventions are rarely called for. Furthermore, due to the unknown etiology behind this disease (autoimmune? infectious?) it is not clear whether the clonality observed amongst the BAL T cells is damaging or beneficial to the patient. Further studies using V-alpha 2.3 CD4 T cells in an attempt to delineate the agent(s) causing their select stimulation may here be the most promising lead for future activities attempting to solve the etiology of sarcoidosis.

In contrast to the above-mentioned diseases we have failed to find any abnormal clonal expansion of T cells in the PBLs of patients suffering from multiple sclerosis (here other groups have reported oligoclonality in cerebrospinal fluid), Sjögren's disease or in SLE patients (data not shown).

DISCUSSION

Immature and mature T cells carrying TcR molecules may both respond to signals through such molecules by positive or negative reactions: expansion and induction of effector cell activities or inhibition of function and physical elimination (for instance, see consequences for responsive T cells making contact with "superantigens" *in vitro* or *in vivo* in mice or man[26,27]). This would accordingly indicate that attempts to eliminate T cells via active or passive immunity directed against TcR associated V-gene epitopes may, if improperly performed, result in the opposite situation, an expansion of exactly the same cells. Different consequences of a supposedly identical signal could depend on, *i.e.*, the stage of maturation and immune activation of the target T cell. Much more work has to be done in experimental systems to define the conditions for a TcR-focused attack to in a predictable manner cause stimulation and activation or elimination and inactivation, respectively. Only clinically extremely dangerous situations would thus at present justify attempts via passive or active immunotherapy to attack a defined TcR-type positive T cell subset. At the same time there are now other really promising leads to a similar kind of selective immunological surgery within the T cell system. Success in treating T cell malignancies and severe autoimmune disorders via focused TcR attacks would first be looked for. If reached in absence of significant side effects such protocols would logically be followed by similar, more preventive measures in less severe autoimmune diseases. Eventually it may be extended to include pretreatment protocols for recipients or donors in transplantation situations. Much of all these therapeutic protocols would have to be tailor-made.

REFERENCES

1. McCONKEY, D. J., S. ORRENIUS & M. JONDAL. 1990. Cellular signalling in programmed cell death (apoptosis). Immunol. Today **11:** 120–123.
2. BLACKMAN, M., J. KAPPLER & P. MARRACK. 1990. The role of the T cell receptor in positive and negative selection of developing cells. Science **248:** 1335–1338.

3. FORD, W. L. Personal communication.
4. MARUCIS-GALESIC, S., D. A. STEPHANY, D. L. LONGO & A. M. KRUISBEEK. 1988. Development of CD4⁻ CD8⁺ cytotoxic T cells requires interactions with class I MHC determinants. Nature 333: 180–183.
5. KRUISBEEK, A. M., J. J. MOND, B. J. FOWLKES, J. A. CARMEN, S. BRIDGES & D. L. LONGO. 1985. Absence of ly2⁻, L3T4⁺ lineage of T cells in mice treated neonatally with anti-I-A correlates with absence of intrathymic I-A-bearing antigen-presenting function. J. Exp. Med. 161: 1029–1047.
6. PATTEN, P., T. YOKOTA, J. ROTHBARD, Y. CHIEN, K. ARAI & M. M. DAVIS. 1984. Structure, expression and divergence of T cell receptor beta-chain variable genes. Nature 312: 40–45.
7. BINZ, H. & H. WIGZELL. 1975. Shared idiotypic determinants on B and T lymphocytes reactive against the same antigenic determinants. III. Physical fractionation of specific immunocompetent T lymphocytes by affinity chromatography using anti-idiotypic antibodies. J. Exp. Med. 142: 1231–1240.
8. BINZ, H. & H. WIGZELL. 1979. Idiotypic determinants on T cell subpopulations. J. Exp. Med. 149: 910–922.
9. ANDERSSON, L. C., H. BINZ & H. WIGZELL. 1976. Specific unresponsiveness to transplantation antigens induced by autoimmunication with syngeneic antigen-specific T lymphoblasts. Nature 264: 778–780.
10. KANAGAWA, O. 1989. In vivo T cell tumor therapy with monoclonal antibody directed to the V beta chain of T antigen receptor. J. Exp. Med. 170: 1513–1519.
11. VANDENBARK, A. A., G. HASHIM & H. OFFNER. 1989. Immunization with a synthetic T cell receptor V-region peptide protects against experimental autoimmune encephalomyelitis. Nature 341: 541–544.
12. Deleted.
13. WILSON, D. B. Personal communication.
14. JANSON, C. H., J. GRUNEWALD, A. ÖSTERBORG, H. DERSIMONIAN, M. BRENNER, H. MELLSTEDT & H. WIGZELL. 1991. Predominant T cell receptor V gene usage in patients with abnormal clones of B cells. Submitted for publication.
15. GRUNEWALD, J., C. H. JANSON & H. WIGZELL. 1990. Biased expression of individual T cell receptor V gene segments in CD4⁺ and CD8⁺ human peripheral blood T lymphocytes. Eur. J. Immunol. In press.
16. CHOI, Y., J. A. LAFFERTY, J. R. CLEMENTS, J. K. TODD, E. W. GELFAND, J. KAPPLER, P. MARRACK & B. L. KOTZIN. 1990. Selective expansion of T cells expressing V beta 2 in toxic shock syndrome. J. Exp. Med. 172: 981–984.
17. JANSON, C. H., M. J. TEHRANI, H. MELLSTEDT & H. WIGZELL. 1987. Three kinds of tumor-unique surface molecules on a human T cell chronic lymphocytic leukemia (T-CLL) detected by monoclonal antibodies. Scand. J. Immunol. 26: 237–246.
18. JANSON, C. H., M. J. TEHRANI, H. MELLSTEDT & H. WIGZELL. 1989. Anti-idiotypic monoclonal antibody to a T-cell chronic lymphatic leukemia. Characterization of the antibody, in vitro effector functions and results of therapy. Cancer Immunol. Immunother. 28: 225–232.
19. LEVY, R. & R. A. MILLER. 1983. Tumor therapy with monoclonal antibodies. Fed. Proc. 42: 2650–2656.
20. MELLSTEDT, H., G. HOLM, D. PETTERSSON, M. BJÖRKHOLM, B. JOHANSSON, C. LINDEMALM, D. PEEST & A. ÅHRE. 1982. T cells in monoclonal gammopathies. Scand. J. Haematol. 29: 57–64.
21. WEN, T., H. MELLSTEDT & H. JONDAL. 1990. Presence of clonal T cell populations in chronic B lymphocytic leukemia and smoldering leukemia. J. Exp. Med. 171: 659–666.
22. GRUNEWALD, J., R. ÅHLBERG, A. K. LEFVERT, H. DERSIMONIAN, H. WIGZELL & C. H. JANSSON. 1991. Restricted V gene usage in peripheral T cells from myastenia gravis patients. Submitted for publication.
23. OKSENBERG, J., M. SHERRITT, A. BEGOVICH, H. ERLICH, C. BERNARD, L. CAVALLI-SFORZA & L. SEIDMAN. 1989. T-cell receptor V alpha and C alpha alleles associated with multiple sclerosis and myastenia gravis. Proc. Nat. Acad. Sci. USA 86: 988–992.

24. VINCENT, A. & J. NEWSOM-DAVIS. 1980. Anti-acetylcholine receptor antibodies. J. Neurol. Neurosurg. Psychiatry **43:** 590–600.
25. GRUNEWALD, J., C. H. JANSON, A. EKLUND, M. ÖRN, U. PERSSON & H. WIGZELL. 1991. Compartmentalization of T lymphocytes with highly restricted TCR V gene usage in BAL from sarcoidosis patients. Submitted for publication.
26. KAWABE, Y. & A. OCHI. 1990. Selective energy of V-beta 8⁺ CD4⁻ T cells in staphylococcus enterotoxin B-primed mice. J. Exp. Med. **172:** 1065–1070.
27. RELLAHAN, B. L., L. A. JONES, A. M. KRUISBEEK, A. M. FRY & L. A. MATIO. 1990. *In vivo* induction of energy in peripheral V-beta 8⁺ T cells by staphylococcal enterotoxin B. J. Exp. Med. **172:** 1091–1100.

Molecular Events in the T Cell-Mediated Suppression of the Immune Response

TOMIO TADA, FEI-YUE HU, HIDEHIRO KISHIMOTO,
MAKOTO FURUTANI-SEIKI, AND YOSHIHIRO ASANO

Department of Immunology
Faculty of Medicine
University of Tokyo
7-3-1 Hongo, Bunkyo-ku
Tokyo 113, Japan

INTRODUCTION

Suppression of immune responses by T cells and T cell products is still a controversial matter. Although the significance of suppression by T cells has been widely accepted in physiologic and autoimmune responses, the existence of the cells that are specialized in suppressing immune responses (suppressor T cells, Ts) has been increasingly questioned. This is mainly due to the difficulty in obtaining T cell lines with stable suppressor functions and in characterizing the soluble mediator (T suppressor factor, TsF) produced by Ts clones. This has also prevented the cloning of the gene encoding TsF. Most of previously published data on Ts and TsF are indeed reproducible, but no further advancement has been made because of the above reasons.

It has recently become possible to establish Ts clones of both CD4+ and CD8+ phenotypes, with which we are now able to re-examine the suppressive interactions between Ts and responding T helper (Th) cells at a subcellular level. We define Ts as *T cells specialized in inhibiting the immune response not by their cytotoxicity for antigen-presenting cells or Th cells, and not by the production of known helper type lymphokines that may be suppressive at certain doses.*[1] We have established several such T cell clones which conform to the above strict criteria. With these T cell clones, we have studied early intracytoplasmic events occurring in the T cell-mediated suppression of target cells, and soluble mediators selectively acting on Th clones that were stimulated by antigen or antibodies against T cell antigen receptor (TcR) complex.

Properties of CD4+ and CD8+ Ts Clones

We have established several IL-2 dependent T cell clones which have definite suppressor activity but not helper and cytotoxic functions.[2,3] CD4+ Ts clones were established in the same way to make Th clones by stimulation of primed spleen cells with antigen (keyhole lympet hemocyanin, KLH; fowl gamma globulin, FGG or bovine αS1 casein) and APC followed by manifestation and maintenance in IL-2-containing medium. Ts clones were selected by their suppressive activity in an *in vitro* Th dependent antibody response and by the lack of helper activity under any *in vitro* conditions. Most of them did not produce IL-2 and

IL-4, while γ interferon (IFNγ) was produced at variable degrees. CD8$^+$ Ts clones were established by a newly devised method where CD4$^+$ T cells were depleted from antigen-primed spleen cells, and the remaining CD8$^+$ T cells were stimulated by antigen and APC followed by expansion with IL-2 containing medium (Hu *et al.*, in preparation). They were cloned by limiting dilution. The established clones have been maintained with occasional stimulation and recloning with antigen and APC in IL-2-containing medium.

TABLE 1 is a partial list of CD4$^+$ and CD8$^+$ Ts clones in comparison with CD4$^+$ Th clones. An I-J^k determinant is generally detected on CD4$^+$ Th and both CD4$^+$ and CD8$^+$ Ts clones if they carry an H-2^k MHC restriction specificity. Most Ts clones produce IFNγ in response to antigen plus APC or Con A, but IFNγ cannot be ascribed to the suppressive activity of these T cell clones, as anti-IFNγ could not block the activity and recombinant IFNγ could not suppress the proliferative response. The role of transforming growth factor (TGFβ) was also excluded from the suppressor function of these clones in the similar manner. Interestingly, all the

TABLE 1. Properties of IL-2-Dependent T Cell Clones

Code	Origin	Type	I-J^k	Specificity	Function	IL2	IFNγ	IL4
2-19-2	B10	CD4	−	A^b + FGG, A^{bm12}	Th	+	+	−
9-16	F$_1$	CD4	+	E^k + KLH	Th	+	+	−
23-1-8	F$_1$ → C3H	CD4	+	A^k + KLH	Th	+	+	−
24-15-1	F$_1$ → B6	CD4	−	A^b	Th	−	ND	+
8-5	F$_1$	CD4	−	A^b + KLH	Th	−	−	+
MS202	C3H	CD4	+	A^k	Th	−	−	+
8-4	F$_1$	CD4	−	A^b + KLH	Ts	−	+	−
9-5	F$_1$	CD4	+	A^k + KLH	Ts	±	+	−
25-11-20	B6 → F$_1$	CD4	+	A^k + KLH	Ts	−	+	−
25-18-5	B6 → F$_1$	CD4	+	E^k + KLH	Ts	±	+	−
3D10*	C3H	CD8	+	A^k + KLH	Ts	−	+	−
13G2*	B6	CD8	−	A^b + casein	Ts	−	+	−
HD4*	C3H	CD8	+	A^k	Ts	−	+	−
HD8*	C3H	CD8	±	A^k	Ts	±	+	−
HD9*	C3H	CD8	+	A^k	Ts	±	+	−

* V$_\beta$8$^+$.

CD8$^+$ Ts clones established independently in different occasions were found to utilize V$_\beta$8, while none of CD4$^+$ clones in the list used this V$_\beta$ gene. The culture supernatant of these clones had no suppressor activity indicating that they do not produce TsF constitutively.

Intracellular Events in T Cell-Mediated Suppression

We have previously reported that CD4$^+$ Ts clones were able to suppress the *in vitro* antibody responses of normal antigen-primed spleen cells or of the mixture of primed B cells and Th clones.[3] The suppression was strictly MHC-restricted in that the identity in the MHC restriction specificities of Ts and Th was definitely required. The mechanism of suppression of antibody response was found to be due to the direct inhibition of Th functions including the IL-2 production. Ts clones were unable to suppress the LPS-induced Ig production.[4]

To study how the Ts suppresses the functions of Th clones, we set up a system where intracellular Ca^{2+} of interacting cells were directly measured by a stopped-flow fluorometry.[5] In brief, antigen-specific MHC-restricted Th clones were labelled with a Ca^{2+}-sensitive fluorophore Fura 2 and admixed with antigen-pulsed syngeneic APC, which resulted in the fluorescence emission from the activated cells. Ts clones preactivated with antigen plus APC were added to this reaction mixture, and the changes in the fluorescence intensity were measured by the stopped-flow fluorometry.

A rapid increase of $[Ca^{2+}]i$ in cloned Th cells was observed within a few second after the antigenic stimulation. This Ca^{2+} response was antigen-specific and dependent on the presence of antigen-pulsed MHC-matched APC. To see the effect of Ts on Th clones, Ts clones were first stimulated with antigen-pulsed APC for 2 min, and were then added to the Fura 2-loaded Th clones, all of which was subsequently activated by the antigen-pulsed APC present in the mixture.

The expected increase of intracellular Ca^{2+} in the Fura 2-loaded Th clone was strongly inhibited by the presence of activated Ts clone. By combinations of Ts and Th clones with different antigen- and MHC-restriction specificities, we found that suppression was, in general, antigen-specific and MHC-restricted. As shown in FIG. 1, KLH plus I-A^k specific Ts clone preactivated for 2 min with antigen pulsed APC could instantly suppress the Ca^{2+} influx of a Th clone from C3H which shared KLH plus I-A^k specificity. If the same Ts clone was added to an I-A^b-restricted KLH-specific Th clone that was subsequently activated with antigen-pulsed B6 APC, the Ca^{2+} response was not instantly suppressed. However, if Ts were preactivated by incubation with C3H APC for 30 min before addition to Th, the increase of $[Ca^{2+}]i$ was substantially suppressed (FIG. 1). The maximum suppressive activity was obtained when Ts clones were preincubated for more than 120 min with antigen and APC. If APC from (B6 × C3H)F_1 was used to stimulate both Ts and MHC-unmatched Th, much shorter time was required for Ts to manifest the suppression in Ca^{2+} response of Th cells (see FIG. 1). If both antigen- and MHC-specificities were unmatched, no detectable suppression was observed.

We examined the inhibition of Ca^{2+} response by combinations of T cell clones with assigned different functions. It was found that all Ts clones would suppress the Ca^{2+} response of antigen- and MHC-matched Th clones. None of Th clones had such an activity to inhibit Ca^{2+} influx of other cells. Ts clones could not suppress the response of other Ts clones. Thus, there is an unidirectional and selective suppression of Th cells by Ts clones.

These results indicated that the $CD4^+$ Ts suppresses the functions of Th clones by inhibiting the early signal transduction involving the influx of Ca^{2+} ion into Th cells. Because of the time required for the suppression in the MHC-unmatched combinations of Ts and Th clones, it was suspected that the effect should be mediated by a soluble factor (TsF) released from Ts, which acts only on the receptor of Th cells present in close proximity.

$CD8^+$ Ts clones also showed a potent inhibitory activity on the antibody response induced with B cells and normal or cloned Th cells. $CD8^+$ clones could strongly inhibit the antigen-induced proliferative response of $CD4^+$ Th clones, while the proliferation induced by Con A or IL-2 was not altered. IL-2 production of Th cells induced by antigenic stimulation was also inhibited by $CD8^+$ T cell clones. The suppression was MHC unrestricted and totally antigen-nonspecific. Interestingly, these $CD8^+$ Ts clones were class II-restricted, and both anti-class II and anti-CD8 antibodies could inhibit the antigen-induced proliferative response of Ts clones. $CD8^+$ Ts clones can also be stimulated by anti-$V_\beta 8$ and anti-CD3 to induce proliferation. No cytotoxic activity against APC and Th cells was detected after antigenic stimulation.

We have attempted to induce soluble mediators from $CD4^+$ and $CD8^+$ Ts clones by stimulation with Con A or antigen plus APC without success. These cells did not produce TsF in the culture supernatant constitutively. However, we have recently found that these cells produce a potent TsF upon stimulation with immobilized anti-CD3. Both $CD4^+$ and $CD8^+$ Ts clones produced TsF within 4–8 hr after stimulation. This condition does not induce such a suppressive molecule

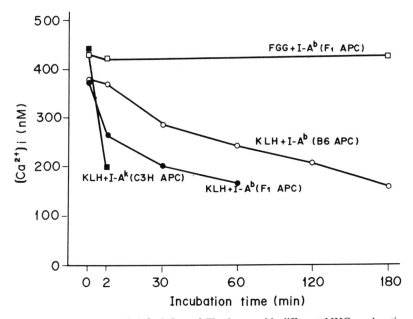

FIGURE 1. Suppression of Ca^{2+} influx of Th clones with different MHC- and antigen-specificities by a Ts clone preactivated for different periods of time with antigen-pulsed APC. Th clones with indicated specificities were loaded with Ca^{2+} sensitive fluorophore Fura 2, and were mixed with a KLH and I-A^k-specific Ts clone which had been preincubated with KLH pulsed APC for different times. Note a strong suppression of Ca^{2+} influx of a Th clone having KLH plus I-A^k specificity by the Ts with the same specificity preactivated only for 2 min (■——■). The responses of a KLH plus I-A^b specific Th clone stimulated by B6 (●——●) or (C3H × B6)F_1 APC (○——○) can be suppressed by the same Ts clone, but it requires a longer preincubation time to activate the Ts clone with KLH plus C3H APC to manifest the suppressive effect. If Th has different antigen (FGG)- and MHC (I-A^b)-specificities (□——□), no suppression was observed.

from any of our $CD4^+$ Th clones of both Th_1 and Th_2 types indicating that the production of TsF is a unique property of Ts clones. TsF from $CD8^+$ Ts clones was able to inhibit the proliferative responses of other T cell clones stimulated with antigen plus APC, anti-TcR$\alpha\beta$ and anti-CD3 monoclonal antibodies. The proliferation induced by Con A and IL-2 was not inhibited by TsF from both $CD4^+$ and $CD8^+$ Ts clones. TsF was also able to inhibit the *in vitro* antibody response in an antigen-nonspecific manner. The characterization of these TsF is now underway.

Agonistic Effect of Anti-I-J Monoclonal Antibody

I-J is an enigmatic molecule that was first determined as a marker of Ts and antigen-specific TsF.[6,7] I-J was believed to be encoded by an MHC gene mapped between I-A and I-E subregions. However, I-J was later found on other cell types too. It has been documented that the I-J identity between Ts and Th was required for successful suppression.[7,8] A controversy started with the discovery that I-J gene was not found at the prescribed position within MHC.[9] In addition, I-J phenotype was found to be adaptively acquired by T cells according to the envi-

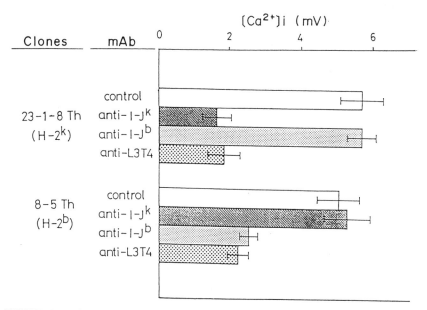

FIGURE 2. Inhibition of antigen-induced increase of [Ca²⁺]i by the treatment of H-2^k- and H-2^b-restricted T cell clones with anti-I-J antibodies. The Th clone 23-1-8 is derived from KLH-primed (C3H × B6)F$_1$ → C3H chimera and restricted to H-2^k. The treatment with anti-I-J^k (JK-10) but not with anti-I-J^b (WF8.D2.4) inhibited the Ca²⁺ response against the subsequent stimulation with KLH and APC. If another Th clone 8-5, derived from (C3H × B6)F$_1$ was treated by the same antibodies, anti-I-J^b but not anti-I-J^k could selectively inhibit the Ca²⁺ response. Since the genotype of these clones is the same, the result indicates that functional I-J phenotypes of these clones are mutually excluded. Some other properties of the anti-I-J-induced suppression of Ca²⁺ responses are discussed in the text.

ronmental MHC when developed in radiation bone marrow chimera.[10] Recently, we determined that I-J is a dimeric glycoprotein composed of 43–45 K glycopeptides on T cell clones.[11] Anti-I-J monoclonal antibody has been found to inhibit the helper activity and antigen-induced proliferative responses of normal T cells as well as CD4$^+$ T cell clones.[1,10,11]

We have tested the effect of anti-I-J on the antigen-induced Ca²⁺ influx of T cell clones by the stopped flow fluorometry as described above. T cell clones were labeled with Fura 2, and were stimulated with antigen plus APC or other stimulators with or without pretreatment with anti-I-J. FIG. 2 shows the result of an experiment where the increase in $[Ca^{2+}]i$ of an I-A^k restricted Th clone 23-1-8 was strongly inhibited by the treatment with anti-I-J^k. The Fura 2-labeled clone was preincubated with anti-I-J or other antibodies, washed, and then stimulated with antigen and APC. The suppression caused by anti-I-J was comparable to that obtained with anti-CD4 mAb. Anti-I-J^b had no effect on this clone with I-A^k restriction. On the other hand, the Ca^{2+} response of I-A^b-restricted Th clone 8-5 was inhibitable by anti-I-J^b but not with anti-I-J^k.

It was further found that the intact anti-I-J, but not the monovalent Fab fragment of anti-I-J, was able to inhibit the antigen-induced Ca^{2+} influx. The addition of anti-mouse Ig antibodies to the cells treated with Fab fragment of anti-I-J resulted in the inhibition of the Ca^{2+} influx. Thus, the inhibitory effect of anti-I-J is not merely a blocking of a site involved in the antigen-recognition but due to the induction of an active intracellular process which is initiated by the ligation of surface I-J molecules.

Furthermore, the inhibitory effect of anti-I-J was directed only to the activation signal induced through the TcR$\alpha\beta$ heterodimer but not through nonspecific receptors. The Ca^{2+} influx caused by the stimulation with antigen plus APC was invariably inhibited, but the response induced by anti-CD3 or by Con A was not inhibited. However, the response induced by an antibody directed to TcR$\alpha\beta$ heterodimer (H57-597, kindly provided by Dr. R. T. Kubo) was inhibitable by the same anti-I-J. These results led us to suspect that anti-I-J act as an agonist to TsF, and that I-J is a receptor-like molecule which transduces a negative signal to inhibit an early cytoplasmic process subsequent to the recognition of antigen via the TcR heterodimer. It is not known whether there is an intermedial messenger between TcR heterodimer and CD3, but the I-J-derived inhibitory signal seems to interfere with the process present in between TcR heterodimer and CD3. This may cause a functional uncoupling of TcR$\alpha\beta$ and CD3. We have recently found that surface I-J molecule is associated with a tyrosine kinase *fyn*. This tyrosine kinase is known to be associated with TcR/CD3 complex too. The antagonistic role of I-J through the activation of *fyn* is now being studied.

DISCUSSION

The availability of CD4$^+$ and CD8$^+$ Ts clones enabled us to study the cellular and molecular events in the T cell-mediated suppression of immune responses. There exist CD4$^+$ and CD8$^+$ T cells that are specialized in the suppression by a noncytotoxic mechanism. The effect is selective and unidirectional from Ts to Th, and Ts cannot suppress the responses of other Ts clones. There is an apparent MHC restriction, but this can be overcome by a preactivation of Ts for a period of time. These results can be best explained by the presence of a soluble mediator that acts on a receptor of target cells of close proximity. Indeed, such TsF is released from Ts clones by stimulation with immobilized anti-CD3. TsF seems to be different from known interleukins, as the conditions to stimulate IL production do not always induce TsF. Anti-I-J mAb behave as an agonist to TsF by inhibiting the antigen-induced responses of CD4$^+$ clones.

The suppression of helper function and proliferative response of CD4$^+$ Th clones was found to be due to the inhibition of early increase of intracellular Ca^{2+} ions which mediates the signal transduction to activate nuclear events. Suppression was highly selective to the TcR-induced signals, and the responses to Con A and IL-2 were not suppressed.

Anti-I-J exerted the similar suppressive effect by crosslinking of surface I-J molecules. I-J molecules are associated with a tyrosine kinase *fyn* which has been known to be bound to TcR/CD3 complex. It is suggested that the crosslinking of I-J molecules will lead to the activation of kinase(s), which make the cells reflectory to further activation signals transduced through TcR/CD3 complex. Apparently, the molecular characterization of both TsF and I-J is definitely necessary to understand the mechanism of suppression.

SUMMARY

To understand the mechanism of T cell-mediated suppression, we have established a number of suppressor T cell (Ts) clones of both $CD4^+$ and $CD8^+$ phenotypes that exert a definite suppressive effect on antigen-induced proliferative response of normal and cloned $CD4^+$ helper T cells (Th). When an antigen-activated Ts clone was added to Th clones that were subsequently stimulated with antigen and APC, the increase of intracellular Ca^{2+} in the latter was greatly inhibited. The suppression was unidirectional where Ts suppressed Th but not vice versa. A Ts clone could not suppress other Ts clones.

Exactly the same suppression of Ca^{2+} response could be induced by the treatment of T cells with an anti-I-J antibody. The anti-I-J suppressed the Ca^{2+} response of Th clones induced by antigen-pulsed APC and anti-TcR$\alpha\beta$ antibody, whereas the responses to anti-CD3 and Con A were not inhibited. The difference in the effect of anti-TcR$\alpha\beta$ and anti-CD3 suggests that the suppression is caused by a functional uncoupling of TcR$\alpha\beta$ and CD3. The stimulation of Ts clones with anti-CD3, on the other hand, induced a unique suppressor factor that potently inhibits the antigen- and anti-TcR induced proliferation of $CD4^+$ Th clones.

REFERENCES

1. TADA, T., Y. ASANO & K. SANO. 1989. Present understanding of suppressor T cells. 26th Forum in Immunology. 1989. Res. Immunol. **140:** 291–294.
2. NAKAYAMA, T., R. T. KUBO, M. KUBO, I. FUJISAWA, H. KISHIMOTO, Y. ASANO & T. TADA. 1988. Epitope associated with MHC restriction site of T cells. IV. I-J epitopes on MHC-restricted cloned T cells. Eur. J. Immunol. **18:** 761–765.
3. ASANO, Y. & R. J. HODES. 1983. T cell regulation of B cell activation. Cloned Lyt-1⁺2⁻ suppressor cells inhibit the major histocompatibility complex-restricted interaction of T helper cells with B cells and/or accessory cells. J. Exp. Med. **158:** 1178–1190.
4. HISATSUNE, T., A. ENOMOTO, K. NISHIJIMA, Y. MINAI, Y. ASANO, T. TADA & S. KAMINOGAWA. 1990. CD8⁺ suppressor T cell clone capable of inhibiting the antigen- and anti-T cell receptor-induced proliferation of Th clones without cytolytic activity. J. Immunol. **145:** 2421–2426.
5. UTSUNOMIYA, N., M. NAKANISHI, Y. ARATA, M. KUBO, Y. ASANO & T. TADA. 1989. Unidirectional inhibition of early signal transduction of helper T cells by cloned suppressor T cells. Int. Immunol. **1:** 460–463.
6. MURPHY, D. B., L. A. HERZENBERG, K. OKUMURA, L. A. HERZENBERG & H. O. McDEVITT. 1976. A new I subregion (I-J) marked by a locus (Ia-4) controlling surface determinants on suppressor T lymphocytes. J. Exp. Med. **144:** 699–712.
7. TADA, T., M. TANIGUCHI & C. S. DAVID. 1976. Properties of the antigen-specific suppressive T cell factor in the regulation of antibody response in the mouse. IV. Special subregion assignment of the gene(s) which codes for the suppressive T cell factor in the H-2 histocompatibility complex. J. Exp. Med. **144:** 713–723.

8. DORF, M. E. & B. BENACERRAF. 1985. I-J as a restriction element in the suppressor T cell system. Immunol. Rev. **83:** 23–40.
9. MURPHY, D. 1987. The I-J puzzle. Ann. Rev. Immunol. **5:** 405–427.
10. ASANO, Y., T. NAKAYAMA, M. KUBO, J. YAGI & T. TADA. 1987. Epitopes associated with MHC restriction site of T cells. III. I-J epitope on MHC-restricted T helper cells. J. Exp. Med. **166:** 1613–1626.
11. NAKAYAMA, T., R. T. KUBO, H. KISHIMOTO, Y. ASANO & T. TADA. 1989. Biochemical identification of I-J as a novel dimeric surface molecule on mouse helper and suppressor T cell clones. Int. Immunol. **1:** 50–55.

The Problems of Presentation of T Cell Receptor Peptides by Activated T Cells[a]

HONG JIANG,[a] ELI SERCARZ,[b] DANUTE NITECKI,[c] AND
BENVENUTO PERNIS[a]

[a]Department of Microbiology and Medicine
College of Physicians and Surgeons
Columbia University
701 W. 168 Street
New York, New York 10032
[b]Department of Microbiology and Molecular Genetics
University of California, Los Angeles School of Medicine
Los Angeles, California 90024-1489
[c]Cetus Corporation
Emeryville, California 94608

INTRODUCTION

There is evidence[1] that cells can process self proteins and present the peptides derived from them coupled to histocompatibility molecules, much in the same way as they do with other endogenously synthesized proteins, like viral antigens.[2]

The MHC molecules to which the self peptides are coupled are as a rule Class I, but in some special cases in which the peptides are derived from immunoglobulins, they can be Class II.[3]

Of special interest is the possibility that peptides derived from the processing of the T cell receptor (TCR) may be generated by the same T cells that synthesize the receptor, and presented coupled to class I MHC (murine T lymphocytes do not express Class II MHC). In fact, such an event, since peptides derived from the hypervariable segments of the TCR are unlikely to be covered by tolerance, might provide a molecular basis for clone-specific interactions between T cells and might provide an explanation of the suppressor function of CD8 T cells. In fact, indirect evidence for suppressor T cells stimulated by TCR peptides has been obtained in experiments in which such peptides provided protection from experimental allergic encephalomyelitis.[4-6]

The Possible Cellular Routes of TCR Processing

It is likely that many self proteins, as many viral proteins, are fragmented in the cytosol and the derived peptides are transferred across the membranes of the endoplasmic reticulum (ER), after which the peptides may bind to the nascent Class I MHC molecules. However, we have no clues to evaluate this possibility for the TCR α and β chains. Actually, since both chains have signal sequences and are co-translationally transferred to the lumen of the ER, it is unlikely that the cytosol is a major site of TCR chain processing.

[a] This work was supported by the Multiple Sclerosis Society PP0112 pilot project grant.

28

On the other hand, it has been established that α and β TCR chains, which are synthesized in excess of the CD3 complex chains γ δ, ε and ζ (zeta) are degraded in the cytoplasm of T cells, actually at least 85% of the newly synthesized TCR α and β chains never reach the cell surface.[7] The degradation of this excess of α and β TCR chains take place in the ER[8,9]; Molecules that escape this and still are not part of the complete multichain receptor ($\alpha\beta$-$\gamma\beta\varepsilon\zeta^2$) are diverted, at a trans-golgi station, to-lysosomes where they are finally degraded.[7] The degradation in the ER can produce peptides which, if they are of the appropriate size and sequence, may bind to the nascent Class I MHC molecules that are being assembled in the E.R itself and from there be transported to the cell membrane as a complex with Class I MHC, in principle capable of being recognized by CD8 cells.

The ER is therefore definitely a potential site of formation of complexes between TCR peptides and Class I MHC (or Class I-MHC-like) molecules that might be involved in immunoregulation. However, it has been shown[10-12] that, in activated T cells, membrane Class I MHC molecules are constitutively endocytosed and recycled through acidic ($\sim$pH 5.2) endosomes. In addition it has been shown that in T lymphoblasts the TCR is also spontaneously endocytosed.[13,14] We therefore wished to investigate if, in activated T cells, Class I MHC molecules and TCR are endocytosed in the same vesicles, since this event might provide an additional site of TCR processing with the possibility that the resulting peptides would combine with recycling Class I MHC molecules in the same endosome. We studied this process in the cells of the encephalitogenic line BML-1.

MATERIALS AND METHODS

Mice

B10PL mice were purchased from the Jackson Laboratory and maintained in the facilities of the medical center of Columbia University.

Monoclonal Antibodies

3–83-P (cross-reactive with H-2^u MHC class I antigen) was obtained from the American Type Culture Collection. F23.1 (reacts with V$\beta_{8.2}$ T cell receptors) was a kind gift from M. Bevan, maintained and subcloned in our laboratory. Both Mabs were purified with a protein A column.

Goat anti-mouse immunoglobulin (Ig) was purified from antiserum as previously described.[10]

Immunofluorescence

Purified antibodies were conjugated to fluorescein isothiocyanate (FITC) or tetramethylrhodamine isothiocyanate (TRITC) by the celite method.[10] FITC and TRITC were purchased from Sigma Chemical Company, St. Louis, MO.

Antigens

Guinea pig myelin basic protein was prepared as previously described.[15] Synthetic peptides corresponding to the encephalitogenic 1–9 acetylated, amino terminal, amino acids of MBP was prepared by D. Nitecki.

Medium

Cultures were incubated in complete IMDM medium (cIMDM) which includes 2 mM glutamine, 100 μg/ml streptomycin, 100 μg/ml penicillin, 5 × 10⁻₅ M 2-mercaptoethanol and 10% fetal calf serum. Mouse Con A supernatant was prepared as described by Ando et al.[16]

T Cell Line BML-1

T cell line BML-1 was maintained according to the procedure of D.G. Ando et al.[16]

Internalization of TCRs Following Anti-TCR Antibody

BML-1 T cells were maintained in mouse Con A supernatant complemented cIMDM for 5 weeks after antigen stimulation, and reincubated with cIMDM containing purified anti-TCR antibody F23.1 (100μg/ml) and 10% con A supernatant for 30 minutes, 1.5 hours, 3 hours and 5.5 hours at 37°C, 5% C02, harvested and washed once with Hank's balanced salt solution (HBSS) containing 5% FCS. For detecting intracellular TCRs, cytocentrifuge smears were prepared, fixed in 95% ethanol for 20 min at -20°C, and stained at room temperature with either TRITC-goat anti-mouse Ig for detecting endocytosed TCRs or F23.1 followed by TRITC-goat anti-mouse Ig for detecting both endocytosed and pre-existing intracellular TCRs. For detecting both intracellular MHC class I antigens and endocytosed TCRs of BML-1 cells, cytocentrifuge smears were stained with TRITC-goat anti-mouse Ig, blocked with 10% normal mouse serum, and restained with FITC conjugated, H-2u MHC class I antigen reactive Mab 3–83-P.

Microscopy

The slides were mounted in elvanol and the cells were viewed with a Leitz Dialux microscope with vertical illumination. The same cells were examined alternatively with a combination of filters and dichroic mirrors specific for fluorescein and those specific for rhodamine. photographs were taken with Kodak Ektachrome Film EES 135 developed for 800 ASA.

RESULTS AND DISCUSSION

The results of a typical experiment are shown in FIGURE 1. FIGURE 1B shows endosomes in BML1 cells containing Class I MHC molecules. This pattern is constitutive and, with some variations, found throughout the period of culture of this cell line. FIGURE 1A, on the other hand, shows endocytosis of TCR molecules that was mainly determined by incubation for 90 minutes with the anti-TCR antibody F23.1. Since this incubation was performed in the presence of Con A supernatant, a condition in which anti-TCR antibodies are known to stimulate T cells, we think that the endocytosis of the TCR was largely the consequence of the stimulation of the cells rather than of the cross-linking of the TCR by the antibody. Actually rapid endocytosis of the TCR has been seen also as a consequence of the stimulation of T cells with other means like phorbol esters[14] or by the mixed lymphocyte reaction (MLR).[17]

The main finding is that the location of the endocytosed TCR coincides almost completely with that of the vesicles containing the recycling Class I MHC molecules. Actually all but one of the endocytic vesicles with TCR are also positive for Class I MHC. On the other side there are a few "extra' Class I containing endosomes that do not show the presence of TCR. This last point is expected on the basis of the extensive constitutive endocytosis of Class I MHC molecules that is occurring in BML-1 cells, and, incidentally, is a good support of the specificity of our immunofluorescence procedure for detecting TCR and Class I MHC independently.

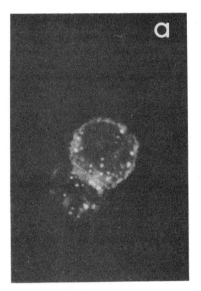 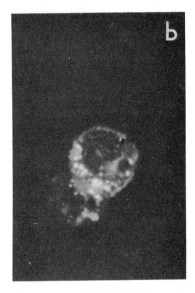

FIGURE 1. (A) BML-1 cells, 2 weeks after last stimulation with BMP 1-9 Nac peptide, incubated for 90 minutes with anti-TCR antibody F23.1 and stained as indicated in Materials and Methods. Illumination for rhodamine visualizes endocytosed TCR. Final magnification was 1000 ×. **(B)** Same cells. Illumination for fluorescein visualizes endocytosed Class I MHC.

We consider, therefore, that we have proved the coexistence, in activated T cells, of TCR and Class I MHC molecules in the same endosomes. The physiological significance of this finding remains to be investigated.

It could be that in the acidic endosomes, the TCR molecules are subject to proteolysis and that peptides are generated that bind to the local MHC Class I molecules that will be recycled to the surface. There is however no proof, so far (F. Carbone, personal communication) that the recycling endosomes of activated T cells are the site of extensive proteolytic activity. In fact, if this were the case one might expect that the Class I MHC molecules, that are quite sensitive to proteolytic enzymes, would at least be cleaved off the membrane of the endosomes. Therefore, we must consider also the possibility that interactions may take place, in the acidic recycling endosomes, between the TCR and Class I MHC molecules, that do not require proteolytic cleavage of either partner. We are now exploring this interesting possibility.

REFERENCES

1. ROTZSCHKE, O., K. FALK, H. J. WALLNY, S. FAATH & H. G. RAMMENSEE. 1990. Science **149:** 283–287.
2. VAN BLEEK, G. M. & S. G. NATHENSON. 1990. Nature **348:** 213–216.
3. WEISS, S. & B. BOGEN. 1991. Cell **64:** 767–774.
4. VANDENBARK, A. A., G. HASHIM & A. HOFFNER 1989. Nature **341:** 541.
5. HOWELL, M. D., S. T. WINTERS, T. OLEE, H. C. POWELL, D. J. CARLO & S. W. BROSTOFF. 1989. Science **246:** 668.
6. OFFNER, H., G. HASHIM & A. VANDENBARK. 1991. Science **251:** 430–432.
7. MINAMI, Y., A. M. WEISSMAN, L. E. SAMELSON & R. KLAUSNER. 1987. Proc. Natl. Acad. Sci. USA **84:** 2688–2692.
8. CHEN, C., J. S. BONIFACINO, L. C. YUAN & R. D. KLAUSNER. 1988. J. Cell Biol. **107:** 2149–2161.
9. BONIFACINO, J. S., C. K. SUZUKI, J. LIPPINCOT-SCHWARTZ, A. M. WEISSMAN & R. KLAUSNER. 1989. J. Cell Biol. **109:** 73–83.
10. TSE, D. & B. PERNIS. 1984. J. Exp. Med. **159:** 193–207.
11. TSE, D. B., C. R. CANTOR, J. MCDOWELL & B. PERNIS. 1986. J. Mol. Cell Immunol. **2:** 315–329.
12. HOCHMAN, J. H., H. JIANG, L. MATYUS, M. EDIDIN & B. PERNIS. 1991. J. Immunol. **146:** 1862–1867.
13. TSE, D. B., M. AL-HAIDERI, B. PERNIS, C. R. CANTOR & C. Y. WANG. 1986. Science **234:** 748–751.
14. KRANGEL, M. S. 1987. J. Exp. Med. **165:** 1141–1159.
15. READHEAD, C., B. POPKO, N. TAKAHASHI, H. D. SHINE, R. A. SAAVEDRA, R. L. SIDMAN & L. E. HOOD. 1987. Cell **48:** 703.
16. ANDO, D. G., J. CLAYTON, D. KONO, J. L. URBAN & E. E. SERCARZ. **1989.** Cell. Immunol. **124:** 132–143.
17. PERNIS, B. & D. TSE. 1985. Dynamics of MHC molecules in lymphoid cells. *In* Cell Biology of the MHC. B. Pernis & H. Vogel, Eds. 153–164. Academic Press. New York.

Accessory Cell-Derived Costimulatory Signals Regulate T Cell Proliferation[a]

KEVIN B. URDAHL, MARC K. JENKINS, AND
STEVEN D. NORTON

Department of Microbiology
University of Minnesota Medical School
Box 196 UMHC
420 Delaware Street S.E.
Minneapolis, Minnesota 55455

INTRODUCTION

Recent evidence indicates that two events must occur at the cell membrane for murine Th1 clones to produce their autocrine growth factor, IL-2.[1] The first is occupancy of the clonally-distributed T cell receptor (TCR) by antigenic peptides bound to class II MHC (Ia) molecules expressed on the surface of antigen-presenting cells (APC).[2] TCR occupancy results in the rapid hydrolysis of phosphatidyl inositol bisphosphate into two second messengers, diacylglycerol and inositol trisphosphate, each associated with distinct biochemical pathways.[3] Diacylglycerol activates protein kinase C and can be mimicked pharmacologically with the phorbol ester, phorbol 12-myristate 13-acetate (PMA). Inositol trisphosphate mediates an increase in cytoplasmic free calcium by regulating calcium channels on both the endoplasmic reticulum and the plasma membrane. TCR occupancy also leads to the activation of tyrosine kinases.[3]

The second requisite signal for IL-2 production is also provided by cell to cell contact between the T cell and the APC.[1] Evidence for this costimulatory signal was originally derived from the observations that although antigenic peptides plus either fixed resting B cells[4] or purified Ia molecule-containing planar membranes;[5] anti-CD3 antibody;[6] or Con A[7] resulted in inositol phosphate production by T cell clones, IL-2 was not produced unless viable accessory cells were present. Splenic low density cells, a mixed population containing activated B cells, macrophages, and dendritic cells, were more potent than resting B cells in providing the costimulatory activity.[8] Once provided, the costimulatory signal did not result in an increase in inositol phosphate production or PKC activation suggesting that a biochemical pathway other than the phosphatidyl inositol pathway was operating.[7] Taking into account all of these observations, a reasonable scenario would be that TCR and costimulatory receptor occupancy engage inositol phospholipid-dependent and -independent biochemical events which in turn induce the synthesis or activation of DNA-binding factors that enhance the transcription of lymphokine genes.[9]

Like murine Th1 clones, human T cell clones require TCR occupancy and costimulatory signals to produce IL-2.[10] Although the cell surface molecules in-

[a] This work was supported by National Institutes of Health Grants AI 27998 and AI 28365 and by a Pew Scholars Award to M.K.J.

33

volved in costimulation have not been identified, CD28 is an attractive candidate for the T cell costimulatory receptor.[11] CD28, a member of the Ig gene superfamily, is a homodimeric integral membrane glycoprotein of 44 Kd expressed on 95% of CD4+ T cells and those CD8+ cells with cytolytic function. Anti-CD28 monoclonal antibodies greatly enhance T cell proliferation in response to PHA or anti-CD3 antibody by a mechanism that does not correlate with increases in intracellular calcium or protein kinase C activation. Here we show that an anti-CD28 monoclonal antibody and accessory cells provide very similar costimulatory signals. This antibody, like accessory cells, restores the ability of antigen-pulsed, costimulation-deficient accessory cells to stimulate proliferation of an antigen-specific T cell line. Furthermore, accessory cells plus PMA, like anti-CD28 plus PMA,[12] drive the cyclosporin A-resistant proliferation of human T cells. These data suggest that the costimulatory signal for T cell activation can be delivered artificially by the binding of an agonistic antibody to CD28, or physiologically by the interaction of CD28 with its natural ligand expressed on the surface of accessory cells.

MATERIALS AND METHODS

Reagents

PMA, paraformaldehyde, and goat anti-mouse IgG antibody were purchased from Sigma Chemical Co. (St. Louis, MO), Fisher Chemical Co. (Fairlawn, NJ), and Caltag (So. San Francisco, CA), respectively. A 1 mg/ml stock solution of PMA was prepared in DMSO. Cyclosporin A, tetanus toxoid, and purified anti-CD28 monoclonal antibody (clone 9.3, mouse IgG2a) were kindly provided by Sandoz (Hanover, NJ), the Massachusetts Public Health Biological Laboratories (Boston, MA), and Oncogen (Seattle, WA), respectively. Anti-CD3 monoclonal antibody (clone OKT-3, mouse IgG2a) was purified from culture supernatant of the OKT-3 hybridoma using protein G-sepharose (Pharmacia Fine Chemicals, Uppsala, Sweden).

Anti-CD3 Immobilization

Tissue culture wells were incubated with 50 μl of 5 μg/ml goat anti-mouse IgG antibody for 1 hour at 37°C, washed three times with PBS, and then incubated with 50 μl of neat OKT3 culture supernatant for 1 hour at 37°C followed by three more PBS washes. When purified OKT3 was used, a 10 μg/ml solution was allowed to incubate for 1 hour at 37°C. The wells were then washed three times with PBS to remove unbound antibody.

Cell Preparation

Peripheral blood mononuclear cells (PBMNC) were isolated from the peripheral blood of healthy adult donors by Ficoll-Hypaque density gradient centrifugation. T cells were purified on Beckman human T cell columns (Somerset, NJ) from PBMNC that had been passed over a G-10 column to remove adherent cells. E− cells were prepared from PBMNC by rosetting out T cells with sheep erythrocytes as described previously.[13] B cells were prepared from T cell-depleted E− cells that had been passed over a G-10 column to remove adherent cells. Adherent cells were prepared by incubating PBMNC on glass petri dishes for 1 hour at 37°C. Nonadherent cells were washed off the plates by vigorous pipetting with RPMI-1640 (Biofluids, Rockville, MD). Adherent cells were then removed using a cell scraper. The tetanus toxoid-specific T cell line, TT-1, was established from the PBMNC of a recently immunized donor. Cells were initially stimulated with 10 μg/ml tetanus toxoid in the complete medium described below. Viable cells were recovered by density gradient centrifugation after 7 days and restimulated with fresh autologous irradiated PBMNC (4,000 R) and 1 μg/ml TT. Two days later 10 U/ml recombinant human IL-2 (Boehringer Mannheim, Indianapolis, IN) was added. After 7–10 days of culture with no further additions the antigen and IL-2 sequence described above (antigen on day 0, IL-2 on day 2, followed by a 7–10 day rest) was repeated. This T cell line has been maintained by this protocol for greater than 3 months. TT-1 cells were rested for at least 7 days following IL-2 addition and repurified by density gradient centrifugation before use in experiments.

T Cell Proliferation and IL-2 Production

Cell cultures were performed in 0.2 ml of Eagle's Hanks Amino Acids medium (Biofluids) supplemented with 10% fetal calf serum, 2 mM glutamine, 100 U/ml streptomycin and penicillin, and 5×10^{-5} M 2-mercaptoethanol in 96 well tissue culture plates. To measure T cell proliferation, T cells, APC (irradiated with either 1,000 or 4,000 R to prevent their proliferation), and various additions were cultured for 72 hours, the last 16 hours in the presence of 1 μCi of ^{3}H-thymidine (ICN, Irvine, CA). At the end of the culture period the cells were harvested onto glass fiber filters using a semiautomated cell harvester (PHD, Cambridge, MA). The incorporation of ^{3}H-thymidine into DNA was quantitated by liquid scintillation counting and used as a measure of T cell proliferation. To measure IL-2 production, supernatants from cultures were removed after 24 hours, serially diluted, and assayed for their ability to support the growth of the IL-2-dependent CTLL line. One unit is defined as the reciprocal dilution of culture supernatant required to yield half maximal CTLL proliferation as assessed by thymidine incorporation during a 24 hour culture period.

Pulsing and Fixation of E⁻ Cells

E⁻ cells (10^7/ml) were pulsed for 2 hours at 37°C with 20 μg/ml tetanus toxoid or medium to allow antigen processing to occur. In some cases the cells were then washed three times in PBS to remove any free toxoid, incubated for 20 minutes at room temperature in 0.15% paraformaldehyde followed by a 30 minute incubation at 37°C in complete media to remove any unreacted paraformaldehyde. Cells were washed several times and diluted in media for use.

RESULTS

Accessory Cell Requirement for Human T Cell Proliferation

Immobilized anti-TCR or anti-CD3 antibodies trigger a similar set of biochemical events in T cells as TCR occupancy by peptide/MHC molecule complexes.[1,3] Previously, we have shown that murine Th1 clones do not produce IL-2 or prolif-

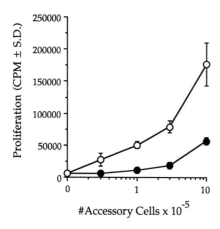

FIGURE 1. Purified human T cells require accessory cells for proliferation in response to immobilized anti-CD3 antibody. Purified T cells (2×10^4) were incubated in duplicate wells coated with 10 μg/ml anti-CD3 mAb (OKT/3) and varying numbers of either adherent cells (*open circles*) or B cells (*closed circles*). Accessory cells were irradiated with 1,000 R, a dose that does not affect the costimulatory capacity of either cell type.[24] T cell proliferation was measured after 72 hours. Results are expressed as the mean CPM ± standard deviation of triplicate determinations.

erate in response to these signals alone, but require additional costimulatory signals from accessory cells.[1] FIGURE 1 shows that this is also true for purified, freshly isolated human T cells. T cell proliferation was not observed in the absence of accessory cells, but increased in a dose-dependent manner as accessory cells were added to the culture. In addition, approximately tenfold more B cells than adherent cells were required to achieve the same degree of proliferation. This costimulatory hierarchy is consistent with that found in the murine system in which macrophages and dendritic cells were more potent in delivering costimulatory signals than resting B cells.[8]

Costimulatory Capacity of Anti-CD28 Antibody

Since both accessory cells and anti-CD28 antibody deliver stimulatory signals to T cells, we tested whether anti-CD28 antibody could substitute for accessory cells and drive proliferation in response to immobilized anti-CD3 antibody. As in the case of purified freshly isolated T cells, immobilized anti-CD3 antibody alone did not stimulate IL-2 production or proliferation by a tetanus-toxoid-specific human T cell line (TABLE 1). When soluble anti-CD28 antibody was added to the culture, however, immobilized anti-CD3 antibody stimulated marked IL-2 pro-

TABLE 1. Immobilized Anti-CD3 Antibody plus Anti-CD28 Antibody Stimulates IL-2 Production and T Cell Proliferation[a]

Stimulus	IL-2 (Units)	Proliferation (CPM)
Medium	<0.5	652
Anti-CD3	<0.5	557
Anti-CD3 + anti-CD28	32	22,132
Anti-CD28	<0.5	628

[a] TT-1 cells (10^4) were stimulated in duplicate microtiter wells. Where indicated, wells were coated with anti-CD3 antibody (OKT/3 culture supernatant) as described in materials and methods and in some cases a 1:1000 dilution of ascitic fluid containing anti-CD28 antibody (9.3) was added. IL-2 levels and T cell proliferation were assayed as described in the materials and methods.

duction and proliferation. Similar results were obtained using T cell-depleted accessory cells (data not shown). Anti-CD28 antibody alone had no measurable effect on the T cells. Therefore, anti-CD28 antibody, like accessory cells, delivers a costimulatory signal to T cells that allows IL-2 production and proliferation in response to immobilized anti-CD3 antibody.

The ability of anti-CD28 antibody to deliver costimulatory signals to T cells was tested further by measuring the proliferative response of a tetanus-toxoid-specific T cell line to stimulation by tetanus toxoid-pulsed, paraformaldehyde-fixed accessory cells in the presence or absence of anti-CD28 antibody. As shown in FIGURE 2, the T cell line proliferated vigorously in response to autologous tetanus toxoid-pulsed, T cell-depleted accessory cells but not in response to un-pulsed accessory cells. Paraformaldehyde fixation of the accessory cells *following*

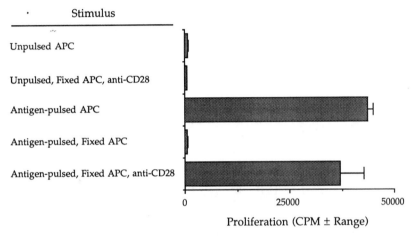

FIGURE 2. Anti-CD28 antibody restores the ability of pulsed, fixed APC to stimulate T cell proliferation. TT-1 cells (2×10^4/well) were incubated with 10^5 E$^-$ cells (unfixed cells were irradiated with 4,000 R). Where indicated, E$^-$ cells were pulsed with 20 μg/ml TT and/or fixed. T cell proliferation was measured after 72 hours. Results are expressed as the mean CPM ± range of duplicate determinations.

the antigen-pulsing step completely abrogated the ability of these cells to stimulate T cell proliferation. Addition of soluble anti-CD28 antibody to the culture restored T cell proliferation in response to the tetanus toxoid-pulsed, fixed accessory cells to the level observed in response to tetanus toxoid-pulsed, unfixed accessory cells. Anti-CD28 antibody alone had no observable effect on T cell proliferation in response to fixed APC that were not prepulsed with antigen. The restoration of the response in an antigen-dependent manner by anti-CD28 antibody demonstrates that fixation of antigen-pulsed APC is not preventing antigen presentation but instead is affecting the costimulatory capacity of the APC. Therefore, anti-CD28 antibody provides a costimulatory signal to T cells not only in response to immobilized anti-CD3 antibody but also when TCR occupancy is delivered by antigenic peptide/MHC molecule complexes.

Comparison of T Cell Proliferation in Response to PMA plus Accessory Cells or Anti-CD28 Antibody

The above results demonstrate that both accessory cells and anti-CD28 antibody can deliver costimulatory signals to T cells. The question remains, however, whether these signals are delivered via the same or different receptor/ligand interactions and biochemical pathways. It has been reported that anti-CD28 antibody plus PMA induces the cyclosporin A-resistant proliferation of human T cells.[12] In addition, PBMNC have been shown to proliferate in response to PMA alone even in the presence of cyclosporin A[14] although purified T cells fail to respond to PMA.[12] Therefore, it is possible that in the presence of PMA the interaction of T cells and accessory cells stimulate cyclosporin A-resistant proliferation through the CD28 molecule. To test this idea, proliferation by freshly isolated, purified T cells in response to PMA plus either accessory cells or anti-CD28 antibody was compared. Anti-CD3 antibody, in the presence of accessory cells, induced a vigorous T cell proliferative response that was exquisitely sensitive to cyclosporin A (FIG. 3). Anti-CD28 antibody plus PMA also resulted in a high level of T cell proliferation, but, in contrast, this proliferation was largely insensitive to cyclosporin A inhibition. Although the degree of proliferation in response to accessory cells plus PMA was less than the response to anti-CD28 antibody plus PMA, it was nonetheless resistant to the inhibitory effects of cyclosporin A. Neither anti-CD28 antibody, nor PMA alone, induced any proliferative response in purified human T cells. These data indicate that in the presence of PMA, accessory cells

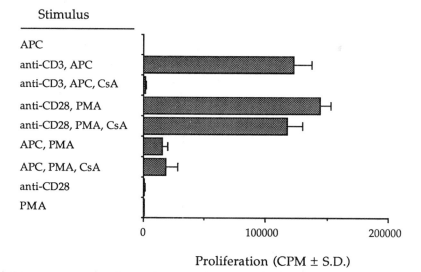

FIGURE 3. Anti-CD28 antibody or accessory cells induce cyclosporin A-resistant T cell proliferation in the presence of PMA. Cultures contained 5×10^4 purified human T cells per well. Where indicated, wells were coated with 10 μg/ml anti-CD3 antibody. Irradiated E⁻ cells (4,000 R, 5×10^4) served as accessory cells. Cyclosporin A (0.5 μg/ml), PMA (1 ng/ml), and anti-CD28 mAb (0.1 μg/ml) were added at the time of culture initiation. T cell proliferation was measured after 24 hours. Results are expressed as the mean CPM ± standard deviation of triplicate determinations.

TABLE 2. Comparison of the Biological Activities of Anti-CD28 mAb and Accessory Cells

Biological Activity	Anti-CD28	Accessory Cells
Augment lymphokine production in response to anti-TCR stimulation	yes	yes
Hierarchy of potency: activated B cells, adherent cells > resting B cells >>> T cells, parenchymal cells	not applicable	yes
Stimulate T cell proliferation in presence of PMA	yes	yes
Proliferation in presence of PMA is cyclosporin A-resistant	yes	yes
Action is not dependent on inositol phospholipid turnover	yes	yes
Stabilize lymphokine mRNAs	yes	unknown
Restore T cell proliferation in response to costimulation-deficient APC	yes	yes

and anti-CD28 antibody activate T cells via a cyclosporin A-resistant biochemical pathway distinct from that induced by the TCR. The fact that anti-CD28 antibody was more effective than accessory cells may be related to the dependence of the latter on cell interaction rather than the rapid binding of a soluble molecule.

DISCUSSION

Much evidence from both human and murine systems now indicates that resting T cells and T cell clones require not only TCR but also costimulatory signals in order to proliferate maximally.[1,7,8,10] In the case of murine IL-4-producing Th2 clones, this costimulatory signal appears to be mediated by the monokine IL-1.[15] In contrast, the molecules involved in costimulation for IL-2-producing cells in man and mouse have not been identified. IL-1 is clearly incapable of providing this signal to murine Th1 clones,[5,8] to some human T cell clones,[10] and to resting human T cell populations when care is taken to remove accessory cells.[16]

What then is the molecular nature of this other costimulatory pathway? Although many have been tested (including interleukins 1–7, interferon-γ, transforming growth factor-β, and crude supernatants from APC cultures), no soluble factor has been shown to replace viable accessory cells.[8] Furthermore, costimulation is not provided when the responding T cells are separated from the accessory cells in the same well using a semipermeable membrane that allows passage of macromoles but prevents cell interaction.[8] These results suggest that costimulation is delivered by physical interaction between T cell and APC.

Does the interaction of CD28 with a ligand expressed on the APC account for this? The observations that: (a) both anti-CD28 antibody and accessory cells provide costimulation to T cells activated with either anti-CD3 antibody or antigen; (b) in the presence of PMA both anti-CD28 antibody and accessory cells stimulate CsA-resistant T cell proliferation; and (c) both anti-CD28 antibody[11,17] and accessory cells[7,10] augment lymphokine production without augmenting intracellular calcium increase all are consistent with this possibility (see TABLE 2). The latter observation suggests that the biological effects of anti-CD28 antibody or accessory cells are mediated through a TCR-independent biochemical pathway. This is supported by the observation that anti-CD28 antibody plus PMA stimulates lymphokine production in a TCR-negative lymphoma cell line.[18] Furthermore, it is particularly striking that in contrast to antibodies against T cell surface molecules that stimulate TCR-dependent proliferation,[11] anti-CD28 antibody plus PMA and accessory cells plus PMA are the only means of stimulating CsA-resistant proliferation described to date.

The immunosuppressive activity of cyclosporin A is mediated by interference with the binding of two DNA binding proteins, NFAT-1 and Oct-1, to regulatory sequences in the IL-2 enhancer.[9] NFAT-1 and Oct-1 appear to be regulated by TCR-mediated calcium increase.[9] Stimulation by PMA and anti-CD28 antibody[17] or accessory cells (data not shown) is not associated with calcium increases and would be predicted to be independent of NFAT-1 and Oct-1 activity. Therefore, perhaps it is not surprising that proliferation in response to PMA plus anti-CD28 antibody or accessory cells is insensitive to cyclosporin A. PMA induces the activity of a third DNA binding protein, AP-1, that is resistant to the effects of cyclosporin A.[9] Signals delivered through CD28 have been shown to contribute to the production of IL-2 by two mechanisms.[11] Initially, anti-CD28 antibody augments IL-2 production by stabilizing IL-2 mRNA without affecting its rate of transcription. Later in the response, anti-CD28 antibody enhances the rate of IL-2 gene transcription as well as stabilizing IL-2 mRNA. Recently, a CD28 responsive element has been localized in the IL-2 enhancer,[19] providing a potential explanation for the enhancement of IL-2 gene transcription by anti-CD28 antibody. Thus, it is possible that high level production of AP-1 and the dual effects of CD28 signalling can activate IL-2 transcription without NFAT-1 or Oct-1 binding. The precise molecular mechanism of costimulation mediated by accessory cells is unknown.

The recent identification of the BB-1/B7 molecule as one ligand for CD28[20] adds further support to the notion that CD28 is a costimulation receptor. BB-1/B7, like CD28, is a member of the Ig gene superfamily.[21] This molecule displays a very restricted pattern of expression: it is absent on resting B cells but is induced upon activation by anti-Ig or lipopolysaccharide; is expressed on some monocytes; and is not expressed on T cells or nonhematopoietic cells.[21,22] As shown in TABLE 2, this pattern is very similar to the quantitative hierarchy of accessory cell potency in providing costimulation. This pattern of expression may also explain the effect of fixation on the delivery of costimulation, i.e., fixation may prevent the induction of BB-1/B7 expression rather than destroy this molecule once expressed. Thus fixed small resting B cells known to be costimulation deficient APC would be incapable of inducing expression of BB-1/B7 upon T cell/APC interaction. A further prediction of this would be that cells that already express BB-1/B7 would retain their ability to deliver costimulation even after they are fixed. Indeed, Weaver et al.[23] have shown that fixation of certain activated accessory cell populations does not prevent their ability to deliver costimulation to Th1 clones.

Occupancy of the TCR in the absence of costimulation induces a state of anergy, or long-term unresponsiveness to subsequent antigenic stimulation. Accessory cells, by providing necessary costimulatory signals, can block the induction of this anergic state. Experiments are currently underway to determine if anti-CD28 antibody can also block the induction of anergy. If so, this would strengthen the correlation between costimulatory signals derived from accessory cells and signals mediated through the CD28 molecule and suggest novel immunosuppressive strategies aimed at disrupting the CD28/BB-1/B7 interaction.

SUMMARY

The costimulatory effects of anti-CD28 antibody or accessory cells on T cells were shown to be very similar. Both stimuli: (a) allowed T cell proliferation and IL-2 production in response to immobilized anti-CD3 antibody or antigen presented by APC whose costimulatory capacity had been damaged by fixation; and (b) stimulated cyclosporin A-resistant T cell proliferation in the presence of a phorbol ester. These similarities raise the possibility that anti-CD28 antibody binding to T cells delivers a costimulatory signal that is normally delivered by the interaction of CD28 with a complementary ligand on APC.

REFERENCES

1. MUELLER, D. L., M. K. JENKINS & R. H. SCHWARTZ. 1989. Clonal expansion versus functional clonal inactivation: a costimulatory signalling pathway determines the outcome of T cell antigen receptor occupancy. Ann. Rev. Immunol. **7**: 445–480.
2. SCHWARTZ, R. H. 1985. T-lymphocyte recognition of antigen in association with products of the major histocompatibility complex. Annu. Rev. Immunol. **3**: 237–261.
3. ASHWELL, J. D. & R. D. KLAUSNER. 1990. Genetic and mutational analysis of the T-cell antigen receptor. Annu. Rev. Immunol. **8**: 139–167.
4. JENKINS, M. K. & R. H. SCHWARTZ. 1987. Antigen presentation by chemically-modified splenocytes induces antigen-specific T cell unresponsiveness *in vitro* and *in vivo*. J. Exp. Med. **165**: 302–319.
5. QUILL, H. & R. H. SCHWARTZ. 1987. Stimulation of normal inducer T cell clones with antigen presented by purified Ia molecules in planar lipid membranes: specific induction of a long-lived state of proliferative nonresponsiveness. J. Immunol. **138**: 3704–3712.
6. JENKINS, M. K., C. CHEN, G. JUNG, D. L. MUELLER & R. H. SCHWARTZ. 1990. Inhibition of antigen-specific proliferation of type 1 murine T cell clones after stimulation with immobilized anti-CD3 monoclonal antibody. J. Immunol. **144**: 16–22.
7. MUELLER, D. L., M. K. JENKINS & R. H. SCHWARTZ. 1989. An accessory cell-derived costimulatory signal acts independently of protein kinase C activation to allow T cell proliferation and prevent the induction of unresponsiveness. J. Immunol. **142**: 2617–2628.
8. JENKINS, M. K., J. D. ASHWELL & R. H. SCHWARTZ. 1988. Allogeneic non-T spleen cells restore the responsiveness of normal T cell clones stimulated with antigen and chemically-modified antigen-presenting cells. J. Immunol. **140**: 3324–3330.
9. CRABTREE, G. R. 1989. Contingent genetic regulatory events in T lymphocyte activation. Science **243**: 355–361.
10. NISBET-BROWN, E. R., J. W. LEE, R. K. CHEUNG & E. W. GELFAND. 1987. Antigen-specific and nonspecific mitogenic signals in the activation of human T cell clones. J. Immunol. **138**: 3713–3719.
11. JUNE, C. H., J. A. LEDBETTER, P. S. LINSLEY & C. B. THOMPSON. 1990. Role of the CD28 receptor in T-cell activation. Immunol. Today **11**: 211–216.
12. JUNE, C. H., J. A. LEDBETTER, M. M. GILLESPIE, T. LINDSTEN & C. B. THOMPSON. 1987. T-cell proliferation involving the CD28 pathway is associated with cyclosporine-resistant interleukin 2 gene expression. Mol. Cell. Biol. **7**: 4472–4481.
13. WAHL, S. M., D. R. ROSENSTREICH & J. J. OPPENHEIM. 1976. Separation of human lymphocytes by E rosette sedimentation. *In* In Vitro Methods in Cell-mediated and Tumor Immunity. B. R. Bloom & J. R. David, Eds. 231–240. Academic Press. New York.
14. ISAKOV, N., M. I. MALLY, W. SCHOLZ & A. ALTMAN. 1987. T lymphocyte activation: the role of protein kinase C and the bifurcating inositol phospholipid signal transduction pathway. Immunol. Rev. **95**: 89–111.

15. LICHTMAN, A. H., E. A. KURT-JONES & A. K. ABBAS. 1987. B-cell stimulatory factor 1 and not IL-2 is the autocrine growth factor for some T helper lymphocytes. Proc. Natl. Acad. Sci. USA **84**: 824–827.

16. UMETSU, D. T., KATZEN, T. CHATILA, R. MILLER, H. H. JABARA, M. MAHER, H. OETTGEN, C. TERHORST & R. S. GEHA. 1987. Requirements for activation of human peripheral blood T cells by mouse monoclonal antibodies to CD3. Clin. Immunol. Immunopathol. **43**: 48–64.

17. LEDBETTER, J. A., M. PARSONS, P. J. MARTIN, J. A. HANSEN, P. S. RABINOVITCH & C. H. JUNE. 1986. Antibody binding to CD5 (Tp67) and Tp44 T cell surface molecules: effects on cyclic nucleotides, cytoplasmic free calcium, and cAMP-mediated suppression. J. Immunol. **137**: 3299–3305.

18. WEISS, A., B. MANGER & J. IMBODEN. 1986. Synergy between the T3/antigen receptor complex and Tp44 in the activation of human T cells. J. Immunol. **137**: 819–825.

19. FRASER, J. D., B. A. IRVING, G. R. CRABTREE & A. WEISS. 1990. CD28 stimulation increases interleukin gene transcription by a pathway distinct from that of the T cell antigen receptor. FASEB J. **4**: A1741.

20. LINSLEY, P. S., E. A. CLARK & J. A. LEDBETTER. 1990. T-cell antigen CD28 mediates adhesion with B cells by interacting with activation antigen B7/BB-1. Proc. Natl. Acad. Sci. USA **87**: 5031–5035.

21. FREEMAN, G. J., A. S. FREEDMAN, J. M. SEGIL, G. LEE, J. F. WHITMAN & L. M. NADLER. 1989. B7, a new member of the Ig superfamily with unique expression on activated and neoplastic B cells. J. Immunol. **143**: 2714–2722.

22. YOKOCHI, T., R. D. HOLLEY & E. A. CLARK. 1982. B lymphoblast antigen (BB-1) expressed on Epstein-Barr virus-activated B cell blasts, B lymphoblastoid cell lines, and Burkitt's lymphomas. J. Immunol. **128**: 823–827.

23. WEAVER, C. T., C. M. HAWRYLOWICZ & E. R. UNANUE. 1988. T helper cell subsets require the expression of distinct costimulatory signals by antigen-presenting cells. Proc. Natl. Acad. Sci. USA **85**: 8181–8185.

24. ASHWELL, J. D., M. K. JENKINS & R. H. SCHWARTZ. 1988. Effect of gamma radiation on resting B lymphocytes. II. Functional characterization of the antigen-presentation defect. J. Immunol. **141**: 2536–2544.

Tum⁻ Antigens, TSTA, and T Cell Immune Surveillance

ALINE VAN PEL, GUY WARNIER, BENOÎT VAN DEN
EYNDE, BERNARD LETHÉ, CHRISTOPHE LURQUIN,
AND THIERRY BOON

Ludwig Institute for Cancer Research
Brussels Branch
Avenue Hippocrate 74, UCL 7459
B-1200 Brussels, Belgium

Tumor-associated transplantation antigens (TATA) are commonly found on rodent tumors induced by oncogenic viruses, chemical carcinogens, and ultraviolet (UV) irradiation.[1-4] In contrast, spontaneous rodent tumors appear to be incapable of eliciting any rejection response in the syngeneic host.[5,6] But further experiments demonstrated that even these tumors express weak TSTA that are recognized by cytolytic T cells (CTL) and are potential targets for immune rejection.[7] In man also, there is good evidence that some tumors carry tumor-associated antigens that are recognized by autologous CTL.[8] However, it is difficult to evaluate to what extent human tumors carry antigens that can be the targets of an autologous rejection response.

What is the molecular nature of TSTA? And what is the relation between their appearance and the tumoral transformation process? These questions are still unanswered because the TSTA, which elicit strong T-cell mediated immune responses, do not stimulate B cells to produce antibodies. It has therefore been impossible to isolate the antigenic molecules by immunoprecipitation. This predicament is not restricted to TSTA: most minor histocompatibility antigens and the male-specific antigen H-Y remain uncharacterized for the same reasons.

We have developed a gene transfection approach aimed at identifying directly the genes that code for this type of antigen and we have applied it to the "tum⁻" transplantation antigens, which are found on mutagenized mouse tumor cells. This methodology also ensured the isolation of the gene coding for a TSTA present on a mouse mastocytoma tumor.

Tum⁻ Variants and Immune Protection Against the Parental Tumor

In vitro mutagen treatment of mouse tumor cell lines generates at extremely high frequency stable immunogenic variants that are rejected by syngeneic mice.[9-11] Since these variants fail to form tumors, they have been named "tum⁻" as opposed to the original "tum⁺" cell line, which forms progressive tumors. This phenomenon has been found on many mouse tumor cell lines of various cell types.[11,12] Most tum⁻ variants express transplantation antigens not found on the tum⁺ cell. The existence of these tum⁻ antigens can be demonstrated *in vivo* by cross-immunization experiments or *in vitro* with cytolytic T lymphocytes[13,14] (FIG. 1).

By rejecting a living inoculum of tum⁻ variant cells, mice acquire a certain degree of resistance against a challenge with the original tumor. This protection is

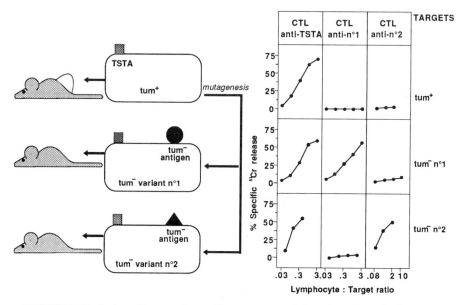

FIGURE 1. Variants and tum⁻ antigens. The percentage of chromium release indicates the percentage of target cells lysed by the lymphocytes.

weak. However, it has long-term effects and it is specific for the parental tumor.[7,10,13] This protective effect was found for tum⁻ variants obtained not only from various weakly immunogenic tumors but most importantly from spontaneous tumors which appear to be devoid of any immunogenicity. Tum⁻ variants have been derived from two spontaneous leukemias obtained by Hewitt in CBA/

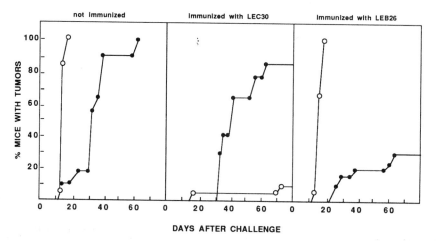

FIGURE 2. Protection against parental LEC and LEB tumor lines. Mice were immunized with tum⁻ variant LEC30 or LEB26. After 32d they were challenged with LEC (O-O) and LEB (●-●) tumor cells.

Ht mice. Some of these variants provide a significant protection against the parental tumors even though they were never adapted to culture. This protection is specific: it applies exclusively to the parental tumor (FIG. 2). With the small reservation that these spontaneous tumors were transplanted many times, these results suggest that spontaneous tumors also carry weak tumor-associated transplantation antigens.

Protection experiments were also realized with mouse teratocarcinoma PCC4.aza1. Some tum⁻ variants like T25 are able to partially protect against the parental tumor, while living tum⁺ cells are unable to confer an immune protection: animals, whose large tumors had been removed by surgery, acquired tumors as readily as control animals when subsequently challenged with tum⁺ cells.

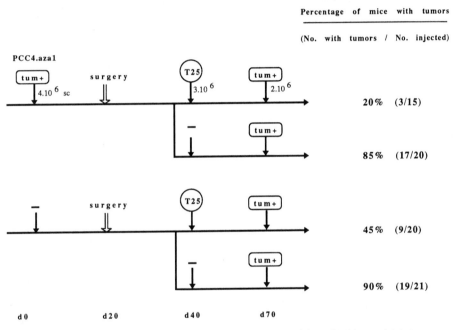

FIGURE 3. Absence of tolerance in mice that have been injected with tum⁺ teratocarcinoma cells. Subcutaneous tumors have been removed by surgery after the injection of tum⁺ cells. Control mice were sham-operated. All mice were immunized with tum⁻ variant T25 and challenged with the original tumor 30d later.

However, such animals had not become tolerant. The subsequent injection of tum⁻ cells still induced partial protection against a challenge with tum⁺ cells (FIG. 3).[15]

Tum⁻ Antigens

We undertook the cloning of the genes coding for tum⁻ antigens on mastocytoma P815, a tumor induced in a DBA/2 mouse with methylcholanthrene. A series of tum⁻ variants were derived by mutagenesis.[16] For most P815 tum⁻ variants, stable DBA/2 CTL clones were obtained that showed a strict specificity for the immunizing variant and thus defined one or several tum⁻ antigens.[17] The diversity of tum⁻ antigens is considerable, since the analysis of 15 P815 tum⁻ variants revealed the existence of a different antigen on each of them.[12] The tum⁻ antigens defined by CTL are relevant to the rejection of the variants, as shown by the correlation between the loss of these antigens and the reversal of the tum⁻ phenotype.[18,19] No antibodies were obtained against these antigens.

To clone the genes that determine the expression of tum⁻ antigens we used an approach based on gene transfection. It involves the use of line P1.HTR, a highly transfectable P815 cell line,[20] and the detection of antigen-expressing transfectants by their ability to stimulate CTL clones directed against the tum⁻ antigen.[21] After transfection of P815 cells with cosmid libraries prepared with the DNA of cells expressing various tum⁻ antigens, we obtained cosmids that were capable of transferring the expression of the tum⁻ antigens. Thus three genes encoding tum⁻ antigens were isolated : P91A, P198 and P35B. From their sequence analysis, we concluded that these genes are completely unrelated and show no similarity with any known gene recorded in data banks (FIG. 4). For each tum⁻ variant, we could also show that the tum⁻ gene differs from the normal allele by one point mutation located in one of the exons.[22-25]

Antigenic Peptides

Considering the overwhelming evidence that T cells recognize short peptides presented by MHC molecules,[26] we examined whether we could also identify a small peptide that would trigger the lysis of P815 cells by anti-tum⁻ CTL. In our search for this peptide we were guided by the location of the tum⁻ mutation. For gene P91A, a short peptide corresponding to the mutant sequence induced the lysis of P1 cells by anti-P91A CTL (FIG. 4). Transfection and peptides studies with H-2^k fibroblasts, which expressed also either K^d, D^d or L^d, demonstrated that antigen P91A is associative with L^d. Antigenic peptides corresponding to the sequence surrounding the tum⁻ mutation were also obtained for genes P35B and P198. They associate with D^d and K^d respectively.

Studies with P91A peptides enabled us to understand the role of the tum⁻ mutation. A priori, the mutation could influence either the production of the antigenic peptide or its ability to associate with the L^d molecule (i.e., the aggretope) or also the epitope presented to T cells by the peptide-MHC complex. Having the antigenic P91A peptide, we prepared the homologous peptide corresponding to the normal allele of the gene. This normal peptide did not induce lysis by anti-P91A CTL, nor did it compete with the mutant peptide. Moreover, we found that the mutant peptide competed effectively to prevent a cytomegalovirus-derived peptide from inducing lysis by CTL directed against a L^d-associative cytomegalovirus antigen. The normal peptide did not compete[23] and we concluded that it does not bind to L^d. This indicates that the P91A tum⁻ mutation generates the aggretope of the antigen, but does not exclude that it also influences the epitope. For antigen P198, the effect of the mutation appears to be different: here a new epitope is introduced on a normal peptide that is already capable of binding to the K^d presenting molecule.

Cloning of a Gene Encoding a Mouse Tumor Rejection Antigen

We have applied our cloning procedure to the isolation of the gene coding for a tumor rejection antigen expressed by tumor P815.[27] As opposed to the tum⁻

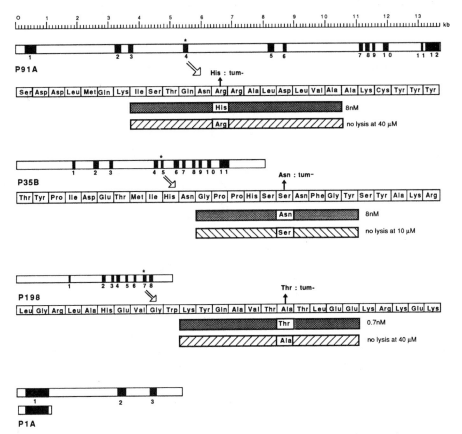

FIGURE 4. Structure of genes P91A, P35B, P198 and P1A and antigenic peptides. *Dark regions* represent exons. The exon containing the tum⁻ mutation is marked by an *asterisk*. Sections of the proteins located around the mutated amino-acid are indicated. Synthetic peptides corresponding to the mutant and normal sequence of the genes are represented by *boxes*. They were tested for their ability to render P1.HTR cells susceptible to lysis by anti-tum⁻ CTL. The concentration indicated to the *right* of each peptide provided 50% of the lysis obtained at saturating concentration of peptide. For P1A, the *box* indicates the sub-genic fragment capable of transferring the expression of antigens P1A and P1B. The antigenic peptides for P1A and P1B are not yet identified.

antigens, these antigens are present on all P815 cells, whether they are muta-genized or not. The study of antigen-loss variants enabled us to identify 4 distinct antigens recognized by different syngeneic CTL clones. They were called P1A, B, C, and D.[28] Antigens P1A and P1B thus defined *in vitro* are relevant *in vivo*, because P815 tumor cells that progressed in mice after nearly complete initial rejection were found to have lost the expression of one or both of these antigens. Antigens P1A and P1B showed linkage, since several antigen-loss variants for P1A were found to have lost P1B concurrently.

For the transfection of antigen P1A, we used as recipient cell a P1A-B-antigen-loss variant selected from line P1.HTR with an anti-P1A CTL clone (P0.HTR).

Transfectants expressing antigens P1A and P1B were obtained with the genomic DNA of P1.HTR. This confirmed the close link between these two antigens. Transfectants were then obtained with a cosmid library made with the DNA of a genomic transfectant. By directly packaging the DNA of one of these cosmid transfectants, we obtained a cosmid that was able to transfect antigens P1A and P1B.

The structure and the complete sequence of gene P1A were then obtained (FIG. 4). They proved completely different from those of the tum⁻ genes and of any known gene reported in data banks.

Transfection studies in H-2^k fibroblasts previously transfected with either K^d, D^d or L^d demonstrated that both P1A and P1B were presented to the CTL by the L^d molecule.

We compared the sequence of this gene, cloned from tumor cells, to the sequence of the equivalent gene cloned from normal cells of the same mouse strain. From a genomic library made with the DNA of normal DBA/2 mouse kidney we isolated the gene homologous to gene P1A. The analysis of this gene revealed that its sequence was identical to the sequence of the tumoral gene. To

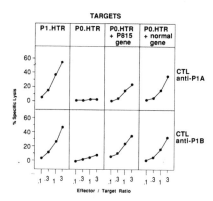

FIGURE 5. Transfection of the P1A gene isolated from normal cells. The P1A gene isolated from a genomic library from normal DBA/2 mouse kidney was transfected in P0.HTR cells. The population of drug-resistant transfectants was tested with the anti-P1A and anti-P1B CTL clones.

confirm this, we transfected this normal gene and found that it transferred the expression of antigens P1A and P1B as efficiently as the gene cloned from P815 cells (FIG. 5). The antigenicity is therefore not the result of a mutation in the tumoral gene, and P1A and P1B are presumably two different peptides derived from the same protein.

The tumor specificity of antigens P1A and P1B can nevertheless be partially explained by the pattern of expression of the gene. Northern blot analysis revealed that the gene was silent in most normal tissues. However, one mast cell line (L138.8A) was found to express high levels of this messenger RNA. This cell line, derived by L. Hültner from bone marrow of BALB/c mice,[29] is cultivated in medium supplemented with IL3. It grew as a permanent line and became spontaneously tumorigenic. Because BALB/c mice and DBA/2 mice express the same H-2 haplotype, we were able to confirm the expression of gene P1A in L138.8A cells by lysis with the anti-P1A and anti-P1B CTL clones: we observed a significant lysis. Other nontransformed mast cell lines on the other hand were negative for P1A expression, so that we do not know whether the expression of the gene is associated to the mast cell lineage at a given stage of its differentiation, or whether it is related to the tumoral transformation. We failed to identify other tumor cell lines expressing messenger RNA for P1A.

Immune Surveillance, Tolerance and Tumor Rejection Antigens

A first conclusion based on the results obtained with the tum⁻ antigens is that mutations throughout all the mammalian genome generate at high efficiency antigenic peptides recognized by T cells, and that this mechanism could account for the presence of specific tumor rejection antigens on carcinogen-induced tumors.

However, the study of antigen P1A clearly showed that gene P1A is identical to its normal counterpart. The apparent tumor specificity of antigen P1A seems to be due to the expression by the tumor of a gene that is silent in most normal cells, rather than to a mutation generating an antigenic peptide. How can the immune system be sensitized against normal peptides without generating an obvious autoimmune pathology? Several hypotheses can be suggested. If the gene encodes an embryonic or oncofetal protein, then the antigen might have disappeared before the establishment of tolerance. If it codes for a differentiation or activation antigen, it may be expressed very transiently by a small number of cells, so that tolerance would not develop. An immune response directed against this antigen may not inflict lasting damage on this differentiation lineage. Finally, tolerance may exist for P1A, and may have been broken because of the simultaneous presence on the P815 tumor of other antigens like C and D. These antigens could indeed be the result of mutations and may therefore be strongly immunogenic like tum⁻ antigens. They could possibly trigger an immune response that would facilitate a response against P1A by a process that would be similar to that accounting for the protection against tum⁺ cells by tum⁻ variants.[7]

REFERENCES

1. GROSS, L. 1943. Intradermal immunization of C3H mice against a sarcoma that originated in an animal of the same line. Cancer Res. **43:** 326.
2. PREHN, R. T. & J. M. MAIN. 1957. Immunity to methylcholanthrene-induced sarcomas. J. Natl. Cancer Inst. **18:** 769.
3. KLEIN, G., H. SJORGEN, E. KLEIN & K. E. HELLSTROM. 1960. Demonstration of resistance against methylcholanthrene-induced sarcomas in the primary autochtonous host. Cancer Res. **20:** 1561.
4. KRIPKE, M. 1974. Antigenicity of murine skin tumors induced by ultraviolet light. J. Natl. Cancer Inst. **53:** 1333.
5. HEWITT, H. B., E. R. BLAKE & A. S. WALDER. 1976. A critique of the evidence for active host defence against cancer based on personal studies of 27 murine tumors of spontaneous origin. Br. J. Cancer **33:** 241.
6. MIDDLE, J. G. & M. J. EMBLETON. 1981. Naturally arising tumors of the inbred WAB/Not rat strain: II. Immunogenicity of transplanted tumors. J. Natl. Cancer Inst. **67:** 637.
7. VAN PEL, A., F. VESSIÈRE & T. BOON. 1983. Protection against two spontaneous mouse leukemias conferred by immunogenic variants obtained by mutagenesis. J. Exp. Med. **157:** 1992.
8. HÉRIN, M., C. LEMOINE, P. WEYNANTS, F. VESSIÈRE, A. VAN PEL, A. KNUTH, R. DEVOS & T. BOON. 1987. Production of stable cytolytic T-cell clones directed against autologous human melanoma. Int. J. Cancer **39:** 390.
9. BOON, T. & O. KELLERMAN. 1977. Rejection by syngeneic mice of cell variants obtained by mutagenesis of a malignant teratocarcinoma cell line. Proc. Natl. Acad. Sci. USA **74:** 272.

10. VAN PEL, A., M. GEORLETTE & T. BOON. 1979. Tumor cell variants obtained by mutagenesis of a Lewis lung carcinoma cell line: immune rejection by syngeneic mice. Proc. Natl. Acad. Sci. USA 76: 5282.
11. FROST, P., R. KERBEL, E. BAUER, R. TARTAMELLA-BIONDO & W. CEFALU. 1983. Mutagen treatments as a mean for selecting immunogenic variants from otherwise poorly immunogenic malignant murine tumors. Cancer Res. 43: 125.
12. BOON, T. 1983. Antigenic tumor cell variants obtained with mutagens. Adv. Cancer Res. 39: 121.
13. BOON, T. & A. VAN PEL. 1978. Teratocarcinoma cell variants rejected by syngeneic mice: protection of mice immunized with these variants against other variants and against the original malignant cell line. Proc. Natl. Acad. Sci. USA 75: 1519.
14. BOON, T., J. VAN SNICK, A. VAN PEL, C. UYTTENHOVE & M. MARCHAND. 1980. Immunogenic variants obtained by mutagenesis of mouse mastocytoma P815. T lymphocyte-mediated cytolysis. J. Exp. Med. 152: 1184.
15. BOON, T., A. VAN PEL & G. WARNIER. Mouse teratocarcinoma cell variants obtained by mutagenesis: rejection by syngeneic mice and immunization against the original tumor cell line. In Protides of Biological Fluids. 27th Colloquium, 1979. Pergamon Press. Oxford and New York.
16. UYTTENHOVE, C., J. VAN SNICK & T. BOON. 1980. Immunogenic variants obtained by mutagenesis of mouse mastocytoma P815. I. Rejection by syngeneic mice. J. Exp. Med. 152: 1175.
17. MARYANSKI, J. L., J. VAN SNICK, J-C. CEROTTINI & T. BOON. 1982. Immunogenic variants obtained by mutagenesis of mouse mastocytoma P815. Clonal analysis of the syngeneic cytolytic T lymphocyte response. Eur. J. Immunol. 12: 401.
18. MARYANSKI, J. L. & T. BOON. 1982. Immunogenic variants obtained by mutagenesis of mouse mastocytoma P815. Analysis of variants-specific antigens by selection of antigen-loss variants with cytolytic T cell clones. Eur. J. Immunol. 12: 406.
19. MARYANSKI, J. L., M. MARCHAND, C. UYTTENHOVE & T. BOON. 1983. Immunogenic variants obtained by mutagenesis of mouse mastocytoma P815. Occasional escape from host rejection due to antigen-loss secondary variants. Int. J. Cancer 31: 119.
20. VAN PEL, A., E. DE PLAEN & T. BOON. 1985. Selection of highly transfectable variant from mouse mastocytoma P815. Somatic Cell Mol. Genet. 11: 467.
21. WÖLFEL, T., A. VAN PEL, E. DE PLAEN, C. LURQUIN, J. L. MARYANSKI & T. BOON. 1987. Immunogenic (tum⁻) variants obtained by mutagenesis of mouse mastocytoma P815. Detection of stable transfectants expressing a tum⁻ antigen with a cytolytic T cell stimulation assay. Immunogenetics 26: 178.
22. DE PLAEN, E., C. LURQUIN, A. VAN PEL, B. MARIAMÉ, J-P. SZIKORA, T. WÖLFEL, C. SIBILLE, P. CHOMEZ & T. BOON. 1988. Immunogenic (tum⁻) variants of mouse tumor P815: cloning of the gene of tum⁻ antigen P91A and identification of the tum⁻ mutation. Proc. Natl. Acad. Sci. USA 85: 2274.
23. LURQUIN, C., A. VAN PEL, B. MARIAMÉ, E. DE PLAEN, J-P. SZIKORA, C. JANSSENS, M. J. REDDEHASE, J. LEJEUNE & T. BOON. 1989. Structure of the gene of tum⁻ transplantation antigen P91A: the mutated exon encodes a peptide recognized with Ld by cytolytic T cells. Cell 58: 293.
24. SZIKORA, J. P., A. VAN PEL, V. BRICHARD, M. ANDRÉ, N. VAN BAREN, P. HENRY, E. DE PLAEN & T. BOON. 1990. Structure of the gene of tum⁻ transplantation antigen P35B: presence of a point mutation in the antigenic allele. EMBO J. 9: 1041.
25. SIBILLE, C., P. CHOMEZ, C. WILDMANN, A. VAN PEL, E. DE PLAEN, J. L. MARYANSKI, V. DE BERGEYCK & T. BOON. 1990. Structure of the gene of tum⁻ transplantation antigen P198: a point mutation generates a new antigenic peptide. J. Exp. Med. 172: 35.
26. TOWNSEND, A. R. M., J. ROTHBARD, F. M. GOTCH, G. BAHADUR, D. WRAITH & A. J. McMICHAEL. 1986. The epitopes of influenza nucleoprotein recognized by cytotoxic T lymphocytes can be defined with short synthetic peptides. Cell 44: 959.
27. VAN DEN EYNDE, B., B. LETHÉ, A. VAN PEL, E. DE PLAEN & T. BOON. 1991. The gene coding for a major tumor rejection antigen of tumor P815 is identical to the normal gene of the syngeneic DBA/2 mice. J. Exp. Med. 173: 1373.

28. UYTTENHOVE, C., J. MARYANSKI & T. BOON. 1983. Escape of mouse mastocytoma P815 after nearly complete rejection is due to antigen-loss variants rather than immunosuppression. J. Exp. Med. **157:** 1040.

29. HÜLTNER, L., J. MOELLER, E. SCHMITT, G. JÄGER, G. REISBACH, J. RING & P. DÖRMER. 1989. Thiol-sensitive mast cell lines derived from mouse bone marrow respond to a mast cell growth-enhancing activity different from both IL3 and IL4. J. Immunol. **142:** 3440.

Thymocyte Activation and Death: a Mechanism for Molding the T Cell Repertoire

CHARLES M. ZACHARCHUK, MLADEN MERĆEP, AND
JONATHAN D. ASHWELL

Biological Response Modifiers Program
National Cancer Institute
National Institutes of Health
Building 10, Room 13N-268
Bethesda, Maryland 20892

INTRODUCTION

Cell death is an integral part of ontogeny. During organogenesis, certain cells within a given lineage are produced and then killed by a process known as programmed cell death (PCD).[1-4] PCD is generally a "suicide," meaning that no other cell type is required for death to occur. The dying cells undergo a distinctive pattern of morphological changes: condensation of the cytoplasm, swelling of the endoplasmic reticulum, clumping of nuclear chromatin, fragmentation of the nucleolus, and plasma membrane blebbing.[5,6] This process has been termed apoptosis, and is easily distinguishable from the other classic type of cell death, necrosis, which is accompanied by cell and mitochondrial swelling and preservation of the nuclear structure. The distinction between PCD and necrosis is important because PCD does not result in an inflammatory or fibrotic response, and thus allows the elimination or remodeling of tissues without damaging "innocent bystander" cells and organ function. Many features are shared between examples of PCD in different experimental systems. For example, PCD is usually manifested hours after the initiating stimulus, and is prevented by reagents such as cycloheximide and actinomycin D, indicating a need for new mRNA and protein synthesis.[5-9] Where tested, there is a requirement for Ca^{2+} in the extracellular medium,[6,10] and cyclosporin A (CsA) prevents the phenomenon.[10,11] Finally the *sine qua non* of PCD is the degradation of nuclear DNA into multimers of 180 to 200 bp fragments, giving a "step ladder" appearance when the DNA is separated on agarose gels. The DNA fragmentation is thought to reflect the activity of one or more so far uncharacterized endonucleases that cleave between nucleosomes.[12] Whether it is the new transcription of endonucleases after the "death signal" is received, the mobilization of regulatory co-factors that control the activity of the nucleases, or the accessibility of DNA as a substrate, that is the controlling step for DNA cleavage is unknown.

PCD has a particular importance for the immune system. Experimental situations that result in programmed cell death in lymphocytes and hematopoietic cells include the withdrawal of cytokine "growth factors" such as IL-2 or colony stimulating factors from dependent cell lines[13,14] and the lysis of target cells by cytotoxic T cells.[15-17] In addition, stimulation of thymocytes via the T cell receptor for antigen (TCR), either *in vivo* or in fetal tissue organ culture, leads to PCD.[4,11,18] This last experimental model is thought to reflect the process of negative selection, in which thymocytes that react with self antigens are deleted, resulting in peripheral tolerance to self antigens.[19] The studies reported in this paper were undertaken to shed light on the issues of how PCD is induced in immature, mature, and transformed T cells, and how PCD is regulated *in vivo* to effect the shaping the T cell antigen-specific repertoire.

MATERIALS AND METHODS

Mice

Balb/c, B10.A, and timed pregnant C57BL/6 (B6) mice were obtained from the Frederick Cancer Research Center (Frederick, MD).

Antibodies

Hamster IgG (HIgG) was purchased from Jackson ImmunoResearch Laboratories, Inc. (West Grove, PA). 145-2C11 (2C11; hamster anti-mouse CD3-ε),[20] H57-597 (H57; hamster anti-mouse TCR $\alpha\beta$),[21] and G7 (rat anti-mouse Thy-1)[22] were produced and purified as described.[23] F23.1 (anti-Vβ8)[24] and RR-4-7(anti-Vβ6)[25] were used as culture supernatants to stain thymocytes. FITC-GK 1.5 (anti-CD4)[26] and biotinylated 2.43 (anti-CD8)[27] were kindly provided by Ada Kruisbeek (NIH, Bethesda, MD). Staphylococcal enterotoxin B (SEB) and dexamethasone (Dex) were purchased from Sigma Chemical Co. (St. Louis, MO). CsA was purchased from Sandoz Inc. (East Hanover, NJ). RU-486 was the generous gift of E. E. Baulieu (Université de Paris-Sud, France). An anti-glucocorticoid receptor (GR) antiserum, aP1, was kindly provided by Bernd Groner (Fridrick Miescher-Institut, Basel, Switzerland).

Culture Medium

2B4.11 cells were maintained in RPMI 1640 (Biofluids Inc., Rockville, MD) supplemented with 10% heat-inactivated fetal calf serum, 4 mM glutamine, 10 U/ml penicillin, 150 μg/ml gentamicin, and 5×10^{-5} M 2-mercaptoethanol (complete medium).

Cells

2B4.11 is a cytochrome *c*-specific T cell hybridoma, a fusion product of the AKR-derived thymoma BW5147 and B10.A splenic T cells.[28] LK 35.2 is MHC class II- and Fc receptor-bearing B cell tumor.[29]

Thymocyte Depletion Assay

Mice were injected i.p. with control HIgG or anti-TCR antibodies in PBS, using a fixed antibody/mouse weight ratio in a given experiment. Twenty-four or

48 hr later the mice were sacrificed and their thymi removed, made into single cell suspensions, and viability determined by trypan blue exclusion. Percent recovery was expressed as the number of thymocytes in treated versus control animals:

$$\frac{\text{average number of viable thymocytes recovered per treated mouse}}{\text{average number of viable thymocytes recovered per hamster IgG-treated mouse}} \times 100$$

For some experiments, timed pregnant B6 mice were used. Day 0 (day of birth) pups were injected within 24 hr of birth. To determine the effects of SEB on $V\beta$ expression, SEB (50 μg SEB/g mouse weight) was either injected i.p. or added at a concentration of 1 to 30 μg/ml to freshly resected thymic lobes, which were then cultured on Nucleopore filters supported by Gelfoam gelatin sponges.[30] After 48 or 24 hr, respectively, the thymocytes were analyzed for $V\beta$ expression by flow cytometry.

Flow Cytometry

Approximately 10^6 thymocytes were stained with FITC-conjugated or biotinylated antibodies (2C11, GK 1.5, and 2.43) or culture supernatants (F23.1 and RR-4-7) followed by phycoerythrin-avidin, FITC-labelled goat anti-mouse, or FITC-goat anti-rat (Jackson ImmunoResearch Laboratories, Inc., West Grove, PA) and analyzed with a FACScan (Becton-Dickinson Immunocytometric Systems, Mountain View, CA).

Measurement of Phosphatidylinositol Hydrolysis

Phosphoinositide hydrolysis was measured as described.[31] Briefly, 2B4.11 cells or thymocytes were labelled with [^{3}H]myo-inositol for 3 hr, washed, and then analyzed in duplicate for inositol phosphates by anion exchange chromatography. Three $\times 10^6$ thymocytes or 10^6 2B4.11 cells were used for each experimental point. Cells were cultured for the indicated times in 10 mM LiCL$_2$ with or without 10^6 LK 35.2 cells. The stimuli were: AlF$_4^-$ (10 μM AlCl$_3$ plus 75 mM NaF), 2C11 (1/40 dilution of culture supernatant), H57 (1/40 dilution of culture supernatant), or G7 (30 μg/ml). When testing the effect of Dex on phosphoinositide hydrolysis, 2B4.11 cells were labelled in the absence or presence of 10^{-6} M Dex, washed, and then cultured with the indicated stimuli for 60 min without or with 10^{-6} M Dex, respectively, before analyzing for inositol phosphates. The mean cpm for each experimental point was divided by the total cpm incorporated by the cells (yielding % labeled phospholipid), and the % labeled phospholipid for control cultures (medium alone) was subtracted from stimulated cultures to obtain Δ % labeled phospholipid.

^{51}Cr Release Assay

Five $\times 10^6$ cells/ml were incubated at 37°C in the presence of 100 μCi of Na$_2$^{51}CrO$_4$ (Amersham Corporation, Arlington Heights, IL). After 2 hr, the cells were washed and placed into 96-well flat bottomed plates (Costar, Cambridge,

MA) in triplicate at a concentration of 3×10^4 cells per well in complete medium. At the indicated times, an aliquot of supernatant was removed and ^{51}Cr release quantitated with a gamma counter (Gamma 5500, Beckman Instruments, Irvine, CA). Specific ^{51}Cr release was calculated with the formula:

percent specific ^{51}Cr release

$$= \frac{\text{experimental release} - \text{spontaneous release}}{\text{maximal release} - \text{spontaneous release}} \times 100$$

Maximal release was determined by lysing the cells with 1% Triton X-100. The standard error of the mean was always <5% for each determination, and spontaneous release was generally 20–30% of maximal release in 12–14 hr assays. In some assays, the experimental release was less than the spontaneous release. This was most frequently seen with Dex or CsA plus cellular activating agents.

Immunoblotting

2B4.11 cells were incubated for 1 hr with 10^{-6} M Dex, 2C11 bound to plastic (20 μg/ml in 100 mm diameter plastic dishes), or in the indicated combinations. Pellets from 20×10^6 cells were ruptured by freeze-thaw lysis and cytoplasmic and nuclear fractions were prepared by centrifugation and then extraction of nuclei with sodium thiocyanate as described.[32] After separation by SDS-polyacrylamide gel electrophoresis, proteins were transferred to nitrocellulose and immunoblotted with aP1. The immunoblots were quantitated by densitometry.

Transfections

The expression vector PBL-CAT$_2$ was obtained from Dr. Warren Leonard (NIH), and PRE-PBL$_7$, which contains 2 copies of the tyrosine aminotransferase gene (TAT) GRE/PRE inserted into PBL-CAT$_2$,[33] was kindly provided by Dr. Bert O'Malley (Baylor College of Medicine, Houston, Texas). 2B4.11 cells were transfected by electroporation as described.[32] After a 2 hr culture in complete medium at 37°C, the cells were cultured under the indicated conditions. After 6 hr, the cells were harvested, washed in cold PBS, lysed by repeated freezing and thawing, and equivalent amounts of cytoplasmic protein (Bio-Rad protein assay, Richmond, CA) were used in a standard chloramphenicol acetyltransferase (CAT) activity assay.[34]

RESULTS

Deletion of Thymocytes In Vivo with Anti-TCR Antibodies

To establish a model system in which to study thymocyte PCD, anti-TCR monoclonal (anti-CD3, 2C11, or anti-$\alpha\beta$, H57) or HIgG control antibodies were injected into 3 to 4 week old Balb/c or B6 mice. Twenty-four hr later total viable thymocyte recovery was determined (TABLE 1). In multiple experiments, 2C11 caused approximately a 70% reduction in viable cell recovery. This value is similar to that reported for the recovery of thymocytes in a thymic organ culture system using the same antibody.[35] Several groups have found that CsA blocks

TABLE 1. Thymocyte Depletion by 2C11 and Effect of CsA[a]

	% Thymocyte Recovery				
	Exp. 1	Exp. 2	Exp. 3	Exp. 4	Mean
No Rx	100	100	100	100	100
HIgG	113	99	102	97	103
CsA	92	64	97	62	79
2C11	32	25	27	32	29
2C11 + CsA	74	61	70	47	63

[a] Balb/c mice (3 to 4 weeks old) were injected i.p. with PBS, 100 μg of HIgG or 2C11, 20 mg/kg of CsA, or the indication combination. Twenty-four hr later thymi were harvested and cell recovery quantitated by trypan blue exclusion.

thymocyte PCD *in vitro*[11] and negative selection *in vivo*.[36,37] Therefore, the effect of CsA on 2C11-induced deletion in this model system was determined. As shown in TABLE 1, CsA alone produced a small decrease in cell yield, an effect that has previously been attributed largely to the loss of CD4$^+$CD8$^-$ and CD4$^-$CD8$^+$ (single positive) thymocytes; this was confirmed in the current studies by staining with fluoresceinated antibodies and analysis by flow cytometry (data not shown). Despite the loss of single positive cells, there was a clear and substantial reversal of total thymocyte (and therefore double positive thymocyte) depletion caused by 2C11. There was a similar depletion of thymocytes with H57 (see below). When the two antibodies were compared on a molar basis, it was found that thymocyte depletion induced by 2C11 was consistently greater than that elicited by H57. A similar finding has been made in a fetal tissue organ culture system.[35]

To identify the cells that were eliminated by anti-TCR treatment, thymocytes from HIgG-treated and H57-treated mice were analyzed by fluoresence flow cytometry for the expression of CD3, CD4, and CD8 (FIG. 1). After antibody treatment, it was the immature, TCR^{low}, CD4$^+$8$^+$ (double positive) cells that were selectively lost, as evidenced by the relative enrichment of TCR^{high} and CD4$^+$CD8$^-$ cells. Although we did not measure PCD directly by DNA fragmentation, after injecting 2C11 *in vivo* Shi et al. were able to observe thymocyte DNA fragmentation, a process that was prevented by co-inoculation with CsA.[11] Taken together, these data support the hypothesis that anti-TCR antibodies initiate PCD in immature, double positive thymocytes, presumably in the same manner as negative selection.

Thymocyte Deletion and Neonatal Tolerance

TCR $\alpha\beta^+$ thymocytes are first detectable on day 17 of fetal life and steadily increase in number thereafter.[38] Since thymocytes in the neonatal period represent cells that have recently acquired sensitivity to antigen, they would appear to offer a rather homogeneous, and largely double positive, population in which to study the process of activation-induced PCD. Therefore, the response to deletional stimuli of thymocytes from newborn mice was compared to that of thymocytes from older animals. B6 mice were injected with the anti-TCR $\alpha\beta$ antibody H57 on the day of birth (day 0) or 1 or 3 weeks after birth (FIG. 2). Because of the dramatic changes in size that take place during the first 3 weeks of life, the inoculum of H57 was adjusted to body weight. Thymi were collected 2 days later and the recovery of viable cells determined by light microscopy and the exclusion

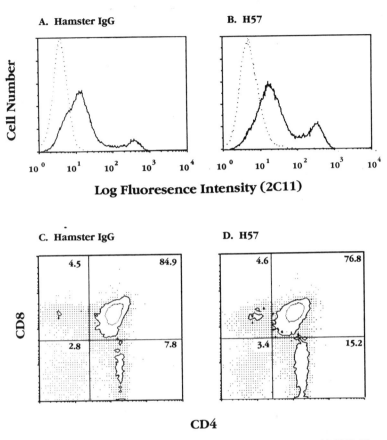

FIGURE 1. Immature thymocytes are depleted after *in vivo* treatment with H57. Three to 4 weeks old C57BL/6 mice were injected with 50 μg of HIgG (panels **(A)** and **(C)**) or H57 (panels **(B)** and **(D)**) i.p. and 48 hr later thymi were removed and separated into single cell suspensions for immunofluoresence staining. The percentage of total thymocytes in each quadrant is indicated. H57 treatment produced a 49% reduction in viable thymocyte recovery in this experiment.

FIGURE 2. Thymocyte depletion by anti-αβ antibodies after birth. C57BL/6 mice were injected with equal amounts of HIgG or H57 (5 or 10 μg/g mouse weight) on day 0 (within 24 hr of birth) or 7 and 21 days after birth. After 48 hr, thymi were harvested and viable cell recovery quantitated by trypan blue exclusion. Percent thymocyte recovery is given as the average of multiple experiments (3 to 8 mice per group) and the error bars represent the standard deviation. Number of experiments: day 0, 4 experiments; day 7, 5 experiments; day 21, 2 experiments).

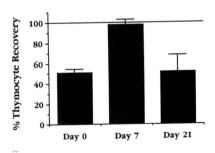

TABLE 2. Effect of SEB on $V\beta8^+$ Thymocytes at Different Days of Ontogeny[a]

	Type of Exp.	Strain	SEB Dose	$\Delta \% V\beta8^+$ Cells		$\Delta \% V\beta6^+$ Cells	
				Day 0	Day 7	Day 0	Day 7
Exp. 1	in vivo	B10.A	50 μg/g	−26%	+9%	+22%	−1%
Exp. 2	in vivo	B10.A	50 μg/g	−29%	−4%	+17%	N.D.
Exp. 3	in vitro	B10.A	1 μg/ml	−38%	−4%	+22%	+7%
Exp. 4	in vitro	C57BL/6	30 μg/ml	−48%	−17%	+23%	+9%

[a] *In vivo* experiments: B10.A mice of the indicated age were injected i.p. with PBS or 50 μg of SEB/g mouse weight. Forty-eight hr later thymi were harvested, separated into a single cell suspension, cultured in complete medium for 4 to 8 hr to allow upregulation of TCR, and then stained for $V\beta$ expression. *In vitro* experiments: freshly resected intact thymic lobes from mice of the indicated strain and age were cultured in complete medium alone or with SEB. After 24 hr the lobes were made into single cell suspensions, cultured for 4 hr, and stained for $V\beta$ expression. The data are expressed as the fraction of $V\beta^+$ cells in the SEB-treated groups compared to the fraction of $V\beta^+$ cells in the control groups.

of trypan blue. Injection of H57 on day 0 consistently resulted in approximately a 50% decrease in viable cell recovery. In contrast, treatment with H57 on day 7 resulted in little or no change in thymocyte number compared to injection with the HIgG control antibody. In separate experiments, treatment with an anti-H-2K^{b}D^b monoclonal antibody, 28-8-6, had little effect on thymocyte recovery on either day 0 or day 7, indicating that mere binding of cell surface molecules by antibody does not cause the loss of thymocytes (data not shown). In contrast to the results obtained with day 7 mice, injection of H57 into mice at 3 weeks of age was once again able to cause a substantial reduction in thymocyte recovery.

Another way to examine the differential susceptibility of neonatal thymocytes is to measure the specific deletion of particular $V\beta$ families in response to "superantigens" such as SEB. Superantigens are thought to bind to conserved regions of $V\beta$ chains and major histocompatibility-encoded class II molecules, and thus to stimulate T cell responses in a fashion similar to that of specific antigens.[39] SEB has been shown to stimulate cells bearing $V\beta3$, $V\beta7$, $V\beta8$, or $V\beta17$, and in thymic organ culture specifically deletes thymocytes bearing these TCRs.[39] Therefore, SEB was injected into day 0 or day 7 B10.A mice and 2 days later the thymi were removed, separated into single cell suspensions and stained for $V\beta$ expression. The data in TABLE 2 show that mice treated with SEB on day 0 exhibited a specific loss of $V\beta8^+$ cells (approximately 25 to 30%). In contrast, SEB caused no significant loss of $V\beta8$ expressing thymocytes in day 7 mice. In keeping with this, $V\beta6^+$ cells, which do not respond to SEB, were reciprocally increased in mice treated on the day of birth; there was no such increase in day 7 animals. To avoid the possible effects that a changing *in vivo* environment might have on these results, *in vitro* experiments were performed in which thymic lobes harvested from day 0 or day 7 animals were cultured in the presence or absence of SEB (TABLE 2, experiments 3 and 4). Once again, there was specific deletion of $V\beta8^+$ cells from the day 0 thymocytes, with little effect on cells from 7 day old animals. A particular virtue of the thymic lobe culture system is that it removes the possibility of thymocyte emigration as an explanation for the SEB-induced deletion. It should be noted that at low concentrations of SEB (1 μg/ml) the specificity of $V\beta$ deletion was absolute, while at higher SEB concentrations (30 μg/ml) there was a small effect on day 7 cells (although there was a much greater effect on day 0 cells). These data, and experiments with high concentrations of

H57 *in vivo* (data not shown), demonstrate that day 0 cells are relatively sensitive, and day 7 thymocytes relatively refractory, to TCR-mediated deletion. The finding that thymocytes from 3 week old animals were once again susceptible to TCR-mediated deletion demonstrates that the inability to delete thymocytes in day 7 mice was not due to incidental effects of the changing size of the thymus or a manifestation of the maturation of stromal thymic elements.

One obvious possible explanation for the different responses of thymocytes at different developmental ages is that their TCRs vary in the quality or quantity of the signals they transduce when occupied or perturbed. Thymocytes from day 0, 1 and 3 week old mice were stained for surface TCR expression. Except for an increase in the number of TCR[high] mature single positive cells with age, the staining profile of the immature TCR[low] cells was virtually identical for day 0, 1 and 3 week old mice (data not shown). One rapid and well characterized second messenger system triggered by TCR perturbation is the hydrolysis of phosphoinositides to diacylglycerol and inositol phosphates.[40] Thymocytes from mice of varying ages were collected and stimulated with H57 or 2C11, using the B cell hybridoma LK 35.2 to provide the Fc receptors necessary for external cross-linking of the antibodies (FIG. 3). Both H57 and 2C11 caused inositol phosphate production. Significantly, the response of day 0, 1 week, and 3 week thymocytes was similar. The H57-induced mobilization of Ca^{2+}, another rapid and sensitive measure of early T cell activation, was also assessed; once again, no difference was found between the three sources of thymocytes.[41] Finally, thymocytes from mice of all ages were equally susceptible to chemicals that are known to cause thymocyte PCD, ionomycin and Dex.[41] Thus, the "defect" in day 7 thymocytes appears to be specific for TCR-initiated PCD pathways. Taken together, these data can be most easily understood if one considers perinatal thymocytes to be a dynamically changing population. These changes are not reflected in the cell surface molecules typically used to assess maturation (*e.g.*, CD3, CD4, and CD8), but rather in the biological responses of these cells to TCR activation signals.

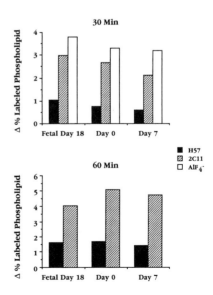

FIGURE 3. Thymocyte anti-TCR-induced phosphoinositide hydrolysis as a function of age. Thymocytes were collected from mice of various ages and inositol phosphate accumulation was measured at the indicated times. [³H]myo-inositol labelling of thymocytes from mice of different ages was comparable (within 10%).

Activation- and Glucocorticoid-Induced PCD

In the last several years we have developed a model system in which to study lymphocyte PCD *in vitro*. Cellular activation of transformed and spontaneously growing T cells, especially T cell hybridomas, causes both lymphokine secretion and inhibition of growth.[28] The latter is the result of two discrete events: a G_1/S cell cycle block and PCD.[23] The cell cycle block occurs within minutes of activation, does not require extracellular Ca^{2+}, and is unaffected by CsA.[10] In contrast, cell death is not detectable until 4 to 6 hr after activation, is accompanied by the classical DNA step ladder appearance on gel electrophoresis, requires mRNA/protein synthesis and extracellular Ca^{2+}, and is prevented by CsA.[9,10] The actual means of activating the T hybridoma cells does not appear to be important in generating either response; growth inhibition and PCD are both elicited by antigen, antibodies to the T cell receptor (TCR), antibodies to activation molecules such as Thy-1, or the combination of phorbol ester and Ca^{2+} ionophore.[10,23] Since T cell hybridomas provide a monoclonal and easily manipulatable source of cells, the mechanisms underlying the activation-induced death of T cell hybridomas have been studied with the assumption that they will shed light upon the more general issue of PCD in negative selection and tolerance induction.

Glucocorticoids are well characterized compounds that lead to PCD in immature, double positive thymocytes.[5,42] The glucocorticoid receptor (GR) belongs to a superfamily that includes, among others, the receptors for steroids, thyroid, and vitamin D hormones.[43] These receptors are composed of discrete functional domains: an N-terminal modulatory portion that appears to be required for maximal hormone activity and tissue specificity, a central "zinc finger" DNA-binding region, and a C-terminal ligand-binding domain. The "unactivated" GR is normally located in the cytoplasm complexed to other proteins, notably the heat shock protein hsp90. It is thought that steroid binding leads to the "activation" of the receptor complex with dissociation of hsp90 and translocation of the occupied receptor to the nucleus. The receptor-steroid complex then binds to glucocorticoid-responsive elements (GREs) that control the expression of target genes.[44] The varied biologic effects of glucocorticoids are modulated by the positive or negative transcriptional control of genes by their GREs.

Studies were undertaken to determine how glucocorticoids might induce PCD in 2B4.11 cells. To determine if the effects of cellular activation and glucocorticoids were additive (suggesting a common pathway) or synergistic (suggesting two independent pathways), the two types of stimulus were added simultaneously (FIG. 4). Surprisingly, the addition of both stimuli resulted in markedly less cell

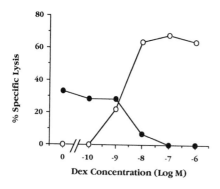

FIGURE 4. Activation- and Dex-induced killing of 2B4.11 are mutually antagonistic. Specific ^{51}Cr release was measured after a 14 hr culture. 2B4.11 cells were incubated with the indicated concentrations of Dex in medium alone (○) or with purified 2C11 (20 μg/ml) bound to plastic (●).

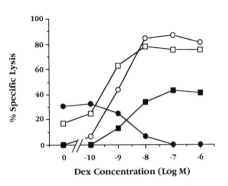

FIGURE 5. CsA reverses the antagonism between activation- and Dex-induced killing. 2B4.11 cells were incubated with the indicated concentrations of Dex in medium alone (○), 2C11 (20 μg/ml) bound to plastic (●), CsA at 100 ng/ml (□), or 2C11 plus CsA (■), and specific ^{51}Cr release was measured 14 hr later.

lysis than when both agents were added independently (FIG. 4, *closed circles*). This phenomenon was confirmed using light microscopy and trypan blue dye exclusion to assess cell viability, as well as a DNA fragmentation assay to directly measure PCD.[32] To further elucidate the nature of the mutual antagonism between Dex and TCR-mediated activation, the effect of CsA was determined (FIG. 5). CsA completely blocked cell death induced by 2C11 stimulation, but did not inhibit Dex-mediated cytotoxicity. In fact, there was a reproducible enhancement of Dex-induced killing; Dex dose-response curves were generally shifted ~3-fold towards lower concentrations of Dex. The addition of CsA to the combination of Dex and 2C11 caused partial reversal of the mutual antagonism, as evidenced by the reappearance of a dose-response relationship for cell lysis with increasing concentrations of Dex. This suggests that both the TCR-mediated negative (PCD) and positive (reversal of Dex-induced PCD) signals are blocked by CsA. In contrast, Dex-initiated events leading to cell death are actually enhanced in the presence of CsA.

A number of different approaches were taken to address the mechanism of the mutual antagonism. First, the effect of Dex treatment on activation-induced signalling molecules and events was studied. To determine if Dex reduced expression of the TCR, thus directly limiting TCR-mediated signalling, 2B4.11 cells were stained with fluoresceinated anti-TCR antibodies after a 4 hr incubation in medium or 10^{-6} M Dex; cell surface TCR levels between the two groups were identical (data not shown). The effect of Dex on phosphoinositide hydrolysis was also ascertained. 2B4.11 cells were incubated with 10^{-6} M Dex for 1 hr, after which time water-soluble inositol phosphate generation was measured in response to stimulation with either 2C11 or G7 (FIG. 6). Dex had no significant effect on TCR-mediated inositol phosphate production. Thus, Dex does not antagonize activation-induced PCD either by regulating TCR expression or by inhibiting TCR-coupled phosphoinositide hydrolysis.

Because most of the important signalling and regulatory steps distal to TCR ligation are not well defined, it was difficult to further evaluate specific models by which Dex might interfere with activation-induced PCD. In contrast, the GR-ligand interaction is well characterized, allowing the exploration in detail of how cellular activation might influence the cellular effects of Dex. Since the translocation of the Dex-GR complex to the nucleus is a prerequisite for its biological activity, the effect of cellular activation on this process was assessed by immunoblotting. After freeze-thaw lysis and centrifugation, control or activated 2B4.11 cells were separated into cytoplasmic and nuclear fractions. Samples were resolved using SDS-polyacrylamide gel electrophoresis, immunoblotted with a

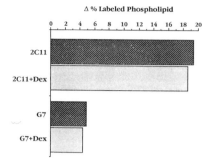

FIGURE 6. Dex does not inhibit activation-induced phosphoinositide hydrolysis. 2B4.11 cells were labelled with [³H]myo-inositol in the absence or presence of 10^{-6} M Dex for 3 hr, washed, and incubated with the indicated activators in the absence or presence of 10^{-6} M Dex for 60 min, at which time inositol phosphates were measured.

specific antiserum to the GR, and quantitated by densitometry. In unactivated cells, the majority of the GR was in the cytoplasmic fraction (FIG. 7). Cellular activation with 2C11 did not cause any significant translocation of the GR to the nucleus. Incubation of 2B4.11 cells with Dex, however, caused the translocation of a significant fraction of the GRs to migrate to the nucleus. Finally, 2C11 activation of 2B4.11 cells did not interfere with the ability of the GR to move to the nuclear fraction in response to Dex. Thus, cell activation had no major effect, either enhancing or inhibitory, on GR translocation.

These results do not exclude the possibility that cellular activation might allow the Dex-GR complex to migrate to the nucleus, but that once there it would be prevented from effectively binding to the critical GREs presumably involved in PCD. Since the relevant genes for PCD that are controlled by GREs are unknown, it was decided to transfect 2B4.11 cells with a plasmid containing two copies of the tyrosine aminotransferase gene GRE (a "classical" GRE) inserted 5′ of a thymidine kinase promoter-driven chloramphenicol acetyltransferase (CAT) gene.[33] By measuring the expression of the CAT reporter gene product, it was possible to determine if TCR-mediated activation inhibited steroid-mediated events up to and including the transcription and translation of a GRE-regulated gene. Transfected 2B4.11 cells exhibited low levels of CAT activity when incubated in medium alone, but exposure to Dex resulted in a 5-fold increase (FIG. 8). Stimulation of 2B4.11 with 2C11 did not cause any increase in CAT activity, nor did it interfere with the Dex-mediated increase in CAT enzyme. In fact, the

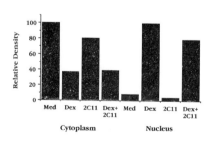

FIGURE 7. Cellular activation has little or no effect on the translocation of the GR from the cytoplasm to the nucleus. 2B4.11 cells were incubated for 1 hr with medium, 10^{-6} M Dex, 2C11 bound to plastic (coated at 20 μg/ml), or in the indicated combinations. Cytoplasmic and nuclear fractions were prepared, separated by SDS-PAGE, and immunoblotted with a specific antiserum to the GR. The immunoblots were quantitated by densitometry. The data are expressed as the relative densities of the 98 kD GR band in the experimental groups, with medium taken as 100% for cytoplasmic fractions, and Dex taken as 100% for nuclear extracts.

combination of 2C11 and Dex paradoxically augmented the CAT activity compared to Dex alone. RU-486 is a potent competitive antagonist of glucocorticoids.[45] RU-486 completely blocks glucocorticoid-induced PCD but has no effect on activation-induced PCD.[32] In FIG. 8 it can be seen that RU-486 blocked the Dex-mediated increase in CAT activity, indicating that the GRE-containing plasmid was responding in an appropriate and physiologic manner. Finally, as shown earlier (FIG. 5), CsA did not interfere with Dex-mediated signalling, and had essentially no effect on the Dex plus 2C11 induction of CAT activity. Taken together, the experiments performed with TCR-activated T cells revealed no direct effects or interference with normal glucocorticoid-induced events that

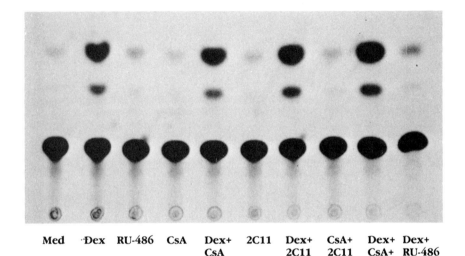

Med	Dex	RU-486	CsA	Dex+ CsA	2C11	Dex+ 2C11	CsA+ 2C11	Dex+ CsA+ 2C11	Dex+ RU-486

FIGURE 8. Activation does not mimic and does not inhibit Dex-driven GRE-mediated CAT transcription. 2B4.11 cells were transfected by electroporation and cultured in medium, Dex (10^{-7} M), RU-486 (10^{-6} M), CsA (100 ng/ml), 2C11 (20 μg/ml) bound to plastic, or in combination, for 6 hr. Equal amounts of cytoplasmic protein were assayed for CAT activity, and acetylated forms of chloramphenicol were separated by TLC. The percent conversion obtained in the 6 hr assay, as measured by scintillation counting of the major monoacetylated species and the unmodified ^{14}C-chloramphenicol, was: medium, 1.1%; Dex, 7.5%; RU-486, 1.2%; CsA, 0.91%; Dex + CsA, 6.5%; 2C11, 0.82%; Dex + 2C11, 11%; CsA + 2C11, 1.1%; Dex + CsA + 2C11, 12%; Dex + RU-486, 1.5%.

could account for the mutual antagonism between the activation- and glucocorticoid-induced pathways leading to PCD. Some of the possible explanations for this phenomenon are considered below.

DISCUSSION

The strikingly different responses to TCR-mediated clonal deletion signals of thymocytes from mice at different stages of ontogeny was unexpected. It is, however, clearly reminiscent of the experimental phenomenon known as neonatal tolerance, first described almost 4 decades ago by Billingham and colleagues.[46] In those studies, mice were injected in utero or after birth with allogeneic cells, and weeks or months later evaluated for allo-specific tolerance. It was found that the earlier the introduction of the allogeneic cells, the more complete the tolerance induced. Indeed, injection on or before fetal day 18 gave the best results, with injection later in development being less efficient and requiring a greater cell inoculum.[47-49] Because of the technical difficulty of in utero injection, neonatal tolerance has been studied almost exclusively in mice injected within the first 24 hours of birth. In recent studies on clonal deletion in this period, MacDonald and co-workers reported that injection of Mls-incompatible spleen cells on day 0 led to the depletion of hydrocortisone-resistant, $CD8^-/V\beta6^+$ thymocytes.[50,51] Our experiments that demonstrate a refractory period 1 week after birth establish the relevance of this to the phenomenon of neonatal tolerance, and strongly indicate that the decreased efficiency of tolerance induction at one week of life is due to a fall off in susceptibility to activation-induced clonal deletion. This is not an irreversible change in the cells that populate the thymus or in the microenvironment, since by 3 weeks of age thymocytes can once again be eliminated by TCR-mediated signalling. It seems reasonable to speculate that we are able to observe these variations in susceptibility to deletion only because early in ontogeny there is a relatively synchronous maturation of a wave of thymocytes, and that later in development (i.e., by 3 weeks), the next wave (or waves) of susceptible cells have populated the thymus. It is also possible that if, as has been suggested,[35,52] there are two $\alpha\beta$ $CD4^+CD8^+$ subsets distinguishable by their capacity for deletion, that by 7 days of age the selectable subset has either been eliminated or has acquired the post-selection phenotype. These data also suggest that the failure of allogeneic cells to induce allogeneic tolerance in older (e.g., 3 week old) mice is not because the thymocytes are refractory to deletional signals, but rather is due to the presence of functionally competent mature peripheral T cells. The response of these T cells to the allogeneic inoculum may diminish or prevent the intrathymic deletion of alloreactive cells. Consistent with this speculation is the finding that allogeneic inoculation of 12 day old mice actually enhanced the subsequent rejection of skin grafts (suggesting that allo-sensitization is dominant over clonal deletion in these animals),[49] and the finding that inoculation of adult mice with Mls-incompatible cells induces $V\beta$-specific thymocyte deletion only if cyclophosphamide is coadministered, to eliminate peripheral, antigen-reactive T cells (i.e., host-vs-graft effector cells).[53]

What is the biochemical or molecular basis for the difference in the activation-induced PCD response between thymocytes of varying ages? Since day 0 and day 7 thymocytes are equally susceptible to killing by Dex or ionomycin, it seems unlikely that there is an inherent resistance to PCD, as has been observed for mature peripheral lymphocytes.[54] Furthermore, neither TCR-mediated phosphoinositide hydrolysis nor Ca^{2+} mobilization appear to be different in thymocytes from day 0, 1 week, or 3 week old mice. There is still the possibility, however, that other signal transduction pathways, such as tyrosine kinase-mediated phosphorylation, differ between these populations. In preliminary experiments, we have observed no marked differences in the structure of the TCR during this period of ontogeny. In particular, no change in the amounts of total cellular TCR ζ or η was observed with anti-ζ precipitated cell lysates resolved by 2-D SDS-PAGE and immunoblotted with an anti-ζ/η-specific serum. Clearly, further investigation will be required to determine the critical differences that result in either the life or death of immature T cells when stimulated via the TCR.

T cell hybridomas have been extremely useful as a model system in which to study activation-induced lymphocyte PCD. Since activation- and glucocorticoid-induced PCD are similar in so many respects, we anticipated that the two pathways might interact prior to nuclear gene activation, and that the two stimuli might be additive or synergistic. In fact, activation- and Dex-induced PCD were found to be quite distinct in several fundamental ways. For example, CsA blocked activation-induced PCD but enhanced Dex-induced killing, while RU-486 had no effect on activation-induced PCD but abrogated the effects of Dex. The two pathways did influence one another in an unexpected way: they were mutually antagonistic. We were unable to demonstrate any antagonism between activation and Dex at any biochemical or molecular steps up to and including the transcription and translation of a GRE-regulated reporter gene. These negative results, however, do not necessarily rule out inhibitory interactions prior to gene transcription. Because the sequence of the GRE that is presumably responsible for the PCD caused by the Dex-GR complex is unknown, a reporter gene construct with a typical "simple" GRE was used for the transfection studies. Other GREs have recently been described, however, notably "negative" GREs (nGREs) that inhibit gene transcription.[55] It is possible, for example, that such a Dex-responsive non-classic negative regulatory element might control the induction of an activation-dependent gene product required for PCD. Other non-classical GREs have been shown to be enhancing or inhibitory, the response depending on the cell studied and the composition of the DNA surrounding the GRE.[55,56] It appears that the transcription factors c-jun and c-fos can physically interact with the GR, which under different conditions can result in either an increase or decrease of GR-GRE activity.[56-58] This latter observation is of particular interest, because c-Fos is induced in 2B4.11 cells after cellular activation (our unpublished observation). These particular models will be tested in the future to determine their relevance to the mutual antagonism between activation- and glucocorticoid-induced PCD.

The observation that cellular activation- and glucocorticoid-induced PCD inhibit one another can serve as the basis for a new model of T cell development (FIG. 9). The bulk of thymocytes die in situ, many of them presumably never having encountered a ligand for their newly rearranged and expressed TCRs.[19] Those that do encounter ligand undergo at least two possible fates: negative selection (presumably if the avidity of the interaction is very high), or positive selection (if the avidity is low to moderate). We propose that immature double positive thymocytes are exposed to either glucocorticoids, or to some similar, and perhaps thymus-specific, signal that initiates the glucocorticoid-induced PCD pathway. Any thymocyte with a nonfunctionally rearranged TCR or with sub-threshold avidity for self antigen/self-MHC will be eliminated by this PCD pathway. Cells that recognize self with low to moderate avidity will be activated. In the presence of glucocorticoids, the activation and glucocorticoid pathways will antagonize each other, leaving a viable, positively selected thymocyte. For cells that recognize self with high avidity, the activation-induced PCD will dominate (as occurs with T cell hybridomas at relatively low levels of Dex and high concentrations of antigen) and negative selection occurs. One virtue of this model is that the same cell can respond either positively or negatively with no change in its differentiation state. Thus, there need be no specific order in the sequence with which positive and negative selection occur (although there might be, due to other factors such as the nature of the antigen or changing levels of the cell surface TCR).[59,60] Future experiments with glucocorticoid analogs and antagonists should shed light on the question of whether glucocorticoids have a role in thymic selection.

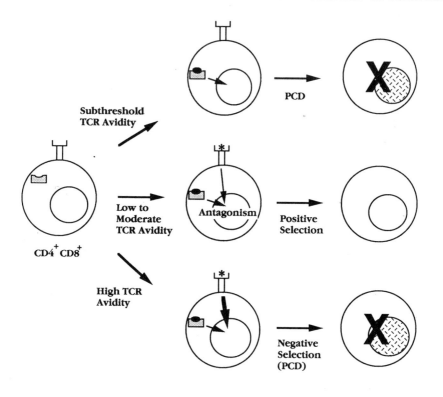

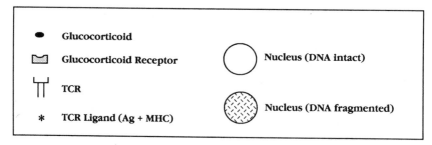

FIGURE 9. Model for thymocyte development. Immature double positive thymocytes express a TCR that recognizes MHC-encoded proteins plus antigen. *Top row:* TCR nonfunctional or of subthreshold avidity; glucocorticoids (or some thymic analog) interacts with the GR and leads to PCD. *Middle row:* TCR of low to moderate avidity for antigen (Ag) + MHC; cellular activation-induced and glucocorticoid-induced signals mutually antagonize the PCD caused by one another, allowing the cell to survive (positive selection). *Bottom row:* TCR of high avidity for Ag + MHC; cellular activation-induced PCD pathway dominates and leads to cell death (negative selection).

SUMMARY

The programmed death of thymocytes and T cells was studied. Injection of anti-TCR antibodies into adult mice caused the specific deletion of CD4$^+$CD8$^+$ thymocytes, an effect that was largely reversed by cyclosporin A. Surprisingly, using either anti-TCR antibodies or superantigens, it was found that the susceptibility of these thymocytes to clonal deletion changed during ontogeny. Double positive thymocytes from newborn and young (3 week old) mice were readily depleted, whereas thymocytes from 1 week old mice were relatively refractory. The differences between these groups could not be accounted for by cell surface TCR expression, TCR-mediated early signal transduction pathways such as phosphoinositide hydrolysis or Ca^{2+} mobilization, or differences in susceptibility to Dex- or ionomycin-induced programmed cell death. These results suggest that there is a relatively synchronous wave of maturing thymocytes that are susceptible to deletional signals during fetal life and shortly after birth, but not 7 days after birth. By 3 weeks of age, the next wave (or waves) of susceptible cells have populated the thymus. These observations closely follow the experimental model known as "neonatal tolerance," and we suggest that the failure to tolerize 1 week old mice in that system reflects an alteration in the cells' susceptibility to clonal deletion. In a separate set of experiments exploring the mechanisms of PCD, it was found that although the activation- and glucocorticoid-induced PCD pathways were distinct (being distinguishable by their sensitivity to CsA and the glucocorticoid antagonist RU-486), they were mutually antagonistic. Attempts to identify the level of the antagonism failed to demonstrate any direct interference between the two stimuli, up to and including the transcription and translation of a GRE-controlled reporter gene. Based upon these observations, we propose the following model of thymocyte development: glucocorticoids eliminate thymocytes with little or no avidity for self; antagonism between glucocorticoids and cellular activation allows thymocytes that recognize self with low or moderate avidity to survive (positive selection); activation of thymocytes that recognize self with high avidity dominates the antagonistic effect of glucocorticoids, leading to PCD (negative selection).

ACKNOWLEDGMENTS

We would like to acknowledge Drs. Pradip K. Chakraborti and S. Stoney Simons, Jr., who collaborated with us on the GR translocation experiment, and with whom we had many stimulating and helpful discussions.

REFERENCES

1. SULSTON, J. E. & H. R. HORVITZ. 1977. Postembryonic cell lineages of the nematode. *Caenorhabditis elegans*. Dev. Biol. **56:** 110–156.
2. CARR, V. M. & S. B. SIMPSON, JR. 1982. Rapid appearance of labeled degenerating cells in the dorsal root ganglia after exposure of chick embryos to tritiated thymidine. Dev. Brain Res. **2:** 57–162.
3. SULSTON, J. M., E. SCHIERENBERG, J. G. WHITE & H. N. THOMSON. 1983. The embryonic cell lineage of the nematode *Caenorhabditis elegans*. Dev. Biol. **100:** 64–119.
4. SMITH, C. A., G. T. WILLIAMS, R. KINGSTON, E. J. JENKINSON & J. J. T. OWEN.

1989. Antibodies to the CD3/T-cell receptor complex induce death by apoptosis in immature T-cells in thymic cultures. Nature **337:** 181–184.

5. WYLLIE, A. H., R. G. MORRIS, A. L. SMITH & D. DUNLOP. 1984. Chromatin cleavage in apoptosis: association with condensed chromatin morphology and dependence on macromolecular synthesis. J. Pathol. **142:** 67–77.

6. DUVALL, E. & A. H. WYLLIE. 1986. Death and the cell. Immunol. Today **7:** 115–119.

7. COHEN, J. J. & R. C. DUKE. 1984. Glucocorticoid activation of a calcium-dependent endonuclease in thymocyte nuclei leads to cell death. J. Immunol. **132:** 38–42.

8. MARTIN, D. P., R. E. SCHMIDT, P. S. DISTEFANO, O. H. LOWRY, J. G. CARTER & E. M. JOHNSON, JR. 1988. Inhibitors of protein synthesis and RNA synthesis prevent neuronal death caused by nerve growth factor deprivation. J. Cell. Biol. **106:** 829–844.

9. UCKER, D., J. D. ASHWELL & G. NICKAS. 1989. Activation-driven T cell death: requirements for *de novo* transcription and translation and association with genome fragmentation. J. Immunol. **143:** 3461–3469.

10. MERĆEP, M., P. D. NOGUCHI & J. D. ASHWELL. 1989. The cell cycle block and lysis of an activated T cell hybridoma are distinct processes with different Ca^{2+} requirements and sensitivity to cyclosporin. A. J. Immunol. **142:** 4085–4092.

11. SHI Y., B. M. SAHAI & D. R. GREEN. 1989. Cyclosporin A inhibits activation-induced cell death in T-cell hybridomas and thymocytes. Nature **339:** 625–626.

12. WYLLIE, A. H. 1980. Glucocorticoid-induced thymocyte apoptosis is associated with endogenous endonuclease activation. Nature **284:** 555–556.

13. DUKE, R. C. & J. J. COHEN. 1986. IL-2 addiction: withdrawal of growth factor activates a suicide program in dependent T cells. Lymphokine Res. **5:** 289–299.

14. WILLIAMS, G. T., C. A. SMITH, E. SPOONCER, T. M. DEXTER & D. R. TAYLOR. 1990. Haemopoietic colony stimulating factors promote cell survival by suppressing apoptosis. Nature **343:** 76–79.

15. DUKE, R. C., R. CHERVANAK & J. J. COHEN. 1983. Endogenous endonuclease-induced DNA fragmentation: an early event in cell-mediated cytolysis. Proc. Natl. Acad. Sci. USA **80:** 6361–6365.

16. RUSSELL, J. H. 1983. Internal disintegration model of cytotoxic lymphocyte-induced target damage. Immunol. Rev. **72:** 97–118.

17. MARTZ, E. & D. M. HOWELL. 1989. CTL: virus control cells first and cytolytic cells second? DNA fragmentation, apoptosis and the prelytic halt hypothesis. Immunol. Today **10:** 79–86.

18. JENKINSON, E. J., R. KINGSTON, C. A. SMITH, G. T. WILLIAMS & J. J. OWEN. Antigen-induced apoptosis in developing T cells: a mechanism for negative selection of the T cell receptor repertoire. 1989. Eur. J. Immunol. **19:** 2175–2177.

19. FOWLKES, B. J. & D. M. PARDOLL. 1989. Molecular and cellular events of T cell development. Adv. Immunol. **44:** 207–264.

20. LEO, O., M. FOO, D. H. SACHS, L. E. SAMELSON & J. A. BLUESTONE. 1987. Identification of a monoclonal antibody specific for a murine T3 polypeptide. Proc. Natl. Acad. Sci. USA **84:** 1374–1378.

21. KUBO, R. T., W. BORN, J. W. KAPPLER, P. MARRACK & M. PIGEON. 1989. Characterization of a monoclonal antibody which detects all murine $\alpha\beta$ T cell receptors. J. Immunol. **142:** 2736–2742.

22. GUNTER, K. C., T. R. MALEK & E. M. SHEVACH. 1986. T cell activating properties of an anti-Thy-1 monoclonal antibody: possible analogy to OKT3/LEU-4. J. Exp. Med. **159:** 709–730.

23. MERĆEP, M., J. A. BLUESTONE, P. D. NOGUCHI & J. D. ASHWELL. 1988. Inhibition of transformed T cell growth in vitro by monoclonal antibodies directed against distinct activating molecules. J. Immunol. **140:** 324–335.

24. STAERZ, U. D., H.-G. RAMMENSEE, J. D. BENEDETTO & M. J. BEVAN. 1985. Characterization of a murine monoclonal antibody specific for an allotypic determinant on T cell antigen receptor. J. Immunol. **134:** 3994–4000.

25. KANAGAWA, O., E. PALMER & J. BILL. 1989. A T cell receptor $V\beta6$ domain that imparts reactivity to the Mls[a] antigen. Cell. Immunol. **119:** 412–426.

26. DIALYNAS, D. P., Z. S. QUAN, K. A. WALL, A. PIEERRES, J. QUINTANS, M. R. LOKEN, M. PIERRES & R. W. FITCH. 1983. Characterization of the murine T cell surface molecule, designated L3T4, identified by the monoclonal antibody GK1.5: similarity of L3T4 to the human Leu-3/T4 molecule. J. Immunol. **131:** 2445–2451.

27. SARMIENTO, M., A. L. GLASEBROOK & F. W. FITCH. 1980. IgG or IgM monoclonal antibodies reactive with different determinants on the molecular complex bearing Lyt 2 antigen block T cell-mediated cytolysis in the absence of complement. J. Immunol. **125:** 2665–2672.

28. ASHWELL, J. D., R. E. CUNNINGHAM, P. D. NOGUCHI & D. HERNANDEZ. 1987. Cell growth cycle block of T cell hybridomas upon activation with antigen. J. Exp. Med. **165:** 173–194.

29. KAPPLER, J., J. WHITE, D. WEGMANN, E. MUSTAIN & P. MARRACK. 1982. Antigen presentation by Ia+ B cell hybridomas to H-2-restricted T cell hybridomas. Proc. Natl. Acad. Sci. USA **79:** 3604–3608.

30. ZUNIGA-PFLUCKER, J. C., S. A. MCCARTHY, M. WESTON, D. L. LONGO, A. SINGER & A. M. KRUISBEEK. 1989. Role of CD4 in thymocyte selection and maturation. J. Exp. Med. **169:** 2085–2096.

31. SUSSMAN, J. J., J. S. BONIFACINO, J. LIPPINCOTT-SCHWARTZ, A. W. WEISSMAN, T. SAITO, R. D. KLAUSNER & J. D. ASHWELL. 1988. Failure to synthesize the T cell CD3-γ chain: structure and function of a partial T cell receptor complex. Cell **52:** 82–95.

32. ZACHARCHUK, C. M., M. MERĆEP, P. K. CHAKRABORTI, S. S. SIMONS, JR. & J. D. ASHWELL. 1990. Programmed T lymphocyte death: cell activation- and steroid-induced pathways are mutually antagonistic. J. Immunol. **145:** 4037–4045.

33. TSAI, S. Y., M.-J. TSAI & B. W. O'MALLEY. 1989. Cooperative binding of steroid hormone receptors contributes to transcriptional synergism at target enhancer elements. Cell **57:** 443–448.

34. SAMBROOK, J., E. F. FRITSCH & T. MANIATIS. 1989. Molecular Cloning: a Laboratory Manual. Cold Spring Harbor Laboratory Press. Cold Spring Harbor, NY.

35. FINKEL, T. H., J. C. CAMBIER, R. T. KUBO, W. K. BORN, P. MARRACK, & J. W. KAPPLER. 1989. The thymus has two functionally distinct populations of immature αβ+ T cells: one population is deleted by ligation of αβTCR. Cell **58:** 1047–1054.

36. GAO, E.-K., D. LO, R. CHENEY, O. KANAGAWA & J. SPRENT. 1988. Abnormal differentiation of thymocytes in mice treated with cyclosporin A. Nature **336:** 176–179.

37. JENKINS, M. K., R. H. SCHWARTZ & D. M. PARDOLL. 1988. Effects of cyclosporine A on T cell development and clonal deletion. Science **241:** 1655–1658.

38. STROMINGER, J. L. 1989. Developmental biology of T cell receptors. Science **244:** 943–950.

39. MARRACK, P. & J. W. KAPPLER. 1990. The Staphylococcal enterotoxins and their relatives. Science **248:** 705–711.

40. WEISS, A., J. IMBODEN, K. HARDY, B. MANGER, C. TERHORST & J. STOBO. 1986. The role of the T3/antigen receptor complex in T-cell activation. Ann. Rev. Immunol. **4:** 593–619.

41. ZACHARCHUK, C. M., M. MERĆEP, J. H. JUNE, A. M. WEISSMAN & J. D. ASHWELL. 1991. Thymocyte susceptibility to clonal deletion varies during ontogeny: implications for neonatal tolerance. J. Immunol. In press.

42. SCREPANTI, I., S. MORRONE, D. MECO, A. SANTONI, A. GULINO, R. PAOLINI, A. CRISANTI, B. J. MATHIESON & L. FRATI. 1989. Steroid sensitivity of thymocyte subpopulations during intrathymic differentiation: effects of 17 β-estradiol and dexamethasone on subsets expressing T cell antigen receptor or IL-2 receptor. J. Immunol. **142:** 3378–3383.

43. EVANS, R. M. 1988. The steroid and thyroid hormone receptor superfamily. Science **240:** 889–895.

44. BEATO, M. 1989. Gene regulation by steroid hormones. Cell **56:** 335–344.

45. BOURGEOIS, S., M. PFAHL & E. E. BAULIEU. 184. DNA binding properties of glucocorticosteroid receptors bound to the steroid antagonist RU-486. EMBO J. **3:** 751–755.

46. BILLINGHAM, R. E., L. BRENT & P. B. MEDAWAR. 1953. 'Actively acquired tolerance' of foreign cells. Nature **172:** 603–606.
47. BILLINGHAM, R. E., L. BRENT & P. B. MEDAWAR. 1956. Quantitative studies of tissue transplantation immunity. III. Actively acquired tolerance. Phil. Trans. Roy. Soc., London, ser. B **239:** 357–414.
48. BILLINGHAM, R. E., V. DEFENDI, W. K. SILVERS & D. STEINMULLER. 1962. Quantitative studies on the induction of tolerance of skin homografts and on runt disease in neonatal rats. J. Natl. Cancer Inst. **28:** 365–435.
49. BRENT, L. & G. GOWLAND. 1960. Cellular dose and age of host in the induction of tolerance. Nature **192:** 1265–1267.
50. MACDONALD, H. R., T. PEDRAZZINI, R. SCHNEIDER, J. A. LOUSI, R. M. ZINKERNAGEL & H. HENGARTNER. 1988. Intrathymic elimination of Mls^a-reactive (Vβ6$^+$) cells during neonatal tolerance induction to Mls^a-encoded antigens. J Exp. Med. **167:** 2005–2010.
51. SCHNEIDER, R., R. K. LEES, T. PEDRAZZINI, R. M. ZINKERNAGEL, H. HENGARTNER & H. R. MACDONALD. 1989. Postnatal disappearance of self-reactive (Vβ6$^+$) cells from the thymus of Mls^a mice: implications for T cell development and autoimmunity. J. Exp. Med. **169:** 2149–2158.
52. FINKEL, T. H., P. MARRACK, J. W. KAPPLER, R. T. KUBO & J. C. CAMBIER. 1989. $\alpha\beta$T cell receptor and CD3 transduce different signals in immature T cells: implications for selection and tolerance. J. Immunol. **142:** 3006–3012.
53. ETO. M., H. MAYUMI, Y. TOMITA, Y. YOSHIKAI, Y. NISHIMURA & K. NOMOTO. 1990. Sequential mechanisms of cyclophosphamide-induced skin allograft tolerance including the intrathymic clonal deletion followed by late breakdown of the clonal deletion. J. Immunol. **145:** 1303–1310.
54. KIZAKI, H., T. TADAKUMA, C. ODAKA, J. MURAMATSU & Y. ISHIMURA. 1989. Activation of a suicide process of thymocytes through DNA fragmentation by calcium ionophores and phorbol esters. J. Immunol. **143:** 1790–1794.
55. SAKAI, D. D., S. HELMS, J. CARLSTEDT-DUKE, J.-A. GUSTAFSSON, F. M. ROTTMAN & K. R. YAMAMOTO. 1988. Hormone-mediated repression: a negative glucocorticoid response element from the bovine prolactin gene. Genes & Dev. **2:** 1144–1154.
56. DIAMOND, M. I., J. N. MINER, S. K. YOSHINAGA & K. R. YAMAMOTO. 1990. Transcription factor interactions: selectors of positive or negative regulation from a single DNA element. Science **249:** 1266–1272.
57. LUCIBELLO, F. C., E. P. SLATER, K. U. JOOSS, M. BEATO & R. MÜLLER. 1990. Mutual transrepression of Fos and the glucocorticoid receptor: involvement of a functional domain in Fos which is absent in FosB. EMBO J. **9:** 2827–2834.
58. YANG-YEN, H.-F., J.-C. CHAMBARD, Y.-L. SUN, T. SMEAL, T. J. SCHMIDT, J. DROUIN & M. KARIN. 1990. Transcriptional interference between c-Jun and the glucocorticoid receptor: mutual inhibition of DNA binding due to direct protein-protein interaction. Cell **62:** 1205–1215.
59. GUIDOS, C. J., J. S. DANSKA, C. G. FATHMAN & I. L. WEISSMAN. 1990. T cell receptor-mediated negative selection of autoreactive T lymphocyte precursors occurs after commitment to the CD4 or CD8 lineages. J. Exp. Med. **172:** 835–845.
60. OHASHI, P. S., H. PIRCHER, K. BURKI, R. M. ZINKERNAGEL & H. HENGARTNER. 1990. Distinct sequence of negative or positive selection implied by thymocyte T-cell receptor densities. Nature **346:** 861–863.

Immunoregulation of Autoimmune Disease by Vaccination with T Cell Receptor Peptides

STEVEN W. BROSTOFF[a] AND MARK D. HOWELL

The Immune Response Corporation
5935 Darwin Court
Carlsbad, California 92008

INTRODUCTION

The major autoimmune diseases, rheumatoid arthritis, multiple sclerosis and Type 1 diabetes, are considered to be T cell-mediated diseases. Since T cells are responsible for the tissue damage in these diseases, T cells can be considered as pathogens. Common pathogens, such as viruses and bacteria, are controlled by vaccines comprised of killed or attenuated pathogens or subunits of these pathogens. In the case of autoimmune T cell pathogens, a killed or attenuated vaccine approach can be used, but would not be commercially feasible because of individual differences in transplantation antigens. Given these differences, T cells from each patient would have to be removed from the body, killed or attenuated and then reinfused back into the patient. Such a procedure would be very costly, time consuming and inefficient. However, a subunit type of therapeutic would be practical. The subunit of the T cell that distinguishes one T cell from another, and therefore, distinguishes the pathogenic T cells from the normal T cells, is the T cell receptor (TCR). A vaccination approach involving the T cell receptor as a subunit is appealing, not only because of its specificity, but because of the opportunity it affords to produce a long lasting immunoregulation, which contrasts with other approaches utilizing monoclonal antibodies, drugs that block the MHC or other antiinflammatories that treat symptoms without affecting the underlying disease process. A focus on the TCR requires that there be restricted usage in the TCR repertoire of autoreactive T cells. In fact, it was the observation of such restricted TCR usage in experimental animals that led directly to the implementation of experiments to test this approach.

During development of the T cell repertoire, various germline gene elements are rearranged to give each T cell its unique α and β chain and its antigen specificity. The α chain is comprised of V, J and C germline elements whereas the β chain has V, D, J and C elements. Although the same germline sequences may be used in T cells of different specificities, the VJα and VDJβ joining regions are unique for each T cell.

[a] S. Brostoff has academic appointments at Medical University of South Carolina, University of California, San Diego and University of California, Irvine.

71

MATERIALS & METHODS

Antigens

Peptides corresponding to rat and mouse T cell receptor sequences were synthesized by solid-phase stepwise elongation on an ABI 430 synthesizer (ABI, Foster City, CA). The peptide sequences used are shown below in TABLE 2. Guinea pig myelin basic protein (MBP) was prepared as described previously.[1]

Vaccination and Challenge

Each antigen was dissolved in saline (1 mg/ml) and emulsified with an equal volume of Freund's complete adjuvant (CFA) containing *Mycobacterium tuberculosis* (10 mg/ml, Difco H37ra). Each animal received intradermal injections containing 50 μg antigen and 500 μg mycobacteria in 0.1 ml divided equally between two footpads. For vaccination with T cell receptor peptides, the injections were given in the hind footpads. After an interval of 30 days the animals were challenged with guinea pig myelin basic protein in the fore footpads.

RESULTS

TABLE 1 illustrates the restricted TCR gene usage of T cells found to cause experimental allergic encephalomyelitis (EAE) in both mice[2,3] and rats.[4,5] As can be seen, Vα2 and Vα4 are used predominantly in both Lewis rats and the two species of mice shown, and these germline elements are rearranged to either Jα31 or Jα39. These Jα regions bear striking sequence homology to each other[6] which makes them a potential focus of attack for developing a regulatory response. Similarly, since the Vβ8.2 TCR germline gene is also used preferentially, this Vβ is another focus, more so than the Jβ region which does not show the same extent of conservation. Although these germline genes are used preferentially in this animal model, the same germline elements might be expected to be used by T cells with specificities for antigens other than the autoantigen in question. Thus, a preferable target would be a sequence specific for the autoreactive T cell. The most specific region would be the VDJ junctional region (the CDR3) of the β chain which also shows sequence conservation in both rat and mouse TCRs.[6]

TABLE 1. T Cell Receptor Gene Usage in EAE

Animal Model	Vα	Jα	Vβ	Jβ	References
PL/J mice	Vα4 (6/6)	Jα31 (5/6)	Vβ8 (6/6)	Jβ2.7 (3/6) Jβ2.3 (2/6) Jβ2.5 (1/6)	2
B10.PL mice	Vα2 (19/33) Vα4 (14/33)	Jα39 (33/33)	Vβ8 (26/33) Vβ13 (7/33)	Jβ2.6 (26/33) Jβ2.2 (7/33)	3
Lewis rats	Vα2 (8/11)	Jα39 (1/1)	Vβ8 (11/11)	Jβ1.1 (1/1)	4
Lewis rats	Vα2 (2/2)	N.D.	Vβ8 (4/4)	Jβ1.3 (3/4) Jβ1.1 (1/4)	5

TABLE 2. Vaccination against EAE with T Cell Receptor Peptides

Vaccination[a]	Dose	No. with Disease No. Tested	Mean[b] Maximum Severity	Mean Onset (Days)	Mean Duration (Days)	No. with Histology No. Tested
None		6/6	3.0	10.5	5.2	
CFA		6/6	2.8	11.5	5.2	
mVDJ	50 μg	2/3	1.7	13.0	2.3	3/3
rVDJ$_9$	50 μg	0/4	0.0	none	0.0	0/4
rVDJ$_8$	50 μg	2/4	1.5	12.5	1.5	2/4
rJαTA39	50 μg	1/3	0.7	15.0	1.7	1/3
rVβ8.2	50 μg	2/3	1.3	13.0	1.7	3/3

[a] Peptide sequences used:

mVDJ	S G D A G G G Y E
rVDJ$_8$	S S D – S S N T E
rVDJ$_9$	A S S D – S S N T E
rJαTA39	R F G A G T R L T V K
rVβ8.2	D M G H G L R L I H Y S Y D V N S T E K

[b] Disease was graded on a 3 point scale as follows:
1. loss of tail tone.
2. hind leg weakness.
3. hind leg paralysis.

In actual practice, targeting either germline regions, such as Vβ8.2 or Jα39, or rearranged VDJβ (CDR3) regions can be effective in preventing EAE[6] as shown in TABLE 2. In our hands, immunization of Lewis rats with guinea pig myelin basic protein produces clinical signs of disease in 10 or 11 days in all animals. The clinical signs last 5–6 days whereupon the animals spontaneously recover. Pretreating with CFA alone had little effect on the disease course. However, as shown in TABLE 2, immunization with a nine amino acid sequence from the rat VDJβ junctional region completely protected rats from EAE. An eight amino acid sequence from this region was effective to a lesser degree. An alteration in disease course and severity was also found using the corresponding sequence found in T cells known to produce EAE in the B10.PL mouse. This mouse sequence shows a significant degree of homology with the rat sequence as shown in TABLE 2. In our hands, both the rJα39 and the rVβ8.2 sequence showed protection, but to a lesser extent than the rVDJ$_9$. It should be noted that Vandenbark and co-workers[7] have reported a Vβ8.2 sequence differing by only one amino acid (an additional glycine at the C-terminus) that provides complete protection in a different substrain of Lewis rats. One region that distinguishes different Vβs from each other is the hypervariable, CDR2 region. The Vβ8.2 sequences used for immunization in both studies were sequences from the Vβ CDR2 region.

DISCUSSION

Proposed Mechanism

The proposed mechanism for protection by T cell receptor vaccination is illustrated in FIGURE 1. The autoreactive T cell, which is a CD4+ lymphocyte,

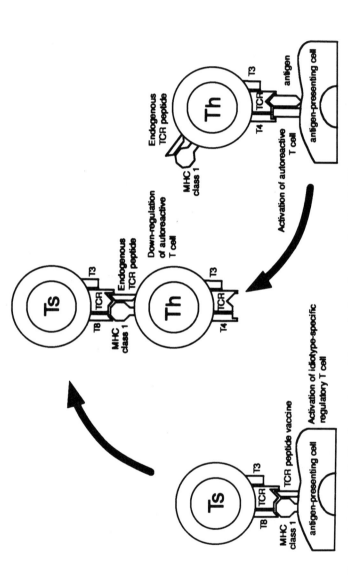

FIGURE 1. Proposed mechanism for T cell receptor peptide vaccination. Autoreactive T cells (Th) not only express TCR on their surface which recognizes antigen in the context of MHC Class II, but also express peptides from the endogenously synthesized TCR on their surface in the context of MHC Class I (*lower right*). Vaccination with TCR peptides produces CD8+ CTLs (Ts) which recognize the TCR peptides in the context of Class I (*lower left*). Autoreactive T cells (Th) which express TCR peptides in the context of MHC Class I on their surface are down regulated or killed by the circulating CD8+ CTLs (Ts) (*middle*).

recognizes MBP in the context of Class II. The limited repertoire of TCR idiotypes that develops uses a germline Vβ8 that is found in very low frequency in the periphery of Lewis rats.[8] Since T cell receptors are endogenously synthesized proteins, it follows that peptides will be produced by proteolytic processing of these proteins and will cycle through the class I MHC on the surface of the CD4+ autoreactive T cell. Such peptide-MHC class I complexes would serve as recognition sites for anticlonotypic cytotoxic T lymphocytes (CTLs). This mechanism is consistent with the existing dogma that T cells recognize peptide antigens in the context of MHC and is more appealing than the intact native TCR itself serving as the idiotype. During immunization with a TCR peptide, the peptide is given in a route designed to stimulate phagocytes and other antigen presenting cells (APCs) in nonphysiologic, high concentrations. Although these are exogenous peptides, a portion of them would be taken up, processed and presented in the context of Class I. There is precedent for this mechanism in a recent report.[9] The CTLs thus generated, that recognize these peptides in the context of Class I, would find their targets on the surface of autoreactive, MBP-specific T cells and kill them. If antibody-mediated downregulation also takes place, we propose the target for this antibody to be the peptide bound by the MHC rather than the intact native T cell receptor. Whether or not this antiidiotypic response is a part of usual regulation of tolerance, as long as it can be induced to downregulate the autoreactive T cells, it becomes a viable long term therapy.

The preferential focus of TCR immunization would be the VDJβ (CDR3) idiotypic determinant on the autoreactive T cell since this region bears the greatest specificity for a given T cell. An alternative focus of TCR immunization would be the Vβ CDR2 region. During development, T cell expressing potentially self-reactive receptors are clonally deleted by a mechanism that results in their death.[10,11] Other potentially autoreactive T cells that escape deletion may be rendered anergic, although they remain physically present in the circulation.[11,12] T cell germline elements that are absent or present at very low levels in the periphery of individuals are thought to include potentially autoreactive T cells that have been either clonally deleted or rendered anergic if they escaped deletion. Thus T cell vaccination of individuals with CDR2 sequences representing germline elements of potentially autoreactive cells, although not as specific as vaccination with CDR3 sequences, nevertheless could prove beneficial by insuring the downregulation of clones that have escaped deletion during development.

Supporting Data

The evidence that the proposed mechanism may be operative has been provided by several observations. The first is the result of a collaboration with Deming Sun who has developed a suppressor line from rats recovered from T cell line-mediated EAE.[13] The suppressor line was propagated with attenuated effector cells and is comprised of anticlonotypic, CD8+ CTLs. These cells can be stimulated by the rVDJ$_9$ but not by the rVβ8.2 or the rJα39 peptides.[14] The second is our ability to show proliferation in response to rVDJ$_9$ in lymphocytes from rats 11 days after immunization with the rVDJ$_9$ peptide. This proliferation takes place only in the presence of IL-2 suggesting that the responding cell is a CD8+ CTL. We can also demonstrate proliferation to rVDJ$_9$, rJα39 and rVβ8.2 in lymphocytes of rats recovered from EAE. Thirdly, antibodies made in rabbits in response to rVDJ$_9$ peptides label cells in a manner different than antibody labelling with monoclonal antibody directed at intact native TCR, but similar to labeling of peptide-pulsed APCs. Finally, preliminary experiments using radiolabelled isolated MHC Class I molecules, in an assay to detect binding to potential Class I epitopes,[15] demonstrate the binding to rVDJ$_9$ in a dose-dependent manner and to a grater degree than the binding to an irrelevant peptide chosen for its characteristics as a T cell epitope.

We have been unable to demonstrate any significant protection using rVβ8.2, rJα39 or rVDJ$_9$ peptides coupled to KLH or ovalbumin and injected with alum in an attempt to develop an antibody response. Hashim and co-workers,[16] however, have reported the presence of antibody resulting from vaccination with TCR peptides and the protective effect of treatment with this antibody. The observation that this latter antibody does not precipitate intact TCR from cells,[17] and the observed staining pattern, is more consistent with the antibody being directed towards the TCR-MHC complex rather than intact native TCR.

The above results are consistent with the proposed mechanism of protection (FIG. 1) and also suggest a role for this mechanism in normal immunoregulation (at least normal recovery in the rat from T cell-mediated EAE). The results also suggest that the VDJβ joining region may be a class I T cell epitope even though its sequence does not fulfill the requirements proposed for T cell epitopes.[18,19] The proposed mechanism is currently being tested by transfecting cells with the appropriate TCR gene and testing whether such cells can be used to immunize against EAE.

TCRs in Human Autoimmune Disease

In order for the above TCR vaccination approach to be useful in human autoimmune disease, restricted TCR gene usage must be observed in such diseases. In recent experiments on rheumatoid arthritis, we have examined by PCR the T cell population infiltrating the synovial tissue of 4 patients. In each case clonal infiltrates of Vβ17+ cells were found among the activated T cell population. Cytotoxic T cell clones reactive with synovial adherent cells were generated from a fifth patient. The majority of these cytotoxic T cells were Vβ17+. Vβ17 is difficult to detect at any level in PBLs of most individuals according to recent studies.[20] Thus this T cell population is a potential target for T cell receptor peptide therapy in rheumatoid arthritis. It is interesting to note that Vβ17 has also been found as a predominant TCR gene in MBP specific clones derived from a patient with multiple sclerosis.[21] MBP is a proposed autoantigen in multiple sclerosis.[22]

SUMMARY

Restricted TCR gene usage in animal models of autoimmune disease has led to strategies for control of these diseases by targeting the idiotypic determinants within the TCR sequence. Rats can be rendered resistant to EAE by immunization with synthetic peptides representing sequences contained within the Vβ, Jα and VDJβ regions of the TCR that are conserved among encephalitogenic T cells. We propose that the mechanism of immunoregulation thus produced results from the stimulation of an anticlonotypic response directed at endogenously synthesized TCR peptides presented by Class I MHC on the surface of the autoreactive T cell, and that this mechanism may be part of the natural immunoregulation of T cell responses. The experimental data demonstrate the utility of this therapeutic approach and its potential for treatment of any pathogenic condition mediated by specific, oligoclonal T cell populations.

REFERENCES

1. BROSTOFF, S. W. & D. W. MASON. 1984. Experimental allergic encephalomyelitis: successful treatment *in vivo* with a monoclonal antibody that recognizes T helper cells. J. Immunol. **133:** 1938–1942.
2. ACHA-ORBEA, HANS, D. J. MITCHELL, L. TIMMERMANN, D. C. WRAITH, G. S. TAUSCH, M. K. WALDOR, S. S. ZAMVIL, H. O. McDEVITT & L. STEINMAN. 1988. Limited heterogeneity of T cell receptors from lymphocytes mediating autoimmune encephalomyelitis allows specific immune intervention. Cell **54:** 263–273.
3. URBAN, J. L., V. KUMAR, D. H. KONO, C. GOMEZ, S.J. HORVATH, J. CLAYTON, D. G. ANDO, E. E. SERCARZ & L. HOOD. 1988. Restricted use of T cell receptor V genes in murine autoimmune encephalomyelitis raises possibilities for antibody therapy. Cell **54:** 577–592.
4. BURNS, F. R., X. LI, N. SHEN, H. OFFNER, Y. K. CHOU, A. A. VANDENBARK & E. HERBER-KATZ. 1989. Both rat and mouse T cell receptors specific for the encephalitogenic determinant of myelin basic protein use similar V α and V β chain genes even though the major histocompatibility complex and encephalitogenic determinants being recognized are different. J. Exp. Med. **169:** 27–39.
5. CHLUBA, J., C. STEEG, A. BECKER, H. WEKERLE & J. T. EPPLEN. 1989. T cell receptor β chain usage in myelin basic protein-specific rat T lymphocytes. Eur. J. Immunol. **19:** 279–284.
6. HOWELL, M. D., S. T. WINTERS, T. OLEE, H. C. POWELL, D. J. CARLO & S. W. BROSTOFF. 1989. Vaccination against experimental allergic encephalomyelitis with T cell receptor peptides. Science **246:** 668–670.
7. VANDENBARK, A. A., G. HASHIM & H. OFFNER. 1989. Immunization with a synthetic T-cell receptor V-region peptide protects against experimental autoimmune encephalomyelitis. Nature **341:** 541–544.
8. GOLD, D. Personal communication.
9. ROCK, K. L., S. GAMBLE & L. ROTHSTEIN. 1990. Presentation of exogenous antigen with class I major histocompatibility complex molecules. Science **249:** 918–921.
10. KAPPLER, J. W., N. ROEHM & P. MARRACK. 1987. T cell tolerance by clonal elimination in the thymus. Cell **49:** 273.
11. SCHWARTZ, R. H. 1989. Acquisition of immunological tolerance. Cell **57:** 1073.
12. MARKMANN, J., D. LO, A. NAJI, R. D. PALMITER, R. L. BRINSTER & E. HEBER-KATZ. 1988. Antigen presenting function of class II MHC expressing pancreatic beta cell. Nature **336:** 476.
13. SUN, D., Y. QIN, J. CHLUBA, J. T. EPPLEN & H. WEKERLE. 1988. Suppression of experimentally induced autoimmune encephalomyelitis by cytolytic T-T cell interactions. Nature **332:** 843–845.
14. D. SUN, S. W. BROSTOFF & M. D. HOWELL. Unpublished data.
15. BOUILLOT, M., J. CHOPPIN, F. CORNILLE, F. MARTINON, T. PAPO, E. GOMARD, M.-C. FOURNIE-ZALUSKI & J.-P. LEVY. 1989. Physical association between MHC class I molecules and immunogenic peptides. Nature **339:** 473–475.
16. HASHIM, G. A., A. A. VANDENBARK, A. B. GALANG, T. DIAMANDUROS, E. CARVALHO, J. SRINIVASAN, R. JONES, M. VAINIENE, W. J. MORRISON & H. OFFNER. 1990. Antibodies specific for Vβ8 peptide suppress experimental autoimmune encephalomyelitis. J. Immunol. **144:** 4621–4627.
17. VANDENBARK, A. A. Personal communication.
18. DELISI, C. & J. A. BERZOFSKY. 1985. T-cell antigenic sites tend to be amphipathic structures. Proc. Natl. Acad. Sci. USA **82:** 118–1135.
19. ROTHBARD, J. & W. TAYLOR. 1988. A sequence common to T cell epitopes. EMBO J. **7:** 93–100.

20. ROSENBERG, W. Presentation at the meeting entitled "T Cells in Health and Disease: Immunity and Tolerance" held at Trinity College, Oxford, September 22–26, 1990.
21. WUCHERPFENNIG, K. W., K. OTA, N. ENDO, J. G. SEIDMAN, A. ROSENZWEIG, H. L. WEINER & D. A. HAFLER. 1990. Shared human T cell receptor Vβ usage to immunodominant regions of myelin basic protein. Science **248:** 1016–1019.
22. ALLEGRETTA, M., J. A. NICKLAS, S. SRIRAM & R. J. ALBERTINI. 1990. T cells responsive to myelin basic protein in patients with multiple sclerosis. Science **247:** 718–721.

Specific Immunoregulation of the Induction and Effector Stages of Relapsing EAE via Neuroantigen-Specific Tolerance Induction

STEPHEN D. MILLER, L. J. TAN, MARY K. KENNEDY,
AND MAURO C. DAL CANTO

Departments of Microbiology-Immunology and Pathology
Northwestern University Medical School
303 E. Chicago Avenue
Chicago, Illinois 60611

INTRODUCTION

Murine relapsing experimental autoimmune encephalomyelitis (R-EAE) is a T cell-mediated autoimmune demyelinating disease of the CNS that can be induced in a variety of ways. Active induction of the disease involves the sensitization of genetically susceptible mice with mouse spinal cord homogenate (MSCH)[1,2,22] or purified myelin proteins, *e.g.*, myelin basic protein (MBP) or proteolipid protein (PLP) in complete Freund's adjuvant (CFA).[3-5] The disease can also be induced by the adoptive transfer of neuroantigen-primed, *in vitro*-activated T-lymphocytes into naive syngeneic recipient mice.[6-8] R-EAE is considered a relevant animal model for multiple sclerosis, a human demyelinating disease of unknown etiology, as the diseases share similarities in clinical course and histopathology.[1,9,10] Clinical signs of R-EAE follow a chronic-unremitting or relapsing-remitting course of ascending paralysis. Pathological changes in the CNS white matter include perivascular mononuclear cellular infiltrates with adjacent areas of acute and chronic demyelination.[2,10]

The fact that R-EAE can be induced both actively and passively, and displays a relapsing course makes it an ideal system to study the efficacy of specific immunoregulation for both prevention and treatment of this clinically relevant autoimmune disease. In this regard our previous studies have demonstrated that neuroantigen-specific tolerance could be induced in SJL/J mice by the i.v. injection of syngeneic splenocytes coupled via carbodiimide (ECDI) with MSCH (MSCH-SP).[11,12] Tolerance was assessed by the failure of the treated mice to develop specific DTH in response to immunization with MSCH, MBP, or PLP in CFA. Mice rendered tolerant to MSCH antigens were specifically protected from the development of clinical and histologic R-EAE induced by sensitization with MSCH/CFA.[11,12] Successful suppression of active R-EAE in mice tolerized after MSCH/CFA immunization and utilization of an adoptive R-EAE system, wherein clinical disease is suppressed in recipients treated i.v. with MSCH-SP up to six days after transfer of MBP-specific T cell blasts, indicated that MSCH-coupled splenocytes could inhibit the *expression* of clinical R-EAE and the accompanying neuroantigen-specific DTH responses.[13]

In the current investigation we addressed the antigen specificity of tolerance induction in both active R-EAE and adoptive R-EAE, by determining the effects of i.v. treatment with splenocytes coupled with MBP, PLP, and their encephalitogenic peptides. In addition, the ability of specific tolerance induction to treat relapsing paralytic episodes was addressed. The results clearly indicate that specific tolerance induction can be induced by small peptides and is effective at both preventing the induction of active R-EAE and in treating established disease. Tolerance induction appears to have the potential for regulating ongoing autoimmune responses without the necessity for eliminating T cell subsets or having previously identified a limited repertoire of autoantigen-specific T cells.

MATERIALS AND METHODS

Mice

Female SJL/J mice, 4–7 weeks old, were purchased from Jackson Laboratories, Bar Harbor, ME. All mice were housed in the Northwestern animal care facility and, except during periods of severe paralysis, were maintained on standard laboratory chow and water *ad libitum*. Paralyzed mice were separated from unaffected mice and were afforded easier access to food and water. Within each experiment, mice were age-matched (generally 8–10 weeks) and from the same shipment.

Antigens

Mouse spinal cords and brains were obtained from various strains of naive mice and were frozen until used for preparation of mouse MBP. Mouse MBP was prepared according to the method of Swanborg et al.[14] Bovine MBP was purchased from Sigma Chemical Co., St. Louis, MO. Water-soluble human and bovine PLP were prepared from chloroform : methanol (2 : 1) extracts of white matter according to the method of Hampson and Poduslo.[15] The chloroform : methanol-soluble PLP was converted to the water-soluble form according to the method of Sherman and Folch-Pi.[16] Mouse spinal cord homogenate (MSCH) and mouse kidney homogenate (MKH) were prepared by homogenizing freshly obtained SJL/J spinal cords or kidneys in distilled water. The homogenates were lyophilized and frozen until use. The following peptides were used in certain experiments: PLP 202–217 (DARMYGVLPWNAFPGK); PLP 141–150 (LGKWLGHPDK); PLP 139–154 (HCLGKWLGHPDKFVGI); PLP 139–151S (HSLGKWLGHPDKF); MBP 91–104 (VTPRTPPPSQGKGR); MBP 84–104 (VHFFKNIVTPRTPPPSQGKGR); and Theiler's murine encephalomyelitis virus (VP2 188–207) (VYPHQILNIRTNTTVDLEVP). Peptides were obtained from the Northwestern University Peptide Synthesis Facility or were the generous gift of Dr. Vince Tuohy, Cleveland Clinic Foundation.

Preparation of Ag-Coupled Splenocytes

RBC-free (Tris-NH$_4$Cl-treated) splenocytes were coupled with protein by the method of Miller et al. using water-soluble 1-ethyl-3-(3-dimethylaminopropyl)-carbodiimide HC1 (ECDI, Calbiochem-Behring Corp., La Jolla, CA).[17] Saline-washed SJL/J splenocytes were pelleted in 50 ml centrifuge tubes and resuspended to a final concentration of 2.5×10^8 cells/ml in saline containing the indicated concentrations of the crude mouse spinal cord or kidney homogenates, purified proteins, or peptides. When necessary, the pH of each solution was adjusted to neutrality. MSCH and MKH/saline preparations were used without separation of the insoluble components. The coupling reaction was initiated by the addition of 0.171 ml of freshly prepared ECDI (150 mg/ml in saline) per ml of cell suspension (final concentration of ECDI: 21.9 mg/ml). Sham-coupled cells were prepared by incubation of splenocytes in saline containing ECDI but no Ag. Following a 1 h incubation at 4°C, the cells were washed three times with Mishell-Dutton balanced salt solution (BSS) and maintained at 4°C until use.

Induction of R-EAE by Active Immunization

Female SJL/J mice were immunized with MSCH in adjuvant (hereafter referred to as MSCH/CFA) according to the method of Brown and McFarlin,[1] with slight modifications. Each mouse received a s.c. injection into the shaved left flank of 0.3 ml of a mixture of 1.0 mg of MSCH in 0.15 ml of PBS and 0.03 mg of *Mycobacterium tuberculosis hominis* H37Ra (Difco) in 0.15 ml of IFA (Difco). Seven days after the first injection, each mouse received a second injection of MSCH/CFA into the shaved right flank. Initial clinical signs of disease were usually observed between days 13 and 25 post-immunization.

Induction of R-EAE by Adoptive Transfer of Sensitized Lymph Node Cells

Female SJL/L mice (10–12 weeks) were immunized with bovine MBP according to the method of Pettinelli and McFarlin.[6] Bovine MBP was dissolved in PBS (8 mg/ml) and emulsified with an equal volume of IFA (Difco) containing 600 μg/ml of *M. tuberculosis hominis* H37Ra (Difco). Each mouse received 0.1 ml of the emulsion (containing 400 μg bovine MBP and 30 μg *M. tuberculosis hominis* H37Ra) which was administered s.c. and distributed over three sites on the shaved flank. Ten days after immunization, the inguinal, axillary, and brachial lymph nodes were removed from sensitized donors and single cell suspensions were prepared. The cells were adjusted to 4×10^6/ml in RPMI 1640 medium (Gibco Laboratories, Grand Island, NY) supplemented with 10% fetal calf serum, 12 mM HEPES, Penicillin G (100 U/ml), streptomycin (100 μg/ml), 2×10^{-3} M glutamine, and 5×10^{-5} M 2-ME containing 65–75 μg/ml bovine MBP. Cells were distributed at 1.5 ml/well into 24 well plates (Falcon 3047) and were incubated at 37°C in a humidified atmosphere containing 5% CO_2, 95% air. Five days later, the cells were harvested on Histopaque (Sigma Chemical Co., St. Louis, MO) density gradients and washed three times in BSS. Recipient mice (10–12 weeks old) were injected i.v. via the lateral tail vein with 0.5 ml of BSS containing 4–5×10^7 viable LNC. Initial clinical signs of disease were usually observed between 6 and 10 days after transfer of the sensitized LNC.

Induction of Tolerance/Desensitization

On the indicated days relative to the immunization with MSCH/CFA or the adoptive transfer of MBP-primed LNC, the indicated number of Ag-coupled splenocytes (in 0.5 ml BSS) were injected i.v. into the lateral tail veins of recipient mice.

Clinical Evaluation

Mice were observed daily for clinical signs of disease until days 30–35 PI or post-transfer; thereafter, mice were observed every 1–5 days for the duration of the experiment. Mice were scored according to their clinical severity as follows: grade 0, no abnormality; grade 1, limp tail; grade 2, limp tail and hind limb weakness (waddling gait); grade 3, partial hind limb paralysis; grade 4, complete hind limb paralysis; and grade 5, moribund. The scores of the asymptomatic mice (score = 0) were included in the calculation of the daily mean clinical score for each group.

Measurement of Ag-specific DTH

DTH responses were quantitated using a 24 h ear swelling assay.[18] On day +12 after the first injection of MSCH/CFA, pre-challenge ear thickness was determined using a Mitutoyo model 7326 engineer's micrometer (Schlesinger's Tools, Brooklyn, NY). Immediately thereafter, DTH responses were elicited by injecting 5–10 μg of Ag (in 10 μl of saline) into the dorsal surface of the ear using a 100 μl Hamilton syringe fitted with a 30 gauge needle. Twenty-four hours after ear challenge, the increase in ear thickness over pre-challenge measurements was determined. Results are expressed in units of 10^{-4} inches $\pm$ SEM. Ear swelling responses were the result of mononuclear cell infiltration and showed typical DTH kinetics (i.e., minimal swelling at 4 h, maximal swelling at 24–48 h).

Statistical Analyses

The Statistical significance of DTH between experimental groups was analyzed using a one-tailed analysis of variance. Group means were compared using the Scheffé multiple comparison test.[19] Comparisons of the percentage of animals showing clinical disease between any two groups of mice were analyzed by X^2 using Fisher's exact probability. Comparisons of the mean day of onset between a single group of mice and the control mice were analyzed by the Student's t test. p values <0.05 were considered significant.

RESULTS

Neuroantigen Specificity of Tolerance Induction on the Development of Clinical Disease and Accompanying Neuroantigen-Specific DTH in Active R-EAE

Our previous work showed that active EAE could be prevented by tolerization with MSCH-SP. To identify which neuroantigen(s) in the crude MSCH preparation were responsible for the induced nonresponsiveness to R-EAE, we asked whether splenocytes coupled with either purified MBP (MBP-SP) or PLP (PLP-SP) could induce Ag-specific nonresponsiveness as assessed by both neuroantigen-specific DTH and clinical signs of disease in mice primed with MSCH/CFA.

Sham-tolerized mice developed significant DTH responses to both MBP and PLP, whereas mice injected with MSCH-coupled splenocytes failed to develop significant DTH to either neuroantigen (FIG. 1a). Mice injected with PLP-coupled splenocytes developed significant MBP-specific DTH, but failed to develop PLP-specific DTH. Conversely, mice injected with MBP-coupled splenocytes developed PLP-specific DTH, but failed to develop MBP-specific DTH. The results thus indicate that a single neuroantigen-specific component of the immune response induced by immunization with mouse spinal cord homogenate can be inhibited by tolerization with splenocytes coupled with the appropriate purified neuroantigen. We next asked whether MBP- or PLP-specific tolerance would be sufficient to prevent the development of MSCH-induced R-EAE (FIG. 1b). Seventy-one percent (17/24) of sham-tolerized mice developed clinical signs of R-EAE. The incidence of disease in mice tolerized with rat MBP was not significantly different from that of the controls (10/20 affected, $p = 0.27$). In contrast, the development of R-EAE was significantly inhibited ($p < 0.001$) in the groups of mice tolerized with MSCH (3/23 affected) or human PLP (2/24 affected). 20–30% of the affected mice in the sham-tolerized control group exhibited relapses and the remainder showed chronic neurologic dysfunction. In contrast, the affected mice in the MSCH- and PLP-tolerized groups exhibited clinical courses of a milder and shorter duration and recovered completely showing no chronic symptoms or relapses out to 100 days post-immunization (data not shown). The data strongly suggest that a PLP-specific immune response is necessary, and may be sufficient, for the development of R-EAE induced by MSCH in SJL/J mice whereas MBP is much weaker in encephalitogenic potential.

Effects of Peptide-Specific Tolerance on Clinical Signs of Active R-EAE

Encephalitogenic regions of both the MBP[20,21] and PLP[22] proteins have recently been identified for the SJL/J mouse. Although MSCH is a complex mixture of neuroantigens, it is possible that within a given mouse strain, the major encephalitogenic component(s) of MSCH consists of a single or a limited number of epitopes of PLP and/or MBP, *i.e.,* immunodominant encephalitogenic epitopes. Thus, the induction of tolerance to encephalitogenic peptides could serve as a feasible approach to prevention of MSCH-induced R-EAE. To address this question, we examined whether the induction of tolerance to the encephalitogenic synthetic peptides of murine PLP or MBP could inhibit the induction of clinical R-EAE (FIG. 2). Mice injected with splenocytes coupled with an irrelevant peptide based on a sequence contained within the VP2 protein of Theiler's murine encephalomyelitis virus (VP2 188–207) or with a nonencephalitogenic PLP peptide (PLP 202–217) were highly susceptible [21/24 (88%) affected] to the development of R-EAE. Mice tolerized with the encephalitogenic PLP peptides 139–151S [14/26 (54%) affected, $p = 0.010$] and PLP 139–154 [5/11 (46%) affected, $p = 0.015$] were significantly resistant to the induction of disease. Similar to the previous experiments utilizing human PLP (FIG. 1), bovine PLP-tolerized mice were highly resistant [2/10 (20%) affected, $p < 0.001$] to MSCH-induced disease. In contrast, tolerization with a third encephalitogenic PLP peptide (PLP 141–150) [10/12 (83%) affected, $p = 0.549$] and with an encephalitogenic determinant of MBP (MBP 91–104) [15/19 (79%) affected, $p = 0.365$] failed to protect SJL/J mice from disease. Thus, tolerance to the major encephalitogenic determinant of PLP, contained within amino acids 139–154, provides significant protection against the induction of active R-EAE induced by a heterogeneous mixture of neuroantigens.

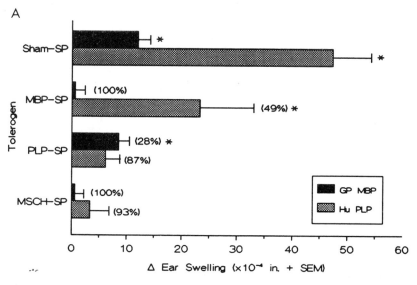

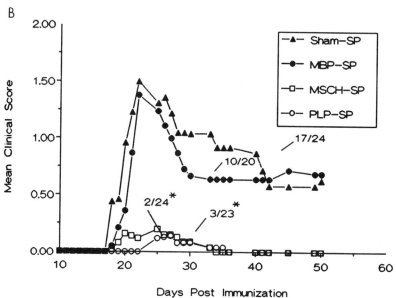

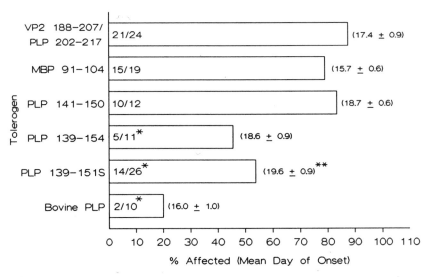

FIGURE 2. Effect of PLP peptide-specific tolerance on the incidence of active R-EAE. In two separate experiments, groups of 10–16 female SJL/J mice were injected i.v. on day −14 with 5×10^7 splenocytes coupled with 0.5 mg/ml bovine PLP, or 400 μM of the following peptides: Theiler's virus VP2 188–207; PLP 202–217, PLP 141–150, PLP 139–154, PLP 139–151S and MBP 91–104. All mice were immunized with MSCH/CFA on days 0 and +7 and observed for clinical signs of disease for 32 days. The percentage of mice showing clinical signs in each treatment group is shown. The numbers in parentheses indicate the mean day of onset of disease. *Indicates percentage of affected mice is significantly below that of the combined VP2 188–207- and PLP 202–217-tolerized controls (p <0.05). **(p <0.01).

FIGURE 1. Neuroantigen-specificity of tolerance induction on the development of clinical disease and accompanying neuroantigen-specific DTH in active R-EAE. **(A)** Groups of 9–15 female SJL/J mice were injected i.v. on day −7 with 7.5×10^7 sham-coupled splenocytes (Sham-SP), or splenocytes coupled via ECDI with 1 mg/ml MSCH (MSCH-SP), purified rat MBP (MBP-SP), or purified human PLP (PLP-SP). All mice were immunized with MSCH/CFA on days 0 and +7. Neuroantigen-specific DTH responses were elicited on day +12 in 4 mice from each group upon challenge with 15 μg guinea pig MBP or 5 μg human PLP and assessed using a 24 hr ear swelling assay. Results are expressed as Δ 24 hr ear swelling responses (background responses of negative control mice subtracted) in units of 10^{-4} inches $\pm$ SEM. Negative control values in unimmunized mice were 24.0 $\pm$ 0.4 for human PLP and 10.6 $\pm$ 2.1 for guinea pig MBP. Percent inhibition of DTH responses as compared to Sham-SP tolerant mice is shown in parentheses. *Indicates DTH responses significantly above (p <0.01) those of negative controls. **(B)** The clinical course of disease was followed in the groups of neuroantigen-tolerized mice described in (A), as well as those from an additional experiment (7–11 mice/group). Pooled results of these two experiments are shown. The number of mice showing clinical signs of disease at any time during the observation period out of the total mice in each group is indicated above the corresponding clinical course. *Indicates percentage of affected mice is significantly below that of the Sham-SP tolerized controls (p <0.001).

Effect of MSCH-Coupled Splenocytes on the Expression of Adoptive R-EAE

Our previous studies have shown that administration of MSCH-coupled splenocytes also inhibited the expression of R-EAE in adoptive recipients of MBP-specific T cells.[13] We next determined the dose-response characteristics and the fine antigen-specificity of inhibition of the effector limb of R-EAE. Groups of 7–9 SJL/J mice received 5×10^7 MBP-sensitized, *in vitro*-activated LNC on day 0. On day +3 the mice were treated with varying numbers of either MSCH-SP (6×10^7, 4×10^7, and 2×10^7) or MBP-SP (4×10^7 and 2×10^7). Recipients of 6×10^7 MKH-SP served as controls. Control animals developed severe paralytic signs which peaked about 10 days post transfer (FIG. 3). In contrast, expression of clinical signs of disease in recipients of $\geq 2 \times 10^7$ MSCH- and MBP-SP were significantly suppressed. The antigen-specificity of this inhibition was next addressed. As seen in FIGURE 4, adoptive R-EAE induced by the transfer of MBP-specific T cells was inhibited by i.v. injection of MBP-SP, but not PLP-SP. Thus, inhibition of expression of clinical signs of disease in adoptive R-EAE is antigen-specific. To determine if this inhibition was associated with presentation of the major encephalitogenic determinant(s) on MBP (contained in the 84–104 peptide),[20,21] the suppressive effects of splenocytes coupled with MBP peptides were compared to those of splenocytes coupled with the intact MBP molecule. As seen

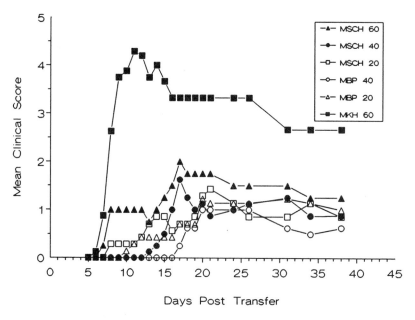

FIGURE 3. Dose-dependency of inhibition of adoptive R-EAE. 5×10^7 bovine MBP-primed LNC were transferred i.v. into syngeneic, naive SJL/J recipients on day 0. On day +3, groups of 7–9 mice each were i.v. injected with either 6×10^7 mouse kidney homogenate-coupled splenocytes (MKH 60); 2×10^7 (MSCH 20), 4×10^7 (MSCH 40) or 6×10^7 (MSCH 60) MSCH—coupled splenocytes; or 2×10^7 (MBP 20) or 4×10^7 (MBP 40) (MBP-coupled splenocytes. Mice in each group were observed for clinical signs of disease for 38 days after LNC transfer. Mean clinical scores of all the mice injected with MSCH-SP or MBP-SP are significantly less ($p < 0.05$) than the MKH-SP control.

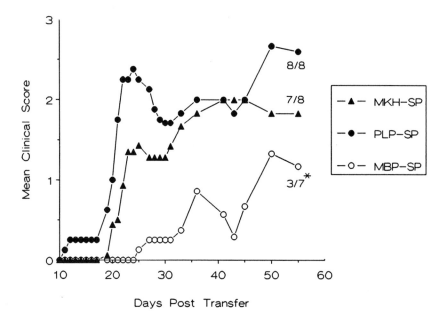

FIGURE 4. Neuroantigen-specificity of inhibition of adoptive R-EAE. 5×10^7 bovine MBP-primed LNC were transferred i.v. into syngeneic, naive SJL/J recipients on day 0. On day +3, groups of 7–8 mice each were i.v. injected with 5×10^7 splenocytes coupled with either mouse kidney homogenate (MKH-SP), proteolipid protein (PLP-SP), or bovine MBP (MBP-SP). Mice in each group were observed for clinical signs of disease for 55 days after LNC transfer. Disease incidence in each group is indicated. *Indicates percentage of affected mice is significantly below that of the MKH-SP treated controls ($p = 0.026$).

in FIGURE 5, the incidence and clinical severity of adoptive R-EAE in mice tolerized with splenocytes coupled with intact bovine MBP were significantly suppressed. Splenocytes coupled with MBP 84–104, but not MBP 91–104 also provided significant protection. Thus, tolerization with the major encephalitogenic epitope of MBP is sufficient to inhibit expression of clinical disease.

Effect of Specific Tolerance Induction of the Clinical Course of Relapses in Adoptive R-EAE

We next asked if specific tolerance induction could be used to alter the course of disease in mice treated after they had experienced their initial paralytic symptoms. A group of 26 SJL/J mice was given 4×10^7 MBP-specific T cells on day 0. The mice showed initial clinical signs of disease beginning 8–10 days later and clinical signs peaked on day 13–14. On day +21, the mice were divided at random into two equal groups of 13. One group was injected with 5×10^7 MKH-SP and the other with 5×10^7 MSCH-coupled splenocytes. The mice were observed for relapses for an additional 60 days. As seen in FIGURE 6A, the mean clinical score of the MSCH-tolerized mice remained constant for the duration of the observation period while that of the controls showed several relapsing episodes. When the

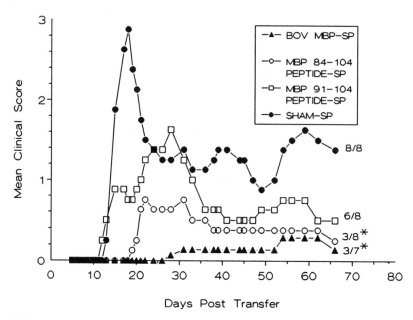

FIGURE 5. Fine specificity of inhibition of adoptive R-EAE using peptide-coupled cells. 4×10^7 bovine MBP-primed LNC were transferred i.v. into syngeneic, naive SJL/J recipients on day 0. On day +3, groups of 7–8 mice each were i.v. injected with 6×10^7 sham-coupled splenocytes or 6×10^7 splenocytes coupled with either intact bovine MBP (BOV MBP-SP), the MBP 84–104 peptide, or the MBP 91–104 peptide. Mice in each group were observed for clinical signs of disease for 66 days after LNC transfer. Disease incidence in each group is indicated. *Indicates percentage of affected mice is significantly below that of the MKH-SP-treated controls ($p < 0.03$).

data is expressed as percentage of mice relapsing (FIGURE 6B), it is apparent that specific tolerance induction significantly ($p = 0.024$) reduced the relapse rate from 69% (9/13 affected) in the control group to 23% (3/13 affected) in the MSCH-tolerant group. Thus, specific tolerance induction appears to be an effective means for treating established autoimmune disease.

DISCUSSION

The present experiments addressed the fine antigen specificity of tolerance induction for both the prevention and treatment of R-EAE. The results show that SJL/J mice tolerant to PLP, or synthetic encephalitogenic peptides of PLP, are resistant to R-EAE induced by immunization with an MSCH emulsion containing MBP, PLP, and other myelin- and nonmyelin-associated neuroantigens. PLP-specific tolerance was as efficient as tolerance induced by MSCH-coupled spleno-cytes (FIG. 1) in preventing the induction of R-EAE and the accompanying neu-roantigen-specific DTH responses.[11] These results are consistent with the hypothesis that immune responses directed toward encephalitogenic region(s) of PLP are of major importance to the pathogenesis of MSCH-induced R-EAE in

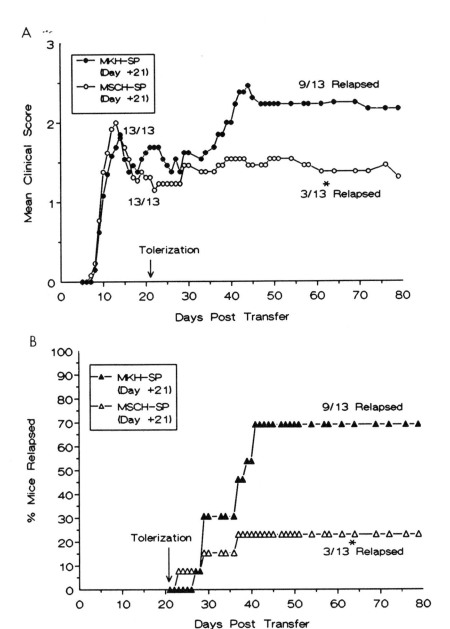

FIGURE 6. Effect of specific tolerance induction on the clinical course of relapses in adoptive R-EAE. 4×10^7 bovine MBP-primed LNC were transferred i.v. into a group of 26 syngeneic, naive SJL/J recipients on day 0. On day +21, 8–10 days after the appearance of initial clinical signs of disease, the mice were randomly divided to two equal groups of 13. The control group was injected with 5×10^7 splenocytes coupled with mouse kidney homogenate (MKH-SP) and the experimental group with 5×10^7 splenocytes coupled with mouse spinal cord homogenate (MSCH-SP). The data is presented as the mean clinical scores of the two groups **(A)** and as the percentage of mice showing clinical relapses **(B)** out to 80 days after LNC transfer. *Indicates percentage of tolerized mice showing clinical relapse is significantly below that of the MKH-SP-injected controls ($p = 0.024$).

SJL/J mice. Tolerance induced by intact PLP was apparently more efficient than that induced by splenocytes coupled with PLP encephalitogenic peptides (FIG. 2). This may indicate the presence of an additional determinant(s) on the PLP molecule (outside of amino acids 139–154) that are encephalitogenic and/or tolerogenic in the SJL mouse. The observation[23] that an encephalitogenic SJL T cell line responded to both PLP and DM-20 (a protein identical to PLP except for a deletion of residues 116–150)[24] supports the possible existence of an additional encephalitogenic determinant(s).

The data also show a differential ability of three PLP peptides, all with known encephalitogenic potential,[22,25] to prevent the induction of R-EAE. Tolerization with PLP 139–151S and PLP 139–154 was found to provide significant protection. However, tolerization with PLP 141–150 (a highly encephalitogenic peptide) failed to prevent induction of R-EAE. This may be related to the observation that amino acid 141 appears to be a critical residue for the encephalitogenic activity of the peptide.[25] The ECDI coupling reaction which catalyzes the formation of peptide bonds may have thus altered or destroyed this critical residue.[26] It could be argued that a similar ECDI-induced alteration of a critical residue of MBP 91–104 may account for the inability of splenocytes coupled with this encephalitogenic peptide to provide protection from MSCH-induced R-EAE. However, we previously showed that mice tolerized to MBP 91–104-coupled splenocytes failed to respond to immunization and ear challenge with MBP 91–104, indicating that tolerance was in fact induced to the unaltered MBP peptide.[12]

In contrast to our ability to prevent the induction of MSCH-induced R-EAE by induction of tolerance to MSCH or PLP, disease prevention in mice pretreated with splenocytes coupled with MBP (FIG. 1a) or the encephalitogenic MBP 91–104 peptide (FIG. 2) were not significantly protected. These results differ from those of Sriram et al., who found that i.v. tolerization of SJL/J mice with splenocytes coupled with mouse MBP (via chromic chloride) prevented the induction of MSCH-induced acute EAE.[27] However, MBP-coupled splenocytes prepared by the ECDI technique, which failed to prevent actively induced R-EAE (FIGS. 1b and 2), suppressed the induction of MBP-specific DTH in mice immunized with either MSCH (FIG. 1a) or MBP (data not shown). Thus, mice developed clinical signs of MSCH-induced active R-EAE in the absence of MBP-specific T cell responses. Regardless of the inability of splenocytes coupled with intact MBP or MBP 91–104 to induce resistance to actively-induced R-EAE, it is clear that PLP appears to be the dominant encephalitogenic (and tolerogenic) component of MSCH as PLP-tolerized mice are protected from the development of R-EAE (FIGS. 1b and 2) despite the presence of an intact MBP-specific immune response (FIG. 1a).

Our previous results showed that i.v. injection of MSCH-SP could inhibit the expression of clinical R-EAE and accompanying neuroantigen-specific DTH responses.[13] In the current study we examined the fine antigen-specificity of inhibition of adoptive R-EAE. It is clear that expression of clinical R-EAE was significantly inhibited in a dose-dependent manner by i.v. tolerization of recipient mice with MSCH- or MBP-coupled splenocytes three days after transfer of 5×10^7 MBP-specific effector T cells (FIG. 3). In contrast to MSCH-induced active R-EAE, treatment with splenocytes coupled with MBP, but not with PLP, were able to suppress expression of clinical signs of adoptive R-EAE mediated by MBP-specific effector T cells (FIG. 4). Interestingly, when the MBP peptide specificity of inhibition of adoptive R-EAE was examined, mice tolerized to MBP 91–104 (which is encephalitogenic in SJL/J mice) were not significantly protected from expression of clinical disease. However, tolerization with the MBP 84–104 peptide, which spans the entire major encephalitogenic region of MBP[20,21] did provide significant protection (FIG. 5). The compilation of a number of experiments indicates that tolerization with MBP 84–104 is generally not as effective as intact MBP in preventing disease expression (data not shown). This may relate to the recent discovery of a minor encephalitogenic MBP epitope in SJL/J mice[28] mapping between amino acids 17 and 27. Preliminary experiments suggest that the mechanism of inhibition of disease expression is due to the induction of energy[17,29] in the transferred MBP-specific effector cells, and not due to alterations in effector cell homing to the CNS or activation of Ts (data not shown).

TABLE 1. Strategies for Regulation of CD4 T Cell-Dependent Responses

Strategy	Comments
I. Anti-MHC Class II and mAb	• blocks Ag presentation
	• Ag-nonspecific
	• more effective on inductive phase of responses
II. Anti-CD4/CD3 mAb	• depletes T cell subsets, receptor modulation, $\pm$ tolerance induction
	• Ag-nonspecific
III. Anti-V_β mAb	• depletes T cells
	• TcR allotype-specific
	• requires prior knowledge of a limited and pre-defined T cell repertoire for Ag
IV. T cell/TcR peptide vaccination	• induction of anti-idiotypic regulatory cells/Ab
	• clonotype/TcR allotype-specific
	• requires isolation of T cell clones specific for a defined Ag from a relatively limited repertoire
V. Epitope competition	• blockage of Ag-specific T cells
	• requires prior knowledge of a limited and pre-defined T cell repertoire for Ag and synthesis of a peptide analog which binds MHC class II with higher affinity than the natural epitope, but does not trigger the T cell
	• requires large amounts of peptide to be effective *in vivo*
VI. Ag (peptide)-coupled syngeneic spleen cells	• deletion/anergy of Ag-specific T cells
	• Ag-specific, long-lasting, efficient
	• does not necessarily require prior knowledge of the specific Ag or epitope
	• efficient at regulating both afferent (induction) and efferent (effector) limbs of the T cell response

The present data also indicate that tolerization with neuroantigen-coupled splenocytes is an effective treatment for established clinical disease. Mice tolerized with MSCH-coupled splenocytes after their initial episode of paralysis (21 days after infusion of effector T cells), were significantly protected from the development of clinical relapses when compared to mice treated with splenocytes coupled with a control kidney homogenate (FIG. 6). In addition, relapses observed in MSCH-tolerized mice were delayed in time and of milder clinical severity than those observed in controls. The ability of tolerance induced by neuroantigen-coupled splenocytes to inhibit expression of initial clinical symptoms, and to treat established disease in the adoptive R-EAE model is relevant to the establishment of therapeutic protocols for treatment of human autoimmune disorders and chronic graft rejection.

TABLE 1 shows a comparison of strategies currently employed for the regulation of CD4-dependent T cell responses. We feel that determinant-specific immune tolerance potentially provides a powerful approach for the prevention[11-13,30,31] and/or treatment (FIG. 6) of autoimmune diseases involving responses to a variety of Ag. Specific tolerance offers several advantages over other strategies of immunoregulation. It does not require nonspecific blockade of antigen presentation with anti-MHC class II monoclonal antibodies. Specific tolerance only targets effector cells bearing clonotypic receptors specific for the autoantigen/autoepitope and thus does not require elimination of entire T cell sets such as depletion with anti-CD4 depletion[32,33] or $V\beta$ subsets[34] which may immunocompromise the host.[35,36] It does not necessarily require that the response to the autoantigen be dominated by a specific epitope(s) within a particular autoantigen[37] or even the identification of the specific autoantigen as evidenced by the demonstration that both active R-EAE (dominated by PLP-specific responses) and adoptive R-EAE (mediated by MBP-specific responses) can be prevented by tolerizing with a homogenate of the target organ, i.e., crude MSCH.[11] Last, it does not require that the response be dominated by a limited repertoire of identifiable autoantigen-specific T cells.[38-41]

SUMMARY

The effects of neuroantigen-specific tolerance on the induction and effector stages of relapsing experimental autoimmune encephalomyelitis (R-EAE) were examined. The incidence of clinical and histologic signs of active MSCH-induced R-EAE, and accompanying neuroantigen-specific DTH responses, were dramatically reduced in SJL/J mice tolerized via the i.v. injection of syngeneic splenocytes coupled with MSCH, PLP, or encephalitogenic PLP peptides 7–14 days before priming. MBP-specific tolerance was not effective in preventing active R-EAE. In contrast to MSCH-induced active R-EAE, treatment of recipient mice with splenocytes coupled with MBP and the encephalitogenic MBP 84–104 peptide, but not with PLP, suppressed of clinical signs of adoptive R-EAE mediated by MBP-specific effector T cells in a dose-dependent manner. Neuroantigen-coupled splenocytes were also efficient in treating established disease as tolerization of SJL/J mice *after* the first incidence of clinical disease significantly reduced the incidence and severity of subsequent paralytic relapses. Antigen-specific tolerance thus provides a powerful approach for the prevention and/or treatment of autoimmune disease.

REFERENCES

1. BROWN, A. M. & D. E. MCFARLIN. 1981. Relapsing experimental allergic encephalomyelitis in the SJL/J mouse. Lab. Invest. **45:** 278–284.
2. LUBLIN, F. D., P. H. MAUER, R. G. BERRY & D. TIPPETT. 1981. Delayed, relapsing experimental allergic encephalomyelitis in mice. J. Immunol. **126:** 819–822.
3. FRITZ, R. B., C.-H. J. CHOU & D. E. MCFARLIN. 1983. Relapsing murine experimental allergic encephalomyelitis induced by myelin basic protein. J. Immunol. **130:** 1024–1026.
4. TROTTER, J. L., H. B. CLARK, K. G. COLLINS, C. L. WEGESCHIEDE & J. D. SCARPELLINI. 1987. Myelin proteolipid protein induces demyelinating disease in mice. J. Neurol. Sci. **79:** 173–188.

5. TABIRA, T. 1988. Autoimmune demyelination in the central nervous system. Ann. N.Y. Acad. Sci. **540:** 187–201.
6. PETTINELLI, C. B. & D. E. MCFARLIN. 1981. Adoptive transfer of experimental allergic encephalomyelitis in SJL/J mice after *in vitro* activation of lymph node cells by myelin basic protein: requirement for Lyt 1^+2^- T lymphocytes. J. Immunol. **127:** 1420–1423.
7. MOKHTARIAN, F., D. E. MCFARLIN & C. S. RAINE. 1984. Adoptive transfer of myelin basic protein-sensitized T cells produces chronic relapsing demyelinating disease in mice. Nature **309:** 356–358.
8. VAN DER VEEN, R. C., J. L. TROTTER, H. B. CLARK & J. A. KAPP. 1989. The adoptive transfer of chronic relapsing experimental allergic encephalomyelitis with lymph node cells sensitized to myelin proteolipid protein. J. Neuroimmunol. **21:** 183–191.
9. LASSMANN, H. & H. M. WISNIEWSKI. 1979. Chronic relapsing experimental allergic encephalomyelitis: clinicopathological comparison with multiple sclerosis. Arch. Neurol. **36:** 490–497.
10. BROWN, A., D. E. MCFARLIN & C. S. RAINE. 1982. Chronic neuropathology of relapsing experimental allergic encephalomyelitis in the mouse. Lab. Invest. **46:** 171–185.
11. KENNEDY, M. K., M. C. DAL CANTO, J. L. TROTTER & S. D. MILLER. 1988. Specific immune regulation of relapsing experimental allergic encephalomyelitis in mice. J. Immunol. **141:** 2986–2993.
12. KENNEDY, M. K., L. J. TAN, M. C. DAL CANTO, V. K. TUOHY, Z. LU, J. L. TROTTER & S. D. MILLER. 1990. Inhibition of murine relapsing experimental autoimmune encephalomyelitis by immune tolerance to proteolipid protein (PLP) and its encephalitogenic peptides. J. Immunol. **144:** 909–915.
13. KENNEDY, M. K., L. J. TAN, M. C. DAL CANTO & S. D. MILLER. 1990. Regulation of the effector stages of experimental autoimmune encephalomyelitis via neuroantigen-specific tolerance induction. J. Immunol. **145:** 117–126.
14. SWANBORG, R. H., J. E. SWIERKOSZ & R. G. SAIEG. 1974. Studies on the species-variability of experimental allergic encephalomyelitis in guinea pigs and rats. J. Immunol. **112:** 594–600.
15. HAMPSON, D. R. & S. E. PODUSLO. 1986. Purification of proteolipid protein and production of specific antiserum. J. Neuroimmunol. **11:** 117–129.
16. SHERMAN, G. & J. FOLCH-PI. 1970. Rotary dispersion and circular dichroism of brain 'proteolipid' protein. J. Neurochem. **17:** 597–605.
17. MILLER, S. D., R. P. WETZIG & H. N. CLAMAN. 1979. The induction of cell-mediated immunity and tolerance with protein antigens coupled to syngeneic lymphoid cells. J. Exp. Med. **149:** 758–773.
18. MILLER, S. D. & M. K. JENKINS. 1986. Detection of suppressor cells and suppressor factors for delayed-type hypersensitivity responses. *In* Handbook of Experimental Immunology, Fourth Edit. D. M. WEIR, L. A. HERZENBERG, C. C. BLACKWELL & L. A. HERZENBERG, Eds. 77.1–77.13. Blackwell Scientific Publications, Ltd. Edinburgh, United Kingdom.
19. ARMITAGE, P. 1971. Statistical Methods of Research. 207–211. John Wiley. New York.
20. KONO, D. H., J. L. URBAN, S. J. HORVATH, D. G. ANDO, R. A. SAAVEDRA & L. HOOD. 1988. Two minor determinants of myelin basic protein induce experimental allergic encephalomyelitis in SJL/J mice. J. Exp. Med. **168:** 213–227.
21. SAKAI, K., S. S. ZAMVIL, D. J. MITCHELL, M. LIM, J. B. ROTHBARD & L. STEINMAN. 1988. Characterization of a major encephalitogenic T cell epitope in SJL/J mice with synthetic oligopeptides of myelin basic protein. J. Neuroimmunol. **19:** 21–32.
22. TUOHY, V. K., Z. LU, R. A. SOBEL, R. A. LAURSEN & M. B. LEES. 1989. Identification of an encephalitogenic determinant of myelin proteolipid protein for SJL mice. J. Immunol. **142:** 1523–1527.
23. SATOH, J., K. SAKAI, M. ENDOH, F. KOIKE, T. KUNISHITA, T. NAMIKAWA, T. YAMAMURA, & T. TABIRA. 1987. Experimental allergic encephalomyelitis mediated by murine encephalitogenic T cell lines specific for myelin proteolipid apoprotein. J. Immunol. **138:** 179–184.
24. NAVE, K.-A., C. LAI, F. E. BLOOM & R. J. MILNER. 1987. Splice site selection in the proteolipid protein (PLP) gene transcript and primary structure of the DM-20 protein of central nervous system myelin. Proc. Natl. Acad. Sci. USA **84:** 5665–5669.

25. SOBEL, R. A., V. K. TUOHY, Z. LU, R. A. LAURSEN & M. B. LEES. 1990. Acute experimental allergic encephalomyelitis in SJL/J mice induced by a synthetic peptide or myelin proteolipid protein. J. Neuropathol. Exp. Neurol. **49:** 468–479.

26. JOHNSON, H. M., K. BRENNER & H. E. HALL. 1966. The use of a water-soluble carbodiimide as a coupling reagent in the passive hemagglutination test. J. Immunol. **97:** 791–796.

27. SRIRAM, S., G. SCHWARTZ & L. STEINMAN. 1983. Administration of myelin basic protein-coupled spleen cells prevents experimental allergic encephalitis. Cell. Immunol. **75:** 378–382.

28. FRITZ, R. B., M. J. SKEEN, C. H. J. CHOU & S. S. ZAMVIL. 1990. Localization of an encephalitogenic epitope for the SJL mouse in the N-terminal region of myelin basic protein. J. Neuroimmunol. **26:** 239–244.

29. JENKINS, M. K. & R. H. SCHARTZ. 1987. Antigen presentation by chemically modified splenocytes induces antigen-specific T cell unresponsiveness *in vitro* and *in vivo*. J. Exp. Med. **165:** 302–319.

30. BRALEY-MULLEN, H., J. G. TOMPSON, G. C. SHARP & M. KYRIAKOS. 1980. Suppression of experimental autoimmune thyroiditis in guinea pigs by pretreatment with thyroglobulin-coupled spleen cells. Cell. Immunol. **51:** 408–413.

31. SCHOEN, R. T., M. I. GREENE & D. E. TRENTHAM. 1982. Antigen-specific suppression of type II collagen-induced arthritis by collagen-coupled spleen cells. J. Immunol. **128:** 717–719.

32. KENNEDY, M. K., R. J. CLATCH, M. C. DAL CANTO, J. L. TROTTER & S. D. MILLER. 1987. Monoclonal antibody-induced inhibition of relapsing EAE in SJL/J mice correlates with inhibition of neuroantigen-specific cell-mediated immune responses. J. Neuroimmunol. **16:** 345–364.

33. WALDOR, M. K., S. SRIRAM, R. HARDY, L. A. HERZENBERG, L. A. HERZENBERG, L. LANIER, M. LIM & L. STEINMAN. 1985. Reversal of experimental allergic encephalomyelitis with monoclonal antibody to a T-cell subset marker. Science **227:** 415–417.

34. ZALLER, D. M., G. OSMAN, O. KANAGAWA & L. HOOD. 1990. Prevention and treatment of experimental allergic encephalomyelitis with T cell receptor Vβ-specific antibodies. J. Exp. Med. **171:** 1943–1955.

35. VOLLMER, T. L., M. K. WALDOR, L. STEINMAN & F. K. CONLEY. 1987. Depletion of T-4+ lymphocytes with monoclonal antibody reactivates toxoplasmosis in the central nervous system: a model of superinfection in AIDS. J. Immunol. **138:** 3737–3741.

36. HAFLER, D. A., J. RITZ, S. F. SCHLOSSMAN & H. L. WEINER. 1988. Anti-CD4 and anti-CD2 monoclonal antibody infusions in subjects with multiple sclerosis: immunosuppressive effects and human anti-mouse responses. J. Immunol. **141:** 131–138.

37. WRAITH, D. C., D. E. SMILEK, D. J. MITCHELL, L. STEINMAN & H. O. McDEVITT. 1989. Antigen recognition in autoimmune encephalitis and the potential for peptide-mediated immunotherapy. Cell **59:** 247–255.

38. ACHA-ORBEA, H., D. J. MITCHELL, L. TIMMERMANN, D. C. WRAITH, G. S. TAUSCH, M. K. WALDOR, S. S. ZAMVIL, H. O. McDEVITT & L. STEINMAN. 1988. Limited heterogeneity of T cell receptors from lymphocytes mediating autoimmune encephalomyelitis allows specific immune intervention. Cell **54:** 263–273.

39. SAKAI, K., A. A. SINHA, D. J. MITCHELL, S. S. ZAMVIL, J. B. ROTHBARD, H. O. McDEVITT & L. STEINMAN. 1988. Involvement of distinct murine T-cell receptors in the autoimmune encephalitogenic response to nested epitopes of myelin basic protein. Proc. Natl. Acad. Sci. USA **85:** 8608–8612.

40. URBAN, J. L., V. KUMAR, D. H. KONO, C. GOMEZ, S. J. HORVATH, J. CLAYTON, D. G. ANDO, E. E. SERCARZ & L. HOOD. 1988. Restricted use of T cell receptor V genes in murine autoimmune encephalomyelitis raises possibilities for antibody therapy. Cell **54:** 577–592.

41. ZAMVIL, S. S., D. J. MITCHELL, N. E. LEE, A. C. MOORE, M. K. WALDOR, K. SAKAI, J. B. ROTHBARD, H. O. McDEVITT, L. STEINMAN & H. ACHA-ORBEA. 1988. Predominant expression of a T cell receptor V_β gene subfamily in autoimmune encephalomyelitis. J. Exp. Med. **167:** 1586–1596.

Inhibition of Antiskin Allograft Immunity Induced by Infusions with Photoinactivated Effector T Lymphocytes (PET Cells). Is *In Vivo* Cell Transferrable?

MARITZA PEREZ, FRANCIS M. LOBO,
YASUHIRO YAMANE, LORI JOHN, CAROLE L. BERGER,
AND RICHARD L. EDELSON

Department of Dermatology
Yale University
New Haven, Connecticut, 06510–8059

and

Department of Dermatology
Columbia University
New York, New York 10032

The selective suppression of aberrant T cell populations is an important goal of immunotherapy. Andersson, Binz and Wigzell[1] have reported that specific immune unresponsiveness can be induced *in vivo* in rodents by immunizing the animal with autologous antigen-specific lymphoblasts obtained after *in vitro* sensitization, if the immunizing cells are emulsified in Freund's complete adjuvant. Thus, autoimmunization against clonotypic determinants, presumably the T cell receptor (TCR) for a potent antigen, may constitute an efficient way of producing specific immune tolerance in immunocompetent adult animals. Animal models of autoreactive disease in which myelin basic protein (MBP)-specific T cell clones[2] induce experimental autoimmune encephalomyelitis in susceptible strains of rodents are examples of such immunotherapeutic intervention. Cohen *et al.*[3] and others[4] have shown that if these pathogenic cloned T cells are passively transferred into syngeneic recipients, the clinical signs of the autoreactive disease are reproduced. However, if the same disease-inducing cloned T cells are extracorporeally attenuated by X-irradiation, mitomycin C or hydrostatic pressure and then intravenously reinfused, they can immunoprotect syngeneic animals in a clonotypic manner against the same autoreactive disease.[2,3,5] Among the obstacles that currently preclude application of that approach to treatment of human diseases caused by pathogenic T cells are the difficulty in identification, isolation, and *in vitro* expansion of such aberrant clones.

We believe we might have overcome those obstacles. We have reported that cutaneous T cell lymphoma (CTCL) patients who received intravenous reinfusion of peripheral blood mononuclear cells that have been extracorporeally exposed to 8-methoxypsoralen (8-MOP) in the presence of ultraviolent A light (UVA) demonstrated a profound and prolonged clinical response which appears to be immunologically mediated.[6] To decipher the mechanism underlying this apparent antimalignant T cell response, we have developed animal models in which potent and

95

defined immunologic responses are expressed in vivo and in which laboratory correlates exist. In such a system involving transplantation of skin across major mouse histocompatability barriers,[7] we have reported that the in vivo and in vitro responses to alloantigen were attenuated in a donor-specific fashion. In that system, splenocytes containing expanded populations of effector T cells mediating the relevant allograft rejection were first treated with 8-MOP/UVA and were then infused into naive syngeneic recipients, which now showed markedly enhanced skin allograft survival. Therefore, infusion of unfractionated populations of autologous mononuclear cells containing an expanded clone(s) of pathogenic T cells immunized against the activity of the same clone(s) if initially extracorporeally altered in an appropriate fashion.

To selectively inhibit the response to alloantigen, we have attempted to exploit the observation that the antigen receptor of effector T cells can be immunogenic and that specific reactions against the TCR can suppress its function.[8,9] In order to inhibit the proliferation of the in vivo expanded effector cells of antialloantigen responses, we selected a pharmacologic method of treating the cells which would permit retention of an intact cell membrane.[10] 8-MOP, a naturally occurring and biologically inert furocoumarin, is transiently transformed by UVA to a state in which it is capable of forming covalent bonds with pyrimidine bases of DNA, leading to crosslinks between complementary DNA strands.[11] The DNA effect induced by 8-MOP is analogous to the chemical impact of a bifunctional alkylating agent like mitomycin C. However, psoralen photoaddition can be more precisely titrated by altering both drug level and UVA intensity. We have previously established conditions for 8-MOP/UVA induced DNA crosslinks to maximally inhibit mitosis of murine T cells while simultaneously sparing the capacity of irradiated mononuclear cells to serve as stimulators[10] in MLC. This requires an irradiance of 1 Joule/cm^2 UVA in the presence of 100 ng/ml of 8-MOP.

This study extends our previous observations[7,12,13] demonstrating that this immunosuppresive response that prolongs skin allograft survival is adoptively transferred into naive syngeneic recipients by radiosensitive Thy-1+, Lyt-2+, L3T4- T lymphocytes.

MATERIALS AND METHODS

Mice

BALB/c (H-2^d, Mls^0), CBA/j (H-2^k, Mls^1) and C57B1/10 (B10, H-2^b, Mls^0) mice were purchased from the Jackson Laboratory, Bar Harbor, ME. All mice were maintained in a specific pathogen-free facility. Female CBA/j mice 4 to 6 wk of age were used as skin transplant donors. Female BALB/c mice 4 to 6 wk. of age were the skin transplant recipients. B10 female mice were the donors of splenocytes used as the irrelevant alloantigen controls in *in vitro* and *in vivo* experiments. All mice used for the following experiments were approximately the same age (aged-matched by not more than 4 weeks).

Skin Transplantation and Preparation of Cell Suspension

The skin grafting was performed following the procedure of Billigham and Medawar,[14] and preparation of cell suspensions has been previously described in detail.[12] Time of maximal antialloantigen response was estimated from the highest cytotoxic response obtained. Therefore, the peak time of rejection was considered to be 8 d post-transplant. Splenocytes obtained at 8 d from these transplanted (sensitized) mice therefore served as a source of the immunizing population of cells (see immunization protocol).

Photoinactivation

Optimal conditions for murine splenocyte photoinactivation with 8-MOP/ UVA, as determined by their proliferative response to non-specific mitogens, has been reported elsewhere.[10]

Immunization Protocol

Recipient mice were injected intravenously in the tail vein with 200 ul of PBS containing $30-50 \times 10^6$ splenocytes from BALB/c mice rejecting a CBA/j skin graft. Among these cells were the *in vivo* expanded clones of T cells mediating CBA/j skin graft rejection, which followed photoinactivation of these cells with 8-MOP. We refer to them as Photoinactivated Effector T or PET cells of allograft rejection. BALB/c recipients were injected once every week for 3 mo with PET cells. Recipient mice were then tested for T cell responsiveness to CBA/j alloantigens in mixed leukocyte culture (MLC), cytotoxicity (CTL), and delayed type hypersensitivity (DTH) assays and challenged with fresh CBA/j skin transplants.

Adoptive Transfer with Lysis of Cell Subsets

Three or six days after the last immunization PET treated and control groups of mice were sacrificed for preparation of spleen cell suspensions. To test for radiosensitivity the spleen cell suspension was X-irradiated with 3200 rads prior to the adoptive transfer. To lyse specific T cell subpopulations, the splenocytes were suspended at $20-25 \times 10^6$ cells/ml in RPMI containing 0.3% BSA and then incubated twice for 90 mins at 4°C with one of the following anti-T cell antibodies at 1:20 dilution from hybridoma supenatant:anti Thy-1.2, anti Lyt-2.2 (Cedar Lane Laboratories, Ontario, Canada) and anti-L3T4 supernatant from hybridoma GK1.5. After centrifugation for 8′ at 1200 rpm, cells were resuspended at $20-25 \times 10^6$ cell/ml in 1:20 dilution of rabbit complement (Low-Tox-M, Cedar Lane Laboratories) in RPMI/0.3% BSA and incubated for 60 min at 37°C. Cell viability was determined by trypan blue exclusion and viable cells separated by fluotation (Lympholyte M, Cedar Lane Lab.). The unlysed cells were washed twice with RPMI/0.3%BSA and resuspended in PBS. Cells from these preparations, each originating from PET-treated or control mice, lacking or not the Thy-1+, Lyt-2+ or L3T4+ lymphocytes were injected into naive BALB/c mice at a concentration of $50-100 \times 10^6$ cells in 200 ul of PBS.

Delayed Type Hypersensitivity Response

DTH assay was performed following the methods of Granstein *et al.*[15] and Van der Kwast *et al.*[16] and largely represent in vivo allogeneic responses to histoincompatible Class II alloantigens.[17] Spleen cell suspensions from CBA/j mice (30–

50×10^6 X-irradiated splenocytes) were injected in the flanks of five naive B10 mice (positive control group) five PET treated BALB/c mice (experimental group 1) and five BALB/c mice treated with photoinactivated naive splenocytes (experimental group 2) six days after the last intravenous treatment with PET cells. After 7 days, elicitation was perfomred by injecting 10×10^6 CBS/j splenocytes in 0.20 ml of PBS subcutaneously in the right hind footpad. After 24 hr, both hind footpads were measured for thickness with a dial caliper (Monostat, Swiss made Fisher scientific, Springfield, NJ). The thickness of the left footpad (noninjected) was subtracted from the right (injected) footpad to measure the DTH response. Percent suppression was calculated by the formula 1-([E-N]/[P-N] $\times$ 100, where E is the measurement obtained from experimental group of mice, N is the negative control and P is the positive control. Determination of specificity of *in vivo* suppression of the DTH response was determined by immunizing and challenging analogous control groups of mice with splenocytes from B10 mice (H-2^b).

Mixed Leukocyte Culture

MLC responses which largely represent the *in vitro* proliferative response to histoincompatible Class II alloantigens[18] were performed following modifications of the methods of Rock et al.[19] and Kruisbeek et al.[20] and are described in detail elsewhere.[7]

Cytotoxicity Assay

Cytotoxicity assays were performed to detect the presence of alloreactive cells primarily responsive to Class I alloantigen disparity[21] and were performed following the methods of Burakoff et al.[22] and Granstein et al.[15] also previously described in detail.[12]

Statistical Analysis

Statistical significance was determined according to Student's *t* test. A *p* value of less than 0.05 was considered significant.

RESULTS

Specific Inhibition of DTH

PET treated and control (mice which received photoinactivated naive T cells or PNT cells) BALB/c mice were tested for response to CBA/j alloantigens after receiving multiple infusions of PET cells. As shown in FIGURE 1a when PET-treated mice were primed and 7 days later challenged with H-2^k, Mls^1 (CBA/j) alloantigen bearing splenocytes a significant suppression of the DTH response (footpad swelling) was demonstrated as compared with positive control mice. However, when BALB/c mice treated with photoinactivated naive cells were primed and 7 days later challenged with the CBA/j alloantigen bearing cells, no

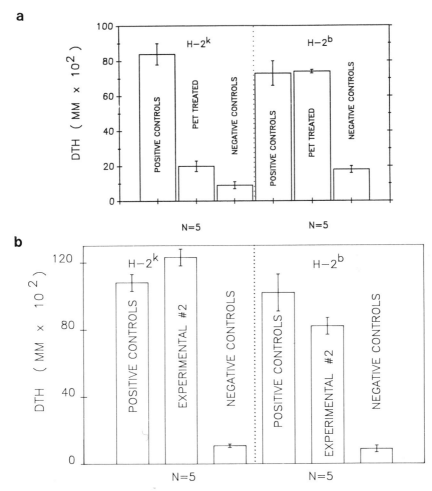

FIGURE 1. (a) Specific inhibition of the DTH response. PET-treated BALB/c mice primed in the flank and footpad challenged with either CBA/j (H-2^k, Mls^1) (*left*) or B10 (H-2^b, Mls^0) (*right*) splenocytes and the measurement of footpad swelling compared to the swelling elicited in positive and negative controls. **(b)** DTH response of experimental control group #2 BALB/c mice that had received iv infusions of 8-MOP-UVA. Photoinactivated syngeneic naive splenocytes were primed in the flank and footpad challenged with splenocytes from either CBA/j (*left*) or B10 (*right*) mice and footpad swelling measurements compared to swelling elicited in control mice.

suppression of DTH response was demonstrated (FIG. Ib). Moreover, no suppression of the DTH response was demonstrated in mice pretreated with either PET cells or with photoinactivated naive cells when they were primed and challenged with splenocytes bearing the unrelated antigen H-2^b, Mls^0 (FIG. 1). Therefore, specificity of the *in vivo* suppression was demonstrated.

Allograft Survival

Balb/c mice which had been repeatedly infused with PET cells recognizing the H-2^k, Mls^1 (CBA/j) alloantigen were challenged with a fresh CBA/j skin graft, the survival of which was clinically and histopathologically followed. Six PET-treated BALB/c female mice received CBA/j skin transplants, in parallel with naive (aged matched +/−3 weeks) BALB/c female mice which also received identical skin grafts. Treated mice continued to receive intravenous PET infusions on a weekly basis, following engraftment.

All *control* naive BALB/c mice demonstrated evidence of rejection by 8 d after transplantation and total necrosis by 12 d after engraftment (TABLE 1). In contrast, none of the PET treated mice demonstrated any clinical evidence of rejections by day 8 after transplantation. Three PET treated mice were sacrificed 18 d post engraftment to evaluate histologically the skin allograft which did not show visual evidence of rejection. Histopathological evaluation revealed epidermotropism of mononuclear cells within a viable epidermis. The surviving PET treated mice were sacrificed at subsequent intervals for histologic evaluation of the graft. Although these mice did not demonstrate visual evidence of rejection at the end of the fifth and seventh week post transplantation, the pathological specimens showed confluent and focal vacuolar basal cell degeneration, and focal areas of mononuclear cell infiltration of engrafted epidermis with a dense dermal mononuclear cell infiltrate. The longest survival of the allograft was 42 d post engraftment. However, five BALB/c mice which had received similar numbers of photoinactivated splenocytes from syngeneic mice rejecting a CBA/j skin graft and then received a skin graft from B10 mice, a distinct strain differing at H-2 and Mls loci demonstrated rejection within 12 days following transplantation (TABLE 1). The histologic evaluation of these skin grafts revealed separation of a necrotic epidermis from the dermis, accompanied by a very dense mononuclear cell infiltrate and thrombus formation within dermal vessels.

Suppression of MLC

BALB/c female mice, intravenously immunized with PET cells obtained from syngeneic mice having rejected primary skin transplants demonstrated highly significant hyporesponsiveness to H-2^k alloantigen in MLC responses (FIG. 2a) without interfering with the response in MLC to unrelated alloantigen H-2^b (FIG. 2b) thus determining the specificity of this hyporesponsiveness. Thus, to determine whether this hyporesponsiveness was the result of deletion or inhibition of the effector cell population by an induced suppressor cell population, a three

TABLE 1. Alloskin Graft Survival. Rejection: Days after Engraftment of Skin Allograft Haplotype

	Graft Donors	
Graft Recipients	CBA/j (H2^k, Mls^1)	B10 (H-2^b, Mls^0)
Naive Balb/c (H-2^d, Mls^0) N = 5	7–8 days	10–12 days
PET Tx Balb/c Mice N = 6	22–42 days	10–12 days

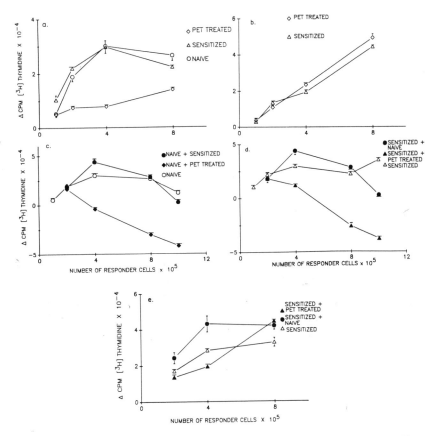

FIGURE 2. Proliferative response in MLC of splenocytes from BALB/c mice. The response of: **(a)** PET-treated BALB/c splenocytes ($\Diamond$) to H-2^k, Mls^1 alloantigen expressed on CBA/j spleen cells compared to the proliferative response of naive ($\bigcirc$) and sensitized ($\triangle$) BALB/c spleen cells; **(b)** PET-treated BALB/c splenocytes ($\Diamond$) to an irrelevant alloantigen H-2^b, Mls^0, expressed on B10 stimulator splenocytes compared to sensitized BALB/c splenocytes ($\triangle$); **(c)** naive BALB/c mice ($\bigcirc$) to H-2^k, Mls^1 alloantigen compared to splenocytes from naive BALB/c mice added in a 1:1 ratio to either sensitized ($\bullet$) BALB/c splenocytes or PET-treated ($\blacklozenge$) BALB/c splenocytes; **(d)** sensitized BALB/c splenocytes ($\triangle$) to H-2^k, Mls^0 compared to sensitized BALB/c splenocytes added 1:1 to either naive ($\bullet$) or PET-treated ($\blacktriangle$) BALB/c splenocytes; and **(e)** sensitized BALB/c splenocytes ($\triangle$) to an irrelevant alloantigen H-2^b, Mls^b compared to sensitized BALB/c splenocytes added in a 1:1 ratio to either naive ($\bullet$) or PET-treated ($\blacktriangle$) BALB/c splenocytes.

party MLC was performed (FIG. 2c and d). However, when splenocytes from naive (FIG. 2c) or skin graft sensitized (FIG. 2d) and PET treated mice were admixed and exposed to x-irradiated cells bearing the relevant antigen H-2^k, Mls^1 (CBA/j) or H-2^{b}Mls^0 (B10) (FIG. 2e), cells bearing irrelevant alloantigens, highly significant suppression in MLC was only observed to the spleen cells expressing the relevant haplotype H-2^k (FIG. 2c and d, $p < 0.001$, FIG. 2e, $p < 0.02$). Therefore, the diminution of MLC reactivity against donor antigens in splenocytes from

PET-treated mice resulted from the presence of a specific inhibitory cell population in these PET treated mice.

Suppression of Cytotoxicity

To evaluate the impact of pretreatment with PET cells on capacity to generate an anti-CBA/j cytotoxic response *in vitro,* cell mediated lympholysis (CML) reactions were generated. Splenocytes from sensitized, naive or PET-treated BALB/c mice were first stimulated in MLC by CBA/j leukocytes (FIG. 3a). As anticipated,

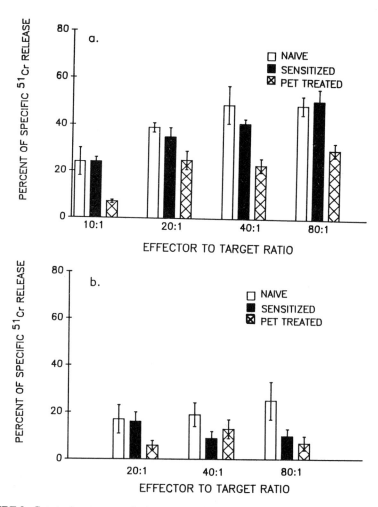

FIGURE 3. Cytotoxic response of splenocytes from BALB/c mice. **(a)** Sensitized BALB/c splenocytes were reexposed *in vitro* to H-2^k, Mls^1 alloantigen. Naive BALB/c and PET-treated mice splenocytes were exposed *in vitro* to H-2^k, Mls^1 alloantigen and all splenocytes tested for lysis of ^{51}Cr labelled CBA/j or **(b)** BALB/c targets at increasing effector to target.

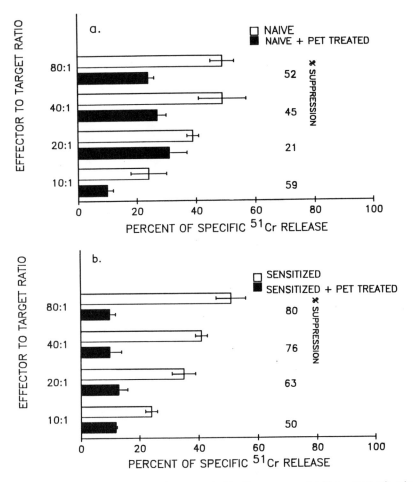

FIGURE 4. Inhibition of the specific cytotoxic T cells response. **(a)** Naive BALB/c mice splenocytes or **(b)** sensitized BALB/c splenocytes exposed to H-2^k, Mls[1] alloantigens *in vitro* and tested for lysis of CBA/j ^{51}Cr labelled targets at increasing effector to target ratios and compared to lysis elicited when cells from PET-treated mice were admixed 1 : 1 to (a) naive BALB/c or (b) sensitized BALB/c mice splenocytes.

a low maximal (25%) specific cytotoxic T cell response was obtained at 80:1 effector:target (E:T) ratio from PET treated BALB/c mice to ^{51}Cr-labelled CBA/j targets and no cytotoxic response was demonstrated to BALB/c ^{51}Cr-labelled targets (FIG. 3b). This response was significantly less than that generated by either naive BALB/c mice at 20, 40, 80:1 E:T ratio ($p < 0.002, 0.005, 0.005$) or sensitized BALB/c mice splenocytes at 10, 20, 80:1 E:T ratio ($p < 0.005, 0.001, 0.001$). As shown in FIGURE 4, highly significant suppression at 40 and 80:1 E:T ratio of the naive (FIG. 4a, $p < 0.02, 0.002$) and at all E:T ratios tested of the sensitized (FIG. 4b, $p < 0.005, 0.005, 0.001, 0.001$) BALB/c cytotoxic T cell response to CBA/j alloantigen was obtained when splenocytes from PET treated BALB/c mice were

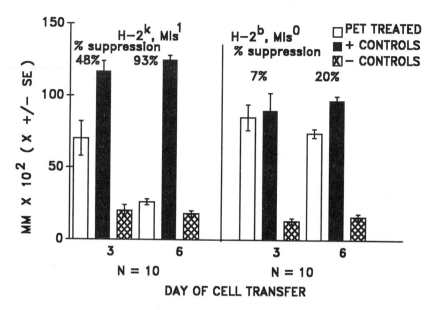

FIGURE 5. Transfer of specific inhibition of the DTH response. Naive BALB/c recipients of spleen cells from PET-treated BALB/c mice (three and six days after treatment) primed in the flank footpad challenged with either CBA/j (relevant) or B10 (irrelevant) splenocytes and the measurement of footpad swelling compared to the swelling elicited in positive and negative controls.

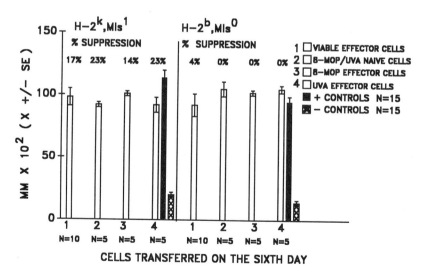

FIGURE 6. DTH response of control mice. Naive BALB/c recipients of spleen cells from different groups of control BALB/c mice (six days after last treatment) primed in the flank and footpad challenged with either CBA/j (relevant) or B10 (irrelevant) splenocytes and the measurement of footpad swelling compared to the swelling elicited in positive and negative controls.

TABLE 2. Skin Allograft Survival

Adoptive Transfer Donor Animals	H-2^k, Mls^1 Days Survival X ± SE	H-2^b, Mls^0 Days Survival X ± SE	p Values
PET-treated cells N = 6	17.50 ± 0.90	9.50 ± 0.68	≤0.0001
Viable effector cells N = 7	8.86 ± 0.70	9.86 ± 1.12	NS
Photoinactivated naive cells N = 6	7.80 ± 0.31	7.67 ± 0.21	NS
8-MOP effector cells N = 8	9.25 ± 0.41	8.80 ± 0.49	NS
UVA effector cells N = 8	9.25 ± 0.49	10.60 ± 0.40	NS
+ control cells	9.25 ± 0.37	10.60 ± 0.25	

added, indicating the presence of potent suppressor cells of the CML response. Therefore, pre-exposure of the mouse immune system to PET cells generated during skin transplant rejection rendered the secondary syngeneic recipient relatively, but not absolutely, tolerant to the alloantigen carried by the transplanted donor used to generate the immunizing effector cell population. Survival time of the grafts was tripled by relevant PET cell infusions and specific suppression of DTH response to alloantigen correlated with prolongation of specific allograft survival.

Adoptive transfer of tolerance for skin allotransplantation was demonstrated by inhibition of the DTH response and prologation of allograft survival in the recipients of the adoptively transferred cell population. As shown in FIGURE 5, 48% of the specific suppression of DTH response was transferred into naive BALB/c recipients when the adoptive transfer was performed in the third day after the last PET treament of the donor BALB/c mice. However, 93% suppression of the DTH response was optimally transferred into BALB/c recipients when adoptive transfer was performed six days after the last PET infusion received by the donor animals. In contrast, no significant suppression of the DTH response (FIG. 6) or prologation of skin allograft survival (TABLE 2) was demonstrated in syngeneic recipients of adoptive transfer from BALB/c mice treated with viable effector cells, photoinactivated naive cells, 8-MOP effector cells and UVA effec-

TABLE 3. Skin Allograft Survival

Adoptive Transfer Donor Animals	H-2^k, Mls^1 Days Survival X ± SE	H-2^b, Mls^0 Days Survival X ± SE	p Values
PET-treated cells N = 6	17.50 ± 0.90	9.50 ± 0.68	≤0.0001
PET-treated cells + THY1 + C' N = 5	11.20 ± 0.58	10.20 ± 0.45	≤0,005
PET-treated cells + Lyt2 + C' N = 5	9.20 ± 0.49	11.25 ± 0.25	NS
PET-treaed cells + L3T4 + C' N = 7	14.70 ± 1.12	10.40 ± 0.25	≤0.0001
+ control cells N = 8	9.25 ± 0.37	10.60 ± 0.25	

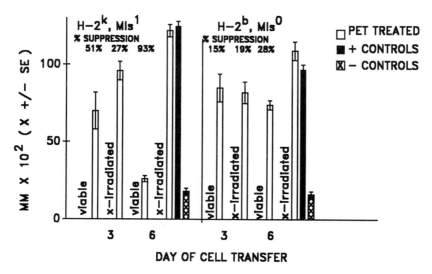

FIGURE 7. Abrogation of inhibition of DTH response by X-irradiation. Naive BALB/c recipients of X-irradiated (3200 rads) or viable spleen cells from PET-treated donors primed in the flank and footpad challenged with either CBA/j (relevant) or B10 (irrelevant) splenocytes and the measurement of footpad swelling compared to the swelling elicited in positive and negative controls.

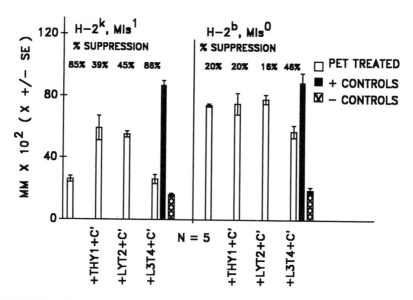

FIGURE 8. Abrogation of inhibition of DTH response by depletion of Thy1+, Lyt2+, L3T4− T lymphocytes. Naive BALB/c recipients of Thy1+, Lyt2+, L3T4+ depleted spleen cells from PET-treated donors primed in the flank and footpad challenged with either CBA/j (relevant) or B10 (irrelevant) splenocytes and the measurement of footpad swelling compared to the swelling elicited in positive and negative controls.

tor cells treated syngeneic mice. Inhibition of the DTH response to the relevant alloantigen was abolished by prior X-irradiation (3200 rads) of the adoptive transfer spleen cell population from the PET-treated BALB/c mice (FIG. 7). Moreover, suppression for the DTH response to the relevant alloantigen was significantly abrogated by the depletion of Thy-1+, Lyt-2+, L3T4- T lymphocytes from the adoptively transferred cell population (FIG. 8). These results correlated with abolishment of skin allograft survival in BALB/c recipients of spleen cells from PET treated mice depleted of Thy-1+, Lyt-2+ T lymphocytes (TABLE 3). Therefore, suppression of skin allograft rejection is adoptively transferrable mainly by radiosensitive Thy-1+, Lyt-2+, L3T4- T lymphocytes.

DISCUSSION

Murine skin transplantation across H-2 barriers results in transplant rejection principally mediated by recipient T lymphocytes[23] with an Lytl+2+[17] and L3T4+ phenotype.[24] In our study, the single, most important result obtained by the infusion of photoinactivated effect T (PET) cells was the significant prolongation of survival of specific allogeneic skin transplants, correlating with the specific suppression of the MLC and CTL responses, the *in vitro* correlates of allograft rejection, and specific suppression of the DTH response. Moreover, this specific suppression of skin allograft rejection was adoptively transferrable mainly by a radiosensitive Thy-1+, Lyt-2+, L3T4- T lymphocytes. That alternation of the very potent immunologic rejection of these transplants could be accomplished without other more standard immunosuppressive therapy and that this attenuation of response was donor specific suggests the induction of highly directed downregulatory signals. Suppression of the DTH response paralleled the skin transplant data and provides a useful and time-saving correlate. Relevant controls indicate the requirement for specifically presensitized cells and the photoinactivation process for this *in vivo* effect. It must be emphasized at this point, that extensive studies by us (Khavari[25]) and Cohen and co-workers[2-4,26] indicate that other methods of effector T cell pretreatment, including glutaraldehyde and mitomycin C, can produce similar effects in other systems and may well do the same in this sytsem. Whereas such other types of extracorporeal manipulations need to be tested, the first and most significant goal has been herein accomplished: the demonstration that survival of allogeneic transplanted skin can be specifically prolonged.

It is noteworthy that in the totally allogeneic model the maximal suppression of the delayed type hypersensitivity response was 84–93%[7] correlating with allograft survival of 42 days, while in the congenic murine model maximal suppression of delayed type hypersensitivity response was 73–75% and graft survival of 22 days.[13] This paradoxical result is of interest, since it suggests that the greater the histocompatability barrier, the greater the downregulatory impact of PET cell treatment. Indeed, the magnitude of the mixed leukocyte culture response from splenocytes of *in vivo* sensitized mice was even greater in the totally allogeneic system and the relative suppressive effect of PET cell treatment on mixed leukocyte culture greater. Therefore, the results suggest that the greater the initial stimulus producing effector T cells, the greater the specific suppression they can produce in a naive syngeneic recipient. Since specific suppression can now be recognized to be superimposed on nonspecific suppression in the congenic system, the vigor of the specific suppression in the total allogeneic system may merely obscure the nonspecific suppression there. Whereas the nonspecific suppression seems not to be relevant to the *in vivo* response to alloantigens, it will be necessary in future experimentation to investigate its impact on weaker antigenic stimuli.

These findings extend those previously reported by our group[7,12,13] and other systems by various investigators[27,28]. Rohowsky and Suciu-Foca[27] have shown that idiotype-like receptors for alloantigens on autologous T lymphoblasts stimulate the autologous mixed leukocyte culture (AMLC) response in resting lymphocytes. In our studies, a substantial increase in the autologous mixed leukocyte culture response has been observed in the splenocytes of PET-treated animals (TABLE 4). Dorsh and Roser[28] demonstrated a rapidly recirculating suppressor T cell population in animals rendered tolerant to alloantigen by transfusions of allogeneic bone marrow cells during neonatal life. These cells are capable of adoptively transferring tolerance, in irradiated syngeneic recipients, to skin transplants bearing the alloantigens to which the original tolerance was induced, without interfering with the rejection of an unrelated skin graft. In a similar fashion we have developed an immunization protocol that induces the production of Lyt-2+ T cells capable of suppressing the MLC, CTL, and DTH responses, prolonging the specific skin allograft survival without interfering with the responses to non relevant alloantigens and adoptively transferring this suppressive response into syngeneic recipients.

TABLE 4. Autologus Mixed Leukocyte Response: cpm [^{3}H]Thymidine (X + SE)

Number of Responder Cells × 10^5 (H-2^d, Mls^b)	H-2 and Mls Haplotype Stimulator Cells (2 × 10^5)	Naive BALB/c Mice (N = 3)	Sensitized BALB/c Mice (N = 3)	Pet-Treated BALB/c Mice (N = 6)
1	H-2^d, Mls^b	250 + 73	281 + 32	4907 + 620
2	H-2^d, Mls^b	806 + 39	1630 + 293	32045 + 3811
4	H-2^d, Mls^b	5577 + 1044	7767 + 715	46820 + 2339
8	H-2^d, Mls^b	14980 + 787	15087 + 627	45147 + 5044

The identity and specific function of these suppressor T cells remains to be established. It will be necessary to determine whether they are Ly2+ suppressor T cells[29] and/or Ly2+ anti-receptor and anti-major histocompatability complex cytotoxic T cells described by Kosmatopoulos *et al.*[30], the CD8+ suppressor T cells[31] or CD8+ autocytotoxic T cells[32] which specifically respond to determinants on the disease-mediating T cell clones and/or the CD4+ and CD8+ anti-ergotypic T cells which respond to non-idiotype determinants expressed on activated T cells.[33]

In our system, photoinactivation with 8-MOP might have been so effective in maximizing the development of a specific inhibitory response to alloantigen, because it has the ability to control two variables (drug dose and UVA energy) which limit the chemical reaction to microseconds.[34] Thus permits meticulous control of the dose-response curve of cellular inactivation to a level not otherwise attainable. Significantly, Lider and Cohen[26] have recently found vaccination to be more effective when the experimental autoimmune encephalomyelitis-inducive T cell clones are inactivated by hydrostatic pressure or chemical cross-linkers prior to vaccination. Also, 8-MOP/UVA pretreatment of cloned anti-basic myelin protein T cells[25] was more effective than X-irradiation, glutaraldehyde or mitomycin C treatment of the same cells for vaccinating rats against the induction of experimental autoimmune encephalomyelitis. Our studies of the suppression of delayed type hypersensitivity response to sheep red blood cells[35] have demonstrated that 8-MOP/UVA treatment of a naive population of splenocytes is ineffective in inducing suppression in a system quite similar to that used in this study, indicating that the presence of expanded population(s) of specific effector T cells is necessary. However, it must be emphasized that 8-MOP/UVA pretreatment of effector cells may be merely one particularly effective means of inducing the observed results.[25,35]

We conclude that it is possible to induce a state of hyporeactivity against a specific and nonspecific set of major histocompatability complex (MHC) antigens. Syngeneic effector cells with specificity for these antigens can be photoinactivated and used as immunogens to induce this hyporesponsive state. This hyporesponsive state is adoptively transferrable mainly by a radiosensitive Thy-1+, Lyt-2+, L3T4- T lymphocytes. Since a method for photoinactivating effector T cells in analogous fashion with the tolerization protocol used here has been successful in the treatment of cutaneous T cell lymphoma,[6] pemphigus vulgaris,[36] scleroderma,[37] rheumatoid arthritis,[38] our treatment may have potential application in the field of transplantation in humans and autoimmune disease.

SUMMARY

We previously reported producing donor-specific tolerance to alloantigens by intravenous exposure to pretreated antidonor T cells. The current study extends that work by adoptively transferring the donor-specific tolerance into naive syngeneic recipients. Eight days after BALB/c mice received histoincompatible CBA/j skin grafts, their splenocytes which included an expanded population of cells mediating rejection were treated with 100 ng/ml 8-methoxypsoralen (8-MOP) photoactivated by 1 Joule/cm^2 of ultraviolet A (UVA) light prior to infusion into naive BALB/c recipients. Whereas 8-MOP itself is biologically inert, photoactivated 8-MOP crosslinks DNA by covalently binding to pyrimidine bases. Recipient BALB/c mice which had been previously demonstrated to be hyporesponsive to CBA/j alloantigens in mixed leukocyte culture (MLC), cytotoxicity (CTL) and *in vivo* delayed type hypersensitivity (DTH) assays were the donors of spleen cells for the adoptive transfer experiments. Fifty to one hundred million viable spleen cells from these pretreated BALB/c mice were transferred into naive syngeneic recipients which then were tested for DTH response and allograft survival to the relevant and irrelevant antigens. The radiosensitivity of this transferrable suppression was evaluated by exposing the adoptively transferred cell population to 3200 rads of C-irradiation prior to cell transfer. The phenotype of the cells transferring this suppressive response was performed by depleting specific populations of cells with monoclonal antibodies prior to cell transfer.

In vivo the DTH response of the pretreated BALB/c mice was specifically suppressed to the relevant alloantigen, correlating with retention of CBA/j skin grafts for up to 42 days post engraftment without visual evidence of rejection, in comparison to control mice complete rejection of the skin graft in less than 8 days. *In vitro*, splenocytes from BALB/c recipients of pretreated syngeneic splenocytes containing large numbers of BALB/c anti-CBA/j T cells proliferated less in MLC and generated lower cytotoxic T cell responses to CBA/j alloantigens than did controls and suppressed the naive and sensitized BALB/c MLC and CTL responses to CBA/j alloantigen.

This specific suppressive response to alloantigen was optimally transferred into syngeneic naive recipients when the adoptive transfer was performed on the sixth day after the last infusion received by the spleen cell donor mice. The adoptive transfer of this suppressive response was abrogated by the prior X-irradiation of the donor spleen cells and significantly abolished by the depletion of Thy-1+, Lyt-2+, L3T4- T lymphocytes. Therefore, specific suppression of the antiskin allograft response induced by infusions of 8-MOP/UVA inactivated spleen cells containing the effector cells of allograft recognition is mainly mediated by radiosensitive, Thy-1+, Lyt-2+, L3T4- T lymphocytes.

REFERENCES

1. ANDERSSON, L. C., H. BINZ & H. WIGZELL. 1976. Specific unresponsiveness to transplantation antigens induced by autoimmunization with syngeneic, antigen specific T lymphoblasts. Nature **264:** 778–779.
2. HOLOSHITZ, J., A. FRENKEL, A. BEN-NUN & I. R. COHEN. 1983. Autoimmune encephalomyelitis (EAE) mediated or prevented by T lymphocyte lines directed against diverse antigenic determinants of myelin basic protein. Vaccination is determinant specific. J. Immunol. **131:** 2810–2813.
3. BEN-NUN, A., W. HARTMUT & I. R. COHEN. 1981. Vaccination against autoimmune encephalomyelitis with T-lymphocyte line cells reactive against myelin basic protein. Nature **292:** 60–61.
4. LEMIRE, J. M. & W. O. WEIGLE. 1988. Passive transfer of experimental allergic encephalomyelitis by myelin basic protein-specific L3T4+ T cell clones possessing several functions. J. Immunol. **137:** 3169–3174.
5. KAKIMOTO, K., M. KATSUKI, T. HIROFUJI, H. IWATA & T. KOGA. 1988. Isolation of T cell line capable of protecting mice against collagen-induced arthritis. J. Immunol. **140:** 78–83.
6. EDELSON, R. L., C. BERGER, F. GASPARRO, B. JEGASOTHY, P. W. HEALD, B. WINTROUB, B. VONDERHEID, R. KNOBLER, K. WOLFF, G. PLEWIG, G. McKIERNAN, I. CHRISTENSEN, M. OSTER, H. HONIGSMANN, H. WILFORD, H. KOKOSCHKA, T. REHLE, M. PEREZ, G. STINGLE & L. LAROCHE. 1987. Treatment of cutaneous T cell lymphoma by extracorporeal photochemotherapy. Preliminary results. N. Engl. J. Med. **316:** 297–303.
7. PEREZ, M., R. EDELSON, L. LAROCHE & C. BERGER. 1989. Inhibition of antiskin allograft immunity by infusions with syngeneic photoinactivated effector lymphocytes. J. Invest. Dermatol. **92:** 669–676.
8. WEBB, S. & J. SPRENT. 1987. Downregulation of T cell responses by antibodies to the T cell receptor. J. Exp. Med. **165:** 584–589.
9. MOHAGHEGHPOUR, N., D. K. DAMLE, S. TAKADA & E. G. ENGLEMAN. 1986. Generation of antigen receptor-specific suppressor T cell clones in man. J. Exp. Med. **164:** 950–955.
10. BERGER, C. L., C. CANTON, J. WELSH, P. DERVAN, T. BEGLEY, S. GRANT, F. P. GASPARRO & R. L. EDELSON. 1985. Comparison of synthetic psoralen derivatives and 8-MOP in the inhibition of lymphocyte proliferation. Ann. N.Y. Acad. Sci. **453:** 80–90.
11. SCOTT, B. R., M. A. PATAK & G. R. MOHN. 1976. Molecular and genetic basis of furocoumarin reactions. Mutat. Res. **39:** 29–74.
12. PEREZ, M. I., R. L. EDELSON, L. JOHN, L. LaROCHE & C. BERGER. 1989. Inhibition of antiskin allograft immunity induced by infusions with photoinactivated effector T lymphocytes (PET cells). Yale J. Biol. Med. **62:** 595–609.
13. PEREZ, M. I., C. BERGER, Y. YAMANE, L. JOHN, L. LaROCHE & R. EDELSON. 1991. Inhibition of antiskin allograft immunity induced by infusions with photoinactivated effector T lymphocytes (PET cells). The congenic model. Transplantation. In press.
14. BILLIGHAM, R. E. & P. B. MEDAWAR. 1951. The technique of free skin grafting in animals. J. Exp. Biol. **28:** 385–399.
15. GRANSTEIN, R. D., C. GOULSTON & G. N. GAULTON. 1986. Prolongation of murine

skin allograft survival by immunologic manipulation with anti-interleukin 2 receptor antibody. J. Immunol. **136:** 898–902.

16. VAN DER KWAST, T. H., T. J. BIANCHI, H. BRIL & R. BENNER. 1981. Suppression anti-graft immunity by preimmunization. Transplant **31:** 79–85.

17. SPRENT, J., J. M. SCHAEFER, D. LO & R. KORNGOLD. 1986. Properties of purified T cell subsets. *In vivo* responses to class I vs class II H-2 differences. J. Exp. Med. **163:** 998–1011.

18. SPRENT, J. & M. SCHAEFER. 1985. Properties of purified T cell subsets. *In vitro* responses to class I vs class II H-2 differences. J. Exp. Med. **162:** 2068–2082.

19. ROCK, K. L., M. C. BARNES, R. N. GERMAIN & B. BENACERRAF. 1983. The role of Ia molecules in the activation of T lympocytes. Ia-restricted recognition of allo K/D antigens is required for Class I MHC-stimulated mixed lymphocyte responses. J. Immunol. **130:** 457–462.

20. KRUISBEEK, A. M., S. BRIDGES, J. CARMEN, D. L. LONGO & J. J. MOND. 1985. *In vitro* treatment of neonatal mice with anti-Ia antibodies interferes with the development of the Class I, Class II and Mls-reactive proliferating T cell subset. J. Immunol. **134:** 3597–3604.

21. BULLER, R. M. L., K. L. HOLMES, A. HUGIN, T. H. FREDERIKSON & H. C. MORSE III. 1987. Induction of cytotoxic T-cell response *in vivo* in the absence of CD4 helper cells. Nature **328:** 77–79.

22. BURACOFF, S. J., R. N. GERMAIN, M. E. DORF & B. BENACERRAF. 1976. Inhibition of cell mediated cytolysis of trinitrophenyl-derivatized target cells by alloantisera directed to the products of the K and D loci of the H-2 complex. Proc. Natl. Acad. Sci. USA **73:** 625–629.

23. WOOD, P. J. & J. W. STREILEIN. 1984. Immunogenetic basis of acquired transplantation tolerance. Transplantation **37:** 223–226.

24. MIZOUCHI, T. S., S. ONO, T. R. MALEK & A. SINGER. 1986. Characterization of two distinct primary T cell populations that secrete IL-2 upon recognition of class I or class II major histocompatibility antigens. J. Exp. Med. **163:** 603–615.

25. KHAVARI, P. A., R. L. EDELSON, O. LIDER, F. P. GALSPARRO, H. L. WEINER & I. R. COHEN. 1988. Specific vaccination against photoinactivated cloned T cells. Clin. Res. **36:** 662a.

26. LIDER, O., T. RESHEF, E. BERAUD, A. BEN-NUN & I. R. COHEN. 1988. Anti-idiotypic network induced by T cell vaccination against experimental autoimmune encephalomyelitis. Science **183:** 181–183.

27. ROHOWSKY, C., N. SUCIU-FOCA, P. KUNG, T. F. TANG, E. REED & D. W. KING. 1983. Suppressor T cells in the autologous MLR with mixed leukocyte culture (MLC)-activated T lymphoblasts. Transplant. Proc. **15:** 765–770.

28. DORSH, S. & B. ROSER. 1977. Recirculating suppressor T cells in transplantation tolerance. J. Exp. Med. **145:** 1144–1157.

29. SY, M. S., M. H. DIETZ, R. N. GERMAIN, B. BENACERRAF & M. I. GREENE. 1980. Antigen and receptor driven regulatory mechanisms. IV. Idiotype bearing I-J+ suppressor T cell factors (TsF) induce second order suppressor T cells (TsF₂) which express anti-idiotypic receptors. J. Exp. Med. **151:** 1183–1195.

30. KOSMATOPOULOS, K., D. S. ALGARA & S. ORBACH-ARBOUYS. 1987. Anti-receptor anti-MHC cytotoxic T lymphocytes: their role in the resistance to graft vs host reaction. J. Immunol. **138:** 1038–1041.

31. ELLERMAN, K. E., J. M. POWERS & S. W. BROSTOFF. 1988. A suppressor T lymphocyte cell line for autoimmune encephalomyelitis. Nature **331:** 265–267.

32. SUN, D., Y. QIN, J. CHLUBA, J. T. EPPLEN & H. WEKERLE. 1988. Suppression of experimentally induced autoimmune encephalomyelitis by cytolytic T cell interactions. Nature **322:** 843–845.

33. LOHSE, A. W., F. MOR, N. KARIN & I. R. COHEN. 1989. Control of experimental autoimmune encephalomyelitis by T cell responding to activated T cells. Science **244:** 820–822.

34. SONG, P. S. & K. J. TAPLEY, JR. 1979. Photochemistry and photobiology of psoralens. Photochem. Photobiol. **29:** 1177–1197.

35. LAROCHE, L., M. I. PEREZ, R. L. EDELSON & C. BERGER. 1987. Induction of tolerance in mice treated with photoinactivated effector cells. Clin. Res. **35:** 698a.
36. ROOK, A., B. V. JEGASTHY, P. W. HEALD et al. 1990. Extracorporeal photochemotherapy for drug-resistant *pemphigus vulgaris*. Ann. Int. Med. **112:** 303–305.
37. ROOK, A. H., B. FREUNDLICH, R. EDELSON et al. 1990. Effective treatment of progressive systemic sclerosis (PSS) with extracorporeal photochemotherapy. Clin. Res. **38:** 420a.
38. MALAWISTA, S., D. TROCK & R. L. EDELSON. Arthritis Rheum. In press.

Antigen-Specific Tolerance Induced by Autoimmunization with Photoinactivated Syngeneic Effector Cells[a]

LILIANE LAROCHE,[b,c] RICHARD L. EDELSON,
MARITZA PEREZ, AND CAROLE L. BERGER[b]

[b]Departments of Dermatology and Pathology
Columbia University
New York, New York 10032

and

Department of Dermatology
Yale University
New Haven, Connecticut 06510

INTRODUCTION

Clinically relevant immunosuppression, induced by cytotoxic drugs, lymphoid irradiation, anti-lymphocyte globulin and thoracic duct drainage, unavoidably introduces nonspecific immunologic effects along with the more desirable inhibition of the particular T cell clones responsible for deleterious reactions.[1-3] A more attractive immunosuppressive therapy would preferentially target those antigen-specific T cells committed to participate in the pathologic process. Such effector T cells have membrane receptors specific to the antigen in association with major histocompatibility complex molecules (reviewed in REF. 4). These T cell antigen receptors are distinctive protein heterodimers which may themselves serve as clone-specific immunogens under certain circumstances[5] and are, therefore, potential targets for directed therapy.

The induction of tolerance by anti-receptor autoimmunity has been reported in several *in vivo* experimental models. Anderson *et al.* have demonstrated that specific unresponsiveness to transplantation antigens may be induced by injection of alloantigen specific blasts generated *in vitro*.[6] These results have been extended to vaccination with inactivated effector T cell clones which mediate autoimmune disease.[7] In these systems, effector cells alone were not immunogenic and required modification or inactivation *in vitro* prior to infusion into recipients. Methods that potentiated immunogenicity of these T cells included the use of complete Freund's adjuvant or X-irradiation.[7-9] These protocols led to specific tolerance in naive immunocompetent recipients. Unfortunately, the requirement for clonal

[a] L.L. was a recipient of an Association pour la Recherche contre le Cancer fellowship. M.P. was a National Institutes of Health (NIH) postdoctoral trainee (5-T-32-ARO). This work was supported by grants from the NIH (CA 20499 and CA 39700), the Matheson Foundation, the Dermatology Foundation (6-41497) and Therakos, Inc.

[c] Present address: Department of Dermatology, Hôpital Avicenne, University of Paris XIII, 125, rue de Stalingrad, 93000 Bobigny, France.

113

expansion of the specific population or the use of adjuvants severely limits their clinical applicability.

A method that may provide a more clinically acceptable means for immune manipulation has been used in the treatment of disseminated cutaneous T cell lymphoma. It consists of the readministration of 8-methoxypsoralen (8-MOP) ultraviolet A (UVA) light-treated autologous pheresis-enriched leukocytes and resulted in profound amelioration and prolonged attenuation or disappearance of the disease process.[10] The long-term clinical improvement, seen in several patients, suggested a host response to distinct antigens expressed on reinfused photomodified lymphocytes, possibly rendered more immunogenic by the procedure. It is noteworthy that these clinical responses were achieved in the absence of *in vitro* manipulations of the patients' cells and were associated with quite limited adverse effects. Based on this clinical trial, we have developed animal models to determine: 1) whether 8-MOP-UVA inactivation of effector T cells provides a means of inducing an autoregulatory host response and 2) whether an immunocompetent host can select a markedly expanded relevant effector T cell population from an unfractionated leukocyte pool. In this context, we asked whether photoinactivated antigen-specific autologous cells can be used as immunogens to render a naive, immunocompetent individual unresponsive to subsequent exposure to the relevant antigen.

We report here that intravenous injections of sheep red blood cell (SRBC) reactive cells from an unfractionated spleen pool photoinactivated *in vitro* can induce a state of selected unresponsiveness to SRBC and suppress an already existing immunity to that antigen. Identical pretreatment of splenocytes from unsensitized mice did not have this effect, indicating that light and photoinactived drug alone are ineffective in this system.

MATERIALS AND METHODS

Mice

Male BALB/c adult mice (6–8 weeks of age) were obtained from the Jackson Laboratory (Bar Harbor, ME).

Antigens and Immunization

Sheep and chicken red blood cells (SRBC, CRBC) were collected and stored in Alsever's solution at 4°C. The RBC were washed 3 times before use and suspended at the appropriate concentration in sterile pyrogen-free phosphate-buffered saline (PBS). Donor mice were intravenously primed with 10^6 RBC, a dose which had previously been shown to induce a T cell response to the exclusion of a demonstrable B cell response.[11] This dose of antigen was also used for the induction of delayed-type hypersensitivity (DTH).

Assay for the DTH Reaction in Sensitized Mice

DTH was measured as described previously.[11] Preliminary experiments were performed to determine the optimal regimen for demonstrating the DTH reaction to RBC. The challenging dose was shown to be subinflammatory in an unprimed animal.[12] The peak of the reaction was determined by a kinetic curve. Four days after immunization with RBC, the mice were challenged with 2.5×10^8 SRBC or 0.25×10^8 CRBC suspended in 50 μl of PBS or saline, injected subcutaneously in the left hind footpad. Footpad swelling was measured 24 hours later with a dial gauge caliper. The results were expressed as the increased thickness of the antigen-injected footpad compared to the saline control. In each experiment, a group of nonimmune mice was tested and the footpad swelling was used as a negative control.

Preparation of Cell Suspensions

Spleens were removed from naive or immune mice 4 days after sensitization. Single cell suspensions were prepared by pressing the spleens through a wire mesh into PBS. Red cells were lysed with 0.83% ammonium chloride. The cells were washed twice and adjusted to the appropriate concentration in PBS. Viability of the cell suspension was determined by trypan blue dye exclusion and found to be at least 90% in all experiments.

In Vitro *Photoactivation of 8-MOP by UVA Light*

8-MOP (Elder Pharmaceutical) was dissolved in 100% ethanol and subsequently in PBS. Purity and concentration of the drug was verified by UV spectroscopy and high-pressure liquid chromatography (personal data). Optimal conditions for the 8-MOP photoactivation had been previously defined by inhibition of the lymphocyte proliferative response to mitogen and alloantigen.[13] Spleen cells were incubated *in vitro* with 100 ng/ml of 8-MOP for 20 minutes in foil-wrapped tubes to allow equilibrium to be established between the psoralen solution and the cells. Cells were deposited into Petri dishes (Falcon) and placed on the irradiation surface. The irradiation unit consisted of six black light fluorescent bulbs (40 BL, Sylvania) emitting broad band UVA energy (320–400 nm). Emission in the UVB range was filtered out by a sheet of window glass. The light dose was monitored by a photometer (International Light, IL 700 A). Spleen cells received a light dose of 1 joule/cm^2 and were washed twice in PBS before injection.

Treatment of Naive Adult Mice

In vitro photoinactivated spleen cells (2 to 5×10^7) from either immune or naive donors were injected into the tail vein of naive adult syngeneic recipients every 7 to 10 days for 8 weeks. Following this treatment, recipient mice were tested for a DTH response.

Transfer of DTH

Twenty-four hours after the DTH reaction, mice were sacrificed, the spleens removed and single cell suspensions prepared. The cells were washed and transferred intravenously into syngeneic recipients. Immediately after cell transfer, mice were challenged in the hind footpad with 2.5×10^8 SRBC.

Statistical Analysis

The statistical significance of the data was determined using the Student t test. A p value of less than 0.05 was considered significant.

RESULTS

Inhibition of the DTH Response to SRBC

The effect of pre-exposure of splenocytes photoinactivated *in vitro* with 8-MOP and UVA on the induction of the DTH reaction to SRBC in adult naive mice was examined. FIGURE 1 shows that mice challenged with SRBC but not sensitized, did not develop a DTH response (negative controls, Group A). Mice that received a priming dose of SRBC and were subsequently challenged in the footpad developed a normal DTH response (positive controls, Group B). Mice treated with photoinactivated nonimmune splenocytes (Group C) and primed and challenged exhibited a normal DTH reaction similar to that observed in the positive controls (Group B). In contrast, treatment with photoinactivated immune

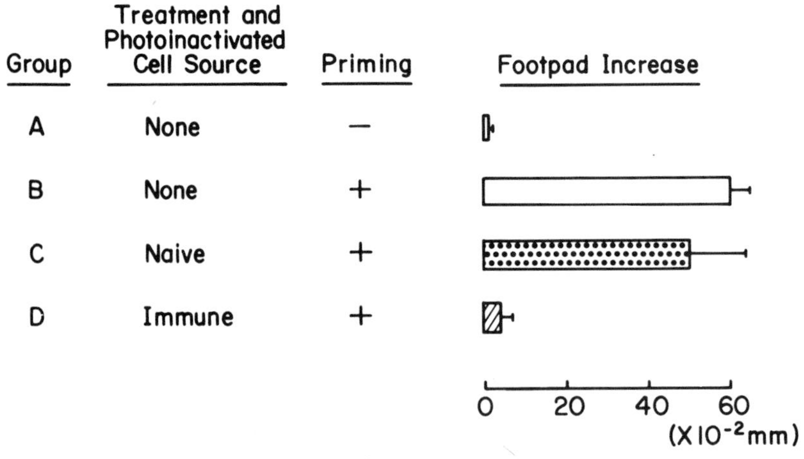

FIGURE 1. Induction of unresponsiveness to SRBC in mice treated with photoinactivated SRBC-reactive cells. To measure the DTH reaction, BALB/c mice were primed intravenously with 10^6 SRBC and then challenged 4 days later by the injection of 2.5×10^8 SRBC into the left hind footpad. Footpad swelling was measured 24 hr later with a dial caliper. Group A mice (negative controls) received only a challenging dose of SRBC. Group B mice (positive controls) were sensitized and challenged with SRBC. Photoinactivated naive splenocytes or splenocytes from 10^6 SRBC-primed mice were treated *in vitro* with 100 ng/ml of 8-MOP for 20 min and irradiated with 1 joule/cm^2 ultraviolet A light. The cells were washed and $2–5 \times 10^7$ photoinactivated splenocytes from naive donors (Group C) or SRBC-primed donors (Group D) were injected into the tail vein of naive syngeneic recipients every 7 to 10 days for 8 weeks. Two days after the sixth treatment, recipient mice were assayed for the T cell response to SRBC, as measured by the DTH reaction. All groups consisted of 5 mice. The results were expressed as increase in footpad thickness. The *bars* represent the arithmetic mean +/− the standard error.

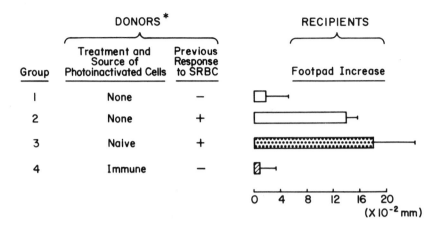

FIGURE 2. Passive transfer of unresponsiveness to normal recipients. Splenocytes (4 × 10[7]) were harvested from the same animals presented in FIGURE 1* and transferred to naive recipients. Group 1 and 2 mice received splenocytes from the negative and positive control animals respectively (Groups A and B respectively, FIG. 1). Group 3 received cells from Group C mice that had been pretreated with photoinactivated naive splenocytes and had a normal DTH response to SRBC (FIG. 1). Group 4 mice were recipients of cells from Group D mice that had been pretreated with antigen-reactive splenocytes and did not develop a DTH reaction when primed and challenged with SRBC. Recipient mice were challenged immediately with 2.5 × 10[8] SRBC. Swelling of the footpad was measured 24 hr later.

splenocytes rendered the mice unresponsive to priming and challenge with SRBC (Group D, $p < 0.001$). The suppression of the DTH response in this group of mice exposed to photoinactivated immune splenocytes was comparable to the degree of footpad swelling observed in the negative controls (Group A).

Adoptive Transfer of Unreactivity to SRBC

To determine whether inhibition of the response to SRBC could be transferred, splenocytes from the same mice previously demonstrated to be unresponsive to SRBC and the controls (FIG. 1) were adoptively transferred to naive syngeneic recipients (FIG. 2). Immediately after transfer, without priming, recipients were challenged in the footpad with SRBC. As expected, transfer of lymphoid cells from the negative control Group A (FIG. 1) resulted in minimal footpad swelling after challenge (Group 1, FIG. 2). Transfer of cells from mice previously shown to be responsive to SRBC (Group B, FIG. 1) resulted in a positive response to the challenge with SRBC (Group 2, FIG. 2) in the naive recipient mice. When cells from the mice treated with photoinactivated naive cells that demonstrated a DTH reaction to priming and challenge with SRBC (Group C, FIG. 1) were injected into naive recipients, they mediated a positive response to SRBC when challenged (Group 3, FIG. 2). In contrast, mice that had received lymphoid cells from animals rendered unresponsive to SRBC (Group D, FIG. 1) by pre-exposure to 8 MOP-UVA inactivated effector cells were unable to develop a significant DTH reaction ($p < 0.001$, Group 4, FIG. 2).

Specificity of Unresponsiveness to SRBC

We next assessed whether unresponsiveness to SRBC was antigen specific using chicken RBC (CRBC) as an unrelated antigen (FIG. 3). Untreated control mice not exposed to SRBC did not develop a DTH reaction when challenged with CRBC (Group A, negative control). Positive control mice were primed and challenged with CRBC and developed a strong DTH response (Group B). In addition, a group of mice primed and challenged to SRBC and responsive to that antigen were subsequently primed and challenged with CRBC. These mice were shown to be normally responsive to the second antigen, CRBC (Group C). Mice which were previously treated with photoinactivated naive splenocytes (Group E) developed a normal DTH response after priming and challenge with CRBC. A group of mice, that had previously been shown to be unresponsive to SRBC after exposure to photoinactivated immune splenocytes, received two additional treatments to maintain unresponsiveness before being assayed for the DTH reaction to CRBC (Group D). The positive DTH response to CRBC, in mice demonstrated to be unresponsive to SRBC, was similar to the response to CRBC elicited in the positive controls. As in Group D, the capacity to respond to CRBC was not inhibited in mice treated with photoinactivated SRBC-immune splenocytes but, in this case, the mice were not exposed to SRBC prior to testing for the response to CRBC (Group F).

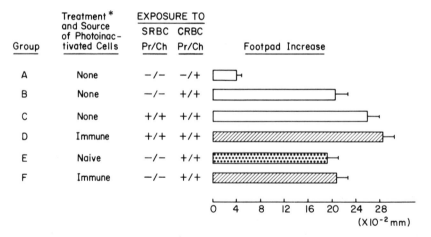

FIGURE 3. Specificity of unresponsiveness to SRBC. In Group A (negative control), mice were not primed (Pr) but only received a challenging (Ch) dose of CRBC. Group B (positive control) was primed and challenged with SRBC before being exposed to CRBC. Group C mice were first primed and challenged with CRBC. Group D mice were rendered unresponsive to SRBC by treatment with photoinactivated SRBC-reactive splenocytes. These mice did not develop a DTH reaction when they were primed and challenged with SRBC. They were treated twice more with photoinactivated effector cells and subsequently primed and challenged with CRBC. Group E mice were pretreated with photoinactivated naive splenocytes and then primed and challenged with CRBC. Group F mice were pre-exposed to photoinactivated SRBC-reactive splenocytes and then primed and challenged with CRBC. The priming dose in all groups of mice was 10^6 CRBC. All groups were challenged in the footpad with 0.25×10^8 CRBC.

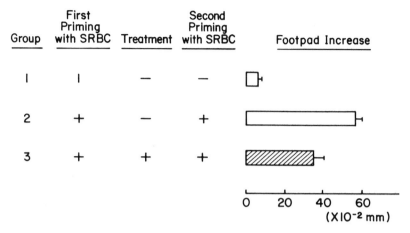

FIGURE 4. Suppression of an established immunity to SRBC. Groups of 4 mice (Groups 2 and 3) were sensitized with 10^6 SRCB. Five days later, group 3 received repetitive injections of 8-MOP and UVA inactivated SRBC primed spleen cells, whereas group 2 did not receive any cell treatment. Following this regimen, both groups were boosted with 10^6 SRBC and tested for DTH reaction on day 3. Group 1 received only the challenging dose of SRBC in the footpad.

Inhibition of an Already Existing Immunity to SRBC

Finally, the possibility that this procedure can abrogate an already existing immunity to SRBC was explored (Fig. 4). Groups of mice were sensitized with SRBC (Groups 2 and 3). Once the T cell immunity to SRBC was established (day 5 after immunization), mice received repetitive treatments with SRBC-sensitized splenocytes photoinactivated *in vitro* with 8-MOP and UVA (Group 3). The positive control group did not receive treatment with cells (Group 2). Both groups were assayed for the secondary DTH reaction to SRBC. The results show that treatment of immune mice with photoinactivated SRBC-reactive cells induces significant ($p < 0.05$) but partial (45% suppression) inhibition of an established immunity to SRBC.

DISCUSSION

The possibility that therapeutically relevant modification of the immune response can be achieved by pre-exposure of the host to extracorporeally photoinactivated effector cells derives from our recent observation that a human T cell malignancy can be meaningfully controlled by reinfusion of autologous neoplastic cells photomodified by 8-MOP-UVA treatment.[10] The specificity of the anti-malignant T cell response was suggested by the absence, in the successfully treated patients, of nonspecific immunosuppression or opportunistic infections.

We hypothesized that a host response against antigenic components of the clonotypic T cell receptor on the reinfused leukemic T cells might have contributed to the long-lasting clinical results. Although the validity of this premise in that clinical setting requires further study, analogous anti-idiotypic maneuvers have been previously demonstrated to control the *in vitro* and *in vivo* growth of B cell tumors.[13,14]

In order to test this concept in an experimental system, it was first necessary to demonstrate that T cell-mediated immune responses could be suppressed by the infusion of antigen-reactive effector cells pretreated with 8-MOP-UVA. In the present study, we provide evidence that a state of specific unresponsiveness, as detected by inhibition of the DTH reaction, was induced by administration of syngeneic photoinactivated effector cells to immunocompetent naive mice. The DTH reaction is a sensitive T cell-mediated *in vivo* assay in which a very small number of anti-SRBC T helper cells have been reported to initiate an inflammatory reaction by recruiting bystander cells to the site of antigen deposition in the skin.[15,16] The dose of SRBC optimal for DTH induction has been demonstrated to be insufficient to elicit B cell activation.[12] Therefore, the regimen used in our study probably evaluated tolerance to a principally T cell-mediated reaction.

The observed suppression of the T cell response to SRBC resulted from a response to the photoinactivated effector T cells and not to a systemic effect of the drug and/or light, since nonimmune splenocytes treated with 8-MOP-UVA and injected into immunologically naive recipients did not inhibit the DTH response to SRBC. Therefore, effector cells preserved in an immunogenic fashion are required for the autoregulatory immune response which we observe. We have also previously shown that UVA alone, at the dose used in the studies (1 joule/cm^2), does not alter the T cell response to mitogens.[10,13] Furthermore, in the experiments reported in this paper, the *in vitro* photoinactivated cells were washed before infusion into mice, thereby removing unbound 8-MOP and any minute residual amounts of free 8-MOP would have been excreted by the recipient within several hours.

The induction of tolerance to SRBC was shown to be antigen specific, since reactivity to an irrelevant antigen (CRBC) was unaltered. The retention of the response to this irrelevant antigen demonstrates that reinfusion of photoinactivated effector cells does not result in generalized immune suppression. It is noteworthy that, in these experiments, the recipient mice were exposed to splenocyte pools in which expanded populations of T cells reactive to SRBC were admixed with presumably smaller numbers of lymphocytes belonging to each of a multiplicity of other unstimulated clones. Therefore, the recipient's immune system was able to discriminate between antigen-reactive cells and the other unrelated cells and specifically suppress the reactivity to SRBC.

The tolerance to SRBC was shown to be transferrable. Naive unprimed recipients of lymphoid cells from unresponsive mice were unable to respond to a challenge with SRBC, while those given lymphoid cells from donors responsive to SRBC were able to mount a normal response to SRBC. The lack of response to SRBC in the unprimed recipient of cells from tolerant mice raises at least two possibilities. Either the effector cells mediating the T cell response to SRBC were not present in the transferred cell population, or a specific suppressor cell subset was present that prevented expression of the DTH reaction. These two possibilities, the role of humoral factors and carry-over of tolerogenic antigen in the antigen presenting cell and the immune lymphocyte populations are currently being studied. However, the transfer of suppression to an unprimed secondary recipient that was fully immunocompetent confirms that generalized immune suppression of the recipient was not required for inhibition of the response to SRBC in our system. Moreover, our tolerance-inducing procedure was also shown to be able to inhibit an already existing immunity to the antigen, favoring the hypothesis of specific suppressor cell induction. This hypothesis is further supported by our results obtained in another experimental model in which an antigen-specific inhibitory cell population was shown to induce tolerance to skin alloantigens.[17]

These experiments demonstrate that it is possible to create a state of specific unresponsiveness to an antigen by pretreating the host with photoinactivated uncloned effector mononuclear cells. Other reported experimental protocols which may mediate similar effects are less clinically feasible, since they rely on isolation and cloning of a known effector cell of an undesirable immune response[7] or require inactivation of the reinfused cells with toxic agents such as complete Freund's adjuvant.[5,18] In contrast, 8-MOP has been widely used clinically in the photochemotherapy of various skin disorders without significant systemic side effects.[19,20] The clinical availability of an 8-MOP-UVA extracorporeal exposure system[10] should allow our tolerance inducing regimen to be readily tested in humans, distinguishing it from the other currently known approaches.

The results of this study have direct implications. First, we have described a new *in vivo* model for inducing tolerance and studying the basic mechanisms involved in this phenomenon. Second, it is likely that the principle(s) demonstrated here will apply to other antigens. Therefore, the clinical availability of such a regimen for 8-MOP-UVA activation in extracorporeally routed human blood offers some exciting therapeutic prospects in the control of undesirable cell clones, such as those expanded in graft rejection, allergy, autoimmune diseases, anti-globulin responses elicited by xenogeneic monoclonal antibodies and malignant lymphocyte proliferations.

SUMMARY

Development of a protocol that could invoke specific suppression of an undesired immune response, while sparing normal immune competence, would be of great clinical value. This report demonstrates that multiple infusions of splenocytes sensitized *in vivo* to sheep red blood cells (SRBC) and photoinactivated *in vitro* with 8-methoxypsoralen and ultraviolet A light can render a syngeneic recipient selectively unresponsive to subsequent challenge with this antigen. Mice treated in this fashion did not develop a T cell-mediated delayed type hypersensitivity (DTH) reaction to SRBC. In contrast, control mice exposed to nonimmune splenocytes pretreated in an identical manner developed a normal DTH response to SRBC, thereby demonstrating that drug and light in the absence of effector T cells were not suppressive. Inhibition of the DTH response was antigen specific, since animals rendered unresponsive to SRBC developed a normal DTH response to chicken red blood cells. Cell transfer experiments demonstrated that unprimed recipients of splenocytes from mice rendered unresponsive to SRBC could not mount a DTH reaction when challenged. Moreover, this procedure can also suppress established immunity to that antigen. The use of photoinactivated syngeneic antigen-reactive effector cells as immunosuppression agents suggests that this method may be clinically useful in inhibiting pathogenic antigen-specific immunologic reactions.

ACKNOWLEDGMENTS

We are indebted to Dr. D. Tripodi for his valuable comments and to Dr. L. Rogozinski for helpful advice during the preparation of the manuscript.

REFERENCES

1. WEIGLE, W. O. 1973. Immunological unresponsiveness. Adv. Immunol. **16:** 61–121.
2. SHELLAM, G. R. 1969. Mechanism of induction of immunological tolerance. VI. Tolerance induction following thoracic duct drainage or treatment with anti-lymphocyte serum. Immunology **17:** 260–280.
3. SLAVIN, S., S. STROBER, Z. FUKS & H. KAPLAN. 1977. Induction of specific tissue transplantation tolerance using fractionated total lymphoid irradiation in adult mice: long-term survival of allogeneic bone marrow and skin grafts. J. Exp. Med. **146:** 34–48.
4. MARRACK, P. & J. KAPPLER. 1987. The T cell receptor. The major histocompatibility complex-restricted antigen receptor on T cells. I. Isolation with monoclonal antibody. Science **238:** 1073–1078.
5. HASKINS, K., R. KUBO, J. WHITE, M. PIGEON, J. KAPPLER & P. MARRACK. 1983. The major histocompatibility complex-restricted antigen receptor on T cells. I. Isolation with a monoclonal antibody. J. Exp. Med. **157:** 1149–1169.
6. ANDERSON, L. C., H. BINZ & H. WIGZELL. 1976. Specific unresponsiveness to transplantation antigens induced by auto-immunization with syngeneic antigen-specific T lymphoblasts. Nature **264:** 778–780.
7. BEN NUN, A., A. WEKERLE & I. R. COHEN. 1981. Vaccination against autoimmune encephalomyelitis using attenuated cells of a T lymphocyte line reactive against myelin basic protein. Nature **292:** 60–61.
8. SCHWARTZ, M., D. NOVICK, D. GIVOL & S. FUCHS. 1978. Induction of anti-idiotypic antibodies by immunization with syngeneic spleen cells educated with acetylcholine receptor. Nature **273:** 543–545.
9. MARON, R., R. ZERUBAVEL, A. FRIEDMAN & I. R. COHEN. 1983. T lymphocyte line specific for thyroglobulin produces or vaccinates autoimmune thyroiditis in mice. J. Immunol. **131:** 2316–2322.
10. EDELSON, R. L., C. BERGER, F. GASPARRO, B. JEGASOTHY, P. HEALD, B. WINTROUB, E. VONDERHEID, R. KNOBLER, K. WOLFF, G. PLEWIG, G. MCKIERNAN, I. CHRISTIENSEN, M. OSTER, H. HONIGSMAN, H. WILFORD, E. KOKOSHKA, T. REHLE, M. PEREZ, G. STINGL & L. LAROCHE. 1987. Treatment of cutaneous T cell lymphoma by extracorporeal photochemotherapy. Preliminary results. N. Engl. J. Med. **316:** 297–303.
11. LAGRANGE, P. H., G. B. MACKANESS & T. E. J. MILLER. 1974. Influence of dose and route of antigen injection on the immunologic induction of T cells. J. Exp. Med. **139:** 528–542.
12. MILON, G., G. MARCHAL, M. SEMAN, P. TRUFFA-BACCHI & V. ZILBERBERG. 1983. Is the delayed-type hypersensitivity observed after a low dose of antigen mediated by helper T cells? J. Immunol. **130:** 1103–1107.
13. BERGER, C. L., C. CANTOR, J. WELSH, P. DERVAN, T. BEGLEY, S. GRANT, F. GASPARRO & R. L. EDELSON. 1986. Comparison of synthetic psoralen derivates and 8-MOP in the inhibition of lymphocyte proliferation. Ann. N.Y. Acad. Sci. **453:** 80–90.
14. KROLICK, K. A., P. C. ISAKSON, J. W. UHR & E. S. VITETTA. 1979. BCL1, a murine model for chronic lymphocytic leukemia: use for the surface immunoglobulin idiotype for the detection and treatment of tumor. Immunol. Rev. **48:** 81–106.
15. MILLER, R. A., D. G. MALONEY, R. WARNER & R. LEVY. 1982. Treatment of B-cell lymphoma with monoclonal anti-idiotype antibody. N. Engl. J. Med. **306:** 517–522.
16. MARCHAL, G., M. SEMAN, G. MILON, P. TRUFFA-BACCHI & V. ZILBERBERG. 1982. Local adoptive transfer of skin delayed-type hypersensitivity initiated by a single T lymphocyte. J. Immunol. **129:** 954–958.
17. PEREZ, M., R. EDELSON, L. LAROCHE & C. BERGER. 1989. Inhibition of antiskin allograft immunity by infusions with syngeneic photoinactivated effector lymphocytes. J. Invest. Dermatol. **92:** 669–676.
18. BINZ, H. & H. WIGZELL. 1979. Induction of specific transplantation tolerance in adult animals. Transplant. Proc. **11:** 914–918.

19. PARRISH, J. A., T. B. FITZPATRICK, L. TANNENBAUM & M. A. PATHAK. 1974. Photochemotherapy of psoriasis with oral methoxsalen and longwave ultraviolet light. N. Engl. J. Med. **291:** 1207–1211.
20. MELSKI, J. W., L. TANNENBAUM, J. A. PARRISH, T. FITZPATRICK, H. L. BLEICH *et al.* 1977. Oral methoxsalen photochemotherapy for the treatment of psoriasis: a cooperative clinical trial. J. Invest. Dermatol. **68:** 328–335.

T Cell Vaccination in Autoimmune Diseases

EVELYNE BERAUD

Laboratoire d'lmmunologie,
Faculté de Médecine La Timone
27 Bd. Jean Moulin
13385 Marseille cedex 5, France

INTRODUCTION

Suppression of experimental autoimmune diseases has been investigated by means of a process termed T cell vaccination. This concept was elaborated by A. Ben-Nun and I. R. Cohen[1] and applied to a variety of experimental autoimmune diseases for some years.[2–4] T cell vaccination may be defined as the administration of T cells under suitable conditions to prevent or to treat autoimmune disease. In the initial experiments, irradiated autoimmune effector T cells were used for vaccination.[1,5] Later on, vaccination was found to be more effective when the T cells were treated by hydrostatic pressure or chemical cross-linkers.[4,6] More recently, untreated autoimmune effector clones could also be used as a vaccine if a dose of cells below the threshold number needed for disease was administered.[7–9] Common to all forms of vaccination is the requirement that the T cells be activated prior to inoculation by incubation with a specific antigen or a T cell mitogen such as concanavalin A (Con A) together with antigen-presenting cells.[10]

The aim of this article is to review information, published or about to be published, illustrating the effectiveness of T cell vaccination and exploring how T cell vaccination might modulate the immune system. Two different models of autoimmune diseases have been studied and the results are summarized in the present paper. Experimental autoimmune encephalomyelitis (EAE) and experimental autoimmune uveitis (EAU) are both organ-specific diseases produced by T lymphocytes. EAE is a paralytic disease of the central nervous system mediated primarily by $V\beta 8+$ cells specific for myelin basic protein.[11–14] EAE is widely regarded as a model for multiple sclerosis. EAU is a disease of the eye characterized by destruction of retinal photoreceptor cells, mediated helper T including $V\beta 8+$ cells[15] specific for retinal antigens (S-Antigen,[16] interphotoreceptor retinoid binding protein (IRBP),[17] and rhodopsin[18]). EAU serves as a model for a variety of human posterior uveitic conditions of an apparently autoimmune nature that are responsive to cyclosporin A therapy (Behçet's disease, Vogt-Koyanagi-Harada's syndrome, birdshot retinochoroidopathy and sympathetic ophthalmia, reviewed in REFS. 19, 20).

Autoimmune T lymphocytes that actually cause EAE and EAU have been grown as lines or clones. Our strategy was to vaccinate rats with a subpathogenic dose of effector T cells from these lines or clones. The results show that resistance to these autoimmune diseases appears to be associated with a combination of anti-idiotypic and anti-ergotypic responses.

124

MATERIALS AND METHODS

Rats

Female inbred Lewis rats, 8–12 weeks old were supplied by the Animal Breeding Center of the Weizmann Institute of Science, Israel; by CSEAL, CNRS, Orleans la Source, France or by Charles River Laboratories Inc., from the facility in Raleigh, North Carolina, USA.

Selection and Maintenance of T Cell Lines

Line Z1a, reactive to BP, was isolated from draining lymph nodes of rats immunized with BP in CFA and maintained as described[5] for several years. Z1a appears to be a clone according to the single rearrangement of its antigen receptor genes. Clone A2b[21] was raised from line A2, a line obtained from rats immunized to *Mycobacterium tuberculosis* (MT) to induce adjuvant arthritis. Clone A2b was found to be arthritogenic in irradiated Lewis rats; line PPD was obtained from rats immunized with PPD. Uveitogenic lines with various degrees of pathogenicity (assessed by the maximal severity of the lesions) were isolated from rats immunized with IRBP-peptides, R4 (sequence 1158–1180, minor pathogenic determinant) and R16 (1177–1191, major pathogenic determinant) in CFA and selected as described in REFERENCES 22 and 16 respectively. Line S-Ag (highly uveitogenic) was obtained from rats immunized with bovine S-Ag and selected for specificity to peptide S35 (which contains the major epitope). Clones were obtained by limiting dilution technique as described elsewhere.[9]

For antigenic or mitogenic activation, the cells (3×10^5/ml) were incubated for 2 to 3 days with an optimal antigen concentration and for 2 days with Con A ($2 \mu g$/ml) in the presence of syngeneic irradiated thymus cells (13×10^6/ml) as accessory cells. On the last day, the lymphoblasts were transferred into a propagation medium (containing T cell growth factors) until the next restimulation or were used to mediate diseases or to vaccinate.

To mediate EAE or EAU, the lymphocytes were collected after antigenic stimulation, washed and, in phosphate buffered saline, injected intravenously or intraperitoneally into Lewis rats.

To vaccinate against EAE or EAU, 1×10^4–5×10^4 living activated lymphoblasts separated by centrifugation on a Ficoll density gradient were injected intravenously or subcutaneously into recipients.

The development of EAE and EAU were monitored clinically; changes in the CNS, in the eye and in the pineal gland were evaluated by histological examination.[23,24]

Lymphocyte Proliferative Assay

Cervical, popliteal and inguinal lymph node cell suspensions were prepared from treated or untreated animals. Lymph node cells were seeded (2×10^5 and 4×10^5/well) in quadruplicate cultures in 96-well microtiter U-shaped plates in stimulation medium.[8] Irradiated (2,500 rads) stimulator cells (2×10^4 and 10×10^4/well) were added to the culture. After 3 days, each well was pulsed with 1 μCi of [3H]-thymidine for an additional 18 h. Results are recorded as counts per minute (cpm).

Analysis of Membrane Markers

Surface cell markers were identified by flow cytometry.[9]

RESULTS

A Subpathogenic Number of Activated Autoimmune Cells Induces Resistance to EAE and EAU

TABLE 1 summarizes the results of four experiments. Lewis rats were inoculated intravenously with 10^4 to 5×10^4 T cells specific for myelin BP or for the ocular antigen, the R16 peptide. The doses were chosen so as not to cause clinical or histological disease. The treated rats, along with naive controls, were then challenged with a pathogenic dose of activated T cells for EAE or EAU, respectively. The results show that the vaccinated rats acquired a significant degree of resistance to the disease. The resistance to adoptive EAE was more striking than that to adoptive EAU. While vaccination did not decrease the incidence of EAU in contrast to EAE, it did reduce the intensity of the lesions by about 50% in the 20 recipients tested.

Vaccination Induces Anti-idiotypic Responses

To detect an immune response against the vaccine cells, the draining popliteal lymph nodes (PLN) and distal cervical lymph nodes (CLN) from vaccinated (in the hind footpad) and unchallenged donors were assayed for T cell proliferation to Z1a or to control clone A2b at different times. Five days after vaccination, the PLN but not the CLN showed a specific response to vaccinating clone Z1a only. By day 11, the response had become systemic (FIG. 1).

LN Cells from Vaccinated Donors Transfer Resistance to EAE

To learn whether the response to Z1a was associated with protection against EAE, the responding PLN were transferred from vaccinated to naive rats on day 6 (FIG. 2). For transfer of resistance, the PLN were excised and the PLN cells

TABLE 1. Low Dose T Cell Vaccination Induces Resistance to Autoimmune Diseases[a]

Autoantigen	Vaccine Cells	Diseases	Protection (%)[b]
Myelin BP	Anti-BP (Z1a)	EAE	85%
IRBP (R16 peptide)	Anti-R16	EAU	53%

[a] Z1a and anti-R16 cells were activated by incubation with Concanavalin A. 10^4 living lymphoblasts were then injected intravenously into naive Lewis rats. Eight to twelve days later, the recipients were challenged for EAE with Z1a line cells (2 to 5 million, intraperitoneally, 16 rats) and for EAU with anti-R16 line cells (2 to 3 million, intraperitoneally, 20 rats, cumulative results of 4 experiments). Clinical and histological EAE and EAU scores were recorded.

[b] Protection (%) was calculated as follows:

$$1 - \frac{\text{severity of disease in vacc. rats}}{\text{severity of disease in unvacc. rats}} \times 100$$

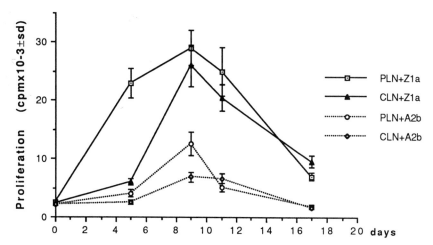

FIGURE 1. Vaccination with Z1a cells induces a specific proliferative response to Z1a cells. Groups of five Lewis rats were vaccinated in the hind footpads by injection of 10^4 activated Z1a cells. At the indicated days, popliteal lymph node (PLN) cells and cervical LN (CLN) cells were assayed for their proliferative response to irradiated (2500 rads) stimulator cells of clone Z1a and clone A2b. The background responses in the absence of stimulators was never more than 2000 cpm.

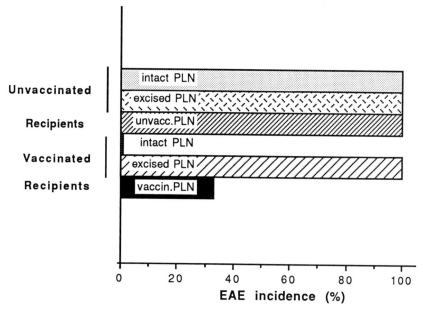

FIGURE 2. Transfer of resistance to EAE with PLN cells. Donor Lewis rats were or were not vaccinated with 10^4 activated Z1a cells in the hind footpad. Six days later, the rats were anesthetized with ether and the draining PLN of some of the rats were excised. The PLN cells were activated by incubation with Con A for 48 h. The activated PLN cells were then transferred intraperitoneally into naive recipient rats (20×10^6 cells/rat). One day later, the vaccinated and unvaccinated controls, the PLN donors and the PLN recipients were challenged with BP-activated Z1a cells to test their susceptibility to EAE.

were activated with mitogen, then inoculated intraperitoneally into naive rats. Control rats either were not vaccinated or were inoculated with mitogen-activated PLN cells from unvaccinated rats. One day later, all the rats were tested for susceptibility to EAE. All of the 12 control rats developed EAE. In contrast, none of the 15 vaccinated rats with intact PLN developed EAE. However, excision of the PLN in all of the 6 vaccinated donors robbed them of their resistance. In

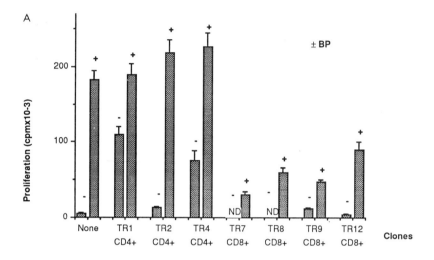

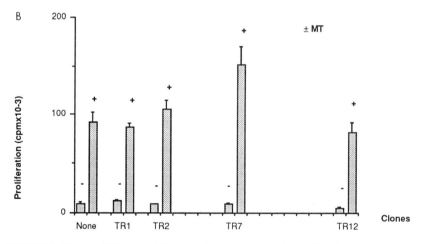

FIGURE 3. Effects of CD4+ and CD8+ anti-Z1a T cells on the proliferation of **(A)** Z1a and **(B)** A2b clones. See legend FIGURE 2; the draining LN were excised and suspensions of lymph node cells (2×10^5/well) were cultured with irradiated Z1a (10^5/well). After 4 days, the blast cells were collected and cloned by limiting dilution. The effect of the anti-Z1a clones on the proliferation of Z1a to myelin BP was examined by culturing Z1a cells in presence of the irradiated anti-Z1a clones. A2b cells were used as control and cultured with or without *Mycobacterium tuberculosis* (MT).

contrast, the naive recipients of these PLN cells acquired a significant measure of resistance (6 rats out of 9 were protected). Thus, the T cell response to Z1a confined to the draining PLN on days 5 and 6 marked the mechanism of resistance.

T Cell Clones Reactive to Z1a Specifically Modulate Z1a Proliferation

PLN cells from vaccinated rats were cloned by limiting dilution technique and stimulated with irradiated Z1a. Four anti-Z1a clones were found by flow cytofluorometry to be positive for OX8 (CD8+) and negative for W3/25 (CD4−). Three clones were composed of cells positive for W3/25 (CD4+) and negative for OX8 (CD8−). FIGURE 3 illustrates the effects of the irradiated CD4+ and CD8+ anti-Z1a cells on the proliferation of Z1a. Two CD4+ helper clones strongly activated Z1a in the absence of BP. In contrast, the four CD8+ cytotoxic/suppressor clones suppressed the response of Z1a to BP by 50 to 80%. No effect on A2b cells could be detected. Thus, both the stimulatory and the suppressive effects were specific for Z1a.

Vaccination with R16 Line Cells Induces Proliferative Response to Activated T Cells

Results summarized in TABLE 1 indicate that vaccination with R16 cells could efficiently protect Lewis rats against adoptive EAU. FIGURE 4 shows that LN from vaccinated animals mounted a proliferative response toward the activated cells used as vaccine. In addition, they reacted clearly and reproducibly to four different activated T cell lines (BP, PPD, R4 and S-Ag/P35 lines) and to normal activated splenocytes (FIGS. 4, 5). Nevertheless, the magnitude of the proliferative responses was higher in the presence of the specific vaccine cells. LN cells from naive rats were used as control responders. None of the irradiated activated T cells could induce a significant proliferation of LN cells. To test whether the activation of the stimulators was a necessary condition for inducing proliferation, the T cell lines were used after antigenic or mitogenic activation and in a resting state. The resting state was monitored by fluorescence analysis for detection of the membrane activation markers. After 7 days in TCGF-medium, the T cell lines used as stimulators did not exhibit detectable amounts of receptor for IL-2 and for transferrin (less than 5% cells were positive for these markers). As expected, the majority (>90%) of antigen or mitogenic-activated T cells did express these markers (results not shown). Two different groups of rats were vaccinated either with R16 cells or with S-Ag/P35 cells. LN cells were tested for their ability to react to irradiated T line cells of various specificities, in an activated or resting state. As was shown in FIGURE 5, LN cells from either vaccinated groups recognized only the activated T cells.

DISCUSSION

The experiments described in this article were undertaken to investigate the mechanism involved in the resistance to experimental autoimmune diseases, such as EAE and EAU, by vaccination with a subpathogenic dose of activated effector T cells.

Stimulators

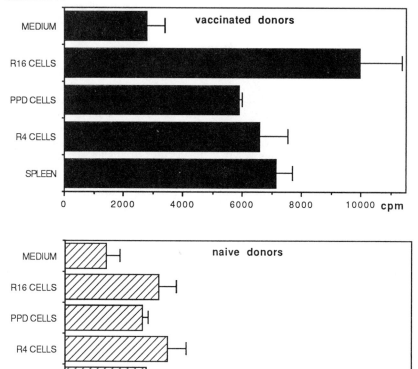

FIGURE 4. Vaccination with R16 line cells induces proliferative responses to activated T cells. Lewis rats were or were not vaccinated with 10^4 R16 cells intravenously, and 9 days later were boosted with 5×10^4 R16 cells in the hind footpad. The cervical, popliteal and inguinal lymph nodes were removed 8 days later. The lymph node cells (4×10^5/well) were assayed for their proliferative responses to activated irradiated R16-cells (1×10^5/well). Con A-activated PPD-cell line, R4-cell line and spleen cells were used as controls.

Resistance could be adoptively transferred from vaccinated to naive syngeneic rats with lymphoid cells. Among the many factors that could account for this phenomenon is immunity directed towards the autoantigen-specific T lymphocytes responsible for producing disease. Compatible with this notion was the finding that vaccinated rats reacted immunologically to the effectors specific for myelin basic protein or retinal antigens. We cloned anti-Z1a cells from the PLN of vaccinated rats and obtained two sets of specific anti-Z1a clones CD4+8− helper T cells and CD4−8+ cytotoxic/suppressor T cells. The observations that Z1a and the anti-Z1a clones stimulated one another is most easily explained by mutual recognition of their receptors. Vaccination induced an immune response which was thought to be an anti-idiotypic response. The demonstration in both rats and mice that encephalitogenic cloned T cells have very restricted receptor variability and the recent successful immunotherapy of EAE with monoclonal antibodies to a shared T cell receptor epitope are consistent with this view.[12,25] Following this lead, Vandenbark et al.[26] and Howel et al.[27] have prevented EAE in rats by immunizing them with synthetic T cell receptor peptides in adjuvant.

Our results, in the EAE model, indicated that the anti-idiotypic lymphoid population was essential for resistance to EAE. The anti-idiotypic response was found in the EAU model as well. Interestingly, in addition to that, another kind of proliferative response toward activated irradiated calls was repeatedly observed. The PLN cells from rats vaccinated with anti-R16 cells recognized activated T cells lacking the receptor for the R16 peptide suggesting that the target structure might be a marker of their state of activation. It has been reported that such cells, termed anti-ergotypic cells, are induced by inoculating animals with activated T cells.[28] In contrast to anti-idiotypic T cells, the anti-ergotypic T cells responded to activated T cells in general without regard for their idiotypic specificities. An anti-ergotypic response thus may combine with an anti-idiotypic T cell response to regulate autoimmunity. It is not clear to what extent these different cell populations participate in the resistance to autoimmune diseases. However, it has been demonstrated that the administration of anti-ergotypic T cells to syngeneic rats protected the rats against EAE. Anti-ergotypic T cells could also be detected after immunization with antigen in vivo, suggesting that they may function physiologically.[28]

Targeting autoimmune cells should be a selective process designed to spare all other elements. In this respect, TCR seems to be the most appropriate target structure. To be successful, the T cells causing the disease must be very homogeneous. There is some evidence that this condition is met in rheumatoid arthritis[29] and possibly in multiple sclerosis.[30,31] Interesting but more speculative is to design peptides that have an agretope (MHC interaction site) allowing them to bind strongly to those MHC molecules that can present autoantigens, thereby blocking the particular subset of MHC molecule.[32,33]

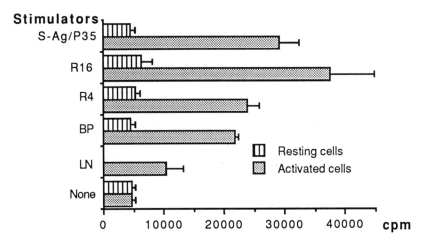

FIGURE 5. Vaccination induces proliferative responses to activated but to resting cells. Ten days after intravenous vaccination, LN cells were tested for their proliferative responses to four different T cell lines in two distinct stages. The stimulators were used after mitogenic activation and after 7 days in TCGF-medium.

In view of the results obtained in the various experimental models of autoimmune diseases, one should be very encouraged in the search for highly specific forms of immune intervention.

SUMMARY

The effectiveness and the mechanism of T cell vaccination were studied in two experimental models of autoimmune disease. The attempt to modulate autoimmune disease via idiotypic regulation of autoreactive antigen-specific T cells was first shown in the rat experimental autoimmune encephalomyelitis (EAE) model where inactivated EAE-inducing T cells could both immunize and protect rats from EAE. We previously reported that low dose T cell vaccination against EAE in Lewis rats was immunologically specific, long lasting and extremely efficient in preventing adoptive transfer of the disease. In experimental autoimmune uveitis (EAU) T cell vaccination was also found to be effective. In both cases, antigen or mitogen activation of the T cells prior to inoculation was required. In the EAE model, T cell vaccination appeared to be associated with two sets of T lymphocytes (CD4+ CD8− helper and CD4− CD8+ cytotoxic/suppressor cells) which were cloned and found to be specifically reactive to the vaccine cells. These anti-idiotypic T cell clones were able to antagonistically modulate the *in vitro* proliferation of encephalitogenic Z1a cells. *In vivo,* transfer of the lymph node cells (from which the anti-idiotypic clones were derived) from vaccinated animals to naive syngeneic recipients conferred resistance to EAE. In the EAU model, we also found a consistent immunological response raised against different activated T cells (four T cell lines with irrelevant specificities and mitogen-activated lymphoid cells) in addition to the anti-idiotypic cells. This response, apparently directed to T cell activation markers, might combine with the anti-idiotypic response to regulate autoimmunity.

ACKNOWLEDGMENTS

This work was done with the collaboration of A. Ben-Nun, O. Lider, T. Reshef, and I. R. Cohen, Department of Cell Biology, Weizmann Institute of Science, Rehovot, Israel; D. Bernard, Laboratoire d'Immunologie, Université de Médecine, Marseille, France; and R. Caspi, C. C. Chan, Y. Gery, S. Kotake, S. Oddo, and R. B. Nussenblatt, Laboratory of Immunology, National Eye Institute, National Institutes of Health, Bethesda, MD.

REFERENCES

1. BEN-NUN, A., H. WEKERLE & I. R. COHEN. 1981. Vaccination against autoimmune encephalomyelitis with T lymphocyte line cells reactive against myelin basic protein. Nature **292:** 60–61.
2. HOLOSHITZ, J., Y. NAPARSTEK, A. BEN-NUN & I. R. COHEN. 1983. Lines of T lymphocytes induce or vaccinate against autoimmune arthritis. Science **219:** 56–58.
3. MARON, R., R. ZERUBAVEL, A. FRIEDMAN & I. R. COHEN. 1983. T lymphocyte line specific for thyroglobulin produces or vaccinates against autoimmune thyroiditis in mice. J. Immunol. **131:** 2316–2321.
4. LIDER, O., N. KARIN, M. SHINITSKY & I. R. COHEN. 1987. Therapeutic vaccination

against adjuvant arthritis using autoimmune T cells treated with hydrostatic pressure. Proc. Natl. Acad. Sci. USA **84:** 4577–4580.

5. BEN-NUN, A. & I. R. COHEN. 1981. Vaccination against autoimmune encephalomyelitis (EAE): attenuated autoimmune T lymphocytes confer resistance to induction of active EAE but not to EAE mediated by the intact lymphocyte line. Eur. J. Immunol. **11:** 949–952.

6. LIDER, O., M. SHINITZKY & I. R. COHEN. 1986. Vaccination against experimental autoimmune diseases using T lymphocytes treated with hydrostatic pressure. Ann. N. Y. Acad. Sci. **475:** 267–273.

7. BERAUD, E., O. LIDER, E. BAHARAV, T. RESHEF & I. R. COHEN. 1989. Vaccination against experimental autoimmune encephalomyelitis using encephalitogenic dose of autoimmune effector cells. (1) Characteristics of vaccination. J. Autoimmunity **2:** 75–86.

8. LIDER, O., E. BERAUD, T. RESHEF, A. FRIEDMAN & I. R. COHEN. 1989. Vaccination against experimental autoimmune encephalomyelitis using a subencephalitogenic dose of autoimmune effector T cells. (2) Induction of a protective anti-idiotypic response. J. Autoimmunity **2:** 87–99.

9. LIDER, O., T. RESHEF, E. BERAUD, A. BEN-NUN & I. R. COHEN. 1988. Anti-idiotypic network induced by T cell vaccination against experimental autoimmune encephalomyelitis. Science **239:** 181–185.

10. NAPARSTEK, Y., A. BEN-NUN, J. HOLOSHITZ, T. RESHEF, A. FRENKEL, M. ROSENBERG & I. R. COHEN. 1983. T lymphocyte lines producing or vaccinating against autoimmune encephalomyelitis (EAE): functional activation induces PNA receptor and accumulation in the brain and thymus of line cells. Eur. J. Immunol. **13:** 418–423.

11. ACHA-ORBEA, H., D. J. MITCHELL, L. TIMMERMAN, D. C. WRAITH, G. S. TAICH, M. K. WALDOR, S. ZAMVIL, H. MCDEVITT & L. STEINMAN. 1988. Limited heterogeneity of T cell receptors from lymphocytes mediating autoimmune encephalomyelitis allows specific murine immune intervention. Cell **54:** 263–273.

12. URBAN, J., V. KUMAR, D. KONO, J. GOMEZ, S. J. HORVATH, J. CLAYTON, D. G. ANDO, E. E. SERCAZ & L. HOOD. 1988. Restricted use of T cell receptor V genes in murine autoimmune encephalomyelitis raises possibilities for antibody therapy. Cell **54:** 577–592.

13. CHLUBA, J., C. STEEG, A. BECKER, H. WEKERLE & J. T. EPPLEN. 1989. T cell receptor β chain usage in myelin basic protein-specific rat T lymphocyte. Eur. J. Immunol. **19:** 279–284.

14. BURNS, F. R., X. LI, N. SHEN, H. OFNER, Y. K. CHOU, A. A. VANDERBARK & E. HEBER-KATZ. 1989. Both rat and mouse T cell receptors specific for the encephalitogenic determinant of myelin basic protein use similar Vα and Vβ chain genes even though the major histocompatibility complex and encephalitogenic determinants being recognized are different. J. Exp. Med. **169:** 27–39.

15. GREGERSON, D., S. P. FLING, C. F. MERRYMAN, X. ZHANG, X. LI & E. HEBER-KATZ. 1990. Conserved T cell receptor v gene usage by uveitogenic T cells. Clin. Immunol. Immunopathol. In press.

16. CASPI, R., F. G. ROGERGE, C. G. MCALLISTER, M. EL-SAIED, T. KUWABARA, I. GERY, E. HANNA & R. B. NUSSENBLATT. 1986. T cell lines mediating experimental autoimmune uveoretinitis (EAU) in the rat. J. Immunol. **136:** 928–933.

17. SANUI, H., T. M. REDMOND, S. KOTAKE, B. WIGGERT, L.-H. HU, H. MARGALIT, J. A. BERZOFSKY, G. J. CHADER & I. GERY. 1989. Identification of an immunodominant and highly immunopathogenic determinant in the retinal interphotoreceptor retinoid-binding protein (IRBP). J. Exp. Med. **169:** 1947–1960.

18. WONG, V. G., W. R. GREEN & P. R. B. MCMASTER. 1977. Rhodopsin and blindness. Trans. Am. Ophthalmol. Soc. **75:** 272–284.

19. GERY, I., M. MOCHIZUCHI & R. B. NUSSENBLATT. 1986. Ocular diseases with presumed retinal/uveal autoimmunity. *In* Progress in Retinal Research. N. Osborne & J. Chader, Eds. Vol. 5: 100–113. Pergamon Press. Oxford and New York.

20. DE SMET, M., J. H. YAMAMOTO, M. MOCHIZUKI, I. GERY, V. K. SINGH, T. SHINOHARA, B. WIGGERT, G. J. CHADER & R. B. NUSSENBLATT. 1990. Cellular immune

responses of patients with uveitis to retinal antigens and their fragments. Am. J. Ophthalmol. **110:** 135–142.

21. HOLOSHITZ, J., A. MATITIAU & I. R. COHEN. 1984. Arthritis induced in rats by cloned T lymphocytes responsive to mycobacteria but not to collagen type II. J. Clin. Invest. **73:** 211–215.

22. HU, L. H., T. M. REDMOND, H. SANUI, T. KUWABARA, C. G. MCALLISTER, B. WIGGERT, G. J. CHADER & I. GERY. 1989. Rat T cell lines specific to nonimmunodominant determinant of a retinal protein (IRBP) produce uveoretinitis and pinealitis. Cell. Immunol. **122:** 251–261.

23. VARRIALE, S., E. BERAUD, D. BRANDLY, J. BARBARIA, M. M. GOLDSTEIN & D. BERNARD. 1989. Regulation of experimental autoimmune encephalomyelitis. Specificity of the "recovery-associated" suppressor cells. J. Neuroimmunol. **22:** 31–40.

24. ROBERGE, F. G., H. LORBERBOUM-GALSKI, P. LE HOANG, M. DE SMET, C. C. CHAN, D. FITZGERALD & I. PASTAN. 1989. Selective immunosuppression of activated T cells with the chimeric toxin IL-2-PE40. Inhibition of experimental uveoretinitis. J. Immunol. **143:** 3498–3502.

25. OWASHI, M., & E. HEBER-KATZ. 1988. Protection from experimental allergic encephalomyelitis conferred by a monoclonal antibody directed against a shared idiotype on rat T cell receptors specific for myelin basic protein. J. Exp. Med. **168:** 2153–2164.

26. VANDENBARK, A., G. HASHIM & H. OFFNER. 1989. Immunization with a synthetic T cell receptor V-region peptide protects against autoimmune encephalomyelitis. Nature **341:** 541–544.

27. HOWELL, M. D., S. T. WINTERS, T. OLEE, H. C. POWELL, D. J. CARLO & W. BROSTOFF. 1989. Vaccination against experimental allergic encephalomyelitis with T cell receptor peptides. Science **246:** 668–670.

28. LHOSE, A., F. MOR, N. KARIN & I. R. COHEN. 1989. Control of experimental autoimmune encephalomyelitis by T cells responding to activated T cell. Science **244:** 820–822.

29. STAMONKOVIC, I., M. STEGANO, K. A. WRIGHT, S. M. KRANE, E. P. AMENTO, R. B. COLVIN, R. J. DUQUESNOY & J. T. KURNICK. 1988. Clonal dominance among T-lymphocyte infiltrates in arthritis. Proc. Natl. Acad. Sci. USA **85:** 1179–1183.

30. HAFLER, D. A., A. D. DUBY, S. J. LEE, D. BENJAMIN, J. G. SEIDMAN & H. L. WEINER. 1988. Oligoclonal T lymphocytes in the cerebrospinal fluid of patients with multiple sclerosis. J. Exp. Med. **167:** 1313–1322.

31. ROTTEVEEL, F. T. M., I. KOKKELINK, H. K. VAN WALBEEK, C. H. POLMAN, J. J. M. VAN DONGEN & C. J. LUCAS. 1987. Analysis of T cell receptor gene rearrangement in T cells from the cerebrospinal fluid of patients with multiple sclerosis. J. Neuroimmunol. **15:** 243–249.

32. TODD, J. A., H. ACHA-ORBEA, J. I. BELL, N. CHAO, Z. FRONEK, C. O. JACOB, M. MCDERMOTT, A. A. SINHA, L. TIMMERMAN, L. STEINMAN & H. O. MCDEVITT. 1988. A molecular basis for MHC class II associated autoimmunity. Science **240:** 1003–1009.

33. ADORINI, L., S. MULLER, F. CARDINAUX, P. V. LEHMAN, F. FALCIONI & Z. A. NAGY. 1988. *In vivo* competition between self peptides and foreign in T cell activation. Nature **334:** 623–625.

Regulatory Interactions among Autologous T Cell Clones

Human Bifunctional T Cell Clones Regulate the Activity of an Autologous T Cell Clone[a]

D. NAOR,[b] G. ESSERY,[c] N. TARCIC,[b] M. KAHAN,[c] AND M. FELDMANN[c]

[b] The Lautenberg Center for General and Tumor Immunology
The Hebrew University–Hadassah Medical School
P.O. Box 1172
Jerusalem 91010, Israel
[c] The Charing Cross Sunley Research Centre
Lurgan Avenue
Hammersmith, London W6 8LW, England

The Controversy of the Suppressor T Cell Concept

The recent debate about suppressor T cells reached a new climax after the publication of Göran Möller's editorial[1] in the *Scandinavian Journal of Immunology:* "Do suppressor T cells exist?" His unequivocal conclusion that "suppressor T cells do not exist" has already prompted contrary responses (see editorials in Scand. J. Immunol., 27: 621–628, 1988). Some of them found, interestingly, conceptual or moral support from the field of Astronomy (but not Astrology). Janeway[2] believes that the missing suppressor cell will be finally found, because the behavior of the other cells of the immune system indicates that they are influenced by additional cells which regulate them, in analogy to the behavior of the visible planets whose orbits are influenced by other, invisible planets. The belief of Tomio Tada[3] in the traditional suppressor cell concept is even stronger, and like Galileo Galilei he states, "Eppure si muove!" (but it still moves). The philosophical point is raised that lack of proof does not constitute disproof.

The suppressor T cell concept that was most popular during the seventies and early eighties has lost credibility as a result of many conflicting observations, some of which have already been listed in Möller's editorial.[1] Thus, suppressor T cells have variously been phenotyped as CD4[+] *e.g.*, REF. 4), CD8[+] (*e.g.*, REF. 5) or double positive (CD4[+]CD8[+], *e.g.*, REF. 6) cells. Some reports indicated that suppressor T cells recognize antigens in association with the major histocompatibility complex (MHC; *e.g.*, REFS. 7, 8); while others implied (*e.g.*, REF. 9) that, like antibodies, they recognize free antigens. B cells,[10] helper T cells[11] and other cells of the hemapoietic system[12] have been implicated as the suppressor T cell targets. Some investigators[13–15] found that "suppression" was in fact mediated by

[a] This work was supported by the Wellcome Trust, ICI plc, BP, Michael and Anna Wix Charitable Trust and the Nuffield Foundation. David Naor holds the Milton Winograd professorial chair of cancer studies.

135

cytotoxic cells. Consequently, the independent status of suppressor T cells has been questioned. However, the difference between suppression and cytotoxicity might be merely semantic, because cytotoxicity is a possible mechanism of suppression. Furthermore, for the sake of simplicity it is, perhaps, better to consider cytolysis and suppression within the same category, because universally accepted discriminatory markers have not yet been established for cells mediating these functions.

The application of molecular biology into T cell research which has clarified many issues, such as the nature of receptors for antigen, has not resolved the problems of the suppressor T cell. Rather it has augmented them as discrepant results were observed. Thus, some authors[16,17] reported that the suppressor T cell antigen receptor expresses both α and β chains, like helper and cytotoxic cells. Other investigators claimed that suppressor T cells delete the β chain gene,[18,19] or do not rearrange it[7] and therefore they cannot express β chains. Others[20] described a suppressor T cell line transcribing the β chain gene but not the α or the γ chain gene, whereas a different line transcribes the β and the γ chain genes. In addition, the J "molecule," initially considered as a suppressor T cell marker,[9] could not be detected in its expected location between $A\beta$ and $E\alpha$ genes, when the mouse MHC was mapped at the DNA level.[21] The confusion is compounded further by the lack of understanding of the mechanism of action of suppressor T cells, and by some of the amazingly complicated, multicellular pathways reported.[22,23]

T Cell Clones Expressing Both Helper and Suppressor Functions

The development of T cell cloning techniques[24] raised new hopes that the suppressor T cell puzzle would be finally resolved. Again the results were disappointing. Whereas some authors characterized suppressor T cell clones by functional (e.g., REF. 25) and molecular biology (e.g., REF. 17) techniques, others[14,26-30] could not find T cell clones committed to a restricted suppression program. On the contrary, they found "bifunctional" T cell clones, which mediated either suppression or help, depending on the experimental conditions. For instance, it has been demonstrated that the number of cloned regulator T cells could affect the immune response of the target cells. A low number of cells (10^2) enhanced the production of anti-sheep red blood cells (SRBC) antibodies by B cells, whereas a high number of cells (10^4) from the same clone suppressed this response by cytolysis.[14] On the other hand, the level of the helper function may dictate the regulatory activity of the cloned T cells. In support of this possibility it has been found that an intensive helper function was suppressed by the cloned T cells, whereas a weak helper function was amplified by the same cells.[29] Another experimental model showed that the polyclonal immunoglobulin production by resting B cells was augmented by cloned T cells, but the same cells suppressed the immunoglobulin synthesis of activated B cells.[28] Similarly, cells of other clones helped the immunoglobulin[26,31] or antibody[30,32] production by resting B cells, whereas activated blast cells were cytolyzed by the same cells. Finally, it has been documented that either helper or cytotoxic functions could be selectively induced in T cell clones, depending on what combination of anti-CD2 monoclonal antibodies (mAbs) was used for stimulating the cloned cells.[33] All the above-described clones share certain properties. First, all express bifunctional regulatory activity. The "decision" as to which function will be potentiated is possibly made either by environmental factors associated with the specific parameters of the experimental design (*e.g.*, REF. 27) or by the activation state of the target cells (*e.g.*, REFS. 26, 28, 34). Secondly, all clones recognize MHC class II products either independently (autoreactive clones; REFS. 4, 28–32), or in conjunction with the inducing antigen,[26] and all express the CD4[+] phenotype. In this respect these bifunctional clones resemble "helper/inducer" cells and are different from the traditional CD8[+] "cytotoxic/suppressor" cells which recognize MHC class I. We believe that these bifunctional clones deserve more attention than that which has been paid to them until now.

Idiotype-Anti-Idiotype-Like Regulatory Interactions between Bifunctional Human T Cell Clones and the Autologous Inducer Clone

Because of our personal interest and involvement in suppressor cell research,[25,35–37], and recognizing the controversy of the suppressor T cell concept, we have decided to re-evaluate the previous suppressor cell dogma, by exploring a human *in vitro* experimental model potentially capable of answering at least some of the questions listed above. The model chosen was to raise autologous clones against a helper clone from human autologous peripheral blood mononuclear (PBM) cells and to explore the specificity of these "anticlones" and their regulatory effect on the inducer clone. This strategy had been used by Lamb and Feidmann in 1982,[25] and reproduced by Engleman's group in 1986.[38]

Peripheral blood mononuclear cells obtained from a JM blood bank donor were incubated with Mx9 (anti-Vβ8 monoclonal antibodies),[39,40] sorted by fluorescence activated cell sorter (FACS) and then cloned with irradiated autologous PBM, anti-Vβ8 and rIL-2 at a ratio of 0.3 cells per well.[41] One of the expanded CD4[+] clones, which proliferated after stimulation with anti-Vβ8 but not with anti-Vβ5 monoclonal antibodies (mAbs) (clone Mx9/9), was employed as the inducer of autologous clones.[34] The PBM of JM were stimulated twice with autologous x-irradiated Mx9/9 cells. The second stimulation was performed in the presence of autologous x-irradiated feeder cells (PBM) and rIL-2. The cells harvested from the second culture were cloned in Terasaki plates at a ratio of 0.3 cells per well in the presence of x-irradiated Mx9/9 cells, autologous x-irradiated feeder cells (PBM) and rIL-2.[34] Of 1440 wells, 70 clones (5%) were recovered, of which 26 clones were successfully "expanded," cryopreserved and finally tested. As indicated by FACS analysis, 25 clones were stained with anti-CD4[+] mAb, and one clone was stained with anti-CD8[+] mAb.[42]

The specificity of the 26 clones was determined by their ability to proliferate after stimulation with the inducer Mx9/9 clone, cells derived from the "sister" clones, unrelated autologous clones (JM6) and allogeneic PBM.[34,42,43] Three types of clones were revealed (summary in TABLE 1). "Type I" clones proliferated in response to the inducer Mx9/9 clone but not when incubated with the other stimulator cells (TABLES 1 and 2). "Type II" clones proliferated when incubated with all stimulator cells, whereas type III clones did not respond to any stimulation (TABLE 1; REFS. 34, 42, 43). Type I clones were the object of our subsequent studies.

The specificity of the anti-Mx9/9 type I clones was stressed by the fact that their cells proliferated after stimulation with cells from the inducer clones Mx9/9 but not after stimulation with cells from the autologous clones A-13 and JM6 (TABLE 2). As indicated earlier, clone JM6 is an autologous T cell clone which recognizes EBV-transformed B cells. Clone A-13 is a sister clone of clone Mx9/9, since it was obtained from the same cloning procedure. Clone A-13 expresses, like

TABLE 1. The Specificity Profile of the Autologous Clones as Indicated by Their Ability (+) or Inability (−) to Proliferate after the Stimulation

| | Stimulators | | | |
Responder Clones	Mx9/9[a]	Sister Clones[b]	JM6[c]	PBM[d]
Type I	+	−	−	−
Type II	+	+	+	+
Type III	−	−	−	−

[a] The autologous inducer clone.
[b] Autologous anti-Mx9/9 clones obtained from the same cloning procedure.
[c] Unrelated autologous clone induced with autologous EBV transformed B cells.
[d] Allogeneic PBM.

clone Mx9/9, the $V\beta8^+$ phenotype (as indicated by FACS analysis) and it proliferated, also like clone Mx9/9, after stimulation with anti-$V\beta8$ but not with anti-$B\beta5$ mAbs. The fact that the anti-Mx9/9 autoreactive clones responded to the inducer clone Mx9/9 but not to the A-13 sister clone excludes the possibility that such anti-Mx9/9 cells recognize mouse IgG, which is possibly absorbed on the T cell surface following the use of anti-$V\beta8$ (the antibody used to stimulate the cells). This finding further suggests that the autoreactive clones recognize an antigen receptor idiotype-like structure of Mx9/9 cells, but $V\beta8$ is not the idiotypic target of that recognition. Surprisingly, we found that whereas Mx9/9 stimulated the proliferation of the specific autoreactive clones this clone failed to be stimulated by them,[34] indicating an unidirectional stimulatory signal (unlike previous work; REF. 25). The proliferative response of the autoreactive type I clones stimulated with Mx9/9 cells varied as the number of the stimulator cells was changed. Each clone demonstrated a distinctive dose-response curve.[34] In addition, none of the specific anti-Mx9/9 autoreactive clones proliferated after stimulation with anti-$V\beta8$ mAb (the specific stimulator of the Mx9/9 clone), whereas Mx9/9 cells proliferated after stimulation with this antibody.[41] Finally, anti-class II and anti-DR, but not anti-DQ mAbs, inhibited the proliferation of the anti-Mx9/9 autoreactive clones after stimulation with Mx9/9 cells.[34] Taken together, these findings suggest that the specific autoreactive clones recognize antigen(s) on the T cell receptor (TCR) of Mx9/9 cells, in association with HLA-DR product. This assumption is based on

TABLE 2. Specificity Analysis of Autoreactive Type I Clones[a]

| | | Stimulators (cpm[b]) | | | | | |
Exp.	Responder Clones	Mx9/9	A-13	JM6	Clone 12	Clone 121	IL-2
1	12	6246		2233	573	1703	27 505
	121	6754		1978	0	410	18 565
	Medium[c]	222		356	262	451	112
2	12	4015	232	142			39 386
	121	5922	449	427			26 915
	Medium[c]	65	415	93			

[a] 1×10^4 cloned cells (responders) were stimulated with 2.5×10^4 irradiated (5000 rad) stimulator cells. The proliferative responses were measured by ^{3}H-thymidine incorporation and they are recorded in the table after substraction of the ^{3}H-thymidine incorporation of responder cells alone.
[b] Standard errors did not exceed 10% of the mean.
[c] ^{3}H-thymidine incorporation of stimulator cells alone.

the fact that type I autoreactive clones recognize the inducing clone Mx9/9, but not other autologous clones, expressing different specificity (JM6) or idiotype-like structure (A-13). The only known differences between these clones and clone Mx9/9 are in the T cell receptor.

The suggestion that the autoreactive anti-Mx9/9 clones interact with the TCR of autologous Mx9/9 cells is supported by another experimental protocol.[44] The experimental approach was based on Cantrell and colleagues'[45] finding, demonstrating a modulation of TCR after treatment with phorbol dibutyrate. Mx9/9 cells were incubated with 10 ng/ml phorbol 12,13-dibutyrate and stained with anti-T3 and anti-Vβ8 fluoresceinated mAbs at different times after the starting of the incubation, in order to analyze by flow fluorocytometry the fate of their receptors. The Mx9/9 cells gradually lost their TCR; after 16 hours of incubation more than 80% of their T3 and Vβ8 TCR components were modulated. Simultaneous FACS analysis of phorbol dibutyrate-treated Mx9/9 cells with other mAbs, also directed against surface molecules, revealed a co-modulation of T4 molecules with the TCR molecules (T3 and Vβ8). In contrast, the expression of Class I and Class II MHC molecules was slightly increased after phorbol dibutyrate treatment and that of IL-2 receptor (IL-2R) was not changed.[44] Cantrell *et al.*[45] proved that phorbol dibutyrate (50 ng/ml)-treated cells responded normally to IL-2. In addition, Saizawa and colleagues[46] demonstrated co-modulation of TCR and CD4 after incubation with anti-TCR mAb and activation of T cells following incubation with an anti-TCR mAb Fab fragment in conjunction with anti-CD4 mAb.

TABLE 3. Summary of JM Clones Phenotype Detected by FACS Analysis

Type I Clones	Phenotypes								
	CD3	CD4	CD8	Vβ8	TCR αβ	TCR γδ	IL-2R	Class I	HLA-DR
12, 17, 18, 111, 121	+	+	−	−	+	−	+	+	+

Mx9/9 cells incubated with different concentrations of phorbol dibutyrate for 16 h were employed to stimulate the anti-Mx9/9 clones, in order to correlate the loss of the TCR complex with the stimulatory capacity of Mx9/9 cells.[44] Mx9/9 cells incubated with 10 ng/ml or more phorbol dibutyrate substantially lost their ability to stimulate the proliferation of the anti-Mx9/9 clones, supporting the suggestion that the T-T interaction is mediated by a receptor recognition.

The FACS contour graphs of the type I autoreactive clones are illustrated in our previous publications,[34,42] and the phenotype of their surface markers are summarized in TABLE 3. The phenotype of JM6 and Mx9/9 clones is identical to that of type I anti-Mx9/9 clones, except that the Mx9/9 clone expresses, in contrast to other clones the Vβ8 chain segment. FACS contour graphs of one representative clone (clone 121) which was stained with WT31 or BMA031 (antiα, β-TCR mAbs) but not with a combination of TiγA and TCRδ1 (anti-γ, δ-TCR mAbs) are demonstrated in FIGURE 1.

The flow cytometry analysis of the cells clearly shows their uniformity and supports their clonal origin. Furthermore, southern blot analysis with a Cβ probe reveals that each one of the analyzed anti-Mx9/9 clones has a distinct rearrangement of its β chain TCR germ line gene[34] indicating that each clone originated from a single cell.

What are the consequences of these clone-anti-clone cellular interactions? To determine whether the anti-Mx9/9 clones regulate the proliferation of the Mx9/9 clone stimulated with anti-Vβ8 mAbs, some of the anti-Mx9/9 type I clones (all CD4[+]) were added, at 1:1 ratio, to microplates coated with anti-Vβ8 mAb and containing Mx9/9 cells. The proliferation of Mx9/9 cells was suppressed by clone 111 and irradiated and unirradiated cells of clone 121.[44] Clone 18 neither suppressed nor enhanced the proliferative response of Mx9/9 cells. When the anti-Mx9/9 clones were subjected to the same assay two months later, no change was observed in their regulatory function.[44] The anti-Mx9/9 clones were maintained in

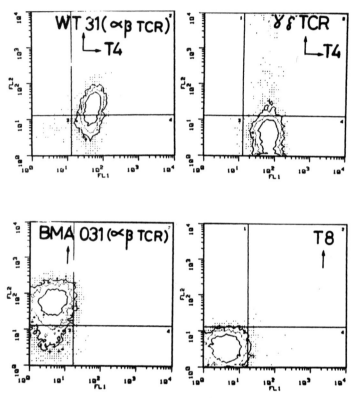

FIGURE 1. Flow cytometric analysis of clone 121. Clone 121 cells were stained directly or indirectly with fluorochromated mAbs directed against TCR, CD4 and CD8 surface molecules. The *horizontal axis* shows the fluoresceinated mAbs while the *vertical axis* shows the fluorescence of phycoerythrin-labeled antibodies. The CD4[+], CD8[−], αβTCR[+] phenotype of the anti-Mx9/9 clone is illustrated.

culture in the presence of autologous feeder cells, IL-2 and OKT3 or anti-Vβ8 mAb for an additional four months and then reassessed. Whereas the phenotypes and the specificity of the anti-Mx9/9 clones remained stable and they were free of mycoplasma, as indicated by sensitive molecular test,[47] a fundamental change was observed in their function. Clone 111, and clone 121 enhanced rather than suppressed the proliferation of Mx9/9 cells stimulated with anti-Vβ8 mAb. In contrast, clone 18, which was functionally silent at the early part of the study exerted an impressive suppressive effect (96% inhibition) at the later stage of the study as indicated by its ability to inhibit the proliferation of Mx9/9 cells stimulated with anti-Vβ8.[44]

We have not been able to precisely define the environmental conditions under which the two antagonistic effects are manifested, but have found that the state of the activation of the target Mx9/9 cells is an important factor.[34] Mx9/9 target cells were prepared in two states of activation. Unrested (activated) Mx9/9 cells were maintained in the culture in the presence of anti-Vβ8 mAb until the time of the assay. Anti-Vβ8 mAb was excluded 48 h before the assay from the culture of the rested (unactivated) Mx9/9 cells. Consequently, the unrested Mx9/9 cells proliferated relatively well after stimulation with anti-Vβ8 (19,000 cpm), whereas the rested Mx9/9 cells proliferated poorly under similar circumstances (3500 cpm). Irradiated (5000 rad) and unirradiated clone 12 cells were added at 1:1 ratios to unrested and rested Mx9/9 cells stimulated with anti-Vβ8 mAb. They suppressed the proliferation of the unrested Mx9/9 cells, but at the same time enhanced the proliferation of the rested mx9/9 cells stimulated with anti-Vβ8 mAb.[34] Whereas the irradiated clone 12 cells affected the proliferation of unrested and rested Mx9/9 cells stimulated with anti-Vβ8 mAb, they did not affect the proliferation of these cells after stimulation with rIL-2[34] indicating the specificity of the regulating effect. The suppression of the unrested clone was not due to adsorption or consumption of IL-2 by IL-2R of the anti-Mx9/9 clones, as it also occurred with irradiated clones which cannot proliferate and thus have limited capacity to absorb IL-2. The enhanced proliferation of rested Mx9/9 cells was induced by both irradiated and unirradiated clone 12 cells, indicating that the effect was not a consequence of mutual proliferative responses of both clones.[34] In conclusion, clone 12 is not committed to a single program; it can either enhance or suppress the response of its target cells, depending on their state of activation.

CONCLUSIONS

Several autoreactive clones which are not committed to a single functional program have been described in both mouse and man.[14,28–32,34] Their activity appears to be controlled by signals delivered from their environment, in particular from the target cells.[26,28–32] These CD4+ cells are probably not related to the veto cells, expressing a variety of T cell markers, presenting various stages of maturation, and committed to a single inhibition program.[48]

At the moment, the signals regulating the effects of these CD4 autoreactive bifunctional clones are not known, although it seems that they are important for dictating the contrasting activities of these cells. The multipotential effects of T cell clones can be envisaged in terms of lymphokine production. Single clones are known to produce multiple lymphokines upon receiving specific or nonspecific stimuli (*e.g.*, REFS. 49, 50). There is also evidence that the molecules released depends on the nature of the inducing stimulus.[51] Furthermore, it has been evidenced that inhibitory (*e.g.*, TGFβ,[52]) and stimulatory lymphokines are produced by the same CD4 cells (our own unpublished data, Grubeck-Loebenstein, Londei and Feldmann). Thus, the potential of a clone to produce both helper and suppressor lymphokines is clear. We do not, at present, know what the antagonistic lymphokines produced by our clones are, but this question will be addressed by our subsequent studies.

Assuming that the cytokine concept is correct, it is conceivable that different antigen-presenting signals delivered from rested or unrested Mx9/9 cells may respectively induce a release of either enhancing or inhibitory cytokines from the anti-Mx9/9 clones. In support of this notion, Eljaafari and colleagues[33] have shown that different second messenger metabolic pathways are triggered when different combination pairs of anti-CD2 mAbs are used for stimulating the corresponding CD2 epitopes of a T cell clone. Consequently, different cytokine or cytokine receptor genes are activated leading to distinct cellular functions (cytotoxicity or help). Alternatively, the anti-Mx9/9 clones may simultaneously release stimulatory and inhibitory cytokines, but the activation state of the target cells may dictate what kind of lymphokine will be accepted.

The "decision" of the bifunctional clones as to which suppression or help will be potentiated is possibly made by variable factors associated with the specific parameters of each experimental design. These parameters include the number of the clone regulator cells added to the indicator system.[14] The level of the immunological response of the target cells,[29] the target cells' antigen specificity,[27] the type of the membrane epitopes of the regulator cells activated by the environmental stimuli[33] and the activation state of the target cells.[26,28,34] The key for identifying the bifunctionality of the clones is possibly associated with the fact that the same clone of cells was tested under different experimental conditions.

Furthermore, our findings provide at least a partial explanation to the controversy of the suppressor cell concept. If the assay system of the regulator cells (or the regulator clone) is kept under stable conditions which provide suppression signal only, the investigator would detect "suppressor cells," whereas the enhancement function of the cells (or the clone) would be missed. It is hard to say how many reported observations of suppressor cell (or helper cell) functions may have been misinterpreted just because the cells or the clones were not tested under a variety of experimental conditions.

T cell lines derived from patients with lymphoma or leukemia and presenting a suppressor function,[37] were considered transformed "suppressor T cells." However, the malignant process may block the enhancement function of the transformed cells while leaving the suppressor function unchanged. This event is not obligatory, since the literature documents[53] at least one case where the leukemic cells of a patient with T cell lymphoma (again, with CD4[+] phenotype) simultaneously exhibited both helper and suppressor functions.

In conclusion, the results presented here support the concept that there are interactions between autologous T cells. They extend previous observations of cells interacting specifically, presumably via their TCR, resulting in inhibitory effects.[25,38] Other examples of T—T interactions, such as T cells acting as antigen presenting cells for other T cells, have been reported (e.g., REFS. 54–56). Existence of L3T4 T cells responding to T cell receptors resembling internal images of self-Ia has also been suggested.[57]

This discussion has limited itself to pointing out that CD4[+] bifunctional cells may explain much of the reported literature on suppression. The function of CD8[+] committed "suppressor cells" is not addressed here, although there are reports that cytotoxic[58,59] and suppressor[38] CD8 cells can be cloned. Therefore, we cannot exclude the possibility that the CD8[+] suppressor cells express restricted committment of inhibition. However, such a possibility must be carefully explored by assessing the suppressor function of CD8[+] cells under a variety of experimental conditions. It is important to understand the full committment of cells with suppressive properties because of the possible importance of suppressor function for regulating autoimmune diseases and other disorders related to the immune system. However, before therapeutic trials are initiated we must ask if it is wise to pursue attempts at therapy, based on immune suppression, with the current gaps in our knowledge.

SUMMARY

In contrast to the ease of cloning and characterizing, at the molecular level, helper and cytotoxic T cells, suppressor T cells remain an enigma, and their existence as discrete entities is being increasingly challenged. Here we review evidence that CD4$^+$ regulatory clones, capable of expressing both helper and suppressor functions, may account for much of the suppressor function. It is suggested that a single T cell clone, depending on the signals it receives from its environment, may release either helper or suppressor cytokines. Studying such clones under defined conditions (providing suppressor signals), may preclude detection of their helper capacity. Since some therapeutic approaches in various human diseases are based on the manipulation of helper and suppressor functions, the question whether committed suppressor cells exist has important practical implications in medicine.

REFERENCES

1. MÖLLER, G. 1988. Do suppressor T cells exist? Scand. J. Immunol. **27:** 247–250.
2. JANEWAY JR., G. A. 1988. Do suppressor T cells exist? A reply. Scand. J. Immunol. **27:** 621–623.
3. TADA, T. 1988. But it still moves! An answer to Professor Goran Möller. Scand. J. Immunol. **27:** 623–624.
4. FARNARIER-SEIDEL, C., S. KAPLANSKI, M-M. GOLSTEIN, E. JANCOVICI, J. SAYAG & R. DEPEIDS. 1983. An OKT4$^+$ T-cell population with suppressor activity in Sézary syndrome. Scand. J. Immunol. **18:** 389–398.
5. THEIN, S. L., D. CATOVSKY, D. OSCIER, J. M. GOLDMAN, H. J. VAN DER REIJDEN, C. J. M. MELEIF, H. C. RUMKE, R. J. M. TEN BERGE & A. E. G. K. R. VON DEM BORNE. 1982. T-chronic lymphocytic leukaemia presenting as primary hypogammaglobulinaemia—evidence of a proliferation of T-suppressor cells. Clin. Exp. Immunol. **47:** 670–676.
6. HOFMAN, F. M., D. SMITH & W. HOCKING. 1982. T cell chronic lymphocytic leukaemia with suppressor phenotype. Clin. Exp. Immunol. **49:** 401–409.
7. BLANCKMEISTER, C. A., K. YAMAMOTO, M. M. DAVIS & G. J. HAMMERLING. 1985. Antigen-specific, I-a-restricted suppressor hybridomas with spontaneous cytolytic activity. Functional properties and lack of rearrangement of the T cell receptor β chain genes. J. Exp. Med. **162:** 851–863.
8. FINNEGAN, A. & R. J. HODES. 1986. Antigen-induced T suppressor cells regulate the autoreactive T helper-B cell interaction. J. Immunol. **136:** 793–797.
9. TADA, T. & K. OKUMURA. 1979. The role of antigen-specific T cell factors in the immune response. Adv. Immunol. **28:** 1–87.
10. MILBURN, G. L. & R. G. LYNCH. 1982. Immunoregulation of murine myeloma *in vitro*. II. Suppression of MOPC-315 immunoglobulin secretion and synthesis by idiotype-specific suppressor T cells. J. Exp. Med. **155:** 852–861.
11. BALLIEUX, R. E. & C. J. HEIJNEN. 1983. Immunoregulatory T cell subpopulations in man: dissection by monoclonal antibodies and Fc-receptors. Immunol. Rev. **74:** 5–28.
12. MANGAN, K. F., B. ZIDAR, R. K. SHADDUCK, Z. ZEIGLER & A. WINKELSTEIN. 1985. Interferon-induced aplasia: evidence for T-cell-mediated suppression of hematopoiesis and recovery after treatment with horse antihuman thymocyte globulin. Am. J. Hematol. **19:** 401–413.
13. HEUER, J., K. BRÜNER, B. OPALKA & E. KÖLSCH. 1982. A cloned T-cell line from a tolerant mouse represents a novel antigen-specific suppressor cell type. Nature **296:** 456–459.
14. CLAYBERGER, C., R. H. DEKRUYFF & H. CANTOR. 1984. Immunoregulatory activities of autoreactive T cells: An 1-A-specific T cell clone mediates both help and suppression of antibody responses. J. Immunol. **132:** 2237–2243.

15. SUN, D., Y. QIN, J. CHLUBA, J. T. EPPLEN & H. WEKERLE. 1988. Suppression of experimentally induced autoimmune encephalomyelitis by cytolytic T-T cell interactions. Nature **332:** 843–845.

16. DE SANTIS, R., D. GIVOL, P-L. HSU, L. ADORINI, G. DORIA & E. APPELLA. 1985. Rearrangement and expression of the α- and β-chain genes of the T-cell antigen receptor in functional murine suppressor T-cell clones. Proc. Natl. Acad. Sci. USA **82:** 8638–8642.

17. MODLIN, R. L., M. B. BRENNER, M. S. KRANGEL, A. D. DUBY & B. R. BLOOM. 1987. T-cell receptors of human suppressor cells. Nature **329:** 541–545.

18. HEDRICK, S. M., R. N. GERMAIN, M. J. BEVAN, M. DORF, I. ENGEL, P. FINK, N. GASCOIGNE, E. HEBER-KATZ, J. KAPP, Y. KAUFMANN, J. KAYE, F. MELCHERS, C. PIERCE, R. H. SCHWARTZ, C. SORENSEN, M. TANIGUCHI & M. M. DAVIS. 1985. Rearrangement and transcription of a T-cell receptor β-chain gene in different T-cell subsets. Proc. Natl. Acad. Sci. USA **82:** 531–535.

19. KRONENBERG, M., J. GOVERMAN, R. HAARS, M. MALISSEN, E. KRAIG, L. PHILLIPS, T. DELOVITCH, N. SUCIU-FOCA & L. HOOD. 1985. Rearrangement and transcription of the β-chain genes of the T-cell antigen receptor in different types of murine lymphocytes. Nature **313:** 647–653.

20. MORI, I., A. F. LECOQ, F. ROBBIATI, E. BARBANTI, M. RIGHI, F. SINIGAGLIA, F. CLEMENTI & P. RICCIARDI-CASTAGNOLI. 1985. Rearrangement and expression of the antigen receptor α, β, and γ genes in suppressor antigen-specific T cell lines. EMBO J. **4:** 2025–2030.

21. STEINMETZ, M., K. MINARD, S. HORVATH, J. MCNICHOLAS, J. SRELINGER, C. WAKE, E. LONG, B. MACH & L. HOOD. 1982. A molecular map of the immune response region from the major histocompatibility complex of the mouse. Nature **300:** 35–42.

22. GREEN, R. D., P. M. FLOOD & R. K. GERSHON. 1983. Immunoregulatory T-cell pathways. Ann. Rev. Immunol. **1:** 439–463.

23. DORF, M. E. & B. BENACERRAF. 1984. Suppressor cells and immunoregulation. Ann. Rev. Immunol. **2:** 127–158.

24. FELDMANN, M. & M. H. SCHREIER, EDS. 1982. Monoclonal T Cells and Their Products. Vol. 5. Lymphokines. Academic Press. New York, NY.

25. LAMB, J. R. & M. FELDMANN. 1982. A human suppressor T cell clone which recognizes an autologous helper T cell clone. Nature **300:** 456–458.

26. TITE, J. P. & C. A. JANEWAY, JR. 1984. Cloned helper T cells can kill B lymphoma cells in the presence of specific antigen: Ia restriction and cognate vs. noncognate interactions in cytolysis. Eur. J. Immunol. **14:** 878–886.

27. CHAMPION, B. R., P. HUTCHINGS, S. DAVIES, S. MARSHALL-CLARKE, A. COOKE & I. M. ROITT. 1986. Helper and suppressor activities of an autoreactive mouse thyroglobulin-specific T-cell clone. Immunology **58:** 51–56.

28. KOTANI, H., H. MITSUYA, R. F. JARRETT, G. C. YENOKIDA, S. P. JAMES & W. STROBER. 1986. An autoreactive T cell clone that can be activated to provide both helper and suppressor function. J. Immunol. **136:** 1951–1959.

29. QUINTÁNS, J., H. SUZUKI, J. A. SOSMAN & P. D. SHAH. 1986. Immunoregulation by T cells. I. Characterization of the IE^k-specific Lbd self-reactive T cell clone that helps, suppresses and contrasuppresses B cell responses. J. Immunol. **136:** 1974–1981.

30. SAITO, K., A. TAMURA, H. NARIMATSU, T. TADAKUMA & M. NAGASHIMA. 1986. Cloned auto-Ia-reactive T cells elicit lichen planus-like lesion in the skin of syngeneic mice. J. Immunol. **137:** 2485–2495.

31. TILKIN, A. F., J. MICHON, D. JUY, M. KAYIBANDA, Y. HENIN, G. STERKERS, H. BETUEL & J. P. LEVY. 1987. Autoreactive T cell clones of MHC class II specificities are produced during responses against foreign antigens in man. J. Immunol. **138:** 674–679.

32. SHIOHARA, T., N. H. RUDDLE, M. HOROWITZ, G. E. MOELLMANN & A. B. LERNER. 1987. Anti-tumor activity of class II MHC antigen-restricted cloned autoreactive T cells. I. Destruction of B16 melanoma cells mediated by bystander cytolysis in vitro. J. Immunol. **138:** 1971–1978.

33. ELJAAFARI, A., C. VAQUERO, J. L. TEILLAUD, G. BISMUTH, C. HIVROZ, I. DORVAL,

A. BERNARD & G. STERKERS. 1990. Helper or cytolytic functions can be selectively induced in bifunctional T cell clones. J. Exp. Med. **172:** 213–218.

34. NAOR, D., G. ESSERY, N. TARCIC, M. KAHAN & M. FELDMANN. 1990. Interactions between autologous T cell clones. Cell. Immunol. **128:** 490–502.

35. TARCIC, N. & D. NAOR. 1982. Delayed-type hypersensitivity induced in immunodeficient mice with syngeneic modified self antigens: a suggestive model of autoimmune response. Eur. J. Immunol. **12:** 961–966.

36. NAOR, D. 1979. Suppressor cells: permitters and promoters of malignancy? Adv. Cancer Res. **29:** 45–125.

37. NAOR, D., B. Y. KLEIN, N. TARCIC & J. S. DUKE-COHAN. 1989. Immunosuppression and Human Malignancy. Humana press, Clifton, NJ.

38. MOHAGHEGHPOUR, M., M. K. DAMLE, S. TAKADA & E.G. ENGLEMAN. 1986. Generation of antigen receptor-specific suppressor T cell clones in man. J. Exp. Med, **164:** 950–955.

39. CARREL, S., P. ISLER, M. SCHREYER, A. VACCA, S. SALVI, L. GIUFFRE & J-P. MACH. 1986. Expression on human thymocytes of the idiotypic structures (Ti) from two leukemia T cell lines Jurkat and HPB-ALL. Eur. J. Immunol. **16:** 649–652.

40. BLANCHARD, D., C. VAN ELS, J. BORST, S. CARREL, A. BOYLSTON, J. E. DE VRIES & H. SPITS. 1987. The role of the T cell receptor CD8 and LFA-1 in different stages of the cytolytic reaction mediated by alloreactive T lymphocyte clones. J. Immunol. **138:** 2417–2421.

41. DE BERARDINIS, P., M. LONDEI, S. CARREL & M. FELDMANN. 1988. Regulation of clonal growth by anti-T-cell receptor antibody-directed lysis. Immunology **64:** 439–443.

42. NAOR, D., G. ESSERY, N. TARCIC, P. DE BERARDINIS, M. KAHAN & M. FELDMANN. 1989. Autoreactivity against class I or class II antigens —immunological downregulation mechanism? Bull. Inst. Pasteur **87:** 3–17.

43. NAOR, D., G. ESSERY, M. KAHAN & M. FELDMANN. 1989. T-cell clone anti-clone interactions. Effects on suppressor and helper activities. J. Autoimmun. 2(Suppl.): 3–14.

44. NAOR, D., G. ESSERY, N. TARCIC, M. KAHAN, J. R. LAMB & M. FELDMANN. 1990. Specific interactions between a human CD4+ clone and autologous CD4+ bifunctional immunoregulatory clones. Immunol. Rev. **116:** 63–83.

45. CANTRELL, D. A., A. A. DAVIES, G. KRISSANSEN & M. J. CRUMPTON. 1986. Interactions between protein kinase C and the T3/T cell antigen receptor complex. *In* Regulation of Immune Gene Expression. M. Feldmann & A. McMichael, Eds. 119–133. Humana Press. Clifton, NJ.

46. SAIZAWA, K., J. ROJO & C. A. JANEWAY, JR. 1987. Evidence for a physical association of CD4 and the CD3 : α : βT-cell receptor. Nature **328:** 260–263.

47. MCGARRITY, G. J. 1982. Detection of mycoplasmal infection of cell cultures. Adv. Cell. Culture **2:** 99–131.

48. MILLER, R. G. 1986. The veto phenomenon and T-cell regulation. Immunol Today **7:** 112–114.

49. MOSMANN, T. R., H. CHERWINSKI, M. W. BOND, M. A. GIEDLIN & R. L. COFFMAN. 1986. Two types of murine helper T-cell clone. I. Definition according to profiles of lymphokine activities and secreted proteins. J. Immunol. **136:** 2348–2357.

50. TURNER, M., M. LONDEI & M. FELDMANN. 1987. Human T cells from autoimmune and normal individuals can produce tumor necrosis factor. Eur. J. Immunol. **17:** 1807–1814.

51. YSSEL, H., J. P. AUBRY, R. DE WAAL MALEFIJT, J. E. DE VRIES & H. SPITS. 1987. Regulation by anti-CD2 monoclonal antibody of the activation of a human T cell clone induced by anti-CD3 or anti-T cell receptor antibodies. J. Immunol. **139:** 2850–2855.

52. KEHRL, J. H., L. M. WAKEFIELD, A. B. ROBERTS, S. JAKOWLEW, M. ALVAREZ-MON, R. DERYNCK, M. B. SPORN & A. S. FAUCI. 1986. Production of transforming growth factor β by human T lymphocytes and its potential role in the regulation of T cell growth. J. Exp. Med. **163:** 1037–1050.

53. YAMADA, Y., T. AMAGASAKI, S. KAMIHIRA, K. KINOSHITA, S. IKEDA, M. KUSANO, J. SUZUYAMA, K. TORIYA, Y. TOMONAGA & M. ICHIMARU. 1985. T lymphomas associated with human T-cell leukemia-lymphoma virus may show phenotypic and functional differences from adult T-cell leukemias. Clin. Immunol. Immunopathol. 36: 306–319.

54. LANZAVECCHIA, A., E. ROOSNEK, T. GREGORY, P. BERMAN & S. ABRIGNANI. 1988. T cells can present antigens such as HIV gp120 targeted to their own surface molecules. Nature 334: 530–532.

55. HEWITT, C. R. A. & M. FELDMANN. 1989. Human T cell clones present antigen. J. Immunol. 142: 1429–1436.

56. OTTENHOFF, T. H. M. AND T. MUTIS. 1990. Specific killing of cytotoxic T cells and antigen-presenting cells by CD4+ cytotoxic T cell clones. A novel potentially immunoregulatory T–T cell interaction in man. J. Exp. Med. 171: 2011–2024.

57. NAGARKATTI, P. S., M. NAGARKATTI & A. M. KAPLAN. 1985. Normal lyt-1+2- T cells have the unique capacity to respond to syngeneic autoreactive T cells. Demonstration of a T cell network. J. Exp. Med. 162: 375–380.

58. MORETTA, A., G. PANTALEO L. MORETTA, J-C. CEROTTINI & M. C. MINGARI. 1983. Direct demonstration of the clonogenic potential of every human peripheral blood T cell. Clonal analysis of HLA-DR expression and cytolytic activity. J. Exp. Med. 157: 743–754.

59. MORETTA, A., G. PANTALEO, M. C. MINGARI, L. MORETTA & J-C. CEROTTINI. 1984. Clonal heterogeneity in the requirement for T3, T4, and T8 molecules in human cytolytic T lymphocyte function. J. Exp. Med. 159: 921–934.

Prospects for Immunotherapy Directed to the T Cell Receptor in Human Autoimmune Disease[a]

LAWRENCE STEINMAN

Departments of Neurology and Neurological Sciences,
Pediatrics, and Genetics
Stanford University School of Medicine
Stanford, California 94305-5235

In an animal model of autoimmune demyelinating disease termed experimental allergic encephalomyelitis (EAE), it has been possible to develop highly selective immunotherapy directed to certain T cell receptor (TcR) variable regions on pathogenic T cells.[1-6] TcR V gene expression appears restricted in a similar manner in myelin basic protein (MBP)-specific T cells in the peripheral blood of multiple sclerosis (MS) patients[7-9] and in T cells in demyelinated plaques in MS brain.[10]

Multiple discrete epitopes of myelin basic protein have been defined in the mouse.[11-17] These epitopes are described in TABLE 1.

Several groups have now identified immunogenic epitopes of MBP in MS patients.[7-9] TcR usage in clones recognizing these MBP epitopes is restricted.[7,8]

The identification of activated T cells in the brain of individuals with MS indicates that these cells are critical in the pathogenesis of the disease. In an attempt to elucidate the nature of the lymphocytic infiltration, we used the polymerase chain reaction (PCR) to amplify T cell antigen receptor $V\alpha$ sequences from transcripts derived from MS brain lesions. In each of three MS brains, only two to four rearranged TcR $V\alpha$ transcripts were detected. $V\alpha$ transcripts encoded by the $V\alpha12.1$ region showed rearrangements to a limited number of $J\alpha$ region segments. These results imply that TcR $V\alpha$ gene expression in MS brain lesions is restricted.

$V\beta$ usage has also been studied in plaques from these patients. $V\beta$ usage included TcR $V\beta$ genes 5.1, 7, and 18. Three $V\beta$ genes were expressed in each of these brains.

In various inbred strains of mice and rats, TcR usage in T cell clones recognizing pathogenic epitopes is highly restricted. TcR gene expression of MBP 1–9 specific T cells has been examined[18] in PL/J mice and (SJL/J × PL/J)F1 mice. These TcR sequences are summarized in TABLE 2.

TcR gene expression for MBP 1–9 specific T cells was examined in another H-2^u strain, B10.PL.[19,20] This strain contains the same major histocompatibility complex (MHC), the H-2^u haplotype, on a B10 background. As in PL/J mice, MBP 1–9 is encephalitogenic in B10.PL and p1–9 specific T cells are restricted by I-A^u.[12] Of 33 MBP 1–9 specific hybridomas, 79% utilized $V\beta8.2$ with $J\beta2.7$ (referred to as $J\beta2.6$ or $J\beta2.7$, depending upon whether or not the sixth J gene of the $J\beta2$ cluster, a pseudogene, is considered in the numerical order),[21,22] and 21%

[a] This work was supported by the National Institutes of Health, the National Multiple Sclerosis Society, and the Phil N. Allen Trust.

147

TABLE 1. Multiple Discrete T Cell Epitopes of Myelin Basic Protein

Peptide	Encephalitogenic Potential	Class II Restriction	Vα	Vβ
p1–11	+	Aα^uAβ^u	Vα4.2 Vα2.3	Vβ8.2 Vβ13
p5–16	–	Aα^uAβ^u, Aα^sAβ^u	ND	Vβ8$^+$
p17–27	ND	Aα^sAβ^s	ND	ND
p35–47	+	Eα^uEβ^u, Eα^uEβ^s	ND	Vβ8$^-$
p89–100	+	Aα^sAβ^s	ND	ND
p89–101	+	Aα^sAβ^s	ND	Vβ17
p96–109	+	Aα^sAβ^s	ND	ND

used Vβ13 with Jβ2.2. Although β chain gene usage was very similar to that seen for PL/J p1-9 specific T cell clones, α chain gene expression was somewhat different. In contrast with the PL/J clones analyzed, all having used Vα4.3, of the B10.PL clones examined, 58% used Vα2.3 and 42% expressed Vα4.2. Both Vα2.3 and Vα4.2 bearing T cell hybridomas utilized the same J gene, Jα39.[19,20]

Within PL/J and B10.PL mice, the expression of TcR genes in the MBP p1–9 specific response is quite strikingly limited. However, when comparing TcR gene expression between these two strains, certain differences were apparent. Even though Vβ8.2 is used to the same extent by both strains, it is unclear why Vα2.3, which was not expressed by any of the PL/J clones, was used more frequently than Vα4 in B10.PL mice. Polymorphic differences in TcR gene expression may exist between these strains. Clones expressing different Vα genes may differ in their p1–9/I-A^u affinity. If so, they may differ in their proliferative capability and/or *in vivo* function.

Despite these differences in TcR V gene usage between PL/J and B10.PL mice, in T cell clones recognizing MBP p1–9 in association with I-A^u, there is a striking conservation of amino acid sequences in the Vα-Jα junction and in the Vβ-Dβ-Jβ junction.[18,20]

TABLE 2. Summary of TcR Sequences

Clone	Vβ	Jβ	Vα	Jα
Group 1				
PJB-20	8.2	2.7	4.3	TA31
PJpR-2.2	8.2	2.7	4.3	TA31
PJpR-6.2	8.2	2.7	4.3	TA31
F$_1$-21	8.2	2.7	4.3	TA31
Group 2				
PJR-25	8.2	2.3	4.3	TA31
PJB-18	8.2	2.3	4.3	TA31
Group 3				
PJpR-7.5	8.2	2.5	4.3	TT11
Group 4				
F$_1$-12	4	2.5	4.3	F$_1$-12

The Encephalitogenic C-Terminus

TcR gene usage in the encephalitogenic T cell response of SJL/J mice to the C-terminus has been examined, although not as extensively as for MBP p–9. The T cell response appears more complex. Three encephalitogenic peptides have been identified, p89–101, p89–100, and p96–109.[13–15] TcR $V\beta$ expression has been examined for T cells that respond to p89–101. Approximately 50% of T cells which proliferate to p89–101 also respond to p89–100. The other 50% require Pro101 for stimulation. TcR $V\beta$ gene expression for these two populations has been examined with a monoclonal antibody that recognizes $V\beta$17, a single gene family, expressed by several I-A$^+$/I-E$^-$ strains, including SJL/J.[23,24] Interestingly, all clones that recognize p89–101, but not 89–100, use TcR $V\beta$17. All clones that proliferate to p89–101 are $V\beta$17$^-$.[13] The TcR $V\beta$(s) expressed by $V\beta$17$^-$ clones is not known at this time. Examination of TcR α chain genes and further analysis of the β chain genes is currently in progress.

Examination of susceptibility to EAE in different strains indicates that MHC genotype, and not TcR repertoire, control susceptibility induced with MBP p89–101. H-2^s (I-A^s) strains, SJL/J and A.SW, and H-2^q (I-A^q) strains, SW/R and B10.T(6R) strains that differ in non-MHC genes, are all susceptible to EAE induced with MBP p89–101. Sequence analyses of Aα[25] and Aβ[26] suggest that I-A^s and I-A^q are very similar. Interestingly, SJL/J and SW/R have deleted approximately 50% of their $V\beta$ genes, including $V\beta$8. However, these two strains express $V\beta$17. In contrast, A.SW and B10.T(6R) express $V\beta$8 but not $V\beta$17. Thus, susceptibility in this case does not correlate with the absence of $V\beta$8 or the expression of $V\beta$17. By examination of transgenic mice expressing various "susceptible" class II genes, it may be possible to assess the relative contribution of MHC and TcR repertoire in individual encephalitogenic responses.

Antibodies to TcR V Region Molecules

The monoclonal antibody (mAb) F23.1 depletes $V\beta$8-positive T cells from the peripheral blood.[27] T cells reactive with mAb F23.1 constitute 25% of the T cells in lymph nodes of normal PL/J mice. In the (PLSJ)F1 mouse this percentage is 14%. The depletion of T cells reactive with mAb F23.1 is 98% complete 3 days after intraperitoneal (ip) administration of a dose of 0.5 mg.[18]

EAE was first induced with T cell clone PJR-25. This clone is fully encephalitogenic, capable of inducing paralysis and demyelination.[11,28] PJR-25 expresses the epitope recognized by mAb F23.1.[29] Therapy was begun 24 hr after the mice first developed paralysis. In two experiments (PLSJ)F1 mice were randomly divided into two groups, with 16 mice each receiving two 100-μg injections of F23.1 ip at 72-hr intervals, while 16 mice received mAb Leu 5b (S5.2), an isotype-matched control reactive with the CD2 antigen (a pan T cell marker on human but not on mouse T cells). Within 2–4 days mice receiving F23.1 showed a marked reversal in their paralysis and 13 out of 16 were completely free of disease 10 days after therapy started. Only one relapse with tail weakness was seen, on day 35, in the animals given mAb F23.1.

Next we tested whether EAE induced with p1–11 in complete Freund's adjuvant (CFA) in (PLSJ)F1 mice could be prevented with mAb F23.1. Immunization with MBP peptide p1–11 in CFA can induce clones which are both F23.1-positive and negative, and which are fully encephalitogenic. Successful prevention of disease with F23.1 would indicate that the F23.1-positive T cell clones predomi-

TABLE 3. Prevention of MBP-Peptide p1–11-Induced EAE with mAb F23.1

Monoclonal Antibody[a]	Incidence[b]	Clinical Disease Mean Onset (Day)
F23.1	1/19	20
S5.2	9/20	15[c]

[a] mAbs F23.1 or S5.2 were given ip (500 μg) on days −1, 1 and 9, where immunization with p1–11 was on day 0.

[b] The ratio of number of paralyzed mice to the total number of mice. All mice were examined through day 40.

[c] The standard deviation was 1.7 days.

nate in the development of disease and that the depletion of these T cell clones *in vivo* would not simply result in an escape to F23.1-negative T cell clones that would cause disease. Results shown in TABLE 3 indicate that whereas 1 of 19 mice receiving mAb F23.1 developed EAE, 9 out of 20 mice given mAb S5.2 became paralyzed ($p < 0.001$). These results serve to indicate that the Vβ8-expressing clones function in the induction of EAE.

(PLSJ)F1 mice were immunized with guinea pig MBP. In (PLSJ)F1 mice there are at least two distinct encephalitogenic epitopes for MBP, p1–11 and p35–47. The response to p35–47 is restricted to I-E^u and involves mostly Vβ8-negative T cells. After paralysis was present, mice were given 0.2 mg ip of the mAb F23.1 or KJ23$_a$, a monoclonal antibody specific for the product of the TcR Vβ17$_a$ gene product.[24,25] KJ23$_a$ prevents EAE induced with T cell lines responsive to MBP p89–101 in the SJL mouse. Of 19 (PLSJ)F1 mice given F23.1, 12 returned to normal within 72 hr, while 21 of 22 mice given KJ23$_a$ had moderate to severe paraplegia after 72 hrs (TABLE 4). Relapses were seen in 5 of 19 F23.1-treated mice in the next 14 days. Thus, treatment with F23.1 reversed EAE in a situation where multiple encephalitogenic epitopes were present. Vβ8-negative T cells capable of responding to MBP p1–11 or p35–47 may have accounted for the relapses seen in the F23.1-treated mice.

In contrast, the SJL(I-A^s) mouse strain recognizes a peptide from MBP (p89–101) with at least three overlapping epitopes. There is evidence for limited TcR gene usage in recognition of one of these epitopes.[14] However, depletion of this subset of T cells did not prevent antigen-induced EAE; elimination of a single Vβ subset, in a polyclonal autoimmune disease such as this, may not be sufficient to prevent or reverse disease. A cocktail of monoclonal antibodies might be necessary.[13]

TABLE 4. Reversal of Guinea Pig MBP-Induced EAE with mAb F23.1

Treatment[a]	Number of Mice with Clinical Symptoms 72 Hr after Treatment[b]			Number of Mice with Clinical Symptoms 14 Days after Treatment			
	None	Mild	Severe	None	Mild	Severe	Deaths
F23.1	12	5	2	14	3	1	1
KJ23a	1	12	9	9	2	7	4

[a] Treatment was begun 24 hr after mice exhibited EAE. At this time the mice were separated randomly into two groups. Mice in each group received one 200 μg ip injection of F23.1 or S5.2. Nineteen mice received F23.1 and 22 mice received KJ23a.

[b] Clinical status was graded as follows: *none,* no neurologic symptoms; *mild,* flaccid tail and/or mild paraparesis; *severe,* severe paraparesis or complete paraplegia.

Vaccination to TcR V Regions

Cohen and associates have shown that it is possible to use autoimmune T cell clones or lines as vaccines to prevent or reverse autoimmune disease. An inoculum of T cell clones below the threshold for triggering disease, or irradiated, fixed, or pressure-treated T cells can serve as vaccines.[30–33] These animals remain free of disease for prolonged times, and EAE could not be induced with T cell lines, with T cell clones, or with MBP in adjuvant. T cell clones specific for EAE-inducing T cells have been isolated from rats that recovered from EAE, suggesting an anti-idiotypic mechanism for protection. These T cell clones are either CD4[+] or CD8[+]. The CD8[+] T cells lyse their targets specifically, and this cytotoxicity is not blockable with anti-CD4, anti-CD8, anti-class I or anti-class II antibodies. Recently, EAE in the Lewis rat was prevented by immunization with a nonapeptide spanning the V-D-J region of $V\beta8$, expressed on about three fourths of T cell clones recognizing encephalitogenic MBP p72–86.[34] Vandenbark and associates protected against EAE with a peptide from the CDR2 region of $V\beta8$.[35]

Thus, the feasibility of highly selective therapies directed to certain TcR's involved in the pathogenesis of EAE has been established. Recent data on TcR gene usage in MS brain lesions and in MBP-specific T cell clones raises the possibility of applying these approaches to humans with MS.

REFERENCES

1. ACHA-ORBEA, H., L. STEINMAN & H. O. MCDEVITT. 1989. T cell receptors in murine autoimmune disease. Annu. Rev. Immunol. 7: 371–405.
2. ZAMVIL, S. & L. STEINMAN. 1990. The T lymphocyte in autoimmune encephalomyelitis. Annu. Rev. Immunol. 8: 579–621.
3. MCDEVITT, H. O., D. C. WRAITH, D. SMILEK, W. LUNDBERG & L. STEINMAN. 1989. Evolution, function and utilization of major histocompatibility complex polymorphism in autoimmune disease. Cold Spring Harbor Symp. Quant. Biol. 853–857.
4. STEINMAN, L. 1991. The development of rational strategies for selective immunotherapy against autoimmune demyelinating disease. Adv. Immunol. In press.
5. STEINMAN, L. Multiple sclerosis and its animal models: the role of the major histocompatibility complex and the T cell receptor repertoire. Springer Semin. Immunopathol. Immunogenet. Autoimmunity. H. O. McDevitt, Ed. In press.
6. WRAITH, D. & L. STEINMAN. New approaches to immunotherapy. Springer Semin. Immunopathol. Immunogenet. Autoimmunity. H. O. McDevitt, Ed. In press.
7. WUCHERPFENNIG, K., K. OTA, N. ENDO, J. G. SEIDMAN, A. ROSENZWEIG, H. L. WEINER & D. A. HAFLER. 1990. Shared human T cell receptor $V\beta$ usage to immunodominant regions of myelin basic protein. Science 248: 1016–1019.
8. OTA, K., M. MATSUI, E. MILDORD, G. MACKIN, H. L. WEINER & D. A. HAFLER. 1990. T cell recognition of an immunodominant myelin basic protein epitope in multiple sclerosis. Nature 346: 183–187.
9. MARTIN, R., D. JARAQUEMADA, M. FLERLAGE, J. RICHERT, J. WHITAKER, E. O. LONG, D. E. MCFARLIN & H. MCFARLAND. 1990. Fine specificity and HLA restriction of MBP-specific cytotoxic T cell lines from MS patients and healthy individuals. J. Immunol. 145: 540–548.
10. OKSENBERG, J. R., S. STUART, A. B. BEGOVICH, R. B. BELL, H. ERLICH, L. STEINMAN & C. C. A. BERNARD. 1990. Limited heterogeneity of rearranged T cell receptor transcripts in brains of multiple sclerosis patients. Nature 345: 344–346.
11. ZAMVIL, S., P. NELSON, D. MITCHELL, R. KNOBLER, R. FRITZ & L. STEINMAN. 1985. Encephalitogenic T cell clones specific for myelin basic protein: an unusual bias in antigen presentation. J. Exp. Med. 162: 2107–2124.
12. ZAMVIL, S. S., D. J. MITCHELL, A. C. MOORE, K. KITAMURA, L. STEINMAN & J.

ROTHBARD. 1986. T cell epitope of the autoantigen myelin basic protein that induces encephalomyelitis. Nature **324:** 258–260.

13. SAKAI, K., A. SINHA, D. J. MITCHELL, S. S. ZAMVIL, H. O. McDEVITT, J. B. ROTHBARD & L. STEINMAN. 1988. Involvement of distinct T cell receptors in the autoimmune encephalitogenic response to nested epitopes of myelin basic protein. Proc. Natl. Acad. Sci. USA **85:** 8608–8612.

14. SAKAI, K., S. S. ZAMVIL, D. J. MITCHELL, M. LIM, J. B. ROTHBARD & L. STEINMAN. 1988. Characterization of a major encephalitogenic T cell epitope in SJL/J mice with synthetic oligopeptides of myelin basic protein. J. Neuroimmunol. **19:** 21–32.

15. KONO, D. H., J. L. URBAN, S. J. HORVATH, D. G. ANDO, R. A. SAAVEDRA & L. HOOD. 1988. Two minor determinants of myelin basic protein induce experimental allergic encephalomyelitis in SJL/J mice. J. Exp. Med. **168:** 213–227.

16. FRITZ, R. B., M. J. SKEEN, C.-H. J. CHOU & S. S. ZAMVIL. Localization of an encephalitogenic epitope for the SJL mouse in the N-terminal region of myelin basic protein. J. Neuroimmunol. In press.

17. SAKAI, K., D. J. MITCHELL, S. J. HODGKINSON, S. S. ZAMVIL, J. B. ROTHBARD & L. STEINMAN. 1989. Prevention of experimental encephalomyelitis with peptides that block interaction of T cells with major histocompatibility complex proteins. Proc Natl. Acad. Sci. USA **86:** 9470–9474.

18. ACHA-ORBEA, H., D. J. MITCHELL, L. TIMMERMAN, D. C. WRAITH, M. K. WALDOR, G. S. TAUSCH, S. S. ZAMVIL, H. O. McDEVITT & L. STEINMAN. 1988. Limited heterogeneity of T cell receptors from lymphocytes mediating autoimmune encephalomyelitis allows specific immune intervention. Cell **54:** 263–273.

19. URBAN, J. L., V. KUMAR, D. H. KONO, C. GOMEZ, S. J. HORVATH, J. CLAYTON, D. G. ANDO, E. E. SERCARZ & L. HOOD. 1988. Restricted use of T cell receptor V genes in murine autoimmune encephalomyelitis raises possibilities for antibody therapy. Cell **54:** 577–592.

20. KUMAR, V., D. H. KONO, J. L. URBAN & L. E. HOOD. 1989. The T cell receptor repertoire and autoimmune diseases. Annu. Rev. Immunol. **7:** 657–682.

21. BURT, D. S., K. H. G. MILLS, J. J. SKEHEL & D. B. THOMAS. 1989. Diversity of the class II (I-I^u/I-E^k)-restricted T cell repertoire and influenza hemaglutinin and antigenic drift. Six nonoverlapping epitopes on HA1 subunit are defined by synthetic peptides. J. Exp. Med. **170:** 383–397.

22. FINK, P. J., L. A. MATIS, D. L. McELLINGOTT, M. BOOKMAN & S. M. HEDRICK. 1986. Correlation between T cell specificity and the structure of the antigen receptor. Nature **32:** 219–226.

23. KAPPLER, J. W., T. WADE, J. WHITE, E. KUSHNIR, M. BLACKMAN, J. BILL, N. ROEHM & P. MARRACK. 1987. A T cell receptor Vβ segment that imparts reactivity to a class II major histocompatibility complex product. Cell **49:** 263–271.

24. KAPPLER, J. W., N. ROEHM & P. MARRACK. 1987. T cell tolerance by clonal elimination in the thymus. Cell **49:** 273–280.

25. BENOIST, C. O., D. J. MATHIS, H. R. KANTER, V. E. WILLIAMS & H. O. McDEVITT. 1983. Regions of allelic hypervariability in the murine Aα immune response gene. Cell **34:** 169–177.

26. ESTESS, P., A. B. BEGOVICH, M. KOO, P. P. JONES & H. O. McDEVITT. 1986. Sequence analysis and structure-function correlations of murine q, k, u, s, and f haplotype I-Aβ cDNA clones. Proc. Natl. Acad. Sci. USA **83:** 3594–3598.

27. BEHLKE, M. A., T. J. HENKEL, S. J. ANDERSON, N. C. LAN, L. HOOD, V. L. BRACIALE, T. J. BRACIALE & D. LOH. 1987. Expression of a murine polyclonal T cell receptor marker correlates with the use of specific members of the Vβ8 gene segment subfamily. J. Exp. Med. **165:** 257–262.

28. ZAMVIL, S., P. NELSON, J. TROTTER, D. MITCHELL, R. KNOBLER, R. FRITZ & L. STEINMAN. 1985. T cell clones specific for myelin basic protein induce chronic relapsing EAE and demyelination. Nature **317:** 355.

29. ZAMVIL, S. S., P. A. NELSON, L. STEINMAN & D. J. MITCHELL. 1989. Treatment of autoimmune encephalomyelitis with an antibody to T cell receptor β chain. In Cellular Basis of Immune Modulation. J. G. Kaplen, D. G. Green & R. C. Bleackley, Eds. 461–464. Alan Liss. New York.

30. BEN-NUN, A., H. WEKERLE & I. R. COHEN. 1981. Vaccination against autoimmune encephalomyelitis with T lymphocyte line reactive against myelin basic protein. Nature 292: 60–61.
31. HOLOSHITZ, J., Y. NAPARSTEK, A. BEN-NUN & I. R. COHEN. 1983. Lines of T lymphocytes induce or vaccinate against autoimmune arthritis. Science 219: 56–58.
32. MARON, R., R. ZERUBAVEL, A. FRIEDMANN & I. R. COHEN. 1983. T lymphocyte line specific for thyroglobulin produces or vaccinates against autoimmune thyroiditis in mice. J. Immunol. 131: 2316–2322.
33. LIDER, O., T. RESHEF, E. BERAUD, A. BEN-NUN & I. R. COHEN. Anti-idiotypic network induced by T cell vaccination against experimental autoimmune encephalomyelitis. Science 239: 181–183.
34. HOWELL, M. D., S. T. WINTERS, T. OLEE, H. C. POWELL, D. J. CARLO & S. BROSTOFF. 1989. Vaccination against experimental allergic encephalomyelitis with T cell receptor peptides. Science 246: 668–670.
35. VANDENBARK, A. A., G. HASHIM & H. OFFNER. 1989. Immunization with a synthetic T cell receptor V-region peptide protects against experimental autoimmune encephalomyelitis. Nature 341: 541–544.

Photopheresis: a Clinically Relevant Immunobiologic Response Modifier

RICHARD L. EDELSON

Department of Dermatology
Yale University School of Medicine
333 Cedar Street
500 LCI
P.O. Box 3333
New Haven, Connecticut 06510-8059

Whereas several presenters at this symposium discuss clinical and basic studies of photopheresis in detail, it is my intention to provide a broad overview of this subject. Photopheresis is an immune response modifier which has shown substantial efficacy in a number of disorders and is distinguished by two attractive features: the relatively limited observed adverse effects and the specificity of control obtained over pathogenic T cell clones.

Evidence has been rapidly accumulating which indicates that the human immune system, even when inundated by very large numbers of disease-provoking T cells, can be immunized against these cells in such a way by photopheresis that certain otherwise progressive disorders can be suppressed and even controlled. By bringing a large number of investigators together who have contributed to this subject, it is hoped that they and others will be further stimulated to contemplate, to investigate and to implement the concept that clinicians may be able to harness the power of the immune system to control serious diseases.

Photopheresis, which is now approved by the Food and Drug Administration for the treatment of cutaneous T cell lymphoma (mycosis fungoides, Sezary syndrome and related presentations), is showing substantial promise in a variety of autoimmune disorders and is operative in over 70 centers in the United States and abroad. Hence, it is appropriate to review its status and to highlight several relevant practical issues. This paper will serve as a clinical update and will summarize our growing knowledge as to how photopheresis works.

At the outset, it would be helpful to briefly discuss the origin of the concept that diseases caused by expanded populations of pathogenic T cells can be effectively treated by extracorporeal photochemotherapy. Since the clinicians who have been using photopheresis have expertise in the relevant disease areas, but may not be experts in experimental immunology, it is appropriate to provide this overview in terms that are readily comprehensible. The papers in this volume by Gasparro, Berger, Perez, Laroche and their co-workers discuss the actual experimentation in greater detail.

This work evolved from an awareness that current approaches to the treatment of disorders of the immune system are often quite nonspecific and toxic. The human body normally regulates the expansion and suppression of each of the several million distinct clones of T cells which form the core of the immune system, clone by clone, permitting the rapid mobilization of those T cells necessary for anti-microbial defenses, but inhibiting the activity of the same cells when their efforts are no longer required. In comparison, our most commonly used tools for treatment of disorders of the lymphocyte or immune system are extremely crude. Corticosteroids, antimetabolites and cyclosporin A do not discriminate between individual clones of pathogenic and benign T cells and lead to many documented side effects. Bioengineered molecules, including monoclonal antibodies and cytokines, will certainly find niches in our therapeutic armamentarium, but as used are generally nonspecific and affect many types of target cells. In short, none of these therapeutic agents approximates the efficiency with which the normal body deals with its own T cells.

Mechanism Underlying Response to Photopheresis

A far more desirable approach would be the development of a way of dealing directly with the clones of T cells which actually cause a disease, while sparing the innocent clones. Studies in experimental animals, largely conducted by Irun Cohen and his colleagues at the Weizmann Institute in Israel over the past decade, suggested that this goal may well be attainable.[1,2] Those researchers found that physically altered pathogenic T cells can be presented to an animal in such a manner that, instead of causing disease, they actually "vaccinate" against the development of the illness. The experimental animal system which they used most extensively is experimental autoimmune encephalomyelitis (EAE).

EAE can be induced in rodents by immunizing them with basic myelin protein extracted from the central nervous system of guinea pigs and presented to the rate in complete Freund's adjuvant, a preparation which markedly enhances efficiency of immunization.[3] Virtually all of the rats so treated develop an acute paralytic syndrome, which is frequently fatal and which is associated with a T cell infiltration of the central nervous system. That the disease is caused by T cells which specifically react against basic myelin protein has been demonstrated by the extraction from affected rats of such T cells, clonal expansion of these cells *in vitro* and introduction of these anti-basic myelin protein T cells into healthy rats. The rat recipients of these anti-basic myelin protein T cells then develop a florid EAE, even though they themselves were not immunized with basic myelin protein.

Cohen's group then made the seminal observation that resistance to the subsequent development of EAE could be induced by first vaccinating potential recipients against the otherwise pathogenic anti-basic myelin protein T cells. This was accomplished by first treating the pathogenic cloned T cells in ways (glutaraldehyde, hydrostatic pressure) that more efficiently exposed cell surface antigens that distinguished the anti-basic myelin protein T cells from other syngeneic T cells. Their data suggested, but did not definitively prove, that the most likely T cell surface structures leading to the observed effects were derived from the T cell receptors (TCR) for specific foreign antigen. T cells react with foreign antigens in a manner analogous to the way that antibodies bind to appropriate antigenic moieties. T cells accomplish this via membrane receptors, unique to each clone of T cells, capable of binding antigens presented in the context of class I or class II histocompatibility molecules. Cells of each T cell clone bear a clone-specific receptor, composed of two disulfide-linked protein chains with distinctive amino acid sequences.[4] The physical properties of these receptors confer specific binding capabilities and permit each of the several million clones of T cells to operate independently.

One of the ways that the normal immune system regulates the proliferation of individual clones of T cells is to single out the T cells on the basis of the T cell receptor for antigen. Antibodies and cellular responses are produced which selectively target the T cell receptor of the relevant T cell clone. Since the TCR of each clone is distinguished by its own distinct amino acid sequence, it is also uniquely antigenic. It appeared that Cohen's team had identified several ways to make the anti-basic myelin protein T cell receptor sufficiently antigenic so that when the treated cells were introduced into rats, the animals developed such a strong clone-specific immunologic response that subsequently infused viable pathogenic T cells of the same clone were either destroyed or inhibited. When these animals were appropriately pretreated, it was not possible to induce in them florid EAE. Since it was possible to induce in them other autoimmune disease by the introduction of different syngeneic clones of T cells, it was clear that the effect was truly clone-specific.

Those studies were of critical importance in clearly demonstrating that it is possible to vaccinate against the activity of pathogenic clones of T cells. However, three major obstacles needed to be negotiated before it would be possible to extend these observations to the treatment of humans with diseases caused by expanded clones of malignant or autoreactive T cells. First, the techniques employed by Cohen's group (glutaraldehyde, hydrostatic pressure) were not readily applicable to reinfusable human blood. Second, patients invariably present with disease, not prior to developing illness. Hence, it needed to be demonstrated that vaccination against T cell activity could be effective even in the face of progressive disease, rather than prophylactically as in the rat system. Finally, in virtually all autoimmune diseases and even in many patients with cutaneous T cell lymphoma, it is not possible to accurately identify or isolate the pathogenic clone(s). Therefore, the only plausible way to proceed was to deal with the intact patient's whole blood in the hope that the pathogenic clone(s) would be sufficiently expanded compared to all other individual clones of normal T cells that *in vitro* cloning would not be required. Fortunately, at least partial solutions to each of these challenges were forthcoming.

The clinically impractical glutaraldehyde and hydrostatic pressure approaches were replaced by use of ultraviolet A (UVA)-activated 8-methoxypsoralen (8-MOP). Several features distinguish psoralen compounds from nearly all other clinically useful drugs.[5,6] First, in the absence of light they are safe and, in fact, without known biologic function. Second, upon activation by ultraviolet energy, they exhibit an exceptional ability to covalently bind to target molecules in a manner which severely interrupts cellular function. Third, the type of ultraviolet energy, ultraviolet A or UVA, which photoactivates psoralens, is capable of passing through clear plate glass and certain plastics and is of lower energy than ultraviolet B, which causes sunburn and generally does not pass through those materials. Fourth, once photoactivated, the transiently energized psoralen molecules remain reactive for microseconds (millionths of a second), long enough to be chemically reactive and short enough so that, for practical purposes, once the light source is turned off, unbound psoralen reverts to its inert form. In essence, psoralens provide the clinician with pharmacologic agents with high chemotherapeutic potency, but only where and when the psoralens come in contact with light of appropriate wavelength. Compounds of this group, therefore, offer a completely directed form of chemotherapy.

In 1953, Lerner and Fitzpatrick demonstrated that a concentrated oral form of 8-methoxypsoralen (8-MOP) had a high therapeutic index.[7] In 1973, Voorhees *et al.* found that topically applied psoralen followed by sunlight improved some patients with psoriasis.[8] Psoriatic epidermal cells actually divide more rapidly than do cells of most cancers but are not malignant, since they do not invade normal tissues and can be returned to normal behavior patterns by effective therapy. In 1974, Parrish and colleagues led a multiinstitutional group which found that orally administered 8-MOP followed by total skin exposure to high intensity UVA was quite effective in clearing extensive psoriatic lesions which had otherwise been quite resistant to other treatments.[9]

During that same period of time, Gilchrest and co-workers found that localized skin lesions of cutaneous T cell lymphoma (CTCL) resolved in response to the same regimen.[10] CTCL is the most common adult malignancy of T lymphocytes and usually has an initial phase characterized by skin lesions containing large numbers of the malignant cells.[11] These clinical observations occurred in the context of a series of laboratory studies which revealed that human T lymphocytes were quite sensitive to the combined effects of 8-MOP and UVA.[12,13] Furthermore, it was known that up to twenty-five percent of the blood supply passes through blood vessels of the skin and that UVA is capable of penetrating the full thickness of the skin, in attenuated amounts. Hence, large numbers of circulating T cells must have been exposed to both UVA and 8-MOP during psoriasis treatments, and yet serious systemic sequelae to the immune system had not been reported. Although approximately two percent of psoriatic patients treated repetitively with UVA and 8-MOP developed low grade skin cancers, no increased numbers of patients with malignancies of white blood cells or increased susceptibility to infection were recognized among the thousands of subjects followed prospectively.

At the same time that the original multicenter trial of photopheresis in the treatment of CTCL was being performed, from 1982 to 1985, the above-mentioned completely independent experimental studies with EAE were being conducted in Cohen's laboratory at the Weitzmann Institute. Our early clinical observations, which will be discussed later in this paper, had indicated quite clearly that the reinfusion of the photodamaged malignant T cells was inducing a response in the patient that was able to target in certain patients the residual malignant cells, while apparently sparing T cells of other normal clones. This suggested to us and to Cohen that the mechanism underlying both his animal and our clinical studies might be the same.

To test this possibility, Khavari from our group spent several months in Israel with Cohen's group comparing 8-MOP's capacity to lead to an effect in his EAE vaccination system with the Weitzmann Institute's glutaraldehyde and hydrostatic pressure approaches.[14] Two syngeneic helper/inducer T cell clones were used: the anti-myelin basic protein (MBP) clone, designated "Zs," which *in vivo* caused EAE, and the A2b anti-tuberculin clone which did not. The only recognized phenotypic difference between cells of these two clones was the composition of their T cell receptors for antigen.

Those studies demonstrated that photoactivated 8-MOP under pharmacologic conditions equivalent to those used in the photopheresis procedure was more efficient than either glutaraldehyde or hydrostatic pressure in vaccinating the rats against the individual T cell clones. After *ex vivo* exposure of the Zs clone to photoactivated 8-MOP and introduction of these otherwise treated T cells to immunologically naive animals, the recipients became resistant to the capacity of viable Zs cells to cause EAE. This resistance substantially exceeded that obtained when the Zs cells were first treated *ex vivo* with glutaraldehyde or hydrostatic pressure. Whereas up to 80 percent of those rats vaccinated with Zs cells pretreated in these other ways succumbed to EAE, none of the animals vaccinated with the 8-MOP pretreated cells did.

The great specificity of the system was further established by the observation that rats vaccinated against isolated cell membranes from 8-MOP-treated Zs T cells developed a delayed hypersensitivity reaction against Zs cells but not against A2b cells. Similarly, rats vaccinated against A2b cell membranes developed a delayed hypersensitivity reaction against only A2b cells.

These findings were provocative, because they suggested that the extraordinarily titratable 8-MOP impact on target cells efficiently altered the exposed cells to initiate a cascade of events culminating in their becoming more immunogenic against their own distinct antigens. Although the precise identification of the mechanisms leading to this effect and the clear identification of the target molecules of the immune response have not yet been accomplished, it is noteworthy that the induced immunologic reaction is able to distinguish between two cell types known only to differ in their T cell receptors. The EAE system is an artificial one, since the disorder is experimentally produced by isolatable T cell clones. In contrast, it is likely that most autoimmune disorders are caused by several clones of T cells, not currently isolatable or even identifiable. Nevertheless, this reductionist system provided strong encouragement to proceed to other experimental models which might have more relevance to the human disease situation.

Carole Berger, Maritza Perez and Liliane Laroche at Columbia and Yale Universities made additional major observations in other experimental systems[15,16] that were subsequently developed and are discussed in detail elsewhere in this volume. They observed that the systemic lupus erythematosus-like disease which spontaneously develops in the inbred strain of MRL mice could be prevented or slowed by vaccinating young mice of that strain, prior to development of disease, with unfractionated 8-MOP/UVA-treated spleen lymphocytes from old diseased mice. These mice are clinically and serologically normal at birth but by early adulthood develop markedly elevated anti-native DNA antibodies, renal disease, splenomegaly and massive lymphadenopathy. Berger and associates found that introduction of 8-MOP/UVA treated cells from diseased adults into young not yet diseased MRL mice prevented development of the anti-DNA antibodies, greatly decreased splenomegaly and lymphadenopathy and significantly prolonged survival times. Similarly, rejection of skin allografts from unrelated mice could be greatly impeded by vaccinating potential recipients with unfractionated 8-MOP/UVA treated splenocytes from animals undergoing rejection of genetically identical skin grafts, while allografts from a third strain of mouse genetically distinct from either of the first two still underwent rapid rejection. In separate experiments, described in this volume by Laroche, a T cell response to sheep erythrocytes was similarly prevented by vaccination with unfractionated splenocytes from animals already manifesting the immunologic response against the same antigen, while the response to the unrelated antigens on chicken erythrocytes was unaffected. In both the allograft and anti-sheep red blood cell systems, the inhibition of the relevant immunologic response was shown to be transferable by T lymphocytes.

The power of this approach to control the anti-allograft or anti-sheep red blood cell reactions was indicated by the capacity of this "T cell vaccination" to occur in the absence of any other manipulation of the immune system. The specificity of the approach was revealed by the limitation of the induced inhibition to the reaction against only the relevant antigens.

The principal importance of these observations was that one could vaccinate against a particular T cell activity without actually isolating or even identifying the clone(s) responsible for the activity. The splenocyte populations in each of these experimental systems contained markedly expanded clones of T cells capable of either causing the lupus-like syndrome, mediating rejection of a particular skin graft or reacting to a certain foreign antigen. The results suggest that even though these expanded T cell clones were admixed with many smaller irrelevant clones, the body was able to selectively react immunologically against the expanded clones. We suggest that sufficient numbers of photoinactivated effector T or "PET" cells had been altered to lead to an immunologic reaction against them after their infusion, while the relatively small numbers of exposed T cells in each of the multitude of irrelevant clones were perhaps below the threshold of the immune system to react to their distinctive membrane antigens. Apparently, the resultant immunologic reaction was also effective against residual cells of the same expanded clone. That likelihood raised the provocative possibility that it might be possible to initiate a similar beneficial immunoregulatory cascade by extracorporeally exposing human blood, containing expanded populations of disease-provoking T cells mixed with a multitude of much smaller clones of passenger normal T cells, to 8-MOP/UVA and then returning the photodamaged white blood cell mix to the patient.

Clinical Trials

The highly refined apparatus necessary to perform this extracorporeal procedure, known now as "photopheresis," was developed by engineers at Therakos, Inc., a subsidiary of Johnson and Johnson, Inc. The procedure involves an initial centrifugation step to enrich for lymphocytes, followed by an ultraviolet exposure step.

Several further developmental steps were required prior to beginning a clinical trial of photopheresis. First, we needed to determine the optimal conditionals for the procedure. Since psoriasis patients readily tolerated blood levels of 50 to 200 nanograms of 8-MOP per milliliter of blood,[9] we elected to administer the drug orally in exactly the same dosage as given them. Having found that cell division by T cells could be almost completely blocked by 1 to 2 joules per square centimeter of UVA energy in the presence of 100 nanograms per milliliter of 8-MOP, we chose to expose the blood cells to this amount of energy.

The weakness of the UVA energy, an advantage in minimizing side effects on other blood components, required an extremely thin blood film in the exposure system: in the currently-used third generation apparatus, blood is passed at a film thickness of only 1 millimeter between two high intensity UVA energy sources, translating to maximal distance between targeted T cells and incident UVA of only 0.5 millimeters. The total volume of patient blood transiently outside the body during the treatment is approximately one unit or 500 milliliters, the same volume which an individual typically donates to a blood bank.

To titrate the amount of UVA impinging on the average T cell passing through the system to that which we had previously determined to be optimal for T cell inactivation, Gasparro and Santella of our group produced monoclonal antibodies which recognized 8-MOP-DNA photoadducts in irradiated cells and permitted their quantification.[17] From predetermined dose-response curves, we found that 150 minutes of UVA exposure in the photopheresis apparatus were necessary to reach our goal of close to 2 joules per square centimeter of irradiation.

In order to justify using such an experimental modality, the first patients treated with this approach needed to fulfill certain requirements. They had to have a seriously debilitating and dangerous disease, unresponsive to standard therapy, caused by circulating T lymphocytes. The disease selected, the leukemic variant of cutaneous T cell lymphoma (CTCL), is characterized by massive expansion of a malignant clone of helper T cells. Those malignant T cells circulate between the skin, which they infiltrate in such a manner that the total surface of that organ is red and swollen, and other body tissues via the blood and lymphatic vessels.[11] This phase of CTCL is not only debilitating but is associated with a median expected survival, when treated by standard means, of less than three years, with patients succumbing to opportunistic infections or destruction of vital organs by the malignant cells, as revealed by a multicenter prospective clinical study.[18]

We used a conservative regimen: photophoresis on two successive days at monthly intervals, a protocol initially intended merely to establish the toxicity of the new procedure. We recognized that such a low frequency of treatments would permit irradiation of less than 10 percent of the total body burden of malignant cells, since so many of them were harbored in the skin and lymphoid tissues, and anticipated that once the safety of the procedure was established we would need to substantially increase the frequency of treatments. It, therefore, astonished us to see that four of the first five patients responded after only 6 to 10 treatments and that eventually the severely involved skin of two of these patients cleared completely. This exceptional level of response, not noted with far more intensive cell removal by standard leukapheresis, extended the experimental rodent studies by suggesting that the body's immunologic response to the reinfused UVA-irradiated T cells was leading to a profound clinical response.

A multiinstitutional study was then organized, with advice from the Food and Drug Administration, to expand the numbers of patients.[19] At the medical centers of Columbia University, University of Pennsylvania, University of California in San Francisco, University of Pittsburgh, Yale University, University of Vienna and University of Düsseldorf, a group of 37 patients with erythrodermic CTCL unresponsive to standard therapy were treated and 27 responded, including 9 with complete or nearly complete clearing of the skin infiltration. Responders included 20 of 26 subjects with histologically demonstrated lymph node involvement.

These clinical responses in a disorder otherwise known to be extremely resistant to conventional chemotherapy were quite noteworthy. Furthermore, as compared to standard chemotherapy, the systemic side effects were minimal and in no instance prevented continuation of the treatments. Approximately 10% of the patients experienced a fever following the reinfusion of the damaged cells, but this febrile response completely resolved within 24 hours. Other problems, often associated with leukapheresis (increased susceptibility to infection and depletion of other blood elements) or with standard chemotherapy of CTCL (bone marrow suppression, hair loss, intestinal bleeding from erosions, severe nausea), were rarely experienced. However, the follow-up period has so far been too short to permit recognition of long-term side effects, and it remains possible that idiosyncratic adverse reactions will be recognized as larger groups of patients are treated now that the procedure has received approval from the FDA for management of advanced CTCL.

The efficacy of photopheresis in management of erythrodermic, and possibly certain plaque stage, CTCL patients, has been confirmed by two independent reports.[20,21] Elsewhere in this volume, Heald reports on our extended experience in CTCL with the modality and provides important survival data. The original multicenter trial revealed the efficacy of photopheresis in inducing prolonged reductions in tumor burdens in responding erythrodermic CTCL patients, but was too short to identify long-term effects. The report of Heald et al. indicates that the survival of the treated erythrodermic patients was doubled, to more than 60 months, over the 30 months obtained from the concurrent prospective Mycosis Fungoides Cooperative Group (MFCG) for the same phase of the disease.[18] Since the erythrodermic CTCL patients admitted to the photopheresis trial were all treatment failures by at least one standard modality and the patients in the MFCG group were not, it appears that the comparison between survival data from the two parallel studies is biased against the photopheresis data, underscoring the significance of the photopheresis findings. This is the first demonstration of prolongation of lifespan in patients with extracutaneous CTCL, since standard chemotherapy and radiotherapy in combination have not increased longevity.[22]

In CTCL patients with tumors or extensive thickly infiltrated plaques, we are now attempting to use photopheresis to maintain post electron beam remissions, since the chemotherapeutic alternatives have quite limited efficacy and major attendant side effects. Prospective analysis of the results obtained in this population of patients will determine whether the optimism generated by our preliminary observations in this clinical situation is warranted.

TABLE 1. Photopheresis Centers

United States

University of Pennsylvania	Yale University
University of California, San Francisco	University of Pittsburgh
Medical College of Wisconsin	Henry Ford Hospital
Boston University	University of Michigan
University of Texas, Dallas	Mayo Clinic
Stanford University	Therapeutic Immunology
M.D. Anderson, Houston	Scripps Clinic
Kenneth Noris Cancer Center	Mt. Sinai, New York
University of Southern California	Ochsner Foundation
University of Indiana	Duke University
University of Iowa	Vanderbilt University
University of Maryland	Morristown Memorial
University of Nebraska	New York University
Columbia University	Thomas Jefferson Hospital
University of Minnesota	Georgetown University
Hemacare	Washington Hospital Center
Hahnemann, Philadelphia	Mt. Sinai, Florida
Huntington Hospital	Oregon University
Cleveland Clinic	University of Cleveland
Cedars Medical Center	Tulane University
Morristown Hospital	Grandview Hospital
Medical University of South Carolina	University of Alabama
Southwest Florida Blood Center	Civitan Blood Center
United Blood Services	United Hospital, ND
Wishard Memorial Hospital	Riverside Hospital, Dayton
Good Samaritan Hospital, Los Angeles	Oklahoma Blood Center
Harper Hospital, Detroit	Loyola University Hospital
Northwestern University, Chicago	University of Utah
Puget Sound Blood Center	Polyclinic Hospital

Overseas

University of Düsseldorf	University of Vienna
Free University of Berlin	RWTH Aachen, Germany
Japanese Cooperative Centers	Hospital Avicenne, Paris
Aachen, West Germany	Ramon Cajal Hospital, Madrid
University of Padova, Italy	St. John's Centre, England
Melbourne Hospital, Australia	

From this initial experience with CTCL, we are able to extend the application of photopheresis to a spectrum of autoreactive disorders. Elsewhere in this volume Rook *et al.* discuss promising preliminary observations in pemphigus vulgaris and in a completed multicenter blinded trial in the progressive systemic sclerosis form of scleroderma. Similarly, Malawista discusses encouraging findings in a preliminary trial in rheumatoid arthritis and Knobler in one in systemic lupus erythematosus. Bisaccia reports positive immunologic alterations in a small group of patients with AIDS-related complex, and Berger discusses experimental and quite preliminary observations in efforts to reverse rejection of transplanted hearts.

Clearly, photopheresis is a biologic response modifier system about which much remains to be learned scientifically and clinically. Yet, the promise of this approach to the treatment of at least certain T cell-mediated disorders has led more than fifty centers in this country to establish operative units (TABLE 1). It will be important to continue to tabulate and interpret the data produced at these centers so that a coordinated effort can be made to determine the overall utility of the treatment. Simultaneously, intensified research into the mechanisms underlying the profound clinical results obtained, despite what must be considered prohibitive immunologic odds against reversing established diseases and T cell clonal activity, is required to discover the most effective, efficient and safe ways to apply the relevant principles.

CONCLUSIONS

Photopheresis is an exciting new immunomodulatory approach to the management of diseases caused by abnormal circulating lymphocytes. Whereas it is already approved by the FDA for management of extensive cutaneous T cell lymphoma and its efficacy in treatment of the cutaneous component of progressive systemic sclerosis is established, its applicability in the treatment of a broad spectrum of other autoimmune diseases will be determined from results of additional clinical trials. The mechanism of action appears to be, at least in large part, an autovaccination against pathogenic clone(s) of T cells. The exciting possibility, therefore, exists that the importance of this new therapeutic modality may substantially increase in the next decade.

SUMMARY

Photopheresis, the process by which peripheral blood is exposed in an extracorporeal flow system to photoactivated 8-methoxypsoralen (8-MOP), is an effective new treatment for certain disorders caused by aberrant T lymphocytes. It has become a standard therapy for advanced cutaneous T cell lymphoma and shows promise in the treatment of four autoimmune disorders (pemphigus vulgaris, the progressive systemic sclerosis form of scleroderma, rheumatoid arthritis, systemic lupus erythematosus) and in reversal of immunologic rejection of transplanted organs. Positive immunologic alterations observed in patients with AIDS-related complex merit further investigation, and preliminary trials in the management of patients with multiple sclerosis, myasthenia gravis and autoimmune insulin-dependent diabetes mellitus have recently been initiated. The inability of the treatment to meaningfully alter the course of the B cell malignancy, chronic lymphocytic leukemia, suggests that B cell proliferations, at least those involving malignant cells, may be more resistant to this treatment. The mechanism of action of photopheresis is likely to be multifaceted, but at least in experimental systems appears to involve an immunization against the pathogenic T cells, in a highly specific manner. Photoactivated 8-MOP initiates a cascade of cellular events by forming covalent photoadducts with nuclear DNA, with cell surface molecules and possibly with other cytoplasmic components of the ultraviolet exposed leukocytes. For reasons not yet clear, exposure of populations of T cells containing expanding a clone(s) of pathogenic T cells to photoactivated 8-MOP alters these cells so that their reinfusion induces a therapeutically significant immunologic reaction that targets unirradiated T cells of the same pathogenic clone(s). It is suggested that the specificity of the induced immunologic reaction may result, in sequence, from the exquisitely titratable damage that 8-MOP inflicts upon cells of the pathogenic clone(s), the return of these cells to an immunocompetent individual, the removal of the photo-damaged cells from the blood by the reticuloendothelial system and the preferential induction of an immune response against cells of the pathologically expanded clone(s).

REFERENCES

1. BEN-NUN, A., H. WEKERLE & I. R. COHEN. 1981. Vaccination against autoimmune encephalomyelitis with T lymphocyte line cells reactive against myelin basic protein. Nature **292:** 60–61.
2. HOLOSHITZ, J., Y. NAPARSTEK, A. BEN-NUN & I. R. COHEN. 1983. Lines of T lymphocytes induce or vaccinate against autoimmune arthritis. Science **219:** 56–58.
3. LIDER, O., T. RESHEF, E. BERAUD, A. BEN-NUN & I. R. COHEN. 1988. Anti-idiotypic network induced by T cell vaccination against experimental autoimmune encephalomyelitis. Science **239:** 181–183.
4. BERGER, C. L., A. EISENBERG, L. SOPER, J. CHOW, J. SIMONE, Y. GAPAS, B. CACCIAPAGLIA, L. BENNETT, R. EDELSON, D. WARBURTON & P. BENN. 1988. Dual genotype in cutaneous T cell lymphoma: immunoglobulin gene rearrangement in clonal T cell malignancy. J. Invest. Dermatol. **90:** 73–77.
5. SONG, P-S. & K. J. TAPLEY. 1979. Photochemistry and photobiology of psoralens. Photochem. Photobiol. **29:** 1177–1197.
6. GASPARRO, F. P. 1988. Psoralen-DNA Photobiology. Vols. 1 and 2. CRC Press. Boca Raton, FL.
7. LERNER, A. B., U. R. DENTON & T. B. FITZPATRICK. 1953. Clinical and experimental studies with 8-methoxypsoralen in vitiligo. J. Invest. Dermatol. **20:** 299–314.
8. VOORHEES, J., J. F. WALTER, W. H. KELSEY & E. E. DUELL. 1973. Psoralen in black light inhibits epidermal DNA-syntheses. Arch. Dermatol. **107:** 861–865.
9. PARRISH, J. A., T. B. FITZPATRICK, L. TANENBAUM & M. A. PATHAK. 1974. Photochemotherapy of psoriasis with oral methoxsalen and longwave ultraviolet light. N. Engl. J. Med. **291:** 1207–1211.
10. GILCHREST, B. A., J. A. PARRISH, L. TANENBAUM, H. A. HAYNES & T. B. FITZPATRICK. 1976. Oral methoxsalen photochemotherapy of mycosis fungoides. Cancer **38:** 683–689.
11. EDELSON, R. 1980. Cutaneous T cell lymphoma (mycosis fungoides, Sezary syndrome and other variants). J. Am. Acad. Dermatol. **2:** 89–10.
12. KRAEMER, K. H. 1982. *In vitro* assay of the effects of psoralen plus ultra-violet radiation in human lymphoid cells. J. Natl. Cancer Inst. **69:** 219–223.
13. MORISON, W., J. A. PARRISH, D. J. MCAULIFFE & R. J. BLOCH. 1981. Sensitivity of immunonuclear cells to PUVA; effect on subsequent stimulation with antigens and an exclusion of frypan blue dyes. Clin. Exp. Dermatol. **6:** 273–277.
14. KHAVARI, P. A., R. L. EDELSON, O. LIDER, F. P. GASPARRO, H. L. WEINER & I. R.

COHEN. 1988. Specific vaccination against photoinactivated cloned T cells. Abstract. Clin. Res. **36:** 662A.

15. PEREZ, M. I., R. L. EDELSON, L. L. LAROCHE & C. L. BERGER. 1989. Inhibition of anti-skin allograft immunity by infusions with syngeneic photoinactivated effector lymphocytes. J. Invest. Dermatol. **92:** 669–676.

16. BERGER, C. L., M. PEREZ, L. LAROCHE & R. EDELSON. 1990. Inhibition of autoimmune disease in a murine model of systemic lupus erythematosus induced by exposure to syngeneic photoinactivated lymphocytes. J. Invest. Dermatol. **94:** 52–57.

17. SANTELLA, R. P., N. DHARMARAJA, F. P. GASPARRO & R. L. EDELSON. 1985. Monoclonal antibodies to DNA modified by 8-methoxysporalen and ultraviolet A light. Nucleic Acids Res. **13:** 2533–2544.

18. LAMBERG, S. I., S. B. GREEN, D. P. BYAR & collaborating centers. 1984. Clinical staging for cutaneous T cell lymphoma. Ann. Intern. Med. **100:** 187–192.

19. EDELSON, R., C. BERGER, F. GUSPARRO, B. JEGASOTHY, P. HEALD, B. WINTROUB, E. VONDERHEID, R. KNOBLER, K. WOLFF, G. PLEWIG, G. McKIERNAN, I. CHRISTENSEN, M. OSTER, H. HONIGSMANN, H. WILFORD, E. KOKOSCHKA, T. REHLE, M. PEREZ, G. STINGL & L. LAROCHE. 1987. Treatment of cutaneous T cell lymphoma by extracorporeal photochemotherapy. N. Engl. J. Med. **316:** 297–303.

20. MARKS, D., S. ROCKMAN, M. OZIEMSKI & R. FOX. 1990. Mechanism of lymphocytotoxicity induced by extracorporeal photochemotherapy for cutaneous T cell lymphoma. J. Clin. Invest. **86:** 2080–2085.

21. ARMUS, S., B. KEYES, C. CAHILL, C. BERGER, D. CRATER, D. SCARBOROUGH, A. KLEINER & E. BISACCIA. 1990. Photopheresis for the treatment of cutaneous T cell lymphoma. J. Am. Acad. Dermatol. **23:** 898–902.

22. DAYE, F., P. BUNN, S. STEINBERG, J. STOCKER, D. IHDE, A. B. FISCHMANN, E. GLATSTEIN, G. SCHECHTER, R. PHELPS, F. FOX, H. PARLETTE, M. ANDERSON & E. SAUSVILLE. 1989. A randomized trial comparing combination electron beam radiation and chemotherapy with topical therapy in the initial treatment of mycosis fungoides. N. Engl. J. Med. **321:** 1784–1790.

Adult T Cell Leukemia/Lymphoma

Perspectives on the Treatment

KAZUNARI YAMAGUCHI,[a] GENGIRO FUTAMI,[b]
TETSUYUKI KIYOKAWA,[b,c] TOSHINORI ISHII,[b]
JOHN R. MURPHY,[c] AND KIYOSHI TAKATSUKI[b]

[a] *Blood Transfusion Service*
and
[b] *Second Department of Internal Medicine*
Kumamoto University Medical School
Kumamoto 860, Japan
[c] *Department of Medicine*
Boston University Hospital
Boston, Massachusetts 02215

Adult T-cell leukemia/lymphoma (ATL) was first discovered and reported in Japan.[1] It has a high incidence in southwest Japan, the Caribbean Islands, and Africa. The retrovirus HTLV-I (human T lymphotropic virus type I) is considered to be related to its etiology.[2,3] In ATL endemic areas, HTLV-I carriers are found at a fairly high percentage even among healthy individuals. ATL has diverse clinical features.

Clinical Features and Classification of ATL

Eight percent of the population over 40 yr old in Kyushu and Okinawa tested positive for HTLV-I antibodies. We studied 187 patients with ATL in Kyushu: 113 males and 74 females, whose age at onset ranged from 27 to 82 yr, with a median of 56 yr.

The predominant physical findings were peripheral lymph node enlargement (72%), hepatomegaly (47%), splenomegaly (26%), and skin lesions (53%). Hypercalcemia (28%) was frequently associated with ATL. White blood cell counts ranged from normal to 500,000. Leukemic cells resembled Sezary cells, having indented or lobulated nuclei. The surface phenotype of ATL cells characterized by monoclonal antibodies was $CD3^+$, $CD4^+$, $CD8^-$ and CD25 (Tac^+).

Anemia and thrombocytopenia were rare. The survival time in acute and lymphoma type ATL ranged from 2 wk to more than 1 yr. The causes of death were pulmonary complications, including *Pneumocystis carinii* pneumonia; hypercalcemia; cryptococcus meningitis; disseminated herpes zoster; and disseminated intravascular coagulopathies.

Pulmonary complication is one of several fatal complications in ATL.[4] Among 29 patients with ATL, pulmonary complications were seen in 26, leukemic pulmonary infiltration in 13, bleeding in 1, interstitial pneumonitis in 1, and pulmonary infection in 13. In 10 of 13 patients with pulmonary infiltration it occurred in the early stage, and 6 of them were diagnosed as having "chronic lung disease" before the diagnosis of ATL. ATL cell infiltration to the lung and fibrosis were confirmed by transbronchial lung biopsy (TBLB). TBLB is useful for lung diagnosis of infiltration or infection.

Another serious complication is hypercalcemia.[5] The incidence of hypercalcemia in patients with ATL is 28% at the time of admission and over 50% during the clinical course. To clarify the mechanism of hypercalcemia, 18 autopsied patients were reviewed clinicopathologically. Eight of nine patients with terminal phase hypercalcemia had osteoclastic bone resorptions. None of the normocalcemic patients had bone resorption. It was concluded that hypercalcemia in ATL was associated with osteoclastic bone resorption. The mechanism of osteoclastic activation in ATL is not clear. Osteoclast activation factors like substance and PTH-related protein (PTH-RP) have been suggested as candidates.[6] Opportunistic infection is also a serious complication.[7]

ATL patients are clinically classified into four types: acute, chronic, smoldering and lymphoma.[8–11] The acute type is the so-called prototypic ATL, which exhibits increased ATL cells, skin lesions, systemic lymphadenopathy, and hepatosplenomegaly. Most of these are resistant to combination chemotherapy using, for example, vincristin, cyclophosphamide, prednisolone, adriamycin and sometimes methotrexate. In general, a poor prognosis is indicated by the elevation of serum lactic dehydrogenase (LDH), calcium and bilirubin as well as by high white blood cell counts. Chronic type ATL patients suffer from increased white blood cell counts, cough, and skin disease. In a few of these patients, slight lymphadenopathy and hepatosplenomegaly are observed, and elevation in serum LDH is also noted, but this is not associated with hypercalcemia or hyperbilirubinemia. Smoldering ATL is characterized by the presence of a few ATL cells (0.5 to 3%) in the peripheral blood for a long period.[8] Patients frequently have skin lesions as premonitory symptoms. The serum LDH values are within normal range and are not associated with hypercalcemia. Lymphadenopathy, hepatosplenomegaly, and bone marrow infiltration are very slight. Smoldering and chronic type ATL often progress to ATL after a long duration. Lymphoma type ATL is characterized by prominent lymphadenopathy. This type has been diagnosed as nonleukemic malignant lymphoma.[10]

Infection with HTLV-I is a direct cause of ATL. Furthermore, infection with this virus can indirectly cause many other diseases via the induction of immunodeficiency, such as chronic lung diseases, opportunistic lung infections, cancer of other organs,[12] monoclonal gammopathy,[13] chronic renal failure,[14] strongyloidiasis,[15] nonspecific dermatomycosis, nonspecific lymph node swelling, and HTLV-I associated myelopathy/tropical spastic paraparesis (HAM/TSP).[16]

Prevention of HTLV-I Infection

To prevent infection with HTLV-I, all samples of donated blood collected at nationwide blood centers were subjected to HTLV-I antibody testing by gelatin particle agglutination beginning in November 1986. From April 1986 to December 1987, sera from patients needing surgery and with hematologic disorders were collected before and after transfusion. Seventy-two of 637 (11.3%) were positive before transfusion. The other 565 patients comprised 412 surgical patients and 153 with hematologic diseases. A transfused unit in our service represents 200 ml. The 565 patients received 7,391 units of red cells, 1,153 units of whole blood and 21,354 units of platelet concentrates. Follow-up periods after transfusion were from 2 to 19 months. None of the recipients seroconverted: some with hematologic disorders received multiple transfusions.[17] A similar test should also be carried out for blood collected within hospitals.

HTLV-I is known to be vertically transmitted from mothers to children.[18] It has been reported that HTLV-I is mainly transmitted from mother to child via breast milk; however, HTLV-I infection has also been reported in children who had not been fed with breast milk, suggesting the possibility of intrauterine and transvaginal infection. To prevent vertical transmission, HTLV-I antibody positive women are now instructed to refrain from breast-feeding in some local communities within the framework of a pilot study. This recommendation will be made on a nationwide level.

Transmission between spouses is transmission between persons of the same generation:[19] hence, there is hardly any risk of ATL onset even when this form of infection occurs. Therefore, to prevent HTLV-I infection in the next generation, HTLV-I antibody positive mothers should refrain from breast-feeding. Although experiments have disclosed that vaccination against HTLV-I is possible, there seems to be no necessity for vaccination.

Treatment of ATL

The results of ATL treatment in the past have been unfavorable. In general, patients with acute and lymphoma type ATL should be treated with combination chemotherapy directed toward achieving a cure. However, those patients showing hypercalcemia, high LDH levels, and an abnormal increase in white blood cells have a 50% survival time of less than 6 mo.[20] Even if aggressive combination chemotherapy such as CHOP, VEPA, or COMLA is given, the prognosis does not improve. Patients often die of severe respiratory infection or hypercalcemia. On the other hand, regardless of treatment, chronic type and smoldering type ATL have a longer course. Aggressive chemotherapy may induce severe respiratory infection. Therefore, an independent treatment protocol for chronic and smoldering type ATL, different from that for acute and lymphoma type ATL, must be established. We are now starting three new treatment protocols.

Deoxycoformycin (DCF) was successfully used as a single agent to treat a patient with acute type ATL, resulting in an apparent long lasting remission.[21] DCF, a nucleoside analogue produced by *Streptomyces antibioticus* or *Aspergillus nidulans,* is a potent tight-binding inhibitor of the enzyme adenosine deaminase (ADA). The therapeutic selectivity of DCF for lymphoid neoplasms was inferred from the preferential lymphoid impairment in congenital ADA deficiency. There are reports about the treatment of B cell malignancies by DCF, and it is now apparent that DCF is effective for some of them, *e.g.,* hairy cell leukemia and B cell prolymphocytic leukemia. Seven patients with ATL refractory to conventional chemotherapy in our hospital were treated with 5 mg/m^2 DCF. Three patients showed a good response, and four were resistant to DCF. Two patients with ATL receiving DCF had a continuous remission without further therapy. Phase II of the clinical study of DCF in Japan was started in 1988.

The second protocol is extracorporeal photochemotherapy. Because the combination of administration of a photoactive drug (8-methoxypsoralen (8-MOP)) and exposure to a long-wave ultraviolet-light system resulted in complete response to psoriasis, this PUVA therapy has been performed in the area of dermatology. Edelson *et al.* developed the technique of extracorporeal photochemotherapy (photopheresis) in which the buffy coat is treated with PUVA before it is returned to the patient. In patients with cutaneous T-cell lymphoma, this therapy resulted in improvement of the disease.[22] We have attempted to apply it to four patients, two with chronic and two with smoldering type ATL. Photopheresis is performed for 2 successive days every 4 weeks, and is repeated for at least four courses. Two patients with chronic ATL had no change in their hematological and serological tests. In 2 patients with smoldering ATL, skin infiltration had begun to disappear and this was associated with changes in the cell surface markers studies. The serial decrease of soluble IL-2 receptor (sIL-2R) levels from 950 to 620 U/ml in one patient was observed after 4 months, and correlated with the number of photopheresis performed. In the other patients, no serial decreases in sIL-2R levels were observed. Concerning the expression of cell surface markers, we observed remarkable changes in at least two patients. Since there was no basic change in the hematological features, the changes in the cell surface marker's expression may be a reliable indicator of the effect of photopheresis. It is still necessary to continue follow-up observations in these patients and to treat a larger number of patients, before definite conclusions can be drawn in the future.[23]

The third protocol is a diphtheria toxin-related interleukin 2 fusion protein (IL-2 toxin) therapy. The inhibitory effect of IL-2 toxin on protein synthesis in ATL cells was examined *in vitro*. Williams *et al.* recently described the genetic construction of chimeric toxin, in which the diphtheria toxin receptor binding domain was genetically replaced with IL-2 sequences.[24] IL-2 toxin has been shown to bind specifically to the high-affinity from of the IL-2 receptor, to be rapidly internalized via receptor-mediated endocytosis, and to inhibit protein synthesis.

Peripheral blood ATL cells from 12 patients (six acute, four chronic and two smoldering) and the lymph node cells from three ATL patients (two acute and one lymphoma) were examined.[25] At a concentration of 10^{-8} M, IL-2 toxin inhibited protein synthesis in ATL cells in six patients of acute type ATL from 20% to 57% compared with the untreated control cultures. It is of interest to note that lymph-node T cells from acute and lymphoma type ATL patients were highly sensitive to IL-2 toxin at a concentration of 10^{-9} M (60 to 98% inhibition). Peripheral blood leukemic from chronic and smoldering type ATL patients were more resistant to the action of IL-2 toxin, and protein synthesis was inhibited by only 1–13%. The cytopathic effects of IL-2 toxin were blocked by the addition of anti CD25 monoclonal antibody, suggesting that the inhibition of protein synthesis in target cells was mediated by the IL-2 receptor (IL-2R). The degree of inhibition of protein synthesis, however, was not closely correlated with the level of expression of CD25 antigen on ATL cells. There was an apparent correlation between the degree of inhibition and the rate of protein synthesis in ATL cells. In addition, we examined the effect of IL-2 toxin on T cells from normal volunteers, lymph-node T cells from a patient with reactive lymphadenopathy following viral infection, and cells from a patient with non-Hodgkin's lymphoma, and found no evidence of nonspecific cytotoxicity. These findings suggest that the high affinity IL-2R present on acute and lymphoma ATL cells may serve as a target for therapy with this recombinant ligand fusion toxin.

Waldmann *et al.* have treated three patients with acute ATL using anti-CD25 antibody and have observed partial remission in one patient.[26] However, the use of monoclonal antibodies, or their corresponding immunotoxins, for the treatment of ATL may have several disadvantages. Monoclonal anti-CD25 is not easily internalized by the IL-2R, thereby suggesting poor clinical efficacy for anti-CD25 based immunotoxins. Moreover, since murine antibodies fail to efficiently bind human complement, cytolysis of leukemia T cells would not be expected following treatment with anti-CD25 monoclonal antibody alone.

For clinical management, patients with acute and lymphoma ATL need intensive chemotherapy (which is generally ineffective), while patients with chronic

ATL are generally not treated until they progress to acute type disease. Since IL-2 toxin is selectively active against high affinity IL-2R positive proliferating T cells, its administration may be a rational approach to the treatment of acute, chronic and lymphoma type ATL.

REFERENCES

1. TAKATSUKI, K., K. YAMAGUCHI, F. KAWANO *et al.* 1985. Clinical diversity in adult T-cell leukemia-lymphoma. Cancer Res. (Suppl.) **45:** 4644–4645.
2. POIESZ, B. J., F. W. RUSCETTI, A. F. FAZDAR *et al.* 1980. Detection and isolation of type C retrovirus particles from fresh and cultured lymphocytes of a patient with cutaneous T-cell lymphoma. Proc. Natl. Acad. Sci. USA **77:** 7415–7419.
3. HINUMA, Y., K. NAGAI, M. HANAOKA *et al.* 1981. Antigen in an adult T-cell leukemia cell line and detection of antibodies to the antigen in human sera. Proc. Natl. Acad. Sci. USA **78:** 6476–6480.
4. YOSHIOKA, R., K. YAMAGUCHI, T. YOSHINAGA *et al.* 1985. Pulmonary complication in patients with adult T-cell leukemia. Cancer **55:** 2491–2494.
5. KIYOKAWA, T., K. YAMAGUCHI, M. TAKEYA *et al.* 1987. Hypercalcemia and osteoclast proliferation in adult T-cell leukemia. Cancer **59:** 1187–1191.
6. WATANABE, T., K. YAMAGUCHI, K. TAKATSUKI, M. OSAME & M. YOSHIDA. 1990. Constitutive expression of parathyroid hormone-related protein gene in human T cell leukemia virus type I (HTLV-I) carriers and adult T cell leukemia patients that can be *trans*-activated by HTLV-I *tax* gene. J. Exp. Med. **172:** 759–765.
7. NAKADA, K., K. YAMAGUCHI, S. FURUGEN *et al.* 1987. Monoclonal integration of HTLV-I proviral DNA in patients with strongloidiasis. Int. J. Cancer **40:** 145–148.
8. YAMAGUCHI, K., H. NISHIMURA, H. KOHROGI *et al.* 1983. A proposal for smoldering T-cell leukemia: a clinicopathologic study of 5 cases. Blood **62:** 757–766.
9. YAMAGUCHI, K., M. SEIKI, M. YOSHIDA *et al.* 1984. The detection of human T-cell leukemia virus proviral DNA and its application for classification and diagnosis of T-cell malignancy. Blood **63:** 1235–1240.
10. YAMAGUCHI, K., R. YOSHIOKA, T. KIYOKAWA *et al.* 1986. Lymphoma type adult T-cell leukemia—a clinicopathologic study of HTLV related T-cell type malignant lymphoma. Hematol. Oncol. **4:** 59–65.
11. KAWANO, F., K. YAMAGUCHI, H. NISHIMURA *et al.* 1985. Variations in the clinical courses of adult T-cell leukemia. Cancer **55:** 851–856.
12. ASOU, N., T. KUMAGAI, S. UEKIHARA *et al.* 1986. HTLV-I seroprevalence in patients with malignancy. Cancer **58:** 903–907.
13. MATSUZAKI, H., K. YAMAGUCHI, T. KAGIMOTO *et al.* 1985. Monoclonal gammopathies in adult T-cell leukemia. Cancer **56:** 1380–1383.
14. LEE, S. Y., K. MATSUSHITA, K. YAMAGUCHI *et al.* 1987. Human T-cell leukemia virus type 1 infection in hemodialysis patients. Cancer **60:** 1474–1478.
15. YAMAGUCHI, K., E. MATUTES, D. CATOVSKY *et al.* 1987. Strongyloides stercoralis as candidate co-factor for HTLV-I induced leukaemogenesis. Lancet **2:** 94.
16. OSAME, M., K. USUKU, S. IZUMO *et al.* 1986. HTLV-I associated myelopathy: a new clinical entigy. Lancet **1:** 1031–1032.
17. NISHIMURA, Y., K. YAMAGUCHI, T. KIYOKAWA *et al.* 1989. Prevention of transmission of human T cell lymphotropic virus type 1 by blood transfusion by screening of donors. Transfusion **29:** 372.
18. HINO, S., K. YAMAGUCHI, S. KATAMINE *et al.* 1985. Mother to child transmission of human T cell leukemia virus type 1. Jpn. J. Cancer Res. **76:** 474–480.
19. MIYAMOTO, Y., K. YAMAGUCHI, H. NISHIMURA *et al.* 1985. Familial adult T cell leukemia. Cancer **55:** 181–185.
20. SHIMOYAMA, M., K. YAMAGUCHI, K. TAKATSUKI *et al.* 1988. Major prognostic factors of adult patients with advanced T-cell lymphoma/leukemia. J. Clin. Oncol. **6:** 1088–1097.

21. YAMAGUCHI, K., K. TAKATSUKI, C. DEARDEN *et al.* 1988. Chemotherapy with deoxy-coformycin in mature T-cell malignancies. *In* Cancer Chemotherapy. K. Kimura *et al.*, Eds. 216–220. Excerpta Medical. Tokyo.

22. EDELSON, R., C. BERGER, F. GASPARRO *et al.* 1987. Treatment of cutaneous T-cell lymphoma by extracorporeal photochemotherapy, preliminary results. N. Engl. J. Med. **6:** 297–303.

23. FUTAMI, G., T. KIYOKAWA, K. YAMAGUCHI *et al.* 1990. Treatment of adult T cell leukemia by extracorporeal photochemotherapy. Leukemia Lymphoma **2:** 195–200.

24. WILLIAMS, D. P., K. PARKER, P. BACHA *et al.* 1987. Diphtheria toxin receptor binding domain substitution with interleukin 2: genetic construction and properties of a diphtheria toxin-related interleukin 2 fusion protein. Protein Eng. **1:** 493–498.

25. KIYOKAWA, T., K. SHIRONO, T. HATTORI *et al.* 1989. Cytotoxicity of interleukin-2 toxin toward lymphocytes from patients with adult T-cell leukemia. Cancer Res. **49:** 4042–4046.

26. WALDMANN, T. A. 1986. The interleukin-2 receptor on malignant cells: a target for diagnosis and therapy. Cell. Immunol. **99:** 53–60.

Photopheresis for Cutaneous T Cell Lymphoma

PETER W. HEALD

Department of Dermatology
Yale University School of Medicine
333 Cedar Street
LCI 500
New Haven, Connecticut 06510

Cutaneous T Cell Lymphoma

The early stages of cutaneous T cell lymphoma (CTCL) are often nondiagnostic erythematous patches which can persist for years or spontaneously resolve.[1] As the cellular infiltrate increases, the lesions become more persistent and indurated. The classical findings on biopsy are atypical lymphocytes infiltrating the dermis, epidermal invasion (epidermotropism), and often clusters of malignant cells in the epidermis (Pautrier microabscesses). The malignant cells express the surface proteins of mature helper T cells and they are functionally active in assays for helper T cell activity on B cells.[2]

Plaque stage disease contains a clonally expanded T cell population. Since every T cell and its progeny will contain their uniquely rearranged T cell receptor gene, a clonal expansion can be detected by studying the DNA isolated from skin biopsies. In benign infiltrates no clones can be detected. In CTCL there are clonal rearrangements which can be detected from patch stage on.[3] Clonality can also be demonstrated and assessed with a series of antibodies which recognize different segments of the variable sections of the beta chain of the T cell receptor. When these antibodies are used to evaluate nonclonal disorders only a few percent of cells react. However, if there is a clonal expansion of cells bearing one of these variable regions, a marked increase in positive cells will be noted. Plaque stage disease has a variable prognosis with a median survival of 8–10 years that is unaffected by therapy.[4,5] Disease progression occurs by way of lymph node involvement, tumor development or peripheral blood involvement.

Progression to peripheral blood involvement may be associated with the clinical findings of erythroderma and diffuse adenopathy. As the disease progresses from limited epidermal to hematogenous involvement there is a failure of a monitoring system which would recognize and destroy circulating abnormal cells. Many patients exhibit the erythroderma stage early before the lymphocyte compartment has been completely taken over by the malignant cells. The increase in the malignant cell population can be seen in increasing CD4/CD8 ratios which reflect both the increase in malignant cells and the diminution in the nonmalignant population. The survival of the erythrodermic state has been estimated as having a median of approximately 30 months.[4,6]

Photopheresis and Erythrodermic CTCL

There have been two large series of erythrodermic CTCL patients treated with photopheresis. The largest was a multicenter international trial of 29 patients[7] first reported in 1987 and again reviewed in a follow-up report in 1990. The second series was a review of 22 erythrodermic patients who had photopheresis at one institution.[8]

Responses to photopheresis were graded into three categories: patients clearing either 75% of their surface involvement, patients improving more than 25% of their involvement but less than 75% and those with less than 25% involvement.

The treatment protocol for CTCL consisted of performing two consecutive photophoresis treatments at four-week intervals. Of the 29 erythrodermic patients in the multicenter study, 24 achieved marked clinical improvement. Seven of the patients cleared over 75% of their skin involvement after 12 months of therapy. Nineteen patients cleared 25–75%, while five patients had less than 25% improvement. Very similar results were seen in the series of 22 patients who received photopheresis as their first line of therapy for erythrodermic CTCL. Complete response was seen in five patients and no response was noted in five patients. Thus, over half of the patients, as in the initial study, achieved an improvement in the quality of life with demonstrable residual disease. It was intriguing that onset of improvement always appeared very gradually. At first there were temporary responses immediately following a two-day cycle of energy. Then, after 4–6 months there was gradually a permanent decrease in erythema, scaling, and pruritis.

The beneficial responses appeared on the head and upper trunk first with a decrease in erythroderma and scaling. As the erythroderma improved in a cephalocaudad manner, patients had less chills and edema. Pruritis and palmo-plantar involvement tended to be the last areas to resolve. As the erythroderma cleared, the patients noticed a return of body hair and the capacity for eccrine sweating. Temperature intolerance and rigors tended to resolve with early signs of improvement.

Those demonstrating marked clinical improvement were maintained on the every-four-week treatment schedule. Their treatments were continued until maximum clearing appeared. An additional six months of therapy after this point was administered to insure the stability of the response. Once stable for this additional six months, patients were then gradually tapered by adding one week per cycle every three cycles. After this had been extended to one cycle of therapy every eight weeks for three times, their therapy was stopped.

Histology

In patients who have achieved clinical remission, biopsies of previously involved skin have revealed surprising findings. The typical pretreatment biopsy showed a heavy lichenoid infiltrate of the upper dermis with epidermotropic abnormal cells. In follow-up biopsies, there is uniform reduction of epidermotropism of malignant cells and depletion of the dermal infiltrate. However there are still atypical mononuclear cells noted in perivascular regions. This finding suggests subsets within the tumor population exhibit differential sensitivities to photopheresis. Presumably the more malignant subclones are preferentially eliminated by photopheresis.

Survival

The long term follow-up of the original 29 erythrodermic patients allowed the investigation of whether photopheresis leads to an improvement in the median survival of patients with this stage of the disease.[9] The observation that photopheresis substantially decreased the severity of skin involvement in erythrodermic CTCL patients[7,8] was encouraging and suggested that survival of these subjects might be prolonged. Previous reports that conventional therapy did not improve survival of CTCL patients[5] would suggest that any improvement in survival would be a significant advance in the treatment or their disease.

The 29 original erythrodermic patients were reviewed and survival determined as a function of duration of time from diagnosis and time from initiation of photopheresis. The median survival of erythrodermic patients is >60 months from the time of diagnosis of the erythrodermic state. It is noteworthy that a genuine median survival for the photopheresis group has not been obtained since more than half of the patients are still alive. Four of the seven complete responders maintained complete remissions. The complete remissions continue to be maintained in 4 patients with durations which still continue to grow from their current lengths of 4, 5(2), and 6 years of disease-free survival. One patient discontinued therapy after 13 cycles of therapy and was in remission for an additional 5 months before he relapsed with lymphoblastic lymphoma invading the bone marrow and lymph nodes. A second patient developed lymphoblastic lymphoma with nodal effacement and cutaneous tumors. The nodal and tumor stage of these two patients did not respond to additional therapy. The four remaining complete responses were maintained after patients had been gradually tapered off photopheresis. By contrast of the five nonresponding patients, only one is still alive, and that patient elected to continue on photopheresis.

The population-based estimate of survival in a tumor registry survey showed patients diagnosed as Sezary syndrome had a median survival from diagnosis of 31 months.[4] Patients in the Mycosis Fungoides Cooperative Group survey with erythrodermic disease had a median survival close to 30 months.[6] The median survival of the photopheresed erythrodermic CTCL patients of greater than 60 months compares quite favorably with the above mentioned studies of erythrodermic patients treated with conventional therapy. The potential significance of the results should be understood by the study having included patients who had failed at least one conventional modality, possibly biasing patient selection to those with an even poorer prognosis. Furthermore, more than half of the photopheresis patients are still alive, so that a true median survival time has not yet been reached.

The prolonged therapeutic effect and the existence of several patients with complete remissions strongly suggests there is a potent host response to the CTCL cells for two major reasons: the usual natural progression of this phase of CTCL was interrupted, and even though only a small fraction of the body's burden of malignant cells were exposed to photoactivated drug and returned to the patient, the remainder of the malignant cell pool diminished remarkably in size.

Multimodality and Multistage Therapy

Those patients with partial responses to photopheresis alone were given adjunctive therapies to look for synergistic therapeutic effects. In addition, the use of photopheresis in the multimodality treatment of tumor stage and markedly leukemic CTCL has demonstrated the ability of this therapy to contribute to improvement in patients with nonerythrodermic CTCL.

Multimodality Therapy

Adjunctive therapy was considered for patients with responses that are incomplete. Methotrexate adjunctive therapy consisted of an initial dose of 15 mg between treatment cycles. If this was well tolerated, the dose was advanced to weekly with no dosing within seven days before or after a cycle of photopheresis. Of the 19 patients followed at one institution, those considered for adjunctive therapy had erythroderma with a stable but not acceptable improvement in response to photopheresis. Repeat skin biopsies were performed to demonstrate disease and to ensure that the patient had not developed tumor or plaque stage which would dictate a change in therapy overall.

In eight patients the test dose of 15 mg methotrexate between two cycles of photopheresis (two weeks after one cycle and before the other) was well tolerated. All eight patients were advanced to the three doses between treatments. Methotrexate led to a complete remission in one, greater than 50% clearing in two, a stabilized pattern in three, and two patients showing no change. The adjunctive use of steroids in photopheresis is best utilized for symptomatic short-term management. All patients had been weaned to an oral prednisone dose of 20 mg every other day or less prior to starting photopheresis.

Tumor Stage

Two patients were treated with photopheresis as the monotherapy for tumor stage disease. The preliminary results of treating tumor stage with photopheresis alone showed that tumors did not resolve within a few months of therapy. Thus, total body electron beam therapy was administered as described in previous studies from this institution.[10] A total dose of 3600 rads was given in 36 sessions. Photopheresis was begun in two of the patients at the commencement of radiation and in 2 additional patients near the end of their radiation. One patient has had a remission of three years duration, another at fourteen months, and the last two at four months. Two additional patients were treated with spot radiotherapy to tumor lesions then begun on nitrogen mustard in conjunction with photopheresis. These two have been on this regimen for four years with one relapse each. The relapse responded to additional radiation therapy.

Markedly Leukemic CTCL

Three patients commenced photopheresis with white blood cell counts of over 35,000 cells/mm[7]. One patient had azathioprine for 18 months, prednisone 20 mg every other day and photopheresis every 4 weeks and he gradually improved. After the white blood cell count was <12,000 the azathioprine was discontinued and the patient maintained a normal white blood cell count along with clinical improvement. The other two patients responded to accelerated treatment regimens of photopheresis every 2 weeks. After attaining a normal range white blood count the photopheresis was performed every 4 weeks.

Side Effects

Since the photoinactivation occurs in the extracorporeal compartment, there were few systemic side effects in the treated subjects. Whereas a minority of the photopheresis patients experienced transiently increased erythroderma following reinfusion of the treated leukocytes, those sequelae frequently associated with systemic chemotherapy, such as bone marrow suppression, hair loss and gastrointestinal erosions, were not encountered. White blood counts were not suppressed, delayed hypersensitivity skin testing was intact, and there is no specific suppression of lymphocyte subsets by therapy.[11]

Mechanism of Action

Understanding the mechanism of action is dependent on the clinical research on patients undergoing therapy, the development of animal models, and a better understanding of the progression of CTCL.

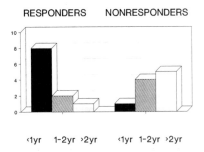

FIGURE 1. The duration between the diagnosis of CTCL and the commencement of therapy (*y-axis*) and responsiveness of photopheresis. On the *left,* each pair is the complete response group; on the *right,* is the nonresponding group.

Responders vs Nonresponders

In both studies of photopheresis therapy, the comparison of the best responding patients to the least responding patients revealed similar findings. The best responders had begun on therapy earlier in the course of their disease (FIG. 1). Thus, since patients appeared to do better when therapy is started earlier in the course of the disease, photopheresis should indeed be considered the first line of therapy for erythrodermic CTCL. The other finding which appeared to correlate with a good response was the presence of suppressor cells in sufficient number. The best responders had a smaller CD4 compartment and larger CD8 compartment when compared to nonresponders (FIG. 2). The latter finding suggested that the CD8 subset size is important as a reflection of immunocompetence, is critical because these cells are the target of therapy and/or that this value inversely correlates with disease progression.

Model for Disease Progression

As the disease progresses from limited epidermal to hematogenous involvement where there is a failure of a monitoring system which would recognize and destroy circulating abnormal cells. Many patients exhibit the erythroderma stage early before the lymphocyte compartment has been completely taken over by the malignant cells. The increase in the malignant cell population can be seen in increasing CD4/CD8 ratios, which reflect both the increase in malignant cells and the withering away of the immunocompetent cells which might be involved in any anti-tumor response. Based on the observations made in the responding and nonresponding patients, it could be postulated that there is a baseline of immunocompetence which is needed to respond to the damaged cells. Since the damaged cell population is less than 15% of the lymphocyte pool, the disappearance of disease in some patients must be the result of an active anti-disease response. Also, since erythrodermic CTCL patients have a presumed failure of the hematogenous based lymphocyte monitoring system, it appears appropriate that the photoinactivated cells are returned to the intravascular compartment.

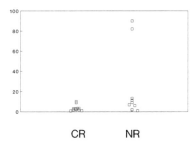

FIGURE 2. Lymphocyte subset ratios were compared between complete responders (*left*) and nonresponders (*right*). The *y-axis* is the ratio of CD4 to CD8 expressing cells.

Modelling Treatment Strategies

The introductory discussion of the components of CTCL leads to the use of this model to develop treatment strategies. After localizing to the skin, the malignancy can progress to compromise longevity by way of the leukemic stage or by developing tumors in the skin, lymph nodes and viscera. These progressions can thus be classified as problems of local autonomous growth (tumors) or of circulating abnormal T-cells.

When the circulating phase of the disease dominates the clinical picture it is detected by peripheral blood studies and/or the presence of erythroderma. The treatment of choice is photopheresis. When white blood cell counts are over 50,000/mm^3, large numbers of circulating cells cen be removed by leukapheresis as a symptomatic adjunct to this therapy.

When the tumorous component dominates the clinical picture there are thick plaques and tumors. The best ablative therapy is radiotherapy to eliminate the lesions. Post-radiotherapy adjunct treatments must be given to attempt to prevent relapse. The maintenance regimens tested to date have been unsuccessful in prolonging survival in this group.[5,10] Based on the low toxicity of photopheresis and its ability to improve survival in erythrodermics, this modality should be utilized as maintenance therapy for tumor patients with radiotherapy-induced remissions.

The inflammatory response which accompanies CTCL produces symptoms which often warrant therapy. With an immunomodulating therapy such as photopheresis the best application of adjunctive therapy is to keep it minimally immunocompromising. Thus, once weekly methotrexate and potentially the interferons are preferred over more aggressive, more immunocompromising regimens with chemotherapeutic agents and corticosteroids.

Therapeutic application of photopheresis technology in the management of the more common patch and plaque stages will follow clinical trials which will attempt to demonstrate efficacy in these stages.

REFERENCES

1. EDELSON, R. 1980. Cutaneous T-cell lymphoma (mycosis fungoides, Sezary syndrome, and other variants). J. Am. Acad. Dermatol. **2:** 89–106.
2. BRODER, S., R. L. EDELSON, M. A. LUTZNER et al. 1976. The Sezary syndrome: malignant proliferation of helper T-cells. J. Clin. Invest. **58:** 1297.
3. WEISS, L. M., E. HU, G. S. WOOD et al. 1985. Clonal rearrangements of T cell receptor genes in mycosis fungoides and dermatopathic lymphadenopathy. N. Engl. J. Med. **313:** 539–544.
4. WEINSTOCK, M. A. & J. W. HOM. 1988. Mycosis fungoides in the United States. Increasing incidence and descriptive epidemiology. J. Am. Med. Assoc. **260:** 42.
5. KAYE, F. J., P. A. BUNN, S. M. STEINBERG et al. 1989. A randomized trial comparing combination electron-beam radiation and chemotherapy with topical therapy in the initial treatment of mycosis fungoides. N. Engl. J. Med. **321:** 1784–1790.
6. LAMBERG, S. I., S. B. GREEN, D. P. BYAR et al. 1979. Status report of 376 mycosis fungoides patients at 4 years: Mycosis Fungoides Cooperative Group. Cancer Treat. Rep. **63:** 701.
7. EDELSON, R. L., C. L. BERGER, F. S. GASPARRO et al. 1987. Treatment of cutaneous T-cell lymphoma with extracorporeal photochemotherapy. N. Engl. J. Med. **316:** 297.
8. HEALD, P., M. PEREZ, I. CHRISTENSEN, G. MCKIENAN & R. EDELSON. 1990. Treatment of cutaneous T-cell lymphoma: the Yale–New Haven Hospital experience. Yale J. Biol. Med.
9. HEALD, P., A. ROOK, M. PEREZ, B. WINTROUB, R. KNOBLER, R. MISCHIG, B. JEGASOTHY, F. GASPARRO, C. BERGER & R. EDELSON. Prolonged survival of erythrodermic cutaneous T-cell lymphoma patients treated with extracorporeal photochemotherapy. Submitted.
10. BRAVERMAN, I. M., N. B. YAGER, M. CHEN, E. C. CHADMAN, W. N. HAIT & T. MAYNARD. 1987. Combined total body electron beam irradiation and chemotherapy for mycosis fungoides. J. Am. Acad. Dermatol. **17:** 40.
11. HEALD, P. & R. EDELSON. 1988. Photopheresis for T-cell mediated diseases. Adv. Dermatol. **3:** 25–40.

Anti-Idiotypic Immunity as a Potential Regulator in Myeloma and Related Diseases

GÖRAN HOLM, SUSANNE BERGENBRANT,
ANN-KARI LEFVERT, QING YI, ANDERS ÖSTERBORG,[a]
AND HÅKAN MELLSTEDT[a]

Department of Medicine
and
[a]Department of Oncology
Karolinska Hospital
Box 60500
S-104 01 Stockholm, Sweden

INTRODUCTION

Multiple myeloma (MM), monoclonal gammopathy of undetermined significance (MGUS) and Waldenstrom's macroglobulinemia (WM) are B cell tumors usually with the clonal immunoglobulin (Ig) appearing as an M-component in the serum. MM is characterized by clonal plasma cells in the bone marrow and by clonal B lymphocytes in various stages of differentiation also present in peripheral blood (for references, see REF. 1). Idiotypic structures of surface-bound clonal Ig may be regarded as tumor-specific antigen which act as a potential target for specific T and B cells in an immune regulation of the tumor cell clone.[2] As a first step in evaluating the role of immune regulation in human monoclonal gammopathies, attention has mainly been paid to the identification of idiotype reactive T and B cells. In addition, efforts to put the composition of various regulatory subsets into the context of prognostically important features of the disease may contribute to the understanding of their regulatory role. The search for anti-idiotypic antibodies in monoclonal gammopathies has been hampered by the heavy antigen load in the blood. However, the production of B cell lines by Epstein-Barr virus (EBV) has allowed the detection of precursor B cells producing antibodies to autologous tumor idiotopes.[3]

In the present paper we summarize recent partly preliminary results indicating the presence of anti-idiotypic B and T cells in patients with MGUS, WM and early MM. The clinical material comprises patients with MGUS, MM and WM from the oncology and hematology departments of Karolinska Hospital. Unless stated otherwise the patients had not been treated with irradiation, cytostatic drugs or corticosteroids before the test.

178

Anti-Idiotypic B Cells

The presence in peripheral blood of B cells with the capacity to produce anti-idiotypic antibodies to the malignant B cell clone has been studied using EBV-induced B cell lines.[4] The clinical material comprised 3 patients with MGUS who had been followed for 5–14 years without progression to MM. Five patients with clinical stage I MM according to Durie and Salmon had no signs of progression during a 1-year follow-up. Three patients with symptomatic clinical stage III MM were tested before the institution of treatment.

Peripheral blood mononuclear cells (PBMC) depleted from T cell after rosetting with neuraminidase-treated sheep red blood cells were incubated for 60 min with EBV, washed and suspended in RPMI 1640 medium with 10% fetal calf serum. The cells were seeded in flat-bottomed microtiter plates and incubated for 10–14 days. At that time cultures from all patients contained IgM-producing colonies in >90% of the wells. The supernatants were screened for IgM antibodies against F(ab')2 fragments of the autologous M-protein using ELISA.

Some results are summarized in TABLE 1. As can be seen the concentrations of anti-id antibodies in supernatants from more than 50 wells were high in MGUS but low or absent in MM clinical stage III. Culture supernatants from clinical stage I MM contained intermediate concentrations. One explanation for this finding is that patients with benign or limited disease have a higher prevalence of blood

TABLE 1. Id-Reactive IgM in Cell Supernatants from EBV-Activated PBL

	Median Absorbance at 405 nM (Range)
MGUS (n = 3)	0.36–0.44
MM stage I (n = 5)	0.10–0.26
MM stage III (n = 3)	0.01–0.03

precursor B cells committed to the production of anti-idiotypic antibodies and susceptible to transformation by EBV. This interpretation is supported by the observation that the number of colonies and the total IgM production in the primary cultures were similar in all groups. Moreover, the nonclonal "background" immunoglobulin concentrations in serum were reduced not only in MM stage III but also in three patients with clinical stage I MM and in one MGUS patient.

Anti-Idiotypic T Cells

The presence of idiotype reactive blood T cells in patients with monoclonal gammopathies was studied by measuring the activation of cells cultivated with autologous M-protein (data to be published). In short, T lymphocytes were enriched to >98% by rosetting with sheep red blood cells followed by lysis of the erythrocytes. The cells were mixed with 10% autologous adherent cells (mainly monocytes) in RPMI medium with 10% immunoglobulin-depleted normal human AB serum and cultivated in microplates for 6–8 days. Stimulation was measured as incorporation of tritiated thymidine into DNA.

In addition, the activation of T lymphocytes was evaluated by enumeration of IFN-gamma and IL-2 producing cells by a modified version of the solid-phase enzyme-linked immunospot (ELISPOT) assay. In short, the wells of 96-well nitro-cellulose microtiter plates were coated with mouse monoclonal anti-human IFN-gamma or IL-2 antibodies. After washing, freshly prepared PBMC (2×10^5 cells/well) with the proper concentration of antigen was added. After incubation at 37°C for 48 hr rabbit polyclonal anti-human IFN-gamma or IL-2 antibodies was added and incubated for 2 hr. Cytokine-producing cells stained with a peroxidase technique were identified and enumerated under a dissection microscope. We here report the results on two patients.

Patient EL had suffered from Waldenström's macroglobulinemia for 16 years. He had been treated with plasmapheresis during the last nine years because of hyperviscosity symptoms. He was tested repeatedly during a 22-month period. During the first 10 months he received no cytostatic treatment (FIG. 1), and his T

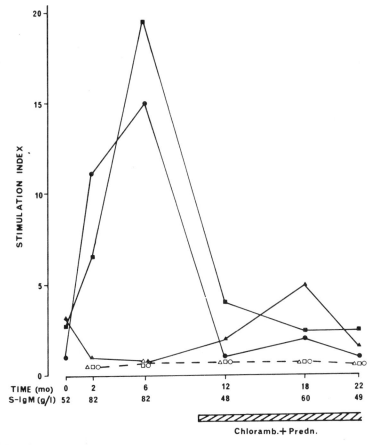

FIGURE 1. DNA synthesis (mean ct/min) in T lymphocytes from patient BL (*filled symbols*) and from one healthy donor (*open symbols*) after activation with 1 (*squares*), 10 (*circles*), 1000 (*triangles*) μg/ml IgG-BL for 6 days. The ct/min values were adjusted for incorporation of thymidine into cells grown in complete medium without IgG-BL. *Hatched area* indicates period of treatment with chlorambucile and prednisolone.

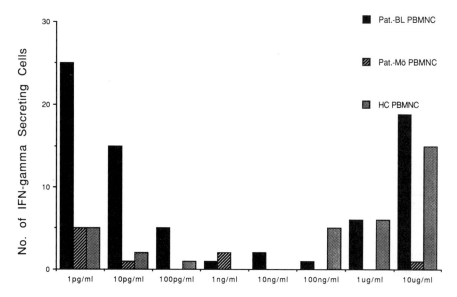

FIGURE 2. IFN-gamma-secreting cells in peripheral blood mononuclear cells from two patients with MGUS (BL and MÖ) and one healthy control after incubation with M component IgG from patient BL. The numbers of spots resulting from cultures with cells incubated in complete medium only were subtracted from the results from incubation with antigen.

cells responded strongly to low concentrations of autologous monoclonal IgM. Lymphocytes from three healthy donors were not stimulated. The T cell activation by low-dose antigen was abolished after institution of cytostatic drugs.

Patient BL is a 43-year-old women with MGUS known about for five years. She has an IgG-1-lambda M-component. There were no signs of progression of the disease during the observation period.

T cells from BL were activated to secretion of IFN-gamma by very low concentrations (1 and 10 pg/ml) of the autologous M-protein (FIG. 2). At such concentrations the reaction was specific, since T cells from another MGUS patient and a healthy control were not stimulated by the same antigen. Moreover, BL cells could not be induced by such low concentrations of another M-protein or by normal IgG (data not shown). High doses of antigen, however, stimulated cytokine production in a nonspecific manner (FIG. 2). The same dose response pattern was noted measuring the single cell production of IL-2. A similar and specific low dose response of BL T lymphocytes to M-protein was noted measuring DNA synthesis on day 6 of culture (data not shown).

Taken together these data demonstrate the presence of T cells reactive to antigenic determinants on the autologous M-protein not shared with normal IgG and IgG M-protein from other donors. Idiotypic epitopes are the most likely targets of T cell recognition in these patients.

T Cell Clones

To approach the question of idiotype-specific T cells and their potential role in human monoclonal gammopathies a series of T cell clones binding the autologous

M component idiotypes were established from peripheral blood of two patients with MM clinical stage I and one MGUS patient.[5] The cultures were started from PBMC using a low dose of antigen (0.1 ng/ml) and serum-free medium (AIM-V, Gibco Lab., Grand Island, NY). The cultures were fed repeatedly with antigen and irradiated autologous monocytes/macrophages. The cells were cloned after 4 weeks. After another 6 weeks' propagation with antigen, IL-2 and feeder cells the clones were tested.

Only cell cultures showing >25% binding of FITC labelled F(ab')2 fragments of the autologous M-protein were considered for further testing (TABLE 2). None of the lines contained B cells as judged from the absence of CD20 staining. Cells from a normal donor cultivated with a IgG M-protein did not result in idiotype-specific T cells. Eleven idiotope binding clones were available for phenotyping with anti-T cell monoclonals. Only one MM clone carried the CD4 marker. The remaining 10 clones were CD8+.

Eleven clones were also tested in a proliferative assay using serum-free medium and irradiated autologous monocytes as feeder cells. In eight of them the presence of autologous IgG M protein resulted in stimulation indices ranging from 1.7 to 7.0. The indices in controls (patient cells with allogeneic M protein or healthy donor T cells grown with M protein) ranged from 0.4 to 1.2.

Earlier studies have reported various T cell abnormalities in human mono-

TABLE 2. Phenotypes of sId+ T Cell Clones

		sId+		
Clone	M-Component	Total	CD3+	CD4+	CD8+
201	auto	69	70	<0.5	75
	homo	9	ND[a]	ND	ND
307	auto	ND	65	6	79
	homo	ND	2	ND	ND

[a] ND, not done.

clonal gammopathies. It is generally agreed upon that there is an imbalance between CD4+ and CD8+ cells with a loss of CD4+ cells and/or an increase of CD8+ cells in MM patients particularly in those with advanced disease.[6] A selective loss of CD4+/CD45R+ suppressor/cytotoxic inducer cells has also been described.[7]

These results lend support to the presence of idiotype-specific T cells in human monoclonal gammopathies. The potential of such cells to participate in regulation of the malignant B cell clone is at present only a matter of speculation. The selection of T cell clones resulted in a clear predominance of idiotope reactive CD8+ cells. Whether this reflects a true predominance of such cells in the blood or is mainly a consequence of their cloning efficiency under the particular conditions used for culture remains to be shown. The murine myeloma system used by Lynch and co-workers (for review, see REF. 8) has clearly revealed the presence of T cells which through an idiotype : anti-idiotype interaction regulate tumor B cells and their immunoglobulin secretion.

Recently, Janson et al.[9] described a clonal expansion of peripheral T cells in MM and MGUS. They examined the alpha/beta V gene distribution in blood CD4+ and CD8+ T cells using monoclonal antibodies to various TCR V region segments. With a panel of eight mAbs covering about one fourth of the TCR repertoire they found that the use of particular V gene segments was increased in

7 of 16 patients as compared with a panel of healthy controls. As an example, 47% of CD8+ cells from one patient reacted with alphaV12.1 antibody. In another 40% CD4+ cells bound betaV8.1 antibody. It is concluded that a clonal expansion of T lymphocytes is a common feature in MM and MGUS. However, the specificity and functional properties of such T cells are not known.

SUMMARY

In this paper some recent and partly preliminary results on anti-idiotypic immunity against clonal B cells in human monoclonal gammopathies are summarized. B cell lines producing antibodies to idiotypic determinants on autologous monoclonal immunoglobulin could be propagated after activation with Epstein-Barr virus of peripheral blood lymphocytes from patients with MGUS and MM clinical stage I but not from untreated persons with advanced MM. Blood T lymphocytes from patients with MGUS and Waldenström's macroglobulinemia were activated to DNA synthesis and production of interleukins by the autologous M protein. In another series of experiments T cell clones raised from patients with MM clinical stage I and MGUS bound F(ab')2 fragments of the autologous M protein and were stimulated to DNA synthesis by the idiotope-bearing protein. Control experiments demonstrated the specificity for idiotypic determinants. Ten of eleven clones were CD4−/CD8+. Finally, using a panel of 8 mAbs to alpha/beta V region epitopes, we noted a clonal expansion of CD4+ and CD8+ T cells in MGUS and MM patients.

REFERENCES

1. MELLSTEDT, H., G. HOLM & M. BJÖRKHOLM. 1984. Multiple myeloma, Waldenström's macroglobulinemia and benign monoclonal gammopathy. Characteristics of the B cell clone, immunoregulatory cell populations and clinical implications. Adv. Cancer Res. **41:** 257–289.
2. LYNCH, R. G., J. R. GRAFF, S. SIRISINHA, E. SIMMS & N. H. EISEN. 1972. Myeloma proteins as tumour-specific transplantation antigens. Proc. Natl. Acad. Sci. USA **69:** 1540–1544.
3. ANDERSSON, M., G. HOLM, A. D. LEFVERT & H. MELLSTEDT. 1989. Anti-idiotypic B-cell lines from a patient with monoclonal gammopathy of undetermined significance. Scand. J. Immunol. **30:** 489–492.
4. BERGENBRANT, S., A. ÖSTERBORG, G. HOLM, H. MELLSTEDT & A. K. LEFVERT. Anti-idiotypic antibodies in patients with monoclonal gammopathies. Relation to tumor load. Submitted.
5. ÖSTERBORG, A., S. BERGENBRANT, G. HOLM, A. K. LEFVERT, M. G. MASUCCI & H. MELLSTEDT. Generation of T cell clones binding F(ab')2 fragments of the idiotypic immunoglobulin in patients with monoclonal gammopathy. Submitted.
6. MELLSTEDT, H., G. HOLM, D. PETTERSSON, M. BJÖRKHOLM, B. JOHANSSON, C. LINDEMALM, D. PEEST & A. ÅHRE. 1982. T cells in monoclonal gammopathies. Scand. J. Haematol. **29:** 57–64.
7. SERRA, H. M., M. J. MANT, B. A. RUETHER, J. A. LEDBETTER & L. M. PILARSKI. 1988. Selective loss of CD4+CD45+ T cells in peripheral blood of multiple myeloma patients. J. Clin. Immunol. **8:** 259–265.
8. LYNCH, R. G. 1987. Immunoglobulin-specific suppressor T cells. Adv. Immunol. **40:** 135–151.
9. JANSON, C. H., J. GRUNEWALD, A. ÖSTERBORG, H. DERSIMONIAN, M. B. BRENNER, H. MELLSTEDT & H. WIGZELL. Predominant T cell receptor V region usage in patients with abnormal clones of B cells. Submitted.

Development of a Treatment Regimen for Human Cytomegalovirus (CMV) Infection in Bone Marrow Transplantation Recipients by Adoptive Transfer of Donor-Derived CMV-Specific T Cell Clones Expanded *In Vitro*[a]

P. D. GREENBERG, P. REUSSER, J. M. GOODRICH, AND
S. R. RIDDELL

Division of Oncology
Fred Hutchinson Cancer Research Center
Seattle, Washington 98104
and
Department of Immunology
Division of Oncology, RM-17
BB1321 Health Sciences Building
University of Washington
Seattle, Washington 98195

INTRODUCTION

Cytomegalovirus (CMV) has an infection prevalence in American adults exceeding 50%. However, it is not generally perceived as a dangerous pathogen since infection of normal immunocompetent hosts typically induces only a mild subclinical syndrome.[1] Similar to other herpes viruses, CMV is not completely eliminated following primary infection, but rather persists for the lifetime of the host in an apparent latent state. The biologic mechanisms operative in maintaining latency are poorly understood, but host immunity to the virus appears to play an essential role in preventing the development of clinical disease resulting from reactivation. Thus, in immunocompromised solid organ and bone marrow transplant recipients, or patients with HIV infection, reactivation of CMV frequently occurs. In this setting, CMV can be highly pathogenic, causing life-threatening and/or severe deep tissue infections, including pneumonia, enteritis, and retinitis.[2-5] Efforts to dissect the role of individual components of the host immune response in controlling the CMV disease that develops in these immunocompromised hosts have suggested that CD8+ CMV- specific cytolytic T cells (Tc) are essential for successful resolution of infection.[6-8] The importance of CD8+ Tc effector cells for controlling CMV infection is also supported by studies in murine models, which have demonstrated that adoptive transfer of CD8+ Tc specific for

[a] This work was supported by Grant CA 18029 from the National Cancer Institute. S. R. Riddell is a Fellow of the Leukemia Society of America.

murine CMV into immunosuppressed mice provides protection from a potentially lethal challenge with the virus.[9–10]

Allogeneic bone marrow transplantation (BMT) offers a unique setting for evaluating T cell immunity to CMV, by permitting analysis of the nature and specificity of the T cell response to CMV present in healthy CMV-seropositive bone marrow donors with latent CMV infection, and comparison of this response both to the response elicited in HLA-matched BMT recipients who successfully control CMV reactivation and to the response in recipients who die of progressive CMV infection. Therefore, studies have been designed to determine if the presence of a CD8$^+$ Tc response in BMT recipients is essential for resistance to life-threatening CMV infection, and to define the specificity for CMV proteins of the immunodominant CD8$^+$ response potentially responsible for maintaining viral latency and preventing clinical reactivation in healthy seropositive individuals. Our plan is to eventually treat immunoincompetent BMT recipients by transfer of CD8$^+$ Tc clones, derived from the bone marrow donor and expanded in vitro prior to adoptive therapy, that are representative of the protective immune response in the normal healthy host. Our results have demonstrated that the presence of a detectable CMV-specific CD8$^+$ Tc response in BMT recipients strongly correlates with resistance to severe CMV infection. Moreover, distinct from the class I-restricted CD8$^+$ Tc responses characterized to other human viral pathogens, CMV-specific CD8$^+$ Tc can lyse target cells infected with CMV prior to viral gene expression. This response may be ideally suited for protecting the latently infected host from episodes of subclinical viral reactivation, and is now being evaluated in studies of adoptive therapy for immunoincompetent BMT recipients to provide protection from the development of clinical disease.

MATERIALS AND METHODS

Patient Population

Cells for these studies were obtained either from healthy volunteers with latent CMV infection, as defined by seropositivity for anti-CMV IgG antibody, or from HLA matched sibling allogeneic BMT donor and recipient pairs in which the donor was CMV seropositive.

Viruses and Cell Lines

AD169 strain CMV was obtained from the American Type Culture Collection and propagated by serial passage on human foreskin fibroblasts. The vaccinia/ CMV immediate early gene recombinant virus was kindly provided by Geoff Smith and J. G. P. Sissons, Cambridge University, England. The construction and characterization of the vac/IE virus has been previously described.[11] Dermal fibroblast lines were established from 3-mm punch skin biopsies obtained from the CMV seropositive individuals in the study population.

Expansion and Cloning of CMV-Specific Tc In Vitro

T cell culture systems developed to generate antigen-specific responses were modified to promote expansion of CMV-specific Tc in vitro.[11] Briefly, fibroblast lines were infected for 8 hours with AD169 strain CMV at a multiplicity of infection of 5, and cultured with PBMC at an R : S ratio of 20 : 1 in RPMI 1640 supplemented with 10% human CMV-seronegative AB serum, 2 mM L-glutamine, and 2.5×10^{-5} M 2-ME. Cultures were restimulated after 7 days with CMV-infected fibroblasts plus autologous irradiated PBMC feeder cells, and fed with 2 U/ml rIL-2 at 2 and 4 days following restimulation.

CD8+ Tc clones were generated from 14-day Tc lines by depleting CD4+ T cells with αCD4 mAb and rabbit complement, and then plating the enriched CD8+ Tc in 96-well plates at 0.3 cells/well with autologous irradiated feeder cells, autologous CMV-infected fibroblasts, and 50 U/ml IL-2. Fourteen days after plating, cells from wells containing proliferating viable cells were transferred to 24-well plates, restimulated every 7 days with CMV-infected fibroblasts and irradiated feeder cells, and fed with 50 U/ml IL-2 at 2 and 4 days after each restimulation.

Cytotoxicity Assay

The cytolytic activity of CMV-specific T cell lines and CD8+ T cell clones was measured in a 4-hour chromium release assay 5 to 7 days following restimulation. Autologous and MHC class I-mismatched fibroblast target cells were labelled overnight with 200 μCi Cr^{51} and infected with CMV for 24 hours at an MOI of 5 to prepare targets expressing all immediate early (IE), early (E), and late (L) CMV genes. Target cells expressing only IE genes were generated by: preincubating cells for 30 minutes with 100 μg/ml of the protein synthesis inhibitor cycloheximide (CHX), infecting with CMV in the presence of CHX for 2 hours to permit transcription but not translation of the IE genes, adding 20 μg/ml Actinomycin D (Act D) to cultures containing CHX for 30 minutes, washing out the CHX with media containing only Act D, and culturing in media with Act D to permit translation of the existing IE mRNA but to prevent transcription of new E and L mRNA, which are dependent on the presence of the regulatory IE proteins. Target cells infected with CMV, but incapable of expressing CMV genes following virion entry, were obtained by preincubating fibroblasts in media with 20 μg/ml Act D, and maintaining the cells in Act D during both infection and the cytotoxicity assay to prevent transcription of any viral mRNA.

RESULTS

CMV-Specific CD8+ Tc Responses in Allogeneic Bone Marrow Donors and Recipients

CMV-specific Tc activity was analyzed in 20 consecutive patients who had CMV seropositive bone marrow donors.[13] Lytic activity for CMV-infected targets was detected in short-term cultures from all 20 marrow donors. In 17/20 donors, depletion of T cell subsets and/or testing against autologous and HLA-mismatched targets demonstrated that target lysis was mediated by HLA-restricted CD8+ T cells (in 3 individuals, the presence of non-specific lytic activity obscured detection of CD8+ CMV-specific Tc).

The presence of CMV-specific Tc, as revealed following short-term lymphocyte cultures, was examined at 1, 2 and 3 months post-BMT in the HLA-matched sibling marrow transplant recipients of these 20 donors. Ten of 20 BMT recipients had no detectable Tc response to CMV during this posttransplant period. By contrast, the remaining 10 of the 20 total BMT recipients had measurable CD8$^+$ Tc within the first 3 months following BMT—with the majority of these responses first detectable at 2 to 3 months post-BMT. The kinetics of the generation of CMV-specific Tc immunity post-BMT in a representative patient is shown in FIGURE 1. A very weak response was detectable 1 month after BMT, the magnitude of this response increased progressively at 2 and 3 months post-BMT, and over the next several months the response achieved levels similar to those observed in the healthy donor.

The clinical courses of these 20 patients were monitored to determine if the presence of CMV-specific CD8$^+$ Tc correlated with protection from CMV disease. Of the 10 patients with detectable Tc, none developed CMV pneumonia. However, of the 10 patients lacking Tc, 6 developed fatal CMV pneumonia. This

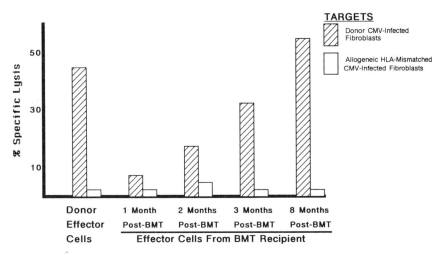

FIGURE 1. Reconstitution of the CMV-specific CTL response after allogeneic BMT. CTL activity was tested after short-term culture (2 stimulation cycles) of PBMC with autologous CMV-infected fibroblast stimulator cells against autologous or HLA-mismatched targets. Cells from the marrow donor were obtained before transplant, and from the patient at 1, 2, 3 and 8 months post-BMT.

incidence of CMV pneumonia in 6/20 (30%) of the total patients is consistent with previous studies of patients with seropositive donors from our center.[3,4,14] Thus, the data suggest that the absence of CMV-specific CD8$^+$ Tc in the first 3 months post-BMT is associated with a markedly increased risk of developing potentially fatal CMV infection.

In Vitro *Cloning and Expansion of CMV-Specific Tc*

These results in immunodeficient BMT recipients implied that specific reconstitution of the CMV-specific Tc response might provide protection from CMV disease. Therefore, a project was initiated to generate CMV-reactive T cells from healthy seropositive HLA-matched bone marrow donors for adoptive transfer into the BMT recipient. CMV-reactive Tc lines were established by repetitive cycles of stimulation with autologous CMV-infected fibroblasts, and tested after a minimum of 4 cycles for lytic activity against autologous, HLA-matched, and HLA-mismatched CMV-infected or uninfected fibroblasts. The majority of T cell lines demonstrated specific lysis of only CMV-infected autologous or HLA-matched targets. However, approximately 25% of these CMV-reactive T cell lines also exhibited lytic activity for uninfected allogeneic targets, suggesting that, as previously demonstrated following stimulation of T cells with other viruses,[15] alloreactive T cells persisted in these CMV-reactive T cell lines. The potential presence of donor T cells not specific for CMV would preclude the adoptive transfer of these T cell lines into the HLA-matched sibling recipient of an allogeneic BMT, because of the risk of inducing graft-versus-host disease. Therefore, it became essential to develop methods for the cloning of individual T cells specific for CMV antigens and for expanding the progeny of these cells to large numbers.

Two methods, as described in Materials and Methods,[12,18] were developed for cloning and expanding CMV-specific T cells to numbers sufficient for adoptive therapy. PBL from seropositive donors were stimulated in vitro with autologous CMV-infected fibroblasts, depleted of $CD4^+$ cells, and then cloned by stimulation in limiting dilution cultures containing IL-2 and filler cells with either CMV-infected fibroblasts or αCD3 mAb to trigger the T cell receptors. The progeny of cells growing under these conditions were expanded for testing and maintained by cyclical periods of stimulation with infected fibroblasts or αCD3 followed by promotion of growth with IL-2. Clones generated by both methods demonstrated specific lytic activity for autologous CMV-infected targets, and did not lyse mismatched or uninfected targets (TABLE 1).

Based on extrapolations from murine models, a cell dose between 10^8 and 10^{10} T cells/m^2 will be required for prophylaxis of CMV infection in humans.[10] Both cloning methods have proved to be efficient for rapid expansion with retention of specificity for CMV yielding adequate T cell numbers for administration of potentially therapeutic doses within 6 to 8 weeks of initiating cloning. Stimulation with αCD3, which does not require autologous infected stimulator cells for clonal expansion, was advantageous in situations in which the availability of fibroblasts was limiting. However, clones grown long-term with αCD3 stimulation exhibited less lytic activity/cell than cells grown with infected fibroblasts, potentially reflecting modulation of the T cell receptor by the mAb. Therefore, whenever possible, the clones used for our studies have been maintained by stimulation with CMV-infected cells.

Nature of the CMV Antigens Recognized by CD8⁺ Tc Clones

CMV contains a large number of proteins that could potentially elicit an immune response. However, CMV persists in the host as a latent virus, and protection from reactivation may require recognition of particular CMV proteins, such as those expressed early following cellular infection and prior to virion assembly. Therefore, the specificity of the CMV-reactive T cell responses present in healthy seropositive individuals was evaluated. Herpes virus genes are divided into 3 major groups based on the kinetics of gene expression:[16] (1) immediate early (IE) genes, which encode regulatory viral proteins; (2) early (E) genes which encode proteins such as the viral DNA polymerase, but require the products of the regulatory IE genes for expression; and (3) late (L) genes, which include the viral structural genes. Target cells expressing only IE genes were established by infecting fibroblasts with CMV in the presence of the protein synthesis inhibitor CHX, which permits transcription but not translation of IE mRNA, followed by addition of Act D and washout of CHX, which permits translation of the already formed IE mRNA but precludes transcription of new mRNA, such as initiation of transcription of the viral E or L genes following expression of the transactivating IE protein.

TABLE 1. MHC Class I Restriction of Representative CMV-Specific Tc Clones Generated with Anti-CD3 or CMV-Infected Fibroblasts

A. Clones Generated with Anti-CD3 mAb Stimulation (Donor TM)[a]

	Target Cell (% Lysis)			
Clone	TM CMV+	TM Mock	CM CMV+	CM Mock
TM 2E9	52	3	0	1
TM 2-24	40	0	0	0
SM 2-19	29	1	1	1
TM 2-30	38	0	1	0
TM 2-21	31	1	1	1
CM Tc line	1	1	49	5

B. Clones Generated with CMV-Infected Fibroblasts (Donor SS)[b]

	Target Cell (% Lysis)			
Clone	SS CMV+	SS Mock	MR CMV+	MR Mock
SS 21D8	61	1	2	0
SS 20D7	60	4	1	0
SS 22D1	52	1	0	0
SS 7D9	30	0	0	1
SS 1G10	31	0	0	0
MR Tc line	9	9	42	0

[a] T cells from short-term CMV-specific Tc line TM were cloned at 0.3 cells/well with autologous irradiated PBL as filler and anti-CD3 mAb as stimulation in media supplemented with 50 U/ml IL-2. Growing clones were assayed at an effector-to-target ratio of 10 : 1 for lysis of Cr^{51}-labelled autologous CMV-infected and mock infected fibroblasts, and class I HLA mismatched CMV-infected and mock infected fibroblasts.

[b] T cells from short-term CMV-specific Tc line SS were cloned at 0.3 cells/well in 96-well round-bottom plates with 2×10^3 autologous CMV-infected fibroblasts/well as stimulator and autologous irradiated feeder cells in media supplemented with 50 U/ml IL-2. Growing clones were assayed at an effector-to-target ratio of 5 : 1 for class I MHC restricted CMV-specific lysis in a 5-hour chromium release assay.

T cell clones from multiple individuals generated in response to CMV-infected stimulator cells recognized target cells treated sequentially with CHX and Act D (TABLE 2). These data were consistent with murine studies demonstrating that IE gene products are a major target for CMV-reactive T cells.[17] However, targets expressing the product of the major CMV-IE gene following infection with a recombinant vaccinia/IE virus were not lysed by the human T cell clones. These results suggested that lysis of CHX/Act D-treated targets by CMV-specific T cell clones did not result form recognition of the major IE protein. Therefore, the requirement for viral gene expression was analyzed by treating targets with Act D throughout the period of infection. Despite the absence of viral gene expression in these cells, as confirmed by Northern blot analysis for IE mRNA and Western blot analysis for IE proteins,[18] targets infected with CMV in the presence of Act D were lysed by the CMV-specific Tc clones (TABLE 3). Thus, viral proteins introduced into the cytoplasm of the target cell following penetration of CMV through the cell membrane and viral uncoating are the targets of the immunodominant host CD8$^+$ T cell response. Processing of these viral proteins occurs in a brefeldin A sensitive pathway (data not shown),[18] as predicted for intracellular proteins either endogenously synthesized or loaded into the cytoplasm of a cell and presented in the context of class I MHC molecules.

Preliminary studies, in which individual CMV genes have been inserted into expression vectors and expressed in targets, have been performed to define the precise CMV proteins recognized by the T cell response to the virus. Targets expressing GB, the major envelope protein, were not lysed by the Tc clones isolated in response to CMV-infected cells. By contrast, targets expressing products of genes encoding tegument proteins were lysed. Thus, these viral proteins, which are contained in the matrix of infectious virions, appear to be introduced into the cytoplasm of target cells in sufficient quantity to render targets susceptible to lysis.

TABLE 2. CMV-Specific Tc Clones from Two Representative Individuals Recognize CMV-Infected Cells Expressing Only the CMV-IE Genes but Do Not Recognize Cells Infected with a Vaccinia-IE Recombinant Virus[a]

A. Donor TM

T Cell Clone	Target Cell (% Lysis)			
	TM Mock	TM CMV	TM CMV(CHX/MTD)	TM Vac/IE
TM 2E9	1	38	32	1
TM 2-24	0	30	26	0
TM 2-19	1	32	28	2

B. Donor SS

T Cell Clone	Target Cell (% Lysis)			
	SS Mock	SS CMV	SS CMV(CHX/ActD)	SS Vac/IE
SS 1G10	0	52	41	1
SS 21E5	1	61	50	2
SS 3D6	2	42	34	1

[a] CMV-specific Tc clones were generated as described in TABLE 1, and assayed in a 4-hour chromium release assay at day 6 of a 7-day restimulation cycle. Target cells were Cr^{51}-labelled autologous fibroblasts either mock infected (Mock); infected with CMV at an MOI of 5 for 24 hours with no metabolic blockade (CMV); pretreated with cycloheximide (100 μg/ml) for 1 hour and infected for 2 hours with CMV, followed by washout of the cycloheximide and addition of Actinomycin D (20 mg/ml) for a further 2-hour incubation prior to use in the 4-hour chromium release assay (CMV-CHX/ActD); or infected with a recombinant vaccinia virus containing an infected CMV-IE gene (vac/IE) at an MOI of 10 for 16 hours. The data is presented for an E/T ratio of 10:1.

TABLE 3. CMV-Specific Tc Clones Lyse CMV-Infected Cells in the Absence of Endogenous Viral Gene Expression[a]

	Target Cell (% Lysis)		
Clone	SS Mock	SS CMV	SS CMV Act D
SS 1G10	0	57	54
SS 21E5	0	77	75
SS 3D6	0	46	47
SS 21G12	1	56	46
SS Tc line	8	61	63

[a] CD8[+] MHC class I restricted CMV-specific T cell clones derived from seropositive donor SS were assayed for lytic activity at day 6 of a 7-day restimulation cycle. Target cells were Cr[51]-labelled autologous fibroblasts either mock infected (Mock), infected with CMV for 4 hours (CMV), or pretreated with Actinomycin D (20 μg/ml) for 1 hour and infected with CMV for 4 hours (CMV-Act D). Targets were plated with effectors at various E/T ratios for 4 hours and % specific release determined. Act D was present in the media throughout the cytolytic assay for lysis of Act D-treated targets. E/T ratio for the data presented is 10 : 1.

Specificity of CMV-Specific Tc for Clinical Isolates of CMV

Isolates of CMV have demonstrated significant genetic variability from each other, although each individual is generally infected with only a single strain.[18] Such viral heterogeneity could interfere with the therapeutic efficacy of adoptively transferred T cell clones. Therefore, to determine if Tc recognize conserved epitopes, Tc clones generated in response to stimulation with laboratory strain AD169 were tested for lysis of targets infected with the Towne laboratory strain or 4 early passage CMV strains isolated from BMT patients. Analysis of restriction endonuclease digests of viral DNA extracted from these viruses demonstrated that all the strains were genetically distinct. Fifteen Tc clones derived from 3 donors were demonstrated to lyse autologous fibroblasts infected with AD169, Towne, or the 4 CMV clinical isolates. Data from 3 representative clones are shown in TABLE 4. The pattern of target lysis was identical for all Tc clones, suggesting that all CMV strains expressed the relevant epitopes. Future studies elucidating the structure-function relationship of these viral proteins should make it possible to determine if the recognition of all isolates by all clones tested reflects an essential function of the portion of the molecule recognized by Tc.

DISCUSSION

Healthy CMV-seropositive patients, who do not develop clinical CMV infection in the absence of immunosuppression, were uniformly found to have in their PBL detectable CD8[+] Tc specific for CMV. However, following elimination of this response as a consequence of ablation of the immune system by high-dose chemoradiotherapy in preparation for BMT, such seropositive individuals are at significant risk for severe CMV infection. Our results demonstrate that a fraction of BMT recipients reconstitute CD8[+] Tc responses to CMV within the first three months following transplant of donor bone marrow, and that the presence of this CMV-specific Tc response strongly correlates with host resistance to the develop-

TABLE 4. Representative CMV-Specific Tc Clones from Donor SS Lyse Cells Infected with Laboratory Strains and Wild Type Isolates of CMV[a]

Cytolytic Effector T Cells	Target Cell (% Lysis)													
	SS Mock	SS AD169	SS Towne	SS 5018	SS 1372	SS 4709	SS 3800	TM Mock	TM AD169	TM Towne	TM 5018	TM 1372	TM 4709	TM 3800
SS 21E5	2	48	37	40	42	31	28	0	0	1	2	0	2	1
SS 1A6	0	55	26	25	30	25	25	0	1	1	2	0	0	1
SS 1G10	2	63	36	33	38	33	20	5	0	2	1	1	0	4
TM Tc line	1	2	2	—	0	—	1	2	26	22	—	16	—	14

[a] Strain AD169 of CMV was obtained from the American Type Tissue Culture Collection and propagated on human foreskin fibroblasts. Supernatant virus was used to infect target fibroblasts at an MOI of 5:1. Strain Towne was kindly provided by Dr. Adam Geballe and used to infect target fibroblasts at an MOI of 5:1. Wild type strains of CMV (5018, 4709, 3800) were isolated from bone marrow transplant recipients and grown on human foreskin fibroblasts. All wild type strains were used in these experiments between passage 4 and 8.

Cytolytic effector T cells were either CD8+ T cell clones derived from donor SS by stimulation with autologous fibroblasts infected with CMV AD169 strain, or a cytolytic T cell line derived from donor TM by repetitive cycles of stimulation with autologous fibroblasts infected with CMV AD169 strain.

Target cells were Cr[51]-labelled autologous (SS) and class I HLA mismatched fibroblasts (TM). Targets were infected with AD169 and Towne strain for 24 hours. To infect with wild type strains, foreskin fibroblasts that showed 4+ cytopathic effect were harvested with trypsin, sonicated or freeze-thawed three times, and plated onto target cells in 6-well plates. To enhance infectivity the plates were centrifuged at 1000 g for 10 minutes. When cultures showed 3–4+ cytopathic effect (usually 72–120 hours post infection), cells were labelled with Cr[51] for use in a 5-hour chromium release assay. Data is shown for an E/T ratio of 10:1.

ment of life-threatening CMV infection. Thus, approaches that augment T cell responses to CMV in patients lacking CMV immunity might provide protection from CMV disease.

There are several methods that could potentially be employed to enhance the immunity of BMT recipients to CMV. However, active immunization of the host is unlikely to be beneficial, since the global immunoincompetence of BMT recipients in the early post-BMT period precludes effective in vivo response. Administration of a large number of CD8$^+$ T cells isolated from the HLA-matched seropositive BM donor could be evaluated, but, in the absence of selection for CMV-reactive cells, the induced T cells would likely contain alloreactive cells that could induce GVHD. Therefore, our laboratory has chosen to examine the potential for generating and transferring donor-derived CD8$^+$ T cell clones that are specific for CMV antigens in the context of an MHC molecule shared by the donor and host. The basis for this approach has been validated by previous studies from our laboratory in murine models demonstrating that adoptively transferred CD8$^+$ T cell clones are effective in the treatment of disseminated virally-induced tumors,[20] as well as studies demonstrating that immunosuppressed mice can be protected from potentially lethal challenge with murine CMV by administration of CMV-specific CD8$^+$ Tc.[9–10]

Our results have demonstrated that human CMV-specific CD8$^+$ T cells can be isolated and cloned *in vitro*. Moreover, the T cell clones can be expanded to numbers sufficient for adoptive therapy by repetitive cycles of stimulation employing either CMV-infected fibroblasts as stimulator cells or αCD3 mAb to crosslink the T cell receptor, with supplementation of cultures with IL-2 as a growth factor. These CD8$^+$ clones retain cytolytic activity and specificity for CMV-infected targets, and can be rested with retention of viability for several weeks in the absence of stimulation (data not shown). The development of this technology has made it possible for us to now initiate a clinical trial for prophylaxis of CMV infection in BMT recipients by adoptive transfer of CMV-specific CD8$^+$ T cell clones derived from the bone marrow donor.

Achieving therapeutic benefit in this trial will be dependent upon the transfer of T cell clones specific for appropriate CMV antigens. Therefore, the nature of the CMV antigens recognized by T cells from healthy seropositive hosts with protective immunity was determined. The results demonstrated that the immunodominant CD8$^+$ Tc response present in such hosts recognizes infected targets prior to expression of CMV genes in the cell. These class I-restricted Tc appear to be specific for viral tegument proteins introduced into the cytoplasm of the cell following viral uncoating. Preliminary studies have demonstrated that CD8$^+$ Tc to other viral proteins, such as IE and GB, can be elicited, but such Tc recognize targets only after the viral gene has been expressed, and are present in very low frequency as compared to the dominant response (data not shown). The presentation and recognition of viral proteins in the context of class I MHC molecules in infected cells in the absence of viral gene expression has not previously been demonstrated to occur in humans following natural infection, although it has been possible to load influenza virus proteins into target cells by chemically blocking the function of the viral neuraminidase.[21]

The generation of a T cell response capable of lysing CMV-infected targets prior to viral gene expression is attractive as a protective response developed by the host, since it permits destruction of infected targets prior to assembly of new infectious virions. Moreover, the transfer of T cell clones recognizing these viral antigens into immunocompromised hosts may be an ideal method to provide protection from CMV disease. The presence of T cells with this specificity as the immunodominant response in healthy seropositive individuals raises theoretical questions about the nature of CMV latency in healthy hosts. The structural viral tegument or capsid proteins that are recognized by these clones would not be expected to be expressed in latently infected cells. Thus, the maintenance of T cell reactivity for such viral proteins in healthy hosts might more likely result from repetitive immune responses to subclinical episodes of viral reactivation rather than a persistent latent state. The necessity for this T cell response to control frequent episodes of usually undiagnosed reactivation may explain why clinical disease occurs so commonly in patients following immunosuppression.

SUMMARY

CMV infection represents a major cause of morbidity and mortality in immunosuppressed bone marrow transplant (BMT) recipients. Life-threatening CMV infection was found to occur only in patients who did not develop a CMV-specific $CD8^+$ Tc response. Therefore, methods to clone and expand CMV-specific Tc were developed to facilitate analysis of the specificity of the $CD8^+$ Tc response to CMV responsible for protective immunity in seropositive donors, and to permit adoptive transfer of in vitro expanded CMV-specific Tc derived from bone marrow donors into immunocompetent HLA-matched BMT recipients to augment resistance to CMV. The immunodominant class I-restricted Tc response present in healthy seropositive individuals was found to be specific for a conserved CMV antigen introduced into the cytoplasm and presented shortly following viral penetration and uncoating, and did not require endogenous viral gene expression and protein synthesis. Thus, the protective immune response to CMV mediates lysis of virally-infected cells prior to virion assembly. Processing of viral proteins and access to presentation in the context of class I MHC molecules immediately following infection of target cells was selective for internal virion proteins, such as the tegument protein pp65. By contrast, presentation by infected cells of GB, the major CMV envelope protein, or IE, the major regulatory protein, was delayed due to a requirement for endogenous synthesis in infected cells, and $CD8^+$ Tc specific for these proteins were detected in low frequency as compared to the immundominant response.

ACKNOWLEDGMENTS

We wish to thank Kathe Watanabe for expert technical assistance and Joanne Factor for assistance in preparation of the manuscript.

REFERENCES

1. Ho, M. 1982. Cytomegalovirus: biology and infection. 309. Plenum Press. New York.
2. PETERSON, P. K., H. H. BALFOUR, JR., S. C. MARKER, D. S. FRYD, R. J. HOWARD & R. L. SIMMONS. 1980. Cytomegalovirus disease in renal allograft recipients: a prospective study of clinical features, risk factors and impact on renal transplantation. Medicine (Baltimore) 59: 283.
3. MEYERS, J. D., N. FLUORNOY & E. D. THOMAS. 1982. Nonbacterial pneumonia after allogeneic marrow transplantation. A review of ten years' experience. Rev. Infect. Dis. 4: 1119.

4. MEYERS, J. D., N. FLUORNOY & E. D. THOMAS. 1986. Risk factors for cytomega-
     lovirus infection after human marrow transplantation. J. Infect. Dis. **153**: 478.

5. JACOBSON, M. A. & J. MILLS. 1988. Serious cytomegalovirus disease in the acquired
     immunodeficiency syndrome (AIDS). Ann. Int. Med. **108**: 585–594.

8. QUINNAN, G. V., N. KIRMANI, A. H. ROOK, J. F. MANISCHEWITZ, L. JACKSON, G.
     MORESCHI, G. W. SANTOS, R. SARAL & W. H. BURNS. 1982. Cytotoxic T cells in
     cytomegalovirus infection: HLA-restricted T lymphocyte and non-T lymphocyte
     cytotoxic responses correlate with recovery from cytomegalovirus in bone marrow
     transplant recipients. N. Engl. J. Med. **307**: 6.

7. OUINNAN, G. V., N. KIRMANI, E. ESKER, R. SARAL, J. F. MANISCHEWITZ, L. ROG-
     ERS, A. H. ROOK, G. W. SANTOS & W. H. BURNS. 1981. HLA-restricted cytotoxic T
     lymphocyte and nonthymic cytotoxic lymphocyte responses to cytomegalovirus in-
     fection of bone marrow transplant recipients. J. Immunol. **126**: 2036.

8. ROOK, A. H., G. V. QUINNAN, W. J. R. FREDERICK, J. F. MANISCHEWITZ, N. KIR-
     MANI, T. DANTZLER, B. B. LEE & G. B. CURRIER. 1984. Importance of cytotoxic
     lymphocytes during cytomegalovirus infection in renal transplant recipients. Am. J.
     Med. **76**: 385.

9. REDDEHASE, M. J., F. WEILAND, K. MUNCH, S. JONJIC, A. LUSKE & U. H. KOS-
     ZINOWSKI. 1985. Interstitial murine cytomegalovirus pneumonia after irradiation:
     characterization of cells that limit viral replication during established infection of
     lungs. J. Virol. **55**: 264.

10. REDDEHASE, M. J., W. MUTTER, K. MUNCH, H. J. BUHRING & U. H. KOSZINOWSKI.
     1987. CD8-positive cytotoxic T lymphocytes specific for murine cytomegalovirus
     immediate-early antigens mediate protective immunity. J. Virol. **61**: 3102.

11. BORYSTEWIRZ, L. K., J. K. HICKLING, S. GRAHAM, J. SINCLAIR, M. P. CRANAGE,
     G. L. SMITH & J. G. P. SISSONS. 1988. Human cytomegalovirus-specific cytotoxic T
     cells: relative frequency of stage-specific CTL recognizing the 72 KD immediate
     early protein and glycoprotein B expressed by recombinant vaccinia viruses. J. Exp.
     Med. **168**: 919.

12. RIDDELL, S. R. & P. D. GREENBERG. 1990. The use of anti-CD3 and anti-CD28 mono-
     clonal antibodies to clone and expand human antigen-specific T cells. J. Immunol.
     Methods **128**: 189.

13. REUSSER, P., S. R. RIDDELL, J. D. MEYERS & P. D. GREENBERG. Cytotoxic T lympho-
     cyte response to cytomegalovirus following human allogeneic bone marrow trans-
     plantation: pattern of recovery and correlation with cytomegalovirus infection and
     disease. Blood. In press.

14. MEYERS, J. D., R. A. BOWDEN & G. W. COUNTS. 1987. Infection after bone marrow
     transplantation. *In* Infections in Transplant Patients. H. Lode, D. Huhn & M.
     Mulzahn, Eds. 17–32. Georg Thieme Verlag. Stuttgart and New York.

15. YANG, Y., P. L. DUNTON, R. R. NAHILL & R. M. WELSH. 1989. Virus-induced
     polyclonal cytotoxic T lymphocyte stimulation. J. Immunol. **142**: 1710–1718.

16. GRIFFITHS, P. D. & J. C. GRUNDY. 1987. Molecular biology and immunology of
     cytomegalovirus. Biochem. J. **241**: 313–324.

17. REDDEHASE, M. J. & U. H. KOSZINOWSKI. 1984. Significance of herpes virus immedi-
     ate early gene expression in cellular immunity to cytomegalovirus infection. Nature
     312: 369–371.

18. RIDDELL, S. R., M. RABIN, A. P. GEBALLE & P. D. GREENBERG. Human cytomega-
     lovirus-specific T lymphocytes recognize infected cells in the absence of viral gene
     expression. J. Immunol. In press.

19. CHOU, S. W. 1986. Acquisition of donor strains of CMV by renal transplant recipients.
     N. Engl. J. Med. **314**: 1418–1423.

20. KLARNET, J. P., L. A. MATIS, D. E. KERN, M. T. MIZUNO, D. J. PEACE, J. A.
     THOMPSON, P. D. GREENBERG & M. A. CHEEVER. 1987. Antigen-driven T cell
     clones can proliferate *in vivo*, eradicate disseminated leukemia and provide specific
     immunologic memory. J. Immunol. **138**: 4012–4017.

21. YEWDELL, J. W., J. R. BENNICK & Y. HOSAKA. 1988. Cells process exogenous pro-
     teins for recognition by cytotoxic T lymphocytes. Science **239**: 637.

T Cell Molecular Targets for Psoralens

MICHELLE S. MALANE AND FRANCIS P. GASPARRO

Photobiology Laboratory
Department of Dermatology
Yale University
333 Cedar Street
New Haven, Connecticut 06510

INTRODUCTION

Psoralens are photoactivatable compounds which have been used as therapeutic agents for skin disorders for centuries. Plant extracts containing psoralens were used in ancient Egypt to treat depigmented skin.[1] In modern times 8-methoxypsoralen (8-MOP) and UVA (PUVA therapy) are used to treat vitiligo,[2] psoriasis[3] and cutaneous T cell lymphoma (CTCL).[4,5] Thirty-five years ago it was demonstrated that UVA-activated psoralens formed photoadducts with DNA. Psoralen research has largely been focused on these DNA effects as the mechanism of action in biological systems. More recently, however, other molecular targets, including proteins and lipids, have been investigated, albeit only to a limited extent. Now with the advent of extracorporeal photochemotherapy for the treatment of cutaneous T cell lymphoma, the elucidation of the molecular events underlying an induced immunologic response has become a new goal. In this paper the effects of 8-MOP on DNA, cell membrane DNA, proteins, and lipids are described. In addition, the possible immunologic mechanisms responsible for the therapeutic effects of 8-MOP and UVA are discussed.

Psoralen—Properties and Characteristics

The furocoumarins (psoralens and angelicins) are a class of tricyclic aromatic compounds formed by the fusion of a furan ring to a coumarin moiety. The linear compound that results is known as a psoralen (FIG. 1, upper). If the 2,3 furan bond is fused to the 7,8 bond of the coumarin, an angular furocoumarin, angelicin, is formed (FIG. 1, lower). The extended aromatic structure of furocoumarins is responsible for their ability to absorb long wavelength ultraviolet A radiation. FIGURE 2 shows the UV spectrum of 8-MOP. Absorption bands near 250 and 300 nm are characteristic of all furocoumarins. It is interesting to note that the optimal wavelengths for activation of 8-MOP (*i.e.,* in the UVA region—320–400 nm) do not coincide with the absorption peak at 300 nm. In fact irradiation of psoralens with 300 nm radiation leads to very efficient photodegradation of the compound. The molecule is inert until exposed to UVA. It then becomes transiently activated into excited states (FIG. 3). Once activated psoralen can react with other compounds creating covalent photoadducts. Photoactivated psoralens can generate a reactive oxygen species, singlet oxygen, which is capable of inducing other biomolecular modifications such as the cross-linking of protein subunits (see below). Alternatively these activated furocoumarins can transfer energy to acceptor

196

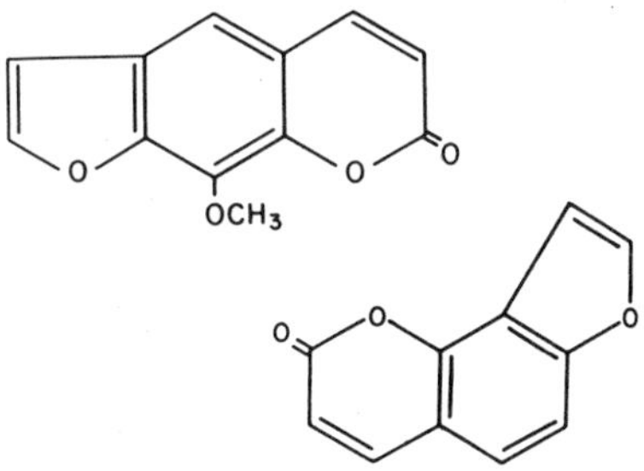

FIGURE 1. Molecular structures: 8-methoxypsoralen (*upper*), angelicin (*lower*).

molecules creating photodynamically active agents. The first noted and most widely studied biomolecular interaction of photoactivated furocoumarins was their interaction with DNA.

Molecular Interactions: DNA

In 1965, Musajo showed that DNA was a target for psoralen photomodification when he discovered the photocycloaddition of psoralen to pyrimidine bases (FIG. 4).[6] Psoralen derivatives can react at either the 3,4 bond of the pyrone ring or the 4',5' bond of the furan ring. The planar structure of these molecules makes them particularly suitable for intercalation with the base pairs found in double helical strands of DNA. In double-stranded DNA the 4',5' monoadduct is the primary photoadduct and with additional exposure to UVA, a second photoreaction can occur at the 3,4 pyrone bond, creating a DNA interstrand crosslink (FIG. 4). Initially it was thought that the cross-links were responsible for "shutting down" the DNA and thus inducing biological effects. However, recent studies have found that certain isomeric furocoumarins or angelicins which are only able to form monoadducts, and not cross-links, also demonstrate therapeutic effects.[7] Thus cross-link formation may not be a necessary condition for biological activity.

The initial studies of the effects of photoactivated psoralen on cells were interpreted in terms of DNA photoadduct formation. Recently, it has been shown that DNA occurs on the surface of cells and specifically on human leukocytes. Bennett showed that leukocytes appear to have a specific DNA binding receptor on the cell surface.[8] This receptor-bound DNA has been studied using selective extraction methods as well as immunofluorescence and radiolabeling assays. Cell

FIGURE 2. Ultraviolet absorption spectrum of 8-methoxypsoralen. Labels indicate regions of UVA activation and the wavelengths responsible for monoadduct (MA) and cross-link (XL) formation.

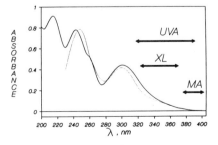

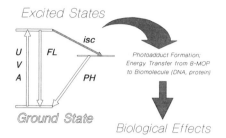

FIGURE 3. 8-MOP energy diagram. UVA activation of 8-methoxypsoralen promotes the molecule to an excited state. UVA: activating radiation; FL, fluorescence; PH, phosphoeresence; isc, intersystem crossing (see text for details).

membrane DNA (cmDNA) can be photomodified by 8-MOP, however, to a lesser extent than chromosomal DNA.[9] One explanation for this could be that interactions between cmDNA and its receptor could limit the access of 8-MOP to base pair intercalation sites. Alternatively, cmDNA could have an unusual base composition which might also alter the extent of 8-MOP intercalation and/or photoreaction.

Molecular Interactions: Proteins

Mechanisms involving either type of DNA may explain many of the mutagenic and cytotoxic effects of psoralens. However, several studies have shown that

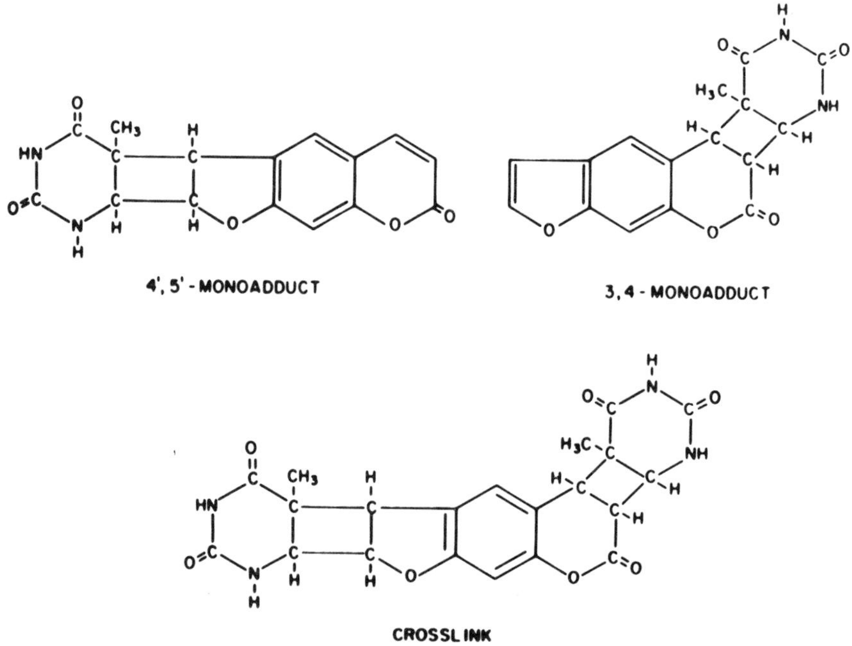

4', 5' - MONOADDUCT   3, 4 - MONOADDUCT

CROSSLINK

FIGURE 4. 8-MOP photoadducts. Photocycloaddition of 8-MOP to pyrimydine bases creates either 3,4 monoadduct (*right top*) or 4',5' monoadducts (*left top*) which with additional exposure to UVA forms interstrand cross-links (*bottom*).

other biological phenomena cannot be linked solely to DNA modification. Some studies have suggested that molecular targets other than DNA play a role in the inhibition of epidermal cell proliferation.[10] Additionally when cells are exposed to psoralens and then analyzed by microspectrofluorometry, the psoralen molecules are found to be distributed throughout the cell and not only in the nucleus.[11] This finding is consistent with recent studies which indicate that other cellular targets such as lipids and proteins can be modified by 8-MOP and UVA.[12]

The effects of UVA-activated psoralens on proteins and amino acids have been the subject of limited investigations.[10,12] No amino acid psoralen photoadduct has been characterized even though psoralen is known to undergo photoaddition reactions with proteins. Megaw performed NMR studies which suggested that the 3,4 and 4',5' positions of 8-MOP and the imidazole moiety of tryptophan were involved in photoadduct formation.[13] Although Megaw suggested that these amino acid adducts may be similar to the cyclobutane type formed with thymidine, detailed structural information was not obtained. The molecular details will no doubt differ from those involving DNA. Thus far, protein photomodification mediated by psoralens appears to proceed in an oxygen dependent fashion. The molecular events include 1) direct binding of the furocoumarin to the protein, 2) cross-linking of protein subunits, and 3) photooxidative processes producing sin-

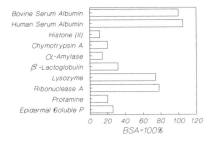

FIGURE 5. Photobinding of 8-MOP to 10 proteins. Extent of binding expressed as a percentage of BSA binding. (Adapted from Megaw et al.[13]).

glet oxygen which can directly modify amino acids. Unfortunately, due to the limited studies that have been performed, the details of the chemical mechanisms, as well as their biological significance, have yet to be elucidated.

One of the earliest described psoralen-mediated protein interactions was that studied by Lerman who characterized damage to human ocular lens tissue.[10] Photoactivated 8-MOP was covalently bound to the lens proteins. In addition, singlet oxygen was implicated in the oxidation of the lens crystallines. Furocoumarins exposed to UVA undergo covalent binding to other proteins such as lysozyme, serum albumin, histone, ribonuclease, glutamate dehydrogenase, enolase, thermolysine and E. coli DNA polymerase 1 (FIG. 5).[14–16] These reactions proceeded in the presence of oxygen but not in its absence except in the case of the DNA polymerase I. For BSA, in addition to photoinduced direct binding of the furocoumarin, it was observed that photolysis or photooxidation of the furocoumarin led to a reactive psoralen intermediate which bound to the protein in the absence of additional UVA exposure.[14] These same investigators also showed that tyrosine was photomodified. Further work by other investigators revealed that there are five amino acids that are particularly sensitive to photooxidation. These photomodified amino acids may be responsible for the photoinactivation of many proteins.[15,16] Veronese determined the amino acid content of lysozyme

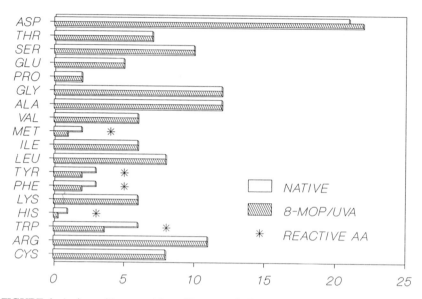

FIGURE 6. Amino acid composition of lysozyme before and after UVA irradiation in the presence of psoralen. Amino acids particularly sensitive to 8-MOP and UVA are indicated with *asterisks*. (Adapted from Yoshikawa *et al.*[14])

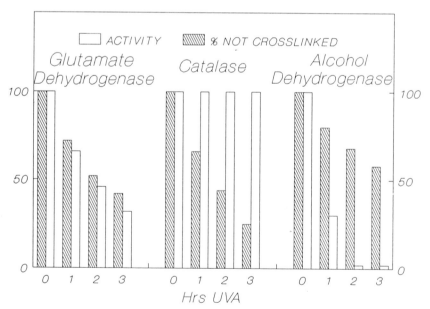

FIGURE 7. Enzymatic activity of proteins after treatment with 8-MOP and UVA. Also shown fraction of uncross-linked protein subunits. (Adapted from Schiavon and Veronese.[17])

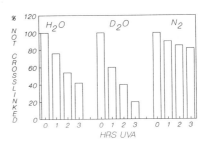

FIGURE 8. Effect of D_2O and N_2 on cross-link formation. (Adapted from Schiavon and Veronese.[17])

before and after UVA irradiation in the presence of psoralen (FIG. 6). They found a close correlation between the ability of the furocoumarins to photoinactivate enzymes and their ability to modify the amino acids histidine, tryptophan, tyrosine, methionine and phenylalanine.[15]

It has also been demonstrated that the exposure of oligomeric enzymes (glutamate dehydrogenase, catalase and alcohol dehydrogenase) to various furocoumarins and UVA irradiation led to extensive intermolecular cross-linking of enzyme subunits. However, as seen in the case of catalase, these cross-links where not necessarily responsible for the inactivation of the enzymes (FIG. 7).[17] In some cases psoralen-mediated cross-linking of polypeptide chains makes enzymes resistant to denaturation.[18] These cross-links may not directly involve the bifunctional furocoumarin moiety. Rather, the cross-links may arise from oxidative processes as a result of singlet oxygen formation.[17] FIGURE 8 shows the effect of two agents, D_2O and N_2, on the oxidative damage induced by 8-MOP and UVA. In the first panel the results of cross-linking in aqueous solutions is shown. In D_2O, more extensive cross-linking was observed as a result of the longer lifetime of singlet oxygen in this solvent. In the third panel the protective effects of N_2 purging is demonstrated.

Molecular Interactions: Lipids

Even more recently discovered are the effects of UVA-activated psoralens on lipids. Furocoumarins have been shown to oxidize unsaturated lipids in a two-step process. A reactive furocoumarin intermediate created by exposure to UVA undergoes an addition reaction to the unsaturated lipid.[10] Oxygen-independent reactions have also been described. Independently, Midden and Dall'Acqua described the covalent binding between furocoumarins and the unsaturated fatty acids linolenic acid and linolenic acid methylester. NMR analysis of the isolated photoadduct revealed a C4-cycloaddition between the 3,4 double bond of psoralen and the central double bond of the unsaturated fatty acid.[19] Photocycloaddition has also been described in the reaction of photoactivated furocoumarin with oleic acid methylester (FIG. 9).[10] Investigators have postulated that inhibition of cell prolif-

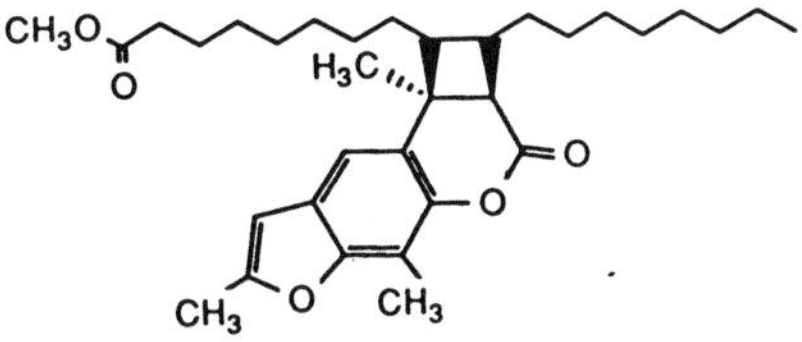

FIGURE 9. Trimethylpsoralen-lipid photoadduct structure. (From Midden.[10] Reprinted by permission from CRC Press.)

eration and altered regulation of metabolism could result from lipid photoadditions and/or oxidations. For example, it was suggested that these photoadducts could inhibit the lipid hydrolysis necessary for activation of protein kinase. In other studies, Beijersbergen showed that 60% of 8-MOP photoadducts formed in the epidermis are covalently bound to lipid, with only 20% bound to nucleic acids and 20% bound to proteins.[12] Thus, reactions involving photoactivated psoralens with lipids may have a significant biological effect.

Treatment of Lymphocytes with 8-MOP and UVA

In 1979 Kraemer demonstrated decreased DNA synthesis in circulating leukocytes of patients treated with PUVA.[20] Studies have since been preformed with lymphocytes *in vitro* where the cells are treated with 8-MOP and UVA.[21,22] DNA photoadducts are formed and can be quantified by scintillation analysis of incorporated [³H]8-MOP (FIG. 10). In addition, nuclear processes represented by tritiated thymidine incorporation can be assessed. These processes are suppressed at relatively low doses of 8-MOP and UVA. These doses were more than ten times less than levels considered lethal. At much greater doses of 8-MOP and UVA the cell membrane is damaged as evidenced by dramatic increases in permeability to trypan blue. The 8-MOP concentrations achieved in patients (double headed arrow in FIGURE 10) and the low effective UVA doses used during photopheresis correspond to doses that are intermediate between the two effects. Therefore, it has been determined that UVA-activated psoralen affects lymphocytes, but the

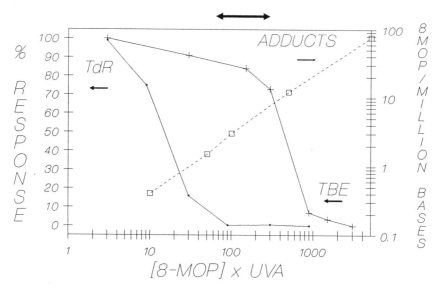

FIGURE 10. Effect of 8-MOP and UVA on lymphocytes. Three parameters are plotted as a function of the combined dose of 8-MOP (ng/ml) and UVA (J/cm²). Tritiated thymidine incorporation (TdR) after PHA stimulation measures the effect of 8-MOP and UVA at nuclear level; Trypan Blue exclusion (TBE) measures membrane integrity; the extent of 8-MOP photoadduct formation over the same dose range is also shown (ADDUCTS).

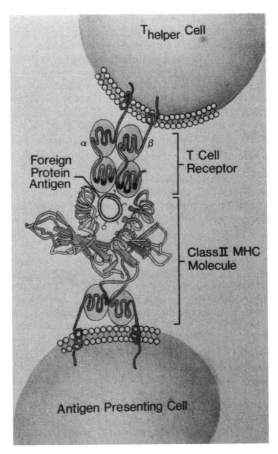

FIGURE 11. Schematic representation of a T cell receptor interacting with a peptide presented by an MHC I element. (From Sinha.[23a] Reprinted by permission from *Science*.)

specific mechanism with the involvement of either DNA, proteins or lipids or some combination of these, remains undetermined.

Among the many cell surface molecules on T lymphocytes one of the most important is its receptor for antigens. T cell receptors recognize "foreign molecules" or antigens when they are on an antigen presenting cell (APC) and associated with surface markers such as the major histocompatability complex (MHC) molecules. The antigen-presenting cell is often a macrophage which has engulfed the foreign protein and enzymatically digested it to a smaller form, an oligopeptide, which is re-presented in association with its cell surface MHC molecule (FIG. 11).[23] The peptides, however, may be either a part of an external foreign protein, as just described, or may be an internally synthesized protein (*e.g.,* viral or tumor specific proteins) which is placed on the cell surface. Modification of T cell components by photoactivated 8-MOP could result in the formation of a new antigenic peptide(s) inducing an immune reaction which may involve the T cell as either the target or the effector cell.

As described above, photoaddition to nuclear DNA is well-characterized. DNA photoadduct effects on cellular function of lymphocytes has been postulated. Whether the effects are secondary to photoaddition with nuclear or cell surface DNA has not been elucidated. Altered cmDNA in its receptor could be perceived as a new antigen leading to an immune response. Alternatively, the modification may indirectly affect other cell surface components such as in Laskin's model described below. Preliminary studies by Perez and Gasparro in an *in vitro* murine model have shown that the treatment of whole T cells with DNase has effects similar to treatment of cells with 8-MOP and UVA.

Perez studied allograft immunity using syngeneic photoinactivated effector lymphocytes and discovered that a temporary suppression of graft rejection could be induced. In that case it was postulated that immunologic reactions against photoaltered T cells were induced and could be directed against distinct antigenic components of the T cell surface, possibly the T cell receptor.[25] The photochemically induced changes in T cell surface components could create antigenic molecules related to photoaltered forms of DNA, protein and/or lipids.

Any surface protein, including specific receptors, could be affected directly by 8-MOP and UVA. If cross-links are formed, protein structure or configuration could change and then possibly render it more antigenic even though the function of the protein might not be altered (see above and FIG. 7). Additionally, the photolysis of specific amino acids and, thus a modification of the protein, could render the protein antigenic and thus lead to an immunological impact. Interestingly, we found that in assessing the amino acid content of variable regions of T cell receptors, the five photosensitive amino acids occurred at a 15% frequency. A less direct effect on receptors has been proposed by Laskin.[25] He noted the existence of a specific binding protein (or receptor) for 8-MOP on the surface of various epidermal cell lines and photobinding of psoralen to this receptor paralleled a decreased rate of cellular proliferation.[26] In his model, the photomodification of a putative psoralen receptor modulates the epidermal growth factor (EGF) receptor by inducing its phosphorylation. If these "psoralen receptors" also occur on circulating T cells, they may not only provide another opportunity for photoactivated 8-MOP to be presented as an "antigenic" component displayed on the cell surface, but may modulate the T cell receptor or other important cell surface receptors as in Laskin's model.

Lipid effects could also be important. One group of investigators found that photoadducts of 8-MOP to unsaturated fatty acids formed when lymphocytes were exposed to 8-MOP and UVA *in vitro*. These effects created changes in the lymphocyte receptor function possibly secondary to membrane damage.[27] Photoaddition to membrane lipids may not only effect its integrity. Membrane photoalterations could possibly expose or produce "new" antigenic species thereby providing non-self or antigenic components.

An immunologic response may occur if the T cell is altered by any of the mechanisms described above or alternatively if the T cell is the effector cell of the process. That is, if other cells are effected in any of the ways stated above then the T cell will recognize these abnormal molecules when presented appropriately. For example, if the peptide in association with the MHC on the antigen presenting cell is modified then the T cell could recognize it in a different way. FIGURE 11 depicts the molecular interactions that must occur for the correct presentation of antigen by an antigen presenting cells. The molecular contacts between these species and the foreign peptide or antigen could create suitable sites for psoralen association and hence possible sites of psoralen photoadduct or psoralen-mediated photooxidative processes.

Photomodification of the MHC molecule itself could alter subsequent T cell interactions. Inspection of the amino acid content of N-terminal region of some prototypical MHC 1 heavy chain amino acids shows a significant number were found to be photoreactive residues (FIG. 12). Treatment of MHC molecules with 8-MOP and UVA under *in vitro* conditions could reveal whether these amino acids are particularly susceptible to photoxidative damage.

Therapeutic Uses of 8-MOP and UVA

PUVA therapy is used in the treatment of psoriasis, vitiligo and CTCL. More recently an extracorporeal form of this phototherapy has been developed and

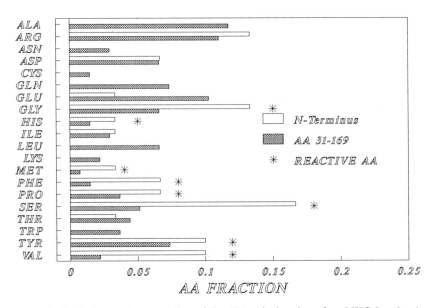

FIGURE 12. Amino acid composition of the N-terminal region of an MHC I molecule. Potentially photoreactive amino acids are indicated with *asterisks*.

used for systemically disseminated CTCL.[5] In this therapy psoralen is orally administered and then a lymphocyte fraction from patient blood is exposed to UVA. Edelson has suggested that the response to this therapy involves an immunologic reaction to the reinfused clonal tumor T cells which restricts the activity of the remaining population of abnormal T cells. In some patients T cell subset analyses revealed persistent decreases in the T4+ and BE2+ cells believed to be responsible for the tumor. Out of the 37 patients completing the study, 27 had an outstanding clinical response and two patients were free of disease for more than two years after treatment was terminated. Several patients have remained free of relapse longer than would be expected if the therapy were based solely on the destruction of existing tumor cells. This suggests an immunological suppression of the malignant cells. Any of the immmunologic mechanisms of action discussed above could be responsible for the therapeutic efficacy of photopheresis.

The progression and dissemination of CTCL may be a result of clinically aggressive subclones of malignant T cells. Thus a specific immunologic mechanism of action similar to the tum$^-$/tum$^+$ transplantation antigens could be involved in the response seen in photopheresis.[28,29] In the tum transplantation antigen system, mutagenization of mouse tumor cells produces tumor cells that acquire the ability to be rejected by the mice. The rejection is secondary to the tumor cell expression of a "new" transplantation antigen which is now recognized by cytotoxic T cells. This new transplanatation antigen is created by a single point mutation causing one amino acid difference in a peptide sequence that binds to the MHC molecule and is recognized by cytotoxic T cells. This process converts the aggressive tumor cell into one that the immune system can recognize. *In vitro* and *in vivo* assays demonstrated that mice immunized with certain tum$^-$ tumor cell variants were then able to mount a cytotoxic response towards the tum$^+$ cells as well. Immunization with the tum- tumor cells generated two distinct populations of cytotoxic lymphocytes—one directed against the tum$^-$ antigen and the other against the common antigen present on the entire tumor cell population (*i.e.,* on both the tum$^-$ and the tum$^+$ cells).[30,31]

In aggressive T cell lymphoma the photoactivated psoralen may be causing a mutation in a gene which leads to a change in a single amino acid in an oligopeptide displayed on the tumor T cell. Alternatively it could lead to the photodestruction of amino acids in tumor-specific proteins on the T cell surface The display of modified proteins or new antigenic epitopes would allow its recognition by the immune system and would lead to the cytolytic elimination of this cell type. In addition, a common tumor antigen may now also be recognized as in the tum transplantation antigen system. This response to the tumor could arrest its progression or perhaps destroy it. As in the tum$^-$ antigen model, the specific antigenic clone(s) created by mutagenizing treatment with 8-MOP and UVA would be responsible for the strength of the immune response against it and thus the subsequent therapeutic response. Experiments in progress will reveal whether 8-MOP and UVA possess this mutagenizing capability.

CONCLUSION

Psoralens are photoactivable compounds which affect a variety of cellular macromolecules leading to photoadduct formation, mutagenesis, inhibition of cell proliferation, altered metabolism and possible cell death. Because psoralens are inert until photoactivated, they are only active at sites simultaneously exposed to UVA. Therefore, they are good candidates as directed therapeutic agents and have been shown to be efficacious in the treatment of psoriasis, vitiligo and CTCL. In the case of CTCL treated with extracorporeal photochemotherapy it appears that an immunologic mechanism may be an important part of the induced responses. A scenario which involves direct effects to the malignant T cell via interactions with its nuclear DNA, cell surface DNA, proteins or lipids rendering it a target for immune surveillance are all possibilities. The precise mechanism(s) leading to the biological responses seen in photopheresis remain to be elucidated.

REFERENCES

1. FITZPATRICK, T. & M. PATHAK. 1959. Historical aspects of methoxsalen and other furocoumarins. J. Invest. Dermatol. **32:** 229–231.

2. LERNER, A., C. DENTON & T. FITZPATRICK. 1953. Clinical and experimental studies with 8-methoxypsoralen in vitiligo. J. Invest. Dermatol. **220:** 299–314.
3. PARRISH, J., T. FITZPATRICK, L. TANNENBAUM & M. PATHAK. 1974. Photochemotherapy of psoriasis with oral methoxsalen and longwave ultraviolet light. N. Engl. J. Med. **291:** 1207–1211.
4. GILCHREST, B. 1979. Methoxsalen photochemotherapy for mycosis fungoides. Cancer Treat. Rep. **63:** 663–667.
5. EDELSON, R., C. BERGER, F. GASPARRO et al. 1987. Treatment of cutaneous T-cell lymphoma by extracorporeal photochemotherapy. N. Engl. J. Med. **316:** 297–303.
6. MUSAJO, L., G. RODIGHIERO & F. DALL'ACQUA. 1965. Evidence of a photoreaction of the photosensitizing furocoumarins with DNA and with pyrimidine nucleosides and nucleotides. Experientia **21:** 24–25.
7. DUBERTRET, L., D. AVERBECK, E. BISAGNI et al. 1985. Photochemotherapy using pyridopsoralens. Biochimie **67:** 417–422.
8. BENNETT, R., G. GABOR & M. MERRITT. 1985. DNA binding to human leukocytes. J. Clin. Invest. **76:** 2182–2190.
9. GASPARRO, F., R. DALL'AMICO, M. O'MALLEY et al. 1990. Cell membrane DNA: a new target for psoralen photoadduct formation. Photochem. Photobiol. **52:** 315–321.
10. MIDDEN, W. 1988. Chemical mechanisms of the bioeffects of furocoumarins: the role of reactions with proteins, lipids, and other cellular constituents. In Psoralen DNA Photobiology. F. Gasparro, Ed. Vol. 2: 1–49. CRC Press. Boca Raton, FL.
11. MORENO, G., C. SALET, C. KOHEN & E. KOHEN. 1982. Penetration and localization of furocoumarins in single living cells studied by microspectrofluorometry. Biochem. Biophys. Acta **721:** 109–111.
12. AVERBECK, D. 1989. Recent advances in psoralen phototoxicity mechanism. Photochem. Photobiol. **50:** 859–882.
13. MEGAW, J., J. LEE & S. LERMAN. 1980. NMR analyses of tryptophan-8-methoxypsoralen photoreaction products formed in the presence of oxygen. Photochem. Photobiol. **32:** 265–269.
14. YOSHIKAWA, K., N. MORI, S. SAKAKIBARA et al. 1979. Photo-conjugation of 8-methoxypsoralen with proteins. Photochem. Photobiol. **29:** 1127–1133.
15. VERONESE, F., O. SCHIAVON, R. BEVILACQUA et al. 1982. Photoinactivation of enzymes by linear and angular furocoumarins. Photochem. Photobiol. **36:** 25–30.
16. GRANGER, M. & C. HELENE. 1983. Photoaddition of 8-methoxypsoralen to E. coli DNA polymerase I. Role of psoralen photoadducts in the photosensitized alterations of POL I enzymatic activities. Photochem. Photobiol. **38:** 563–568.
17. SCHIAVON O. & F. VERONESE. 1986. Extensive crosslinking between subunits of oligomeric proteins induced by furocoumarins plus UV-A irradation. Photochem. Photobiol. **43:** 243–246.
18. KLIBANOV, A. 1979. Enzyme stabilization by immobilization. Anal. Biochem. **93:** 1–25.
19. CAFFIERI, S., D. VEDALDI, A. DAGA & F. DALL'ACQUA. 1989. Photosensitizing furocoumarins: photocycloaddition to unsaturated fatty acids. In Psoralens: Past, Present and Future of Photochemoprotection and other Biological Activities. T. Fitzpatrick, P. Forlot, M. Pathak & F. Urbach, Eds. 137–143. John Libbey Eurotext. Montrouge, France.
20. KRAEMER, K., H. WATERS, O. ELLINGSON & K. TARONE. 1979. Psoralen plus ultraviolet radiation-induced inhibition of DNA synthesis and viability in human lymphoid cells in vitro. Photochem. Photobiol. **30:** 263–270.
21. GASPARRO, F. 1990. Psoralen photobiology and photochemotherapy: perspectives and prospects. In Future Directions and Applications of Photodynamic Therapy. C. Gomer, Ed. Vol. IS6: 195–204. SPIE Institute. Bellingham, WA.
22. BEVILACQUA, P., R. EDELSON & F. GASPARRO. 1991. HPLC analysis of 8-methoxypsoralen monoadducts and cross-links in lymphocytes and keratinocytes. J. Invest. Dermatol. **97:** 151–155.
23. GREY, H., A. SETTE & S. BUSS. 1989. How T cells see antigen. Sci. Am. **261:** 56–64.
23a. SINHA, A. A. 1990. Autoimmune diseases: the failure of self tolerance. Science **248:** 1380–1388.

24. PEREZ, M., R. EDELSON, L. LAROCHE & C. BERGER. 1989. Inhibition of antiskin allograft immunity by infusions with syngeneic photoinactivated effector lymphocytes. J. Invest. Dermatol. **92:** 669–676.
25. LASKIN, J. & D. LASKIN. 1988. Role of psoralen receptors in growth regulation. *In* Psoralen DNA Photobiology. F. Gasparro, Ed. Vol. 2: 135–148. CRC Press. Boca Raton, FL.
26. LASKIN, J., E. LEE, E. YURKOW *et al.* 1985. A possible mechanism of psoralen phototoxicity not involving direction interaction with DNA. Proc. Natl. Acad. Sci. USA **82:** 6158–6162.
27. CAFFIERI, S., Z. ZAREBSKA & F. DALL'ACQUA. 1990. Lymphocyte damage by furocoumarin and UVA radiation. In press.
28. SIBILLE, C., P. CHOMEZ, C. WILDMANN *et al.* 1990. Structure of the gene of tum⁻ transplantation antigen P198: a point mutation generates a new antigenic peptide. J. Exp. Med. **172:** 35–45.
29. LURQUIN, C., A. VAN PEL, B. MARIAME *et al.* 1989. Structure of the gene of tum⁻ transplantation antigen P91A: a mutated exon encodes a peptide recognized with L^d by cytolytic T cells. Cell **58:** 293–303.
30. UYTTENHOVE, C., J. VAN SNICK & T. BOON. 1980. Immunogenic variants obtained by mutagenesis of mouse mastocytoma P815: rejection by syngeneic mice. J. Exp. Med. **152:** 1175–1183.
31. BOON, T., J. VAN SNICK, A. VAN PEL *et al.* 1980. Immunogenic variants obtained by mutagenesis of mouse mastocytoma P815: T cell lymphocyte-mediated cytolysis. J. Exp. Med. **152:** 1184–1193.

Photopheresis in the Treatment of Autoimmune Disease: Experience with *Pemphigus vulgaris* and Systemic Sclerosis

ALAIN H. ROOK

Department of Dermatology
Hospital of the University of Pennsylvania
3400 Spruce Street
Philadelphia, Pennsylvania 19104

Following the initial demonstration by Edelson and colleagues that approximately 75 percent of individuals with the Sezary form of cutaneous T cell lymphoma experienced improvement during treatment with photopheresis,[1] pilot studies were developed to explore the safety and benefit of this therapy for autoimmune disease. The recent completion of phase I studies for pemphigus vulgaris, rheumatoid arthritis, systemic lupus erythematosus and systemic sclerosis have yielded data suggesting that photopheresis can be both beneficial and safe in the management of these complex medical conditions.[2-4] This review will summarize our experience with photopheresis in the treatment of pemphigus vulgaris and systemic sclerosis.

Pemphigus vulgaris

Pemphigus vulgaris is an autoimmune blistering disease that is characterized by the production of abnormal immunoglobulin G antibodies that possess specificity for determinants on the cell surface of keratinocytes.[5] The clinical features typically involve the formation of blisters and erosions on mucosal and cutaneous surfaces. Before the availability of corticosteroids, more than 80 percent of patients with Pemphigus vulgaris died from their disease.[6] Presently, the majority of patients can have disease manifestations controlled with the use of corticosteroids and immunosuppressive agents. Nevertheless, disease relapses are common, often requiring long term treatment with high doses of these medications which can result in serious side effects.

In view of these observations, a pilot study was undertaken to examine whether photopheresis could benefit patients who had chronic pemphigus vulgaris that was relatively resistant to conventional therapy.[2] Four patients with histologically confirmed *Pemphigus vulgaris* were entered into this study (TABLE 1). Their mean duration of disease was 3.5 years (range 1 to 6 years) requiring chronic therapy with azathioprine and high doses of prednisone in an effort to maintain disease control. Despite this therapy, active blister formation was extensive and persistent. In addition, all four manifested high serum titers of antiepidermal cell antibodies.

Therapy with photopheresis was initiated at a frequency of two successive days of treatment at four-week intervals. Within the first six months of treatment, all patients had improved clinically (TABLE 1). Subsequent rapid tapering of other

TABLE 1. Clinal Course Antibody Titers and Drug Therapy in *Pemphigus* Patients

Patient (Disease Duration and Extent)	Month of Therapy (Photochemotherapy plus Prednisone and Azathioprine or Prednisone Alone)										
	Baseline	6	12	18	24	25	26	30	36	42	48
Patient 1 (4 yrs; mouth, face, trunk extremities)											
Activity[a]	++++	+	++	+	++	++	++++	+	0	0	0
Antibody titer	1/320	1/160	1/640	1/80	1/80	1/2560	1/2560	1/320	0	0	0
Drug therapy	100/150	15/50	20/50	10/50	10/50	50/150[b]	80/150[b]	50	20	20	0
Patient 2 (3 yrs; mouth, face, trunk)											
Activity	++++	0	+	+	++			++	++	+	
Antibody titer	1/1280	not done	1/80	0	1/160			1/320	1/80	1/160	
Drug therapy	100/100	0	40[c]	5[c]	30[c]			20[c]	10[c]	15[c]	
Patient 3 (6 yrs; mouth, face, vagina)											
Activity	++++	+	++++	+	+			+	0	0	
Antibody titer	1/320	1/80	1/640	1/160	1/40			1/40	1/40	not done	
Drug therapy	120	10[c]	50	15	7.5[c]			5[c]	0	0	
Patient 4 (1 yr; face, trunk)											
Activity	++++	++	+	++	++++						
Antibody titer	1/640	1/640	1/80	1/160	1/160						
Drug therapy	80/100	80/100	40/100	40/100	100/100						

[a] Represents percent of initial disease activity at initiation of extracorporeal photochemotherapy with 4+ equivalent to 100%.
[b] Patient 1 at months 25 to 30 received prednisone and cyclophosphamide; otherwise drug treatment consisted of prednisone and azathioprine or prednisone alone in all patients.
[c] Administration of prednisone at this time was every other day.

medications along with a decrease in photopheresis treatments to less than an every-four-week regimen appeared to coincide with worsening of skin lesions in two patients during months six to twelve of therapy. The reinstitution of a more aggressive photopheresis regimen consisting of treatments on alternate weeks in one and every three to four weeks in the other resulted in clearing of skin lesions in these two individuals. Generally, a significant drop in auto-antibody titer was observed concurrently with clinical improvement.

Ultimately, three of four patients participating in this study developed a complete response to photopheresis therapy. The responses were characterized by a complete remission lasting a mean of 19.3 months (range 7 to 36 months) permitting discontinuation of other medications in two and the tapering of prednisone and azathioprine from 100 mg and 150 mg, respectively, to 10 mg of prednisone alone in the third patient. Disease relapses in the three responded promptly to the resumption of photopheresis with the rapid reinduction of remission after only three to four monthly cycles of photopheresis.

During the course of this study, minimal adverse effects of the treatment were observed. One episode of hypotension occurred which was attributed to a vasovagal reaction. It is noteworthy that there was no clinical evidence of treatment-induced immune deficiency, such as the occurrence of opportunistic infections. Thus, in this trial, photopheresis was an extremely well tolerated alternative to conventional immunosuppressive drugs. Above all, photopheresis appeared to achieve the induction of a remission in patients whose clinical course had been refractory to conventional therapy.

Systemic Sclerosis

Systemic sclerosis is an autoimmune disorder characterized by excessive deposition of collagen within the skin and frequently within visceral organs.[7] The precise mechanisms underlying the pathogenesis of systemic sclerosis are currently incompletely understood. Nevertheless, substantial evidence has recently emerged supporting the belief that abnormal immune activation is an important factor leading to augmented collagen synthesis.[8,9] Peripheral blood mononuclear cells are spontaneously releasing cytokines such as interleukin 2 and interleukin 6. Moreover, clinically involved tissues manifest an increased number of infiltrating, activated helper T lymphocytes which can be found to be producing transforming growth factor β which is a potent inducer of collagen synthesis.

Recently, the prognosis of patients with systemic sclerosis has been related to the extent and rapidity of progression of skin thickening.[10] Barnett and colleagues have noted that diffuse skin involvement extending beyond the arms to encompass the trunk within one year of disease onset is an indicator of poor prognosis and has been associated with a ten-year survival of only 20 percent.[10] It must also be stressed that even for patients with sclerosis limited to the hands, substantial functional disability can occur due to the development of contractures.

Since photopheresis had been previously demonstrated to be a well tolerated therapy, and because it may more specifically target activated T lymphocytes which are present in abundance within the peripheral blood of patients with systemic sclerosis, a pilot study was initially performed to determine the safety of this treatment for severe systemic sclerosis.[4] The first patient treated was a 60-year-old male with a six-month history of diffuse cutaneous thickening as well as pulmonary and renal involvement. Photopheresis administered on two successive days every four weeks resulted in the prompt reversal of all disease manifestations. This included the complete disappearance of microangiopathic hemolysis and proteinuria of 1300 mg/24 h. Furthermore, his response has been maintained, without adverse effects of treatment, during four years of follow-up therapy. Treatment of a second patient with extensive skin involvement was also associated with significant skin softening. Again, no adverse effects of treatment were observed.

These initial findings resulted in the development of a multicenter, randomized, single-blinded clinical trial to examine the efficacy of photopheresis for patients with recent onset systemic sclerosis. Individuals were selected for this study on the basis of having progressive skin thickening during the preceding six months. Thus, 79 patients with recent onset disease (mean symptom duration was 1.83 years; mean duration of skin thickening was 1.22 years) were randomized to receive either photopheresis or D-penicillamine. Patients with advanced renal (serum creatinine greater than 3.0 mg/dl) or pulmonary involvement (carbon monoxide diffusing capacity or DLco less than 50% of normal) were excluded because of concern that they might not be able to complete the clinical trial. The study was designed to compare the use of photopheresis in the treatment of systemic sclerosis to that of D-penicillamine. Patients randomized to photopheresis received two consecutive daily treatments every four weeks. Patients randomized to D-penicillamine were to receive a daily dose of 750 mg for a minimum of six months. The dose was increased by 250 mg every two months until a daily dose of 750 mg was reached. Patients receiving a stable dose of D-penicillamine not exceeding 500 mg per day for less than six months were permitted entry into the study. For those not on D-penicillamine, a dose of 250 mg was given for two months and then the dose was increased by increments of 250 mg every two months, until a daily dose of 750 mg was attained. Patients on D-penicillamine who were randomized to the photopheresis arm discontinued their medication at the time of randomization which occurred at least one week prior to initiation of photopheresis.

All blinded examiners participating in this study were trained at a single center (University of Pittsburgh). The severity of each patient's skin was assessed by rating the thickness of the skin on a 0 to 3+ scale in 15 areas of the body. A rating of zero meant the skin was normal, one represented minimal involvement, while three meant there was severe thickening or hide-bound skin, and two was intermediate between one and three. Thus, when summed up for all 15 body areas, the possible skin severity (thickness) scores ranged from 0 to 45. The area of skin involvement was recorded on a body diagram, and the percentage of surface area involved was then determined by use of a digital planimeter. Possible area scores ranged from 0 to 100%. A change in the skin score during treatment was considered to be clinically relevant if it differed by at least 15% from baseline. This was felt to ensure that random changes due to observor variability were excluded. Additional parameters of disease activity that were evaluated included changes in pulmonary involvement. Pulmonary function testing was performed at baseline, and at six, nine and 12 months of follow-up. Skin biopsies were also obtained at baseline and at 6 and 12 months. Blood levels of 8-methoxypsoralen were monitored throughout the study to ensure adequate absorption.

At the commencement of the trial, seventy-nine patients were randomized to receive either photopheresis or D-penicillamine. Sixty-three individuals initiated therapy, while 56 received six full months of treatment (31 on photopheresis and 25 on D-penicillamine) and 47 received 10 months of treatment (29 on photopheresis and 18 on D-penicillamine). The demographic features for the two treatment groups were similar at baseline in regard to mean duration of disease, mean skin severity score, mean percent area of skin involvement and previous administration of D-penicillamine.

Following six months of treatment, 21 of 31 (68%) patients treated with photopheresis and 8 of 25 (32%) on D-penicillamine had experienced at least a 15% improvement in their skin severity score (TABLE 2). Worsening of skin severity score by at least 15% occurred in 3 of 31 (9.7%) photopheresis patients and 8 of 25 (32%) of those who received D-penicillamine. Thus, the proportion of patients responding at the six month treatment interval was significantly greater ($p = 0.02$; ordered chi square test) in the photopheresis arm than in the D-penicillamine arm.

At the 10-month treatment interval, 20 of 29 (69%) patients who received photopheresis improved by at least 15% and 3 of 29 (10%) worsened by at least 15%. For those who remained on D-penicillamine for 10 full months, 9 of 18 (50%) patients improved by at least 15% and 3 of 18 (16.6%) had worsened after 10 months of treatment (TABLE 2). It should be emphasized, nevertheless, that among the seven patients within the D-penicillamine arm who discontinued treatment between six and ten months of therapy, five were experiencing at least 15% worsening in their skin severity score at the time of treatment cessation. There-

TABLE 2. Change in Severity Scores During Treatment

Treatment Group	Evaluation Interval			
	6 Month		10 Month	
	Improved ≥15%	Worse ≥15%	Improved ≥15%	Worse ≥15%
Photochemotherapy	21/31(68%)[a]	3/31(10%)	20/29(69%)	3/29(10%)
D-penicillamine	8/25(32%)	8/25(32%)	9/18(50%)	3/18(16%)[b,c]

[a] The proportion of patients responding to therapy at six months was significantly greater ($p = 0.02$) in the photochemotherapy arm than in the D-penicillamine arm.

[b] Five out of seven patients who dropped out between six and ten months of therapy within the penicillamine arm had more than 15% worsening from baseline in their severity score at the time of drop-out.

[c] Patients not shown had less than 15% change in their skin severity score during therapy.

fore, 8 of 25 (32%) D-penicillamine-treated patients had actually worsened by the 10 month evaluation point.

Standardized measurements of the change in oral aperture and right and left hand closure were also evaluated by blinded examiners after six and ten months of treatment. Mean oral aperture measurements among patients who received six months of photopheresis were significantly improved from baseline at the six-month treatment interval ($p = 0.01$). The mean of each of the three parameters was significantly improved from baseline at the 10-month treatment interval for this treatment group. These parameters of disease were not significantly improved after either six or ten months of therapy among those individuals who received D-penicillamine.

Since randomization into this trial was permitted if patients had taken a subtherapeutic dose of D-penicillamine for less than six months, an analysis was performed to determine if there was a relationship between recent exposure to this drug and response. A three-way analysis of variance was performed on the arithmetic differences from baseline for the six-month observations. No significant difference was detected between the recent and nonrecent D-penicillamine exposure groups for skin severity ($p = 0.931$). Moreover, no significant interaction was detected between D-penicillamine exposure and type of treatment for skin severity ($p = 0.782$). The results of these analyses suggest that exposure to D-penicillamine was not a major factor responsible for the observed treatment effect.

In addition to assessment of skin thickening, pulmonary function tests were evaluated at baseline and after 6, 9, and 12 months of treatment. For the 29 patients who received photopheresis, three experienced significant improvement in carbon monoxide diffusing capacity, six had significant worsening, and 20 were unchanged. Among the 18 patients who received 10 full months of D-penicillamine, three had significant improvement in this parameter, 10 were unchanged, and five had significant worsening. Thus, for the 47 patients completing 10 months of therapy, the DLco was largely unchanged in both treatment groups during 12 months of observation.

Skin biopsies were also obtained from adjacent sites at baseline and at six and 12 months of follow-up. The thickness of dermal collagen was evaluated by a

TABLE 3. Adverse Effects by Treatment Group

Treatment	Adverse Effect	Number[a]
D-penicillamine	myopathy	1
	proteinuria	4
	fever	1
	oral ulcers	2
	renal failure	1
	nausea	1
	elevated transaminases	1
Photochemotherapy	nausea	2
	hemolysis	1
	hypotension	1
	vasovagal reaction	1
	clotted device	3
	thrombocytopenia	1

[a] Adverse experiences required permanent discontinuation of treatment in six cases on D-penicillamine and zero cases in the photochemotherapy arm during 10 months of observation.

single pathologist through use of a computer-assisted image analyzer. In 75 percent of cases, the direction of the change in thickness of the dermal layer corresponded to the clinical change in skin thickness documented by the blinded examiner. The most frequently observed histologic changes were a decrease in the degree of "compactness" of the dermal collagen bundles and a decrease in the thickness of the dermal layer among patients who experienced clinical improvement.

Adverse effects of photopheresis were minimal during the course of this trial (TABLE 3). No patients were required to permanently discontinue this therapy due to the adverse effects associated with treatment. In contrast, six individuals (24%) taking D-penicillamine were required to permanently discontinue this therapy due to serious adverse effects of this drug (TABLE 3).

The results of this trial have demonstrated that photopheresis is an extremely well tolerated therapy that can induce significant skin softening in the majority of patients with recent onset systemic sclerosis. Furthermore, the cessation of disease progression and clinical improvement occurred within a reasonably short period of time. These results are remarkable in view of the observation that most of the study participants had extensive, progressive disease that placed them within a poor prognostic category. In contrast to the results obtained with photopheresis, a much smaller proportion of the D-penicillamine-treated patients experienced clinical improvement and had a much higher frequency of adverse events in response to treatment during the same period of observation.

It is noteworthy that, in addition to skin softening, significant improvement in hand closure and oral aperture measurements were also observed among individuals who received photopheresis, but not among those treated with D-penicillamine. Decreased mobility of the hands and mouth can produce substantial disability. Clearly, small improvements in these parameters can have a significant impact on the ability of a patient to function in the workplace and even to feed themselves.

Photopheresis has now been demonstrated to produce clinical benefit for a diverse number of autoimmune diseases characterized by disordered T cell regulation. Elsewhere in this symposium, specific mechanisms of action of photopheresis are described using relevant animal models of autoimmunity. In regard to human autoimmunity, we suspect that the development of heightened suppressor T cell activity may blunt the ongoing autoreactive process. Moreover, recent findings within our laboratory indicate that a particular pattern of cytokine induction may occur that may have a salutary effect with respect to the pathogenesis of systemic sclerosis.[11] For example, photopheresis appears to be a potent inducer of tumor necrosis factor production by monocytes. This particular cytokine can inhibit collagen synthesis by fibroblasts.[12] Thus, in addition to producing an immunization effect against clones of autoreactive T cells, as observed by Khavari *et al.*,[13] and Perez and colleagues,[14] photopheresis also appears to be responsible for the induction of soluble immune mediators which can have a therapeutic adjuvant effect for a number of disease states.

The implication that photopheresis may have multiple modes of action is important in regard to the future optimization of its therapeutic effects. Combinations of therapies may prove to be more advantageous once the mechanisms are fully understood. For instance, our experience has suggested that the addition of interferon alfa to photopheresis may provide a further benefit for patients with cutaneous T cell lymphoma who have a particularly poor prognosis.[15] In the same light, addition of interferon gamma, which has been demonstrated to inhibit collagen synthesis,[16] is theoretically feasible for patients with systemic sclerosis. It is clear that a more comprehensive understanding of this novel and well tolerated therapy will permit us to successfully apply photopheresis to the treatment of a variety of complex medical conditions.

REFERENCES

1. EDELSON, R., C. BERGER, F. GASPARRO et al. 1987. Treatment of cutaneous T-cell lymphoma by extracorporeal photochemotherapy: preliminary results. N. Engl. J. Med. **316:** 297–303.
2. ROOK, A. H., B. V. JEGASOTHY, P. HEALD et al. 1990. Extracorporeal photochemotherapy for drug resistant *Pemphigus vulgaris*. Ann. Intern. Med. **112:** 303–305.
3. MALAWISTA, S., D. TROCK & R. EDELSON. 1991. Treatment of rheumatoid arthritis by extracorporeal photochemotherapy: a pilot study. Arthritis Rheum. In press.
4. ROOK, A. H., B. FREUNDLICH, G. T. NAHASS et al. 1989. Treatment of autoimmune disease with extracorporeal photochemotherapy: progressive systemic sclerosis. Yale J. Biol. Med. **62:** 639–645.

5. STANLEY, J. R., L. KOULU & C. THIVOLET. 1984. Distinction between epidermal antigens binding *Pemphigus vulgaris* and *Pemphigus foliaceus* autoantibodies. J. Clin. Invest. **74:** 313–320.
6. LEVER, W. F. & J. H. TALBOTT. 1942. Pemphigus. A clinical analysis and follow-up study of sixty-two patients. Arch. Derm. **46:** 348–357.
7. LEROY, E. C. 1988. Systemic sclerosis (scleroderma). *In* Cecil Textbook of Medicine, 18th Edit. J. B. Wyngaarden & L. H. Smith, Jr., Eds. 2018–2024. W. B. Saunders. Philadelphia.
8. KAHALEH, M. B., & E. C. LEROY. 1989. Interleukin-2 in scleroderma: correlation of serum level with extent of skin involvement and disease duration. Ann. Intern. Med. **110:** 446–450.
9. FREUNDLICH, B. & S. A. JIMENEZ. 1987. Phenotype of peripheral blood lymphocytes in patients with progressive systemic sclerosis: activated T lymphocytes and the effect of penicillamine therapy. Clin. Exp. Immunol. **9:** 375–384.
10. BARNETT, A. J., M. H. MILLER & G. O. LITTLEJOHN. 1988. A survival study of patients with scleroderma diagnosed over 30 years (1953–1983): the value of a simple cutaneous classification in the early stages of the disease. J. Rheumatol. **15:** 276–283.
11. VOWELS, B. R., M. CASSIN, M. BOUFAL, L. WALSH & A. H. ROOK. 1991. Extracorporeal photochemotherapy induces production of tumor necrosis factor and IL-6 by adherent peripheral blood mononuclear cells. J. Invest. Dermatol. In press.
12. KAHARI, V. M., Y. Q. CHEN, M. W. SU, F. RAMIREZ & J. UITTO. 1990. Tumor necrosis factor alfa and interferon gamma suppress the activation of human type I collagen gene expression by transforming growth factor beta1. J. Clin. Invest. **86:** 1489–1495.
13. KHAVARI, P. A., R. L. EDELSON, O. LIDER, F. P. GASPARRO, H. L. WEINER & I. R. COHEN. 1988. Specific vaccination against photoinactivated cloned T cells. Clin. Res. **36:** 662.
14. PEREZ, M., R. EDELSON, L. LAROCHE & C. BERGER. 1989. Inhibition of antiskin allograft immunity by infusions with syngeneic photoinactivated effector lymphocytes. J. Invest. Dermatol. **92:** 669–676.
15. ROOK, A. H., M. PRYSTOWSKY, M. CASSIN, M. BOUFAL & S. R. LESSIN. Combined therapy of the Sezary syndrome with extracorporeal photochemotherapy and low dose interferon-alfa: clinical, molecular and immunologic observations. Arch. Dermatol. In press.
16. KAHAN, A., B. ARMOR, C. J. MENKES & G. STRAUCH. 1989. Recombinant interferon gamma in the treatment of systemic sclerosis. Am. J. Med. **87:** 273–277.

Photopheresis for Rheumatoid Arthritis[a]

STEPHEN E. MALAWISTA, DAVID TROCK, AND
RICHARD L. EDELSON

Section of Rheumatology
Department of Internal Medicine
Department of Dermatology
and
General Clinical Research Center
Yale University School of Medicine
333 Cedar Street
New Haven, Connecticut 06510-8056

The naturally occurring photoactive compound 8-methoxypsoralen (8-MOP) binds covalently to pyrimidine bases of DNA when activated by ultraviolet A (UVA) energy.[2] For the hyperproliferative epidermal disease psoriasis vulgaris, oral administration of 8-MOP followed by exposure of involved skin to UVA has been efficacious, without significant systemic toxicity.[3] The *extracorporeal* exposure of peripheral blood leukocytes to UVA and 8-MOP is of proven value in erythrodermic cutaneous T cell lymphoma (CTCL).[4] Since the large majority of malignant cells are in the skin and lymphoid tissue in that condition, and therefore not treated directly, it is likely that the eventual clearing of tumor is mediated by an immunologic reaction to the reinfused psoralen-injured cells. Because there is no evidence of generalized immunosuppression in the treated CTCL patients, the host response appears to be directed primarily against the malignant clone. Studies in experimental animal systems support this formulation by demonstrating that intravenous infusion of psoralen-damaged syngeneic T cells leads to subsequent selective suppression of the activity of the parent clones.[5,6]

We were struck by the potential implications of such a therapy for "rheumatic" or "autoimmune" diseases such as rheumatoid arthritis, in which non-monoclonal, presumably pathogenic, activated T cells do appear to circulate,[7] but for which inciting antigens or organisms have not been identified. Extracorporeal photochemotherapy (ECP; photopheresis) might be a way of inducing a rather specific, host-directed, immune regulation of pathogenic oligoclonally expanded T cells, without one having first to identify either the cells themselves or the antigens to which they are responding. In that context we initiated a pilot study of ECP in seven patients with various presentations of rheumatoid arthritis.

METHODS

Patient Population

The seven patients, all of whom satisfied the 1987 revised criteria for rheumatoid arthritis of the American Rheumatism Association (now the American Col-

[a] Supported in part by grants from the National Institutes of Health (AM 10493, AM 07107, CA 43058, and AR 07016) and by Therakos, Inc. An expanded version of this work has appeared.[1]

TABLE 1. Patient Population[a]

Pt. No.	Sex	Age	Onset of Symptoms	Diagnosis of R.A.	A.M. Stiffness, Min	Sed Rate MM/HR	R.F. Titer	Previous Treatment*	Study Treatment**
1.	F	43	11/86	4/88	60	50	2,560	Prednisone 40 mg/d tapered over 3 mos N, S, IB	Piroxicam 20 mg/d
2.	F	43	12/82	2/83	10	55	320	Gold Prednisone 2 mg/d N, P, S, D, K	Diclofenac 200 mg/d
3.	M	55	6/74	8/74	60	50	2,560	Gold IB	Prednisone 5 mg/d Methotrexate 7.5 mg/w IB 2.4 g/d
4.	M	65	10/74	1/75	120	34	10,200	Gold Penicillamine Plaquenil Methotrexate Synovectomy, L knee; R hip replacement P, IB, N	Prednisone 5 mg/d Ecotrin 1.2 g/d
5.	M	30	11/81	2/82	300	74	2,560	Gold Penicillamine Sulfasalazine Plaquenil IB, S, P	Prednisone 10 mg/d Methotrexate 15 mg Im/w
6.	M	55	9/82	2/83	30	68	(NEG)***	Gold Penicillamine Plaquenil B, IB, IN, P	Naproxyn 1 g/d ASA 1.8 g/d
7.	M	53	9/58	2/59	90	19	1,280	Gold Penicillamine Methotrexate Plaquenil IB, IN, S, P	Prednisone 10 mg/d Naproxyn 1 g/d

* B, Benoxaprofen (Oraflex); D, Diflunisal (Dolobid); IB, Ibuprofen (Motrin); IN, Indomethacin (Indocin); K, Ketoprofen (Orudis); N, Naproxyn (Naprosyn); P, Piroxicam (Feldene); S, Sulindac (Clinoril); Diclofenac (Voltaren).

** Oral route, except as noted.

*** Psoriasis since 1982.

[a] From Malawista et al.[1] Reprinted by permission from Arthritis and Rheumatism.

lege of Rheumatology),[8] were a deliberately diverse group in terms of duration and severity of disease and previous treatment (TABLE 1). For entry they were required to have six tender joints or three swollen joints despite therapy with nonsteroidal antiinflammatory drugs (NSAIDs). They were not to have received antimalarial drugs, gold salts, sulfasalazine, or D-penicillamine for at least 4 weeks, or azathioprine or cyclophosphamide for at least 6 weeks, before entrance into the study. Throughout the study, articular symptoms were to continue to be managed by the patient's private rheumatologist, with NSAIDs, analgesics, rest, physical therapy, maintenance of established low-dose methotrexate therapy, low-dose prednisone therapy to a maximum of 10 mg daily or 20 mg every other day (maintained if possible at the entry dosage), intraarticular injection of corticosteroids (large joints, when necessary), or hospitalization.

Procedure

The instrument used (Therakos, West Chester, PA) integrates an initial discontinuous leukopheresis step with subsequent exposure to ultraviolet light in a single apparatus. The procedure involves pooling 240 ml of leukocyte-enriched blood with 300 ml of the patient's plasma (removed two hours after ingestion of 0.6 mg of methoxsalen per kilogram of body weight [Oxsoralen, Elder, Bryan, OH]) and 200 ml of sterile normal saline, yielding a final hematocrit of 6.4 ± 1.7% (mean ± SD) and containing about 30% of the number of lymphocytes in the patient's bloodstream. The total volume is then passed as a 1-mm film through a six-chambered disposable sterile cassette, in order to expose it to ultraviolet A energy, delivered by a fluorescent source. Lethal damage to lymphocytes requires a concentration of 50 ng of methoxsalen per milliliter (this minimal level is confirmed in each patient's serum[9] before the initial treatment) in the presence of 1 to 2 J of ultraviolet A per square centimeter.[10] After exposure, the irradiated cells are returned to the patient.

Study Design

ECP was to be given over a period of 6 months, initially on two consecutive days per month. After three months, at the investigator's discretion, the frequency of the two treatments could be increased to biweekly. Improvement for a given clinical index was defined as a 30% decrease in its value, sustained for at least two successive measurements.

Assessments of Disease Activity

All measurements were made at a baseline visit, at each visit for ECP, and at a follow-up visit after about one year. Our primary parameters in evaluating patients with arthritis were the joint count and the joint score. Thirty-eight joints were evaluated,[11] including both interphalangeal joints of the thumbs; 8 proximal interphalangeal joints of the hands; 10 metacarpophalangeal and 10 metatarsophalangeal joints; and both wrists, elbows, ankles, and knees. *Joint count:* each joint was assigned one point for swelling or tenderness (maximum count, 38). *Joint score:* each joint was assigned a numerical score for tenderness: 0, not tender; 1, mildly tender; and 2, obviously tender so that the patient withdrew or winced (maximum score, 76). Note: Particularly in Patients 2, 5, and 7, the joint counts and especially joint scores just before the first ECP treatment (time zero) were higher than at baseline (BL). To be conservative, we compared each patient's final measurement with his baseline value.

We also used several secondary parameters of efficacy, including *grip strength* (mm Hg) in each hand, using a sphygmomanometer with its cuff inflated to 20 mm Hg; *fifty-foot walking time* (sec); *ring size,* as mean circumference (mm) of the proximal interphalangeal joints of the hands, measured with an arthrocircameter;[12] duration of *morning stiffness* (min; 60 min is considered significant); *physician's assessment,* starting at a score of 3, where on successive visits 1 is much better than at last visit, 2, better, 3, unchanged, 4, worse, and 5, much worse; patient's assessment of pain on a 100-mm horizontal *visual analogue scale;*[13] an *activities-of-daily-living scale* of nine questions[13] (maximum score, 36); the titer of serum rheumatoid factor (*RF titer*); a Westergren erythrocyte sedimentation rate (*ESR;* mm/hr); and a serum *C-reactive protein* (CRP; ng/ml). CRP was quantified by radial immunodiffusion (LC-Partigen, Behring Diagnostics, Somerville, NJ) in stored serum samples run simultaneously.

Statistical Analysis

To evaluate changes in joint counts in this small sample, we employed two statistical approaches; in both of them every point contributed to the analysis. First, we used a "repeated-measures" analysis of variance[14] to examine changes over time in all seven patients. Second, having identified (by inspection) an apparent breakpoint after which four patients appeared to respond, we examined mean slopes—*i.e.,* mean change in joint count or score per day—both over the entire study period, and before and after the apparent breakpoint. We divided the mean slope by the standard error of the mean, and used a *t* test to determine if the slope was significantly different from zero. We performed these analyses both for all seven patients, and for the four apparent responders. For joint scores we used the Wilcoxon rank sum test.

RESULTS AND DISCUSSION

In this pilot study of seven patients with rheumatoid arthritis in whom our primary measure of improvement was the condition of their joints, Patients 1–3 improved during ECP, Patient 4 improved by definition (just), but not sufficiently to be deemed a clinical success, and Patients 5–7 did not improve (FIG. 1).

On repeated-measures statistical analysis using all seven patients, we found significant changes over time in joint counts ($p < 0.001$). On mean-slope analysis of joint counts (TABLE 2), the slopes were significantly different from zero after an apparent breakpoint between 12 and 16 weeks, and not before; this was so whether the analysis employed all seven patients or only the four apparent responders. For joint scores, which required a nonparametric test, differences in initial and final values were not statistically significant ($p \geq 0.10$ for all), despite the similarity of the mean slopes to those for the joint counts (TABLE 2).

Supporting the improvement in joint measurements are improvements in grip strength (Patients 2 and 4), fifty-foot walking time (Patient 2), morning stiffness (Patient 1; that of Patient 2 was already less than one hour at baseline and did not

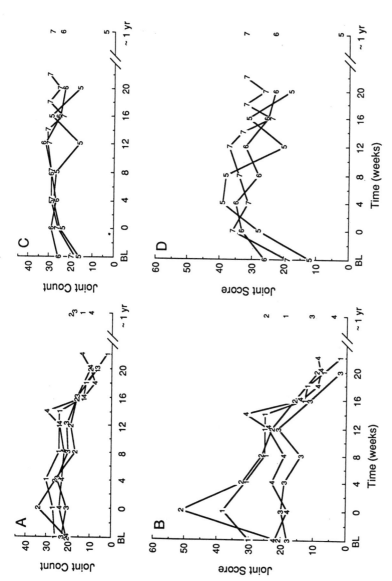

FIGURE 1. Joint counts and scores of 7 patients with rheumatoid arthritis. The 4 patients who fulfilled the criteria for improvement are depicted at *left* (**A** & **B**), the 3 who did not, at *right* (**C** & **D**). Measurements were made at baseline (BL), on each admission for extracorporeal photochemotherapy, and at follow-up after approximately one year. Note that in those who improved, the definitive decreases in joint counts and scores were focused in time, 12 to 16 weeks after onset of therapy. When ECP was stopped, Patients 1–3 maintained their improved status for 2 to 3 months (not shown). (From Malawista *et al.*[1] Reprinted by permission from *Arthritis and Rheumatism.*)

TABLE 2. Mean-Slope Analysis of Joint Counts and Scores[a]

	Mean Slope (p)		
	Total Period	Before Breakpoint	After Breakpoint
All seven patients			
Joint count	−0.05 (0.06)	0.01 (0.67)	−0.22 (0.01)
Joint score	−0.07	0.01	−0.27
Four apparent responders			
Joint count	−0.09 (0.01)	−0.02 (0.50)	−0.26 (0.01)
Joint score	−0.12	−0.02	−0.33

[a] From Malawista et al.[1] Reprinted by permission from *Arthritis and Rheumatism*.

deteriorate), physician's assessment (Patients 1 and 2), visual analogue scale (Patients 2 and 3), activities-of-daily-living scale (Patient 2), ESR (Patient 2), and concomitantly measured values for serial CRP (Patients 2 and 3 [that of Patient 1 began and remained low]; TABLE 3). *None* of these measures improved during ECP in Patients 5–7, except for a single ESR in Patient 5 and serial CRP in Patient 6 (the latter inexplicably, since nothing else supported the early decline). RF titer did not change significantly in anyone, and ring size, which, like fifty-foot walking time, may be one of the least useful measures of disease activity,[15] was of no use. These results are summarized in TABLE 4.

During the follow-up period, the two improved patients who received no additional therapy (Patients 1 and 2) deteriorated in joint counts and scores and in physician's assessment; in addition, Patient 1 developed new nodules about her fingers and her RF titer rose to 20,500, and Patient 2 also regressed in grip strength in both hands, visual analogue scale, and activities-of-daily-living scale. Conversely, on alternative therapy during the follow-up period, Patient 5, who had not improved during ECP, improved in all parameters except fifty-foot walking time (where he nevertheless regained the loss experienced during ECP), and Patient 4, who had improved only modestly during ECP, improved in joint score, grip strength in both hands, physician's assessment, visual analogue scale, and CRP. Thus, it appears that individuals who respond not at all or minimally to ECP may still be treated successfully by other means.

Toxicity during the study was essentially nil. In 102 treatment sessions among the seven patients, Patient 1, during her initial ECP (of 18 such sessions), experi-

TABLE 3. C-Reactive Protein (mg/dl)[a]

Pt. No.	Week				~1 Year
	BL	12	16	20	
1.	0.6	1.2	0.6	<0.5	<0.5
2.	2.2	1.5	0.7	1.2	1.4
3.	5.6	2.1	2.6	2.9	1.5*
4.	1.3	3.6	6.1	6.1	<0.5*
5.	1.6	2.7	8.3	12.7	7.4*
6.	12.3	5.0	5.4	ND	5.4*
7.	2.0	7.8	8.3	7.4/5.9**	ND

* New therapy since end of treatment period.
** 18 wks./22 wks.; 20 wks. not done, BL, baseline; ND, not done
[a] From Malawista et al.[1] Reprinted by permission from *Arthritis and Rheumatism*.

enced a single episode of hypotension during leukopheresis that responded rapidly to reinfusion of plasma. Over the six months of observation we saw none of the complications of established therapies for rheumatoid arthritis—*e.g.*, in gut, skin, blood, liver, or kidney.

Although only a larger, longer, and properly controlled study will show definitively what ECP can do for rheumatoid arthritis, there are indications in the current work that the observed responses, beyond their occurrence some years into the illness (TABLE 1), are due neither to chance nor to a placebo effect. Again, for both joint counts and joint scores, there appears to be a breakpoint for the apparent responders, noted on inspection and confirmed by mean-slopes analysis, that occurred between 12 and 16 weeks after the first ECP treatment (FIG. 1, A & B). The fact that the response is so focused in time, along with the long delay of its onset three to four months into treatment, recalls established second-line anti-rheumatic agents such as parenteral gold salts, and argues against chance or placebo effect. Similarly, during the follow-up period, Patients 1, 2, and 3 re-

TABLE 4. Estimations of Improvement[a]

Measure	Patient						
	1	2	3	4	5	6	7
Joint count	+	+	+	+	−	−	−
Joint score	+	+	+	+	−	−	−
Grip strength	−	+	−	+	−	−	−
Fifty-foot walk	−	+	−	−	−	−	−
Ring size	−	−	−	−	−	−	−
Morning stiffness	+	−*	−	−	−	−*	−
Physician's assmt.	+	+	−	−	−	−	−
Vis. analogue scale	−	+	+	−	−	−	−
ADL scale	−	+	−	−	−	−	−
RF titer	−	−	−	−	−	−	−
ESR	−	+	−	−	+†	−	−
CRP	−°	+	+	−	−	+	−

* Initial and subsequent values all <60 min.
† At 5 mos; the 4 previous monthly readings were all > initial reading.
° Initial and subsequent values were all low.
[a] From Malawista *et al.*[1] Reprinted by permission from Arthritis and Rheumatism.

mained stable for 2 to 3 months without alteration in their baseline therapy. The delayed deterioration in the conditions of Patients 1 and 2 (who continued not to receive alternative therapy) also mitigates against chance or placebo effect.

Although the precise mechanism of action of ECP is unclear, evidence continues to accumulate that points to an immune mechanism, beyond the clinical results in patients with cutaneous T cell lymphoma.[4] In mice, the rejection of highly immunogenic allogeneic skin grafts has been greatly retarded in a donor-strain-specific fashion by reinfusion of anti-graft effector T cells treated with 8-MOP/UVA.[5] Similarly, the development of high titers of anti-native-DNA antibodies, hepatosplenomegaly, and premature death in the MRL murine model of lupus were substantially slowed by the reinfusion of 8-MOP/UVA-treated splenocytes from old, diseased mice into young syngeneic mice not yet exhibiting florid disease.[6] In humans, three of four patients with pemphigus vulgaris, a disorder in which anti-epidermal antibodies cause a severe blistering skin disease, responded to ECP.[16]

For this preliminary study, we deliberately cast a wide net clinically, in terms both of type and severity of illness, and of current and previous treatment history (which are, of course, related); our purpose was not to miss a potentially responsive subset of rheumatoid arthritis (TABLE 1). If the mechanism of action of ECP is indeed immune-mediated, then the concomitant use of immunosuppressive agents is of some concern. Although our numbers are small, it is perhaps worth noting that the two patients who improved the most were taking only NSAIDs concomitantly (the only other such individual, Patient 6, was also the only one who was seronegative and had psoriasis; psoriatic arthritis has recently been found to respond only slightly, if at all, to ECP[17]). All the other patients were taking either low-dose prednisone (Patients 4 and 7) or both prednisone and methotrexate (Patients 3 and 5). Alternatively, the patients taking concomitant immunosuppressive drugs may have been doing so because they had a form of disease more difficult to treat by *any* modality; their previous treatment histories (TABLE 1) support this view. Nevertheless, in future studies the issue of concomitant therapy needs to be addressed.

A second issue that merits further study concerns dosage schedules. We chose the current one because of its success in cutaneous T cell lymphoma, where the kinetics and numbers of the circulating malignant target cells may be quite different from those of the putative pathogenic T cells in rheumatoid arthritis. In the current study, because of a general lack of response at 12 weeks, we increased the frequency of treatments to biweekly in three patients (Patients 1, 4, and 7), two of whom eventually had apparent responses to therapy. However, because all four apparent responders began to improve by 16 weeks, the value of the increased frequency of treatment is moot.

Finally, the prolonged clinical stability of Patients 1, 2, and 3 after cessation of ECP is also instructive for future studies in which, instead of stopping ECP After an apparent response has occurred, we will increase the interval between treatments, aiming for the minimum maintenance dosage. A regimen requiring only several treatments a year would make highly attractive a treatment that, at least in the short run, appears less toxic than any currently established therapy for rheumatoid arthritis, including nonsteriodal antiinflammatory drugs.

SUMMARY

For rheumatoid arthritis, an effective therapy with minimal toxicity would be welcome. In a six-month pilot study of seven patients with a variety of presentations and previous treatments, we tested a therapy involving the extracorporeal photoactivation of biologically inert methoxsalen (8-methoxypsoralen) by ultraviolet A energy to a form that covalently cross-links lymphocyte DNA; the injured cells are returned to the patient. Prior experimental studies had indicated that this regimen produces an immune reaction against antigens on treated T Cells, and a clinical trial in cutaneous T cell lymphoma had been successful. The current patients were treated on two successive days monthly (or, later on, biweekly). Between 12 and 16 weeks of therapy there appeared to be a breakpoint after which joint counts and joint scores of four patients began to improve. In three of them, these measures eventually diminished by mean values of 71% and 80%, respectively, of their baseline values, along with variable improvement in less direct indicators of clinical response. The joints of the fourth patient improved modestly (by 33% and 59%, respectively, of baselines) but he required alternative therapy, and those of the remaining three patients did not improve. Mean slopes for the joint counts were significantly different from zero after the apparent breakpoint (but not before), whether one examined the four apparent responders ($p = 0.01$) or the entire group of seven ($p = 0.01$). After completion of therapy, there was also a delay, of two to three months, in the clinical deterioration of those who had improved. There was only one mechanical adverse effect—a single episode of transient hypotension in 102 treatment sessions—and no toxic ones.

This preliminary study suggests that extracorporeal photochemotherapy may be effective at least in the short term in certain patients with rheumatoid arthritis, with less apparent toxicity than that of any of the drugs currently used for this disorder. It deserves further evaluation.

REFERENCES

1. MALAWISTA, S. E., D. TROCK & R. EDELSON. 1991. Treatment of rheumatoid arthritis by extracorporeal photochemotherapy. Arthritis Rheum. **38:** 646–654.
2. SCOTT, B. R., M. A. PATHAK & G. R. MOHN. 1976. Molecular and genetic basis of furocoumarin reactions. Mutat. Res. **39:** 29–74.
3. PARRISH, J.A., T. B. FITZPATRICK, L. TANENBAUM & M. A. PATHAK. 1976. Photochemotherapy of psoriasis with oral methoxsalen and longwave ultraviolet light. N. Engl. J. Med. **291:** 1207–1211.
4. EDELSON, R. L., C. BERGER, F. GASPARRO, B. JEGASOTHY, P. HEALD, B. WINTROUB, E. VONDERHEID, R. KNOBLER, K. WOLFF, G. PLEWIG, G. MCKIERNAN, I. CHRISTIANSEN, M. OSTER, H. HONIGSMANN, H. WILFORD, E. KOKOSCHKA, T. REHLE, M. PEREZ, G. STINGL & L. LAROCHE. 1987. Treatment of cutaneous T-cell lymphoma by extracorporeal photochemotherapy. N. Engl. J. Med. **316:** 297–303.
5. PEREZ, M. I., R. EDELSON, L. LAROCHE & C. BERGER. 1989. Inhibition of antiskin allograft immunity by infusions with syngeneic photoinactivated effector lymphocytes. J. Invest, Dermatol. **92:** 669–676.
6. BERGER, C. L., M. PEREZ, L. LAROCHE & R. EDELSON. 1990. Inhibition of autoimmune disease in a murine model of systemic lupus erythematosus induced by exposure to syngeneic photoinactivated lymphocytes. J. Invest. Dermatol. **94:** 52–57.
7. HARRIS, E. D., JR. 1990. Rheumatoid arthritis: pathophysiology and implications for therapy. N. Engl. J. Med. **322:** 1277–1289.
8. ARNETT, F. C., S. M. EDWORTHY, D. A. BLOCH, D. J. MCSHANE, J. F. FRIESE, N. S. COOPER, L. A. HEALEY, S. R. KAPLAN, M. H. LIANG, H. S. LUTHRA, T. A. MEDSGSER, D. M. MITCHELL, D. H. NEUSTADT, R. S. PINALS, J. G. SHALLER, J. T. SHARP, R. I. WILDER & G. G. HUNDER. 1988. The American Rheumatism Association 1987 revised criteria for the classification of rheumatoid arthritis. Arthritis Rheum. **31:** 315–324.
9. PUGLISI, C. V., A. J. DE SILVA & J. C. MEYER. 1977. Determination of 8-methoxypsoralen, a photoactive compound, in blood by high pressure liquid chromatography. Anal. Lett. **10:** 39–50.
10. BERGER, C. L., C. CANTOR, J. WELSH, P. DERVAN, T. BEGLEY, S. GRANT, F. P. GASPARRO & R. L. EDELSON. 1985. Comparison of synthetic psoralen derivatives and 8-MOP in the inhibition of lymphocyte proliferation. Ann. N.Y. Acad. Sci. **453:** 80–90.
11. EGGER, M. J., D. A. HUTH, J. R. WARD, J. C. READING & H. J. WILLIAMS. 1985. Reduced joint count indices in the evaluation of rheumatoid arthritis. Arthritis Rheum. **28:** 613–619.
12. WILKENS, R. F., J. E. GLEICHERT & E. T. GADE. 1973. Proximal interphalangeal joint measurement by arthrocircameter. Ann. Rheum. Dis. **32:** 585–586.
13. CALLAHAN, L. F., R. H. BROOKS, J. A. SUMMEY & T. PINCUS. 1987. Quantitative pain assessment for routine care of rheumatoid arthritis patients, using a pain scale based on activities of daily living and a visual analog pain scale. Arthritis Rheum. **30:** 630–636.

14. FLEISS, J. L. 1986. The Design and Analysis of Clinical Experiments. John Wiley and Sons. New York.
15. ANDERSON, J. J., D. T. FELSON, R. F. MEENAN & H. J. WILLIAMS. 1989. Which traditional measures should be used in rheumatoid arthritis clinical trials? Arthritis Rheum. **32:** 1093–1099.
16. ROOK, A. H., B. V. JEGASOTHY, P. HEALD, G. T. NAHASS, C. DITRE, W. K. WITMER, G. S. LAZARUS & R. L. EDELSON. 1990. Extracorporeal photochemotherapy for drug-resistant pemphigus vulgaris. Ann. Int. Med. **112:** 303–305.
17. WILFERT, H., H. HONIGSMANN, G. STEINER, J. SMOLEN & K. WOLFF. 1990. Treatment of psoriatic arthritis by extracorporeal photochemotherapy. Br. J. Dermatol. **122:** 225–232.

Antigen-Driven Peripheral Immune Tolerance

Suppression of Organ-Specific Autoimmune Diseases by Oral Administration of Autoantigens

HOWARD L. WEINER, Z. JENNY ZHANG,
SAMIA J. KHOURY, ARIEL MILLER,
AHMAD AL-SABBAGH, STALEY A. BROD, OFER LIDER,
PAUL HIGGINS, RAYMOND SOBEL,
ROBERT B. NUSSENBLATT, AND DAVID A. HAFLER

Center for Neurologic Diseases
Brigham and Women's Hospital and Harvard Medical School
75 Francis Street
Boston, Massachusetts 02115
and
Laboratory of Immunology
National Eye Institute
National Institutes of Health
Bethesda, Maryland 20205

One of the primary goals in developing effective therapy for autoimmune diseases is to specifically suppress autoreactive immune processes without affecting the remainder of the immune system. Autoimmune diseases involve the presence of autoreactive clones that have not been deleted in the thymus and thus these cells must be inactivated in the periphery. We have been investigating antigen-driven peripheral immune tolerance as a means to suppress autoimmune processes using the oral route of antigen-exposure to the immune system because of its inherent clinical applicability. An effective and long-recognized method of inducing immunologic tolerance is the oral administration of antigen, which was first demonstrated by Wells for hen's egg protein.[1] The mechanism by which orally administered antigen induces tolerance most probably relates to the interaction of protein antigens with gut-associated lymphoid tissue (GALT) and the subsequent generation of regulatory or suppressor T cells.[2] The two primary points of contact of orally administered antigen are Peyer's patches and gut epithelial cells, the latter of which overlie intraepithelial lymphocytes. Investigators have reported that specific suppressor cells can be found in the Peyer's patches following oral administration of antigen and that such cells then migrate systemically.[2] Intestinal epithelial cells express class II antigens on their surface and thus have the capacity to function as antigen-presenting cells.[3] Furthermore, it has been shown that human gut epithelial cells preferentially stimulate CD8+ cells *in vitro* which can function to suppress *in vitro* immune responses.[4] Although most investigators have reported that the generation of antigen-specific suppressor T cells is the primary mechanism responsible for mediating oral tolerance, other reported mechanisms include antiidiotypic antibodies, immune complexes and biologically filtered antigen (reviewed in REF. 5).

In order to test whether feeding an autoantigen could suppress an experimental autoimmune disease, the Lewis rat model of experimental autoimmune encephalomyelitis (EAE) was studied.[6] Animals were fed increasing amounts of myelin basic protein (MBP), either once or three times prior to immunization with MBP in complete Freund's adjuvant. With increasing dosages, the incidence and severity of disease was suppressed. In addition, proliferative responses of lymph node cells to MBP was also suppressed. Antibody responses to MBP were decreased but not as dramatically as proliferative responses. Thus, it appears that oral tolerance to MBP preferentially suppresses cellular immune responses. EAE is associated with inflammatory cells that accumulate in the central nervous system. In animals fed myelin basic protein, there was a marked decrease in the number of cells infiltrating the nervous system. In order to determine the length of protection following feeding, animals were fed three times prior to immunization and then immunized at weekly intervals. Animals were protected for approximately 2–3 months after this feeding regimen.

It is known that there are specific regions of MBP that are encephalitogenic in the Lewis rat. In order to determine whether nonencephalitogenic portions of MBP could suppress EAE, both fragments of MBP and synthetic peptides were orally administered.[6] Suppression of disease occurred by feeding fragments or synthetic peptides prior to immunization with BP/CFA. There was some suggestion that nonencephalogenic fragments were more potent in generating suppression than encephalitogenic fragments, although more investigation is needed in this area. We also noted that feeding bovine MBP was able to suppress EAE in the Lewis Rat and in the strain 13 guinea pig, showing cross-species tolerization.[7] Nonetheless in a series of pilot experiments, it appears that homologous MBP is a more potent oral tolerogen for EAE than heterologous MBP.[8]

The majority of studies related to mechanisms of oral tolerance suggest that active suppression is generated following exposure of antigen via the gut.[5] In order to test this mechanism in the EAE model, mesenteric lymph nodes and spleen cells were adoptively transferred from animals fed myelin basic protein into naive animals that were then immunized with MBP/CFA. We found that protection could be adoptively transferred and that such protection was dependent on CD8+ T cells.[9] Splenic and mesenteric T cells from fed animals were also able to suppress both *in vitro* proliferative responses and antibody production by MBP-primed popliteal lymph node cells. *In vitro* suppression was also mediated by CD8+ T cells. The suppression was antigen specific in that adding T cells from animals fed MBP suppressed MBP responses, but not responses to mycobacteria. Recent experiments from our laboratory suggest, however, that *in vitro* antigen-specific suppression involves triggering of suppressor T cells by antigen with the release of antigen nonspecific soluble suppressor factors (Miller and Weiner, unpublished).

EAE in the Lewis rat is usually an acute monophasic illness. In order for oral administration of autoantigens to have clinical applicability, it must be effective in patients in whom the disease process has expressed itself and in whom activated autoreactive cells already exist. Thus, experiments were performed in relapsing models of EAE.[7] A relapsing Lewis rat model of EAE occurs following injection of spinal cord homogenate plus adjuvant. Feeding MBP to animals following recovery from their first attack significantly suppressed the second attack and decreased histologic manifestations of the disease. In addition, cell-mediated immunity as measured by DTH and anti-myelin antibody responses were also suppressed. A more chronic model of EAE occurs in the strain 13 guinea pig. In a series of experiments, guinea pigs were injected with white matter homogenate plus adjuvant and upon recovering from the first attack, were fed 10 mg of bovine myelin or BSA, three times weekly over a three-month period. In animals fed the bovine myelin preparation there was a diminution in frequency of attacks, and a decrease in demyelination in the spinal cord and certain portions of the white matter. These results demonstrate that oral administration of myelin antigens can suppress chronic relapsing EAE and have direct relevance to the therapy of human demyelinating disorders such as multiple sclerosis.

The generation of an immune response in animals often requires concomitant administration of an adjuvant to enhance antibody production and to generate T cell-mediated responses. Antigens administered per os generally result in systemic hyporesponsiveness even though there may be local stimulation of IgA antibody.[5] We thus initiated a series of experiments to determine whether a tolerogenic adjuvant could be found for oral tolerance to MBP. It has been suggested that colonization of the gastrointestinal tract by LPS-producing bacteria is one of the requirements for oral tolerization as LPS converts germ-free mice to sensitivity to oral tolerance induction.[10] Furthermore, LPS-nonresponsive C3H/HeJ mice are unable to be orally tolerized to sheep red blood cells,[11,12] and LPS and dextran sulfate have been reported to enhance oral tolerance for DTH responses to picryl chloride in mice,[13] although LPS did not affect DTH responses to ovalbumin.[14] We found that the oral administration of LPS enhanced the suppressive effects of myelin basic protein on EAE.[15] LPS given without MBP had no effect on EAE and LPS given subcutaneously with orally administered MBP tended to abrogate oral tolerance. The enhanced suppression of EAE associated with oral administration of LPS was also associated with a decrease in DTH responses to MBP, but not with decreased anti-MBP antibody responses. Further experiments demonstrated that it was the lipid A moiety of LPS that was active in enhancing oral tolerance to MBP in the EAE model.[15] The mechanism of action of LPS is unknown but presumably relates to enhanced generation of cellular suppressive mechanisms by gut associated lymphoid tissue.

In addition to oral exposure to antigen, the body is constantly exposed to inhaled antigen which contacts the mucosal immune system at the level of the bronchial associated lymphoid tissue. In order to determine the effect of this route of antigen exposure on EAE, MBP was aerosolized to Lewis rats on days -10, -7, -5, -3 prior to immunization with MBP in Freund's adjuvant and on days 0, $+2$, $+4$ following immunization. Five ml of PBS containing 5 mg/ml of MBP was aerosoled to a group of 5 rats in an airtight plastic cage over a 10-minute period. Aerosolization of MBP completely abrogated clinical EAE: incidence in controls, 20/20; in treated group, 0/20. CNS inflammation and DTH and antibody responses to MBP were also significantly reduced in aerosol-treated animals. Aerosolization of histone, a basic protein of similar weight to MBP had no effect. Disease was also suppressed with one aerosol treatment on day -3. Aerosolization was more effective than oral administration of MBP over a wide dose range (0.005–5 mg) suggesting that protection via aerosolization was not merely secondary to gastric absorption of aerosolized antigen. Splenic T cells isolated from aerosoled animals adoptively transferred protection to naive animals immunized with MBP. Aerosolization of MBP to animals with relapsing EAE after recovery from the first attack decreased subsequent attack severity, and MBP antibody and DTH responses. Thus, aerosolization of an autoantigen is a highly potent method to downregulate an experimental T cell-mediated autoimmune disease and suggests that exposure of antigen to lung mucosal surfaces preferentially generates immunologic tolerance.[16]

In order to further assess oral tolerization as a method to treat autoimmune diseases, studies were performed in experimental autoimmune uveitis and in adjuvant arthritis. Oral administration of S-antigen (S-Ag), which is a retinal autoantigen that induces experimental autoimmune uveoretinitis (EAU), prevented or markedly diminished the clinical appearance of S-Ag-induced disease as measured by ocular inflammation.[17] Furthermore oral administration of S-Ag also markedly diminished uveitis induced by the uveitogenic M and N fragments of the S-Ag. Oral administration of S-Ag did not prevent MBP-induced EAE. *In vitro* studies demonstrated a significant decrease in proliferative responses to the S-Ag in lymph node cells draining the site of immunization from fed versus nonfed animals. Furthermore the addition of splenocytes from S-Ag-fed animals to cultures of a CD4+ S-Ag-specific cell line profoundly suppressed the cell line's response to the S-Ag, whereas these splenocytes had no effect on a PPD-specific cell line. The antigen-specific *in vitro* suppression was blocked by anti-CD8 antibody demonstrating that suppression was dependent on CD8+ T cells.

Oral tolerance was also tested in the adjuvant arthritis model. Previous investigators have demonstrated suppression of collagen-induced arthritis by feeding collagen type II.[18,19] We studied adjuvant arthritis (AA), another well-characterized and more fulminant form of experimental arthritis.[20] Adjuvant arthritis is induced by injection of Mycobacterium tuberculosis (MT) into the base of the tail. Attempts to suppress adjuvant arthritis by oral administration of MT were not successful. Nonetheless we found that oral administration of chicken collagen type II (CII) given at a dose of 3 μg per feeding on days -7, -5, and -2 before disease induction consistently suppressed the development of AA. A decrease in delay-type hypersensitivity responses to CII was also observed that correlated with suppression to AA. AA was optimally suppressed by 3 and 30 μg CII, variably by 300 μg, and not by 0.3 μg or 1 mg. Oral administration of collagen type I also suppressed AA; only minimal effects were seen with collagen type III. Suppression was antigen specific in that feeding collagen type II did not suppress EAE, and feeding MBP did not suppress AA. Suppression of AA could be adoptively transferred by T cells from CII-fed animals and could be obtained when CII was fed after disease onset. These results suggest that autoimmunity to CII has a pathogenic role in AA and raises the possibility that cross-reactive epitopes exist between collagen type II and MT.

In summary, we have found that the oral administration of autoantigens suppresses experimental autoimmune diseases (EAE, EAU, AA) in a disease- and antigen-specific manner. Our results are consistent with those of other investigators who have also shown suppression of EAE by oral administration of MBP[21] and of collagen-induced arthritis by oral administration of CII.[18,19] Suppression can be adoptively transferred by CD8+ T cells in EAE and T cells in AA. In EAE and EAU, CD8+ T cells from fed animals suppress antigen-specific proliferative responses *in vitro,* and nonencephalitogenic fragments of MBP suppress EAE when given orally. Chronic relapsing EAE can be suppressed by oral administration of myelin antigens after disease expression and AA can be suppressed when CII is fed after disease onset. LPS given orally enhances oral tolerance to MBP in EAE, and aerosol administration of MBP suppresses EAE.

Based on these results, clinical trials are planned to test oral tolerance as a means to treat human disease states. A double-blind trial using a myelin antigen preparation is currently in progress in 30 patients with early relapsing remitting multiple sclerosis at the Brigham and Women's Hospital in Boston. In addition, trials are planned in rheumatoid arthritis utilizing orally administered collagen type II (David Trentham, Beth Israel Hospital, Boston) and in uveitis using S-antigen (Robert Nussenblatt, National Eye Institute, NIH).

Note added in proof: We have recently defined that the mechanism by which CD8+ T cells suppress following oral tolerance is via the release of TGFB after antigen triggering (Miller *et al.*, J. Exp. Med. 174: 791, 1991 and Miller *et al.*, PNAS, in press). Also we have found suppression of diabetes in the NOD mouse by oral tolerization to insulin (Zang *et al.*, PNAS, in press, Nov. 1991).

REFERENCES

1. WELLS, H. 1911. Studies on the chemistry of anaphylaxis. III. Experiments with isolated proteins, especially those of hen's egg. J. Infect. Dis. 9: 147.
2. MATTINGLY, J. & B. WAKSMAN. 1978. Immunologic suppression after oral administration of antigen. I. Specific suppressor cells found in rat Peyer's patches after oral administration of sheep erythrocytes and their systemic migration. J. Immunol. 121: 1878.
3. SANTOS, L. M. B., O. LIDER, J. AUDETTE, S. J. KHOURY & H. L. WEINER. 1990. Characterization of immunomodulatory properties and accessory cell function of small intestinal epithelial cells. Cell. Immunol. 127: 26–34.
4. MAYER, L. & R. SHLIEN. 1987. Evidence for function of Ia molecules on gut epithelial cells in man. J. Exp. Med. 166: 1471.
5. MOWAT, A. 1987. The regulation of immune responses to dietary protein antigens. Immunol. Today 8: 193.
6. HIGGINS, P. J. & H. L. WEINER. 1988. Suppression of experimental autoimmune encephalomyelitis by oral administration of myelin basic protein and its fragments. J. Immunol. 140: 440–445.
7. BROD, S. A., A. AL-SABBAGH, R. A. SOBEL, D. A. HAFLER & H. L. WEINER. Suppression of experimental autoimmune encephalomyelitis by oral administration of myelin antigens. IV. Suppression of chronic relapsing disease in the Lewis rat and strain 13 guinea pig. Ann. Neurol. In press.
8. MILLER, A., O. LIDER, S. J. KHOURY & H. L. WEINER. 1990. Oral tolerance induced by myelin basic protein from different species in the Lewis rat EAE model. Neurol. (Abstr.) 40(Suppl. 1): 217.
9. LIDER, O., L. M. B. SANTOS, C. S. Y. LEE, P. J. HIGGINS & H. L. WEINER. 1989. Suppression of experimental autoimmune encephalomyelitis by oral administration of myelin basic protein. II. Suppression of disease and *in vitro* immune responses is mediated by antigen-specific CD8+ T lymphocytes. J. Immunol. 142: 748–752.
10. WANNEMUEHLER, M. J., H. KIYONO, J. L. BABB, S. M. MICHALEK & J. R. MCGHEE. 1982. Lipopolysaccharide (LPS) regulation of the immune response: LPS converts germfree mice to sensitivity to oral tolerance induction. J. Immunol. 129:959–965.
11. KIYONO, J. R. MCGHEE, M. J. WANNEMUEHLER & S. M. MICHALEK. 1982. Lack of oral tolerance in C3H/HeJ mice. J. Exp. Med. 155: 605–610.
12. MICHALEK, S. M., H. KIYONO, M. J. WANNEMUEHLER, L. M. MOSTELLER & J. R. MCGHEE. 1982. Lipopolysaccharide (LPS) regulation of the immune response: LPS influence on oral tolerance induction. J. Immunol. 128: 1992
13. NEWBY, T. J., C. R. STOKES & F. J. BOURNE. 1980. Effects of feeding bacterial lipopolysaccharide and dextran sulphate on the development of oral tolerance to contact sensitizing agents. J. Immunol. 41: 617–621.
14. MOWAT, A. M., M. J. THOMAS, S. MACKENZIE & D. M. V. PARROTT. 1986. Divergent effects of bacterial lipopolysaccharide on immunity to orally administered protein and particulate antigens in mice. Immunology 58: 677.
15. KHOURY, S. J., O. LIDER, A. AL-SABBAGH & H. L. WEINER. 1990. Suppression of experimental autoimmune encephalomyelitis by oral administration of myelin basic protein. III. Synergistic effect of lipopolysaccharide. Cell. Immunol. 131: 302–310.
16. WEINER, H. L., A. AL-SABBAGH & R. SOBEL. 1990. Antigen driven peripheral immune tolerance: suppression of experimental autoimmune encephalomyelitis (EAE) by aerosol administration of myelin basic protein. FASEB J. (Abstr.) 4(7): 2102.
17. NUSSENBLATT, R. B., R. R. CASPI, R. MAHDI, C.-C. CHAN, R. ROBERGE, O. LIDER &

H. L. WEINER. 1990. Inhibition of S-antigen induced experimental autoimmune uveoretinitis by oral induction of tolerance with S-antigen. J. Immunol. **144:** 1689–1695.

18. NAGLER-ANDERSON, C., L. A. BOBER, M. E. ROBINSON, G. W. SISKIND & G. J. THORBECKE. 1986. Suppression of type II collagen-induced arthritis by intragastric administration of soluble type II collagen. Proc. Natl. Acad. Sci. USA 83:7443.

19. THOMPSON, H. S. G. & N. A. STAINES. 1986. Gastric administration of type II collagen delays the onset and severity of collagen-induced arthritis in rats. Clin. Exp. Immunol. **64:** 581.

20. ZHANG, J. Z., C. S. Y. LEE, O. LIDER & H. L. WEINER. 1990. Suppression of adjuvant arthritis in Lewis rats by oral administration of type II collagen. J. Immunol. **145:** 2489–2493.

21. BITAR, D. M. & C. C. WHITACRE. 1988. Suppression of experimental autoimmune encephalomyelitis by the oral administration of myelin basic protein. Cell. Immunol. **112:** 364.

Immunotoxins and Cytokine Toxin Fusion Proteins[a]

TERRY B. STROM,[b] PAIGE L. ANDERSON,[c]
VICKI E. RUBIN-KELLEY,[d] DIANE P. WILLIAMS,[c]
TETSUYUKI KIYOKAWA,[c] AND
JOHN R. MURPHY[c]

[b]Department of Medicine
Beth Israel Hospital
Harvard Medical School
330 Brookline Avenue
Boston, Massachusetts 02215

[c]Evans Department of Clinical Research
and
Department of Medicine
University Hospital
Boston University Medical Center
Boston, Massachusetts 02118

[d]Department of Medicine
Brigham and Women's Hospital
Harvard Medical School
Boston, Massachusetts 02115

Rat anti-mouse and mouse anti-rat pan-T cell, anti-CD4, and anti-CD25 (interleuken-2 receptor) monoclonal antibodies (mAbs) exert remarkable immunosuppressive effects in murine transplant and autoimmune models whereas only select rodent anti-human mAbs can exert immunosuppression in clinical practice. While graft tolerance is readily achieved with these anti-T cell mAbs in the rodent, immunosuppression, but not tolerance, is noted with clinical application of very select anti-T cell mAbs. One of the reasons for the failure of mAb treatment in clinical practice to live up to expectations may be the failure of the constant, *e.g.* Fc, region of most murine mAbs to kill human target cells in the treated human host. These antibodies do not fix human complement or activate human Fc receptor positive cytolytic cells. As a consequence, clinical application of the first generation rodent anti-human mAbs does not destroy the targeted human cells, while *in vivo* treatment with mouse anti-rat or rat anti-mouse mAbs frequently destroys the targeted rodent cell population. It is not surprising that to date the most successful first generation mAbs in clinical practice target functionally important domains of vitally important T cell surface proteins, *e.g.*, the T cell antigen/CD3 complex or the IL-2 receptor, since these mAbs probably function as receptor site blockers. Hence, efforts now are proceeding in many quarters to use genetic engineering strategies to replace the constant regions of murine antibodies with human Fc region sequences in order to produce mAbs that will lyse the

---

[a] Preparation of this review was supported in part by Public Health Service Grants R01 CA-41746 and U01 CA-48626 from the National Cancer Institute, and R01 AI-22882 from the National Institute of Allergy and Infectious Diseases.

targeted human cell *in vivo*. An alternative strategy, the subject of this brief review, is to fashion "magic bullet' hybrid toxins.

The great German scientist Paul Ehrlich first suggested that *Zauberkugeln, i.e.*, "magic bullet" hybrid molecules, consisting of cell-specific antibodies linked to a toxin (immunotoxin) be constructed for therapeutic purposes. He envisioned that immunotoxins could be used as magic bullets to destroy a highly selective population of target cells. In recent years, advances in understanding and mapping the functional domains of select toxins has fostered cognate development of a new generation of immunotoxins and fusion protein hybrid toxins for potential use as therapies in transplantation, autoimmunity, AIDS, and cancer.

Immunotoxins

Each mature holotoxin used in the construction of hybrid molecules possesses at least three functionally specialized domains that i) bind to specific target cell surface receptors; ii) translocate the toxin into the appropriate subcellular compartment; and iii) enzymatically intoxicate the target cell.[1,2] An enzymatically active domain, the toxophore, is responsible for catalyzing the chemical reaction that intoxicates the target cell. In the case of diphtheria toxin (FIG. 1) the enzymatically active core is an ADP-ribosyltransferase which targets elongation factor-2 (EF-2). EF-2 is an essential element in the translational apparatus of the cell. Following ADP-ribosylation, EF-2 is inactivated and the cell dies as a consequence of a failure to manufacture new cellular proteins. Another domain functions as a receptor binding element and is responsible for the binding of the toxin to specific eukaryotic cell surface receptors (FIG. 1). The third domain, the translocating element, enables the intact toxin to traverse the target cell membrane, thereby gaining access of the toxin to the endosome and subsequent delivery of the toxophore to the cytosol.[1,2]

Some efforts to construct hybrid toxin molecules have utilized full length diphtheria toxin (DT) (FIG. 1). These DT hybrids are potent but lack exquisite specificity for the desired target cell since the receptor binding domain of DT is retained. As a consequence, these hybrid immunotoxins can bind to desired target cells via the antigen binding domain of the antibody or nonspecifically via the receptor binding domain of DT. These hybrid molecules are ill-suited for clinical use because of nonspecific toxicity that results from failure to eliminate or inactivate the receptor binding domain of DT. Mutant DTs, such as CRM 45, lacking the receptor binding domain can be used to construct chemically linked immunotoxins insofar as the enzymatically active core and translocating domains are retained; nonetheless, the resulting chemically cross-linked immunotoxins are often less potent, albeit less dangerous, than chimers using whole length DT.

Pseudomonas exotoxin A (PE), made by pseudomonas aeroginosa, while structurally unrelated to DT, is in many ways the mirror image of DT. The enzymatically active domain of PE is situated near the C-terminus while the receptor binding domain is housed at the N-terminus.[1] The central portion of the PE molecule, like the DT, possesses the translocating element. DT and PE intoxicate target cells through a common mode of action. Like DT, PE is an ADP-ribosyltransferase which binds to and inactivates EF-2 thereby blocking the translational apparatus of the target cell. The intoxicated target cell dies as a consequence of a failure to express cellular proteins. Indiscriminate cellular targeting of PE can be obviated by chemically reacting PE with 2-iminothiolane resulting in loss of function of the receptor binding domain. Thus, at least in theory, 2-iminothiolane-treated PE can be used to construct specificity targeted chemically linked PE immunotoxins.

Ricin, a plant toxin, is a heterodimer. The A-chain enzymatically directly inactivates the ribosome, thereby blocking protein synthesis of the target cell. The ricin B-chain bears both the receptor binding and translocation activities. Many workers have constructed immunotoxins with isolated ricin A-chains since non-specific cellular targeting with undesired binding of the receptor binding domain element located on the B-chain is avoided. Regrettably these ricin-A immunotoxins are often not nearly as potent as whole ricin-based hybrids insofar as the translocating element is also positioned on the B-chain. Recently an intact, chemically treated ricin has been constructed in which the receptor binding domain has

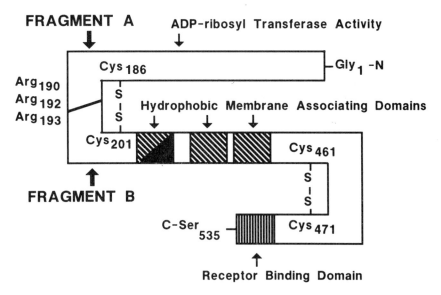

FIGURE 1. Diphtheria toxin. Diphtheria toxin possesses three functional domains: the enzymatically active (ADP-ribosyltransferaseactive) toxophore, a translocating domain, and a receptor binding domain. An additional feature of note is a protease sensitive region within the stretch of amino acids that subtend the first disulfide loop. Proteolytic nicking off the toxin at this site results in separation of the fragment A from fragment B.

been chemically blocked. It is hoped but not proven that the blocked ricin immunotoxins may prove as potent as intact ricin-based immunotoxins.

Biochemical Coupling of Toxin Hybrids

Often antibody or other targeting ligands are coupled to whole ricin or the enzymatically active ricin A-chain by creation of a disulfide bond. Whole ricin conjugates are potent but often mediate indiscriminate binding owing to the binding capacity of the B-chain. Ricin A-chain conjugates are often (but not always) far less potent than whole ricin.

DT- and PE-hybrid toxins have also been constructed by introduction of sulf-hydryl groups and creation of disulfide bonds. As noted previously mutant DT proteins, lacking the receptor binding domain, or 2-iminothiolane-treated PE, "blocked PE," can be used to mitigate against indiscriminate cellular targeting.

Several chemically coupled immunotoxins have been used to deplete T cells from bone marrow transplants because T cells are responsible for mounting graft vs host reactions. DT, whole ricin, and ricin A-chain have each been chemically linked to pan-T cell antibodies for this purpose in clinical bond marrow transplantation although *ex vivo* T cell depletion can also be effectively achieved with conventional antibodies plus complement or lectin-binding columns.

An anti-CD5 whole ricin immunotoxin is currently being tested in the clinic for treatment of advanced graft vs host disease. Partial, but meaningful (2 clinical grades), remissions have been obtained in 70% of treated patients. Plans to test this molecule for less virulent forms of graft vs host disease and as an antirejection treatment in organ transplantation and in drug resistant autoimmune processes are underway. An immunotoxin utilizing blocked ricin is being administered for treatment of B cell lymphomas, but a blocked ricin immunotoxin has not yet been deployed as an immunosuppressive drug. Treatment with both ricin-based immunotoxins has been associated with hepatotoxicity. It is not certain as to whether this is due to liberation of ricin as a consequence of lability of the chemically cross-linked chimeric molecule. In the case of chemically modified "blocked" ricin, it is possible that chemical modification (glycosylation) of the receptor binding domain, which allows specific cell targeting *in vitro,* may not remain stably glycosylated *in vivo.* Should the chemical blockade of the receptor binding domain prove labile *in vivo,* hepatotoxicity and other nonspecific cytotoxicity would be expected.

Recombinant Cytokine-Toxin Fusion Proteins

Within the last three years, the design and genetic construction of eukaryotic cell surface receptor specific toxins has become a reality. A detailed understanding of the structure/function relationships of both DT and PE, the nucleic acid sequence of their respective structural genes, as well as the technical ability to precisely construct recombinant toxin-related peptide fusion proteins has allowed the development of a number of unique receptor-specific cytotoxins.

The genetic replacement of either the native diphtheria toxin or *Pseudomonas* exotoxin A receptor binding domain with eukaryotic cell receptor-specific cytokine, polypeptide hormones or growth factors has resulted in the development of a new class of biological response modifiers—the fusion toxin.[3,4,6,16–18] The first of these fusion toxins, DAB_{486}-IL-2, is currently in human Phase I clinical trials and the early results clearly demonstrate that this molecule is safe, well-tolerated, and biologically active in the elimination of high affinity IL-2 receptor positive leukemia and lymphoma cells without adverse side effect (LeMaistre, personal communication). DAB_{486}-IL-2 is a bipartite fusion protein composed of diphtheria toxin fragment A and fragment B sequences to Ala^{486} linked to Pro^2 through Thr^{133} of human interleukin-2 (IL-2)[4] (FIG. 2). This chimeric protein is the product of a genetic fusion between a truncated gene (FIG. 3) encoding fragment A and the membrane associating domains of fragment B of diphtheria toxin and a synthetic gene encoding human IL-2.[19] DAB_{486}-IL-2 has been shown to selectively bind to high affinity IL-2 receptors, be internalized by receptor-mediated endocytosis, and facilitate the delivery of diphtheria toxin fragment A to the cytosol of target

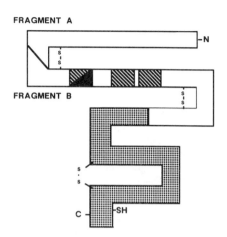

FIGURE 2. DAB$_{486}$-IL-2 toxin. The DAB$_{486}$-IL-2 fusion protein is composed of the entire diphtheria toxin toxophore (fragment A), a truncated fragment B component, lacking the receptor binding domain, and human Il-2.

cells bearing high affinity IL-2 receptors.[5,7] Recent studies have defined the minimal size of fragment B that is required to deliver fragment A across the endocytic vesicle membrane in target cells, and defined the site of proteolytic processing involved in the release of fragment A from the intact fusion toxin molecule.[20,21]

In an attempt to broaden the scope of the fusion toxin technology, we have recently focused our attention on the development of tripartite proteins in which diphtheria toxin fragment A sequences are being substituted with a variety of active polypeptides. While the application of protein engineering to the development of new biologicals is in its infancy, it is now clear that one can design and genetically construct a wide variety of fusion toxins that are extraordinarily selective and potent in the elimination of receptor-bearing target cells. Indeed, the early results from human Phase I/II clinical trials of DAB$_{486}$-IL-2 suggest that the fusion toxin technology will play an important role in the development of new biological agents for the treatment of specific human hemopoietic malignancies.

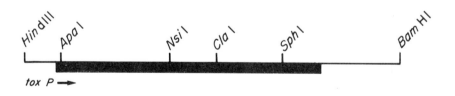

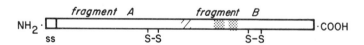

FIGURE 3. Genetic construction of DAB$_{486}$-IL-2 was achieved through a fusion of a cDNA encoding a truncated diphtheria toxin gene, lacking the codons for the receptor binding domain and a synthetic cDNA encoding human interleukin-2.

Diphtheria Toxin

As outlined previously, biochemical and genetic analyses of diphtheria toxin have clearly shown that the toxin molecule is composed of at least three functional domains: (i) the enzymatically active fragment A, (ii) the membrane associating domains and (iii) receptor binding domain of fragment B (FIG. 1). Moreover, each domain of diphtheria toxin has been shown to play an essential role in the intoxication of intact sensitive eukaryotic cells.[22] In mature form, diphtheria toxin is a single polypeptide chain of 585 amino acids in length (FIG. 1), and contains four cysteine residues which form two disulfide bridges: Cys^{186}–Cys^{201} and Cys^{461}–Cys^{471}.[23–25] The fourteen amino acid loop subtended by the first disulfide bridge contains three arginine residues (Arg^{190}, Arg^{192}, and Arg^{193}) and this loop is extremely sensitive to proteolytic attack by serine proteases. Upon trypsin "nicking" and reduction of the first disulfide bridge, diphtheria toxin can be separated under denaturing conditions into two polypeptide fragments.[26,27] Fragment A, the N-terminal 21.1 kDa polypeptide, carries the catalytic centers for the nicotinamide adenine dinucleotide (NAD+) dependent adenosine diphosphoribosylation (ADPR) of eukaryotic EF-2.[28] The B fragment of diphtheria toxin, the 37.1 Kda polypeptide, carries at least two functional domains: the hydrophobic membrane associating domains which are responsible for the translocation of fragment A through the cell membrane and into the cytosol,[29] and the native diphtheria toxin receptor binding domain.[28] The toxin receptor binding domain has been recently located at the extreme C-terminal end of the toxin molecule.[30,31]

Interactions between diphtheria toxin and toxin-sensitive eukaryotic cells involve (i) the binding of intact toxin to the cell surface receptor,[32] (ii) internalization of bound toxin by receptor-mediated endocytosis into acidification competent vesicles,[33] and upon "nicking" of the toxin in this acidic environment [pH 5.3–5.1],[32,34] (iii) insertion of the hydrophobic domain(s) into the vesicle membrane,[35,36] thereby facilitating the (iv) delivery of fragment A to the cytosol. Once delivered to the cytosol, fragment A catalyzed ADP-ribosylation of EF-2 abolishes cellular protein synthesis and as a result leads to the death of the cell. Yamaizumi *et al.*[37] have demonstrated that a *single* molecule of fragment A delivered to the cytosol of a cell is sufficient to be lethal for that cell.

Since structure/function analysis of diphtheria toxin has shown that the toxin's receptor binding domain of diphtheria toxin is positioned at the C-terminal end of the molecule, and that the first step in the intoxication process involves the binding of diphtheria toxin to its receptor, we reasoned several years ago that the replacement of the receptor binding domain with either a cytokine, polypeptide hormone or cell specific growth factor should result in the formation of *new* toxins. Moreover, the cellular target of these new toxins should be determined by the polypeptide hormone or growth factor used in its construction.[3,4] Unlike the immunotoxins (*i.e.,* fragments of microbial or plant toxins cross-linked to monoclonal antibodies), we chose to assemble these chimeric toxins at the level of the gene rather than by chemically coupling the toxophore with the ligand. The assembly of these fusion toxins at the level of the gene allows for (i) the precise linkage of the two components through a peptide bond, (ii) the modification of that structure through recombinant DNA techniques, and (iii) the production of the fusion toxins in recombinant *Escherichia coli.*

Thus, the approach that we have taken toward the development of targeted cytotoxins is fundamentally different from that of the immunotoxins. Rather than chemically cross-linking the toxophore and ligand components through a disulfide bond, we have employed protein and genetic engineering methods to create gene fusions whose chimeric products are joined by a peptide bond at a defined site. The precision of the genetic fusion strategy enables the assembly of isomeric fusion proteins, while chemical cross-linking yields racemic mixtures. Moreover, following interaction with cell surface receptors, the genetically engineered fusion toxins would be expected to be internalized by receptor-mediated endocytosis which would deliver the toxin to the acidic environment of the endosome and facilitate the delivery of the ADP-ribosyltransferase to the cytosol. As previously noted, monoclonal antibodies can insure the delivery of immunotoxins to the cell surface; however, they do not provide assured delivery of the toxophore to either the endosome or the cytosol. Moreover, cytokines, polypeptide hormones and growth factors bind to their target receptor proteins with a higher binding affinity than mAbs. Hence, it is likely that cytokine toxin hybrids will possess a greater therapeutic "window" than conventional immunotoxins. Therefore, rather than to employ mAbs as the cellular targeting component, we have used cytokines and growth factors whose receptors are known to undergo receptor-mediated endocytosis. Since cytokines and growth factors are known to be internalized into vesicles that become acidified, we reasoned that the internalization of a given toxin-related fusion protein should follow the same route of entry into the cell as diphtheria toxin itself.

IL-2-Toxin (DAB$_{486}$-IL-2)

Williams *et al.*[4] described the genetic construction and properties of a fusion toxin that was assembled from a truncated form of diphtheria toxin and human interleukin-2 (IL-2), DAB$_{486}$-IL-2. In this construct, the 3'-end of the *tox* structural gene encoding the C-terminal receptor binding domain of diphtheria toxin was removed and replaced by a synthetic gene encoding amino acids 2 through 133 of mature human IL-2 (FIG. 2). Since the native diphtheria toxin receptor binding domain was replaced with IL-2 sequences, the resulting fusion toxin is directed towards cells bearing the IL-2 receptor. Importantly, cells which lacked the IL-2 receptor were found to be resistant to the inhibitory action of DAB$_{486}$-IL-2. Bacha *et al.*[5] have confirmed and extended these initial observations and have shown that the cytotoxic action of this fusion toxin is mediated through the IL-2 receptor and can be blocked by excess free recombinant IL-2, as well as by antibodies that bind to the p55 subunit (alpha chain) of the IL-2 receptor. Moreover, since lysozomatrophic agents (*e.g.*, chloroquine) also block the cytotoxic action of DAB$_{486}$-IL-2, it is apparent that the fusion toxin must pass through an acidic compartment in order to deliver its ADP-ribosyltransferase to the cytosol of target cells. Bacha *et al.*[5] also demonstrated that inhibition of protein synthesis in target cells was, in fact, due to the specific ADP-ribosylation of elongation factor 2 in the target cell cytosol. Thus the cytotoxic action of DAB$_{486}$-IL-2 (i) is directed through the IL-2 receptor, (ii) requires passage through an acidic compartment in a manner analogous to native diphtheria toxin, and (iii) catalyzes the ADP-ribosylation of elongation factor 2 in a manner indistinguishable from that of native diphtheria toxin fragment A.

More recently, Walz *et al.*[38] demonstrated that the sequential events following the binding of DAB$_{486}$-IL-2 to the IL-2 receptor on PHA-activated T cells reflects both the IL-2 and the ADP-ribosyltransferase components of the fusion toxin. In a manner identical to native IL-2, DAB$_{486}$-IL-2 was found to stimulate the expression of c-*myc*, interferon gamma, IL-2 receptor, and IL-2 mRNA's for the first seven hours of exposure. However, after 7 hours' exposure the action of the fusion toxin is analogous to that of cycloheximide—an inhibitor of protein synthesis. By this time, the effects of inhibition of protein synthesis by the ADP-ribosylation of elongation factor 2 predominate and the steady state levels of c-*myc* and IL-2 receptor mRNA are decreased. Importantly, Walz et al.[38] have demonstrated that the ADP-ribosyltransferase defective mutant DA(197)B$_{486}$-IL-2 does not inhibit protein synthesis and is capable of signal transduction in PHA-activated T cells. This study has demonstrated that the functional activity of each of DAB$_{486}$-IL-2's component parts is retained: (i) interaction of the fusion toxin with the IL-2 receptor results in signal transduction, and (ii) the delivery of the ADP-ribosyltransferase to the cytosol results in an inhibition of protein synthesis and elicits a series of effects which are similar to those imposed by cycloheximide.

It is well known that the high affinity form of the IL-2 receptor is composed of at least two subunits: a low affinity 55 kDa glycoprotein (p55, alpha chain) and an intermediate affinity 75 kDa glycoprotein (p75, beta chain).[39–44] Moreover, it is known that both the high affinity (p55 + p75) and p75 intermediate affinity receptor, but not the p55 low affinity IL-2 receptor, undergo accelerated internalization after binding native IL-2.[43–46] Based on these observations, Waters et al.[7] have examined the receptor binding requirements of DAB$_{486}$-IL-2 for the efficient intoxication of target cells. Dose response analysis of high, intermediate, and low affinity IL-2 receptor bearing cells demonstrates that only cell lines which bear the high affinity form of the IL-2 receptor are sensitive to the cytotoxic action of DAB$_{486}$-IL-2 (IC$_{50}$ $\leq 10^{-10}$ M). In marked contrast, cell lines which bear either isolated p55 chains or p75 chains are resistant to the action of the fusion toxin and require exposure to ca. 1,000-fold higher concentrations (IC$_{50}$ $\geq 1 \times 10^{-7}$ M) of DAB$_{486}$-IL-2.

Since peripheral blood mononuclear cells (PBMC) with natural killer (NK) activity have been reported to bear only the p75 subunit of the IL-2 receptor on the cell surface and these cells are responsive to IL-2 and appear to be precursors of lymphokine activated killer (LAK) cell activity, Waters et al.[7] examined the effect of DAB$_{486}$-IL-2 on NK cell activity. In these experiments, PBMC from healthy donors were cultured in the presence or absence of IL-2 and DAB$_{486}$-IL-2 and the subsequent NK cell activity was measured using NK sensitive K562 target cells in a 4 hour [^{51}Cr]-release assay. Anti-CD3-induced T cell cytotoxicity was measured in the same assay using an anti-CD3 mAb-producing target cell line. The concentrations of DAB$_{486}$-IL-2 greater than 10^{-7} M are required to inhibit NK cell activity. Thus, human peripheral blood monocytes with NK activity are as resistant to the action of DAB$_{486}$-IL-2 as continuous cell lines which bear only the p75 subunit of the IL-2 receptor.

Weissman et al.[45] have shown that the p55 subunit of the IL-2 receptor does not mediate efficient internalization of bound [^{125}I]-labeled IL-2. By comparison, native IL-2 bound to the p75 subunit of the receptor is known to be internalized as rapidly as the high affinity receptor (t½ = 15 min).[47] Since intermediate affinity p75$^+$, p55$^-$ bearing cell lines were resistant to the action of DAB$_{486}$-IL-2, we reasoned that this resistance was due to altered binding of the fusion toxin to this subunit of the receptor. Waters et al.[7] have also determined the receptor binding properties of DAB$_{486}$-IL-2 by competitive displacement experiments using [^{125}I]-labeled IL-2. Approximately 200-fold higher concentrations of DAB$_{486}$-IL-2 are required to displace radiolabeled IL-2 from the high affinity (p55 + p75) receptor. It is of interest to note that only 18-fold higher concentrations of DAB$_{486}$-IL-2 than native IL-2 are required to displace radiolabeled ligand from the p55 subunit; whereas, 120-fold higher concentrations are required for the p75 subunit.

These receptor binding experiments strongly suggest that the relative resistance of intermediate affinity IL-2 receptor bearing cells to the cytotoxic action of DAB_{486}-IL-2 is due to altered binding to the p75 subunit of the receptor. Although both the p75 and the high affinity heterodimer share the common property of rapidly internalizing bound ligand, IL-2 binding to cells bearing the intermediate affinity receptor site is characterized by slow kinetics of association/dissociation. In contrast, the high affinity receptor displays the fast "on" rate of p55 and the slow "off" rate of p75.[48,49] Thus, an alteration in DAB_{486}-IL-2 binding to the p75 subunit may more dramatically influence the kinetics of this fusion toxin's binding to the intermediate vis-à-vis high affinity receptor. Clearly, the results of the competitive displacement studies described by Waters *et al.*[7] are consistent with this interpretation. As determined by the concentration of fusion toxin required to inhibit radiolabeled IL-2 binding, it is evident that DAB_{486}-IL-2 displays altered binding to *both* subunits of the IL-2 receptor; however, binding to the p75 subunit appears to be more significantly affected than binding to the p55 subunit.

Since Collins *et al.*[50] have reported that the N-terminal sequences of native IL-2, particularly Asp^{20}, are essential for binding to the p75 subunit of the IL-2 receptor, it is likely that the altered binding of DAB_{486}-IL-2 to this subunit results from stearic constraints imposed on the fusion toxin: p75 IL-2 receptor interaction. In the case of DAB_{486}-IL-2, human IL-2 sequences are fused to the C-terminal end of a truncated form of the toxin. Therefore, the fusion junction between diphtheria toxin-related and IL-2 sequences are likely to place Asp^{20} (Asp^{505} in DAB_{486}-IL-2) in an internal or less favorable position to bind to the p75 subunit. Consistent with this interpretation are the results of Lorberboum-Galski *et al.*[51] who have described the cytotoxic action of an analogous fusion toxin composed of a truncated form of *Pseudomonas* exotoxin-A and IL-2, IL-2-PE40. In this instance, cells which express the high affinity form of the IL-2 receptor have been found to be only 8–20 times more sensitive to the cytotoxic action of IL-2-PE40 than cell lines which express either intermediate or low affinity IL-2 receptors. Moreover, only 6-fold differences in binding to the p75 subunit were reported for IL-2-PE40 relative to native IL-2. In the case of IL-2-PE40, the fusion junction between the two proteins occurs at the C-terminal end of IL-2 and the N-terminus of PE40. Since the N-terminus of this fusion toxin consists of IL-2 sequences, Asp^{20} is likely to be more available for binding to the p75 subunit of the receptor than Asp^{505} in DAB_{486}-IL-2. The observed cytotoxicity of this fusion toxin for p75 only bearing cells supports this hypothesis.

Williams *et al.*[20] have demonstrated that the in-frame deletion of 97 amino acids from Thr^{387} to His^{485} of DAB_{486}-IL-2 increases both the potency ($IC_{50} \approx 2 - 5 \times 10^{-11}$ M) and the apparent dissociation constant (K_d) of the resulting DAB_{389}-IL-2 for high affinity IL-2 receptor bearing T cells (FIG. 4). In marked contrast, the deletion of an additional 94 amino acids (Asp^{291} to Gly^{483}) results in a greater than 1,000-fold loss of cytotoxic potency in the fusion toxin DAB_{295}-IL-2. It is important to note that the structural regions between Asp^{291} and Gly^{483} include the hydrophobic putative membrane spanning helical regions of fragment B that have been postulated to facilitate the delivery of fragment A across the endocytic vesicle membrane.[29] The results of experiments described by Williams *et al.*[20] strongly suggest that the putative membrane-spanning helices of fragment B are essential in the intoxication process.

In addition, Williams *et al.*[20] have shown that the amphipathic membrane surface binding region of fragment B contained between Asn^{204} and Ile^{290} is also essential to the cytotoxicity of the DAB-IL-2 fusion toxins. It is important to note that the genetic deletion of this region of fragment B in both DAB $(205-289)_{486}$-IL-2 and DAB$(205-289)_{389}$-IL-2 also decreases biologic activity of the fusion toxin by ca. 1,000-fold. Most interestingly, these in-frame internal deletion mutations also effect the apparent K_d of the fusion toxin for the high affinity IL-2 receptor. Since the region that has been deleted carries an amphipathic domain(s),[52] it is reasonable to postulate that this region of fragment B associates with the T cell membrane surface forming a nonspecific secondary binding event and appears to stabilize the interaction of the fusion toxin with the target cell surface.

We have analyzed the primary amino acid sequence of DAB$_{486}$-IL-2 and DAB$_{389}$-IL-2 fusion toxins for predicted secondary structure using the PC GENE software (Intelligenetics, Mountain View, CA). In particular, the FLEXPRO program of Karplus and Schulz[53] was used to predict the flexibility of the DAB-IL-2 fusion toxins at each point of their sequence. This algorithm calculates the theoretical flexibility of the peptide chain at each amino acid and is measured from the average value of the atomic temperature factor (B value) of the alpha carbon atom, as affected by the adjacent amino acids. The "neighbor-correlated" average of normalized B values for each amino was found from a set of proteins whose

FRAGMENT A

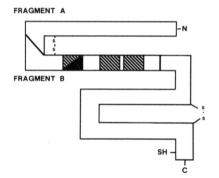

FIGURE 4. DAB$_{389}$-IL-2 toxin. The DAB$_{389}$-IL-2 fusion protein was created by deleting the codons for the second disulfide loop of diphtheria toxin from the DAB$_{486}$ construct. This streamlined molecule is a more efficient toxin than DAB$_{386}$-IL-2.

three-dimensional structural was known. The predicted flexibility at an amino acid is the weighted sum of the normalized B values (taking account of neighbors) of the seven amino acids closest to that point in the sequences.

It is of particular interest to note that this analysis of the DAB-IL-2 toxins has revealed a common predicted "most" flexible region—amino acids 1 through 10 of human IL-2. Since this region was also found to be unordered in the 3A crystal structure of IL-2,[54] we postulated that the apparent flexibility of this region of the fusion toxin might allow for some degree of mobility of the IL-2 component with respect to the diphtheria toxin-related sequences. Were this the case, duplication of the flexible region might result in a fusion toxin with increased receptor binding affinity and potency. In order to test this hypothesis, we (Kiyokawa and Murphy, unpublished) have genetically constructed mutants of DAB$_{486}$-IL-2 and DAB$_{389}$-IL-2 in which amino acids 2 through 8 of IL-2 were duplicated at the fusion junction. These constructions were made by cloning a 33-mer oligonucleotide linker encoding amino acids 2 through 8 of IL-2 into the unique *Sph*I site which defines the fusion junction between diphtheria toxin-related and IL-2 sequences. It should be noted that codon usage in the linker was changed with respect to that already present in the DAB_{486}-IL-2 structural gene in order to insure genetic stability of the insert.

The dose response curve of the duplication mutant DAB_{389}-(1–10)IL-2 on high affinity IL-2 receptor bearing HUT 102 6/TG cells reveals that the IC_{50} for DAB_{389}-(1–10)IL-2 (6×10^{-12} M) is 40- to 60-fold higher than that of DAB_{486}-IL-2 and approximately 10-fold higher than DAB_{389}-IL-2. These studies clearly demonstrate that the application of protein engineering methodologies towards the development of second and third generation DAB-IL-2 fusion toxins will result in variants with increased biologic potency.

Tripartite Fusion Toxins: Shiga-A-DT"B"-IL-2

We (Anderson, Itoh, Nishibuchi, Takeda, and Murphy, in preparation) have selected the A chain of Shiga-like toxin to replace diphtheria toxin fragment A in the construction of the first tripartite toxin for the following reasons: (i) both Shiga-like A and diphtheria fragment A are similar in molecular mass, (ii) the introduction of a single molecule of Shiga-like A chain to the cytosol of a target cell will result in an irreversible inhibition of protein synthesis, and, as a result, the measurement of biologic activity of the tripartite fusion would be both convenient and sensitive, and (iii) the modification of the gene for Shiga-like A chain required to construct the tripartite fusion toxin gene is straightforward and could be readily accomplished.

The gene for Shiga-like toxin has recently been cloned and sequenced.[55,56] Shiga-like toxin is composed of an A subunit (32,225 Da) that is noncovalently bound to a pentameric B subunit (7,961 Da). The A subunit of Shiga-like toxin contains a single disulfide bridge that subtends a protease sensitive loop. Upon trypsin nicking in A1 and A2 fragment are released. The A1 fragment of Shiga-like toxin has been shown to be an enzyme which specifically cleaves the N-glycosidic bond at adenine 4325 in the 28S ribosomal RNA. Thus, Shiga-like toxin inhibits protein synthesis in a manner that is identical to that of the plant toxin ricin.[57] It should be noted that the isolated chains of Shiga-like toxin, like those of diphtheria toxin, are *not* toxic for intact eukaryotic cells.

Biochemical/genetic analysis of DAB_{486}-IL-2 mutants has recently shown that fragment A *must* be released from the fusion toxin in order to intoxicate target lymphocytes. Williams *et al.*[21] have found that the substitution of Arg194 with Gly results in an approximate 5,000-fold loss of cytotoxic potency of the fusion toxin. Interestingly, pre-nicking the mutant fusion toxin with trypsin restores full biologic activity. These results suggest that DAB_{486}-IL-2 binds to the IL-2 receptor, and is then *processed* by a cellular protease at Arg194 in order to release fragment A which is then delivered to the cytosol. These results strongly suggest that an intact disulfide bridge between Cys^{187} and Cys^{202} in DAB486-IL-2 is essential for full biologic activity.

As a result of these observations, we have developed a vector for the genetic construction of the tripartite fusion toxin which retains the $Cys^{187} : Cys^{202}$ disulfide bond. We have taken advantage of a unique *Nsi*I restriction endonuclease site that is positioned at Cys^{202} and the *Nco*I site that contains the ATG of the translational initiation signal at the beginning of fragment A. Following digestion of plasmid pABI6508 with *Nsi*I and *Nco*I, we have cloned an *NSI*I-*Apa*I-*Nco*I linker that restores the genetic information encoding the $Cys^{187} : Cys^{202}$ disulfide loop. The modified plasmid has been designated pPA101. Importantly, this linker also introduces a unique *Apa*I site immediately upstream of Cys^{187}. As a result,

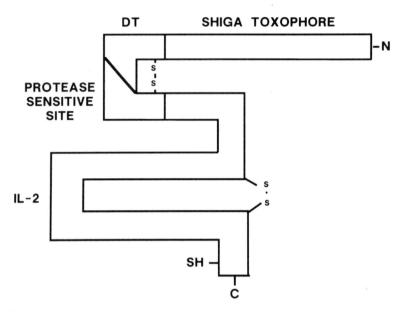

FIGURE 5. Tripartite-IL-2 toxin. A tripartite toxin was created by genetically fusing: 1) a Shiga-like A domain, 2) to the protease sensitive first disulfide loop of diphtheria toxin, 3) to interleukin-2.

any gene that can be modified at its 5′ end by the introduction of an *Nco*I site, and at its 3′ end by the introduction of an *Apa*I site can be inserted into pPA101 giving rise to a tripartite fusion gene.

We have modified the structural gene for Shiga-like toxin A chain by the introduction of a 5′ linker and a 3′ linker. The modified gene for Shiga-like A chain was then introduced into the sites of pPA101 (Anderson and Murphy, unpublished). Following growth and expression of the tripartite toxin gene, the Shiga-like A-DT″B″-IL-2 fusion toxin was purified by immunoaffinity chromatography on an anti-IL-2 matrix (FIG. 5). The tripartite toxin can be readily purified to apparent homogeneity by immunoaffinity chromatography followed by HPLC chromatography. Furthermore, the tripartite fusion toxin has been shown to carry determinants that are reactive on immunoblots probed with anti-Shiga-like A, anti-IL-2, and anti-diphtheria toxin sera. Thus, the three domains of the tripartite toxin fold in such a way as to present their own unique and characteristic immunodominant epitopes. Most exciting, however, is the observation that the tripartite toxin is biologically active against high affinity IL-2 receptor bearing T lymphocytes. It should be noted that the biological activity of the tripartite toxin can be specifically blocked with either excess IL-2 or monoclonal antibody to the IL-2 binding domain of the p55 subunit of the IL-2 receptor. These results demonstrate that the action of this fusion toxin is mediated through the IL-2 receptor. It is notable that both diphtheria toxin and shiga toxin intoxicate target cells by poisoning the translational apparatus of the target cell. However, these toxins target different molecules. Diphtheria toxin inactivates EF-2 while shiga toxin directly targets the ribosome. Although as yet unproven, we believe it likely that combined treatment with diphtheria toxin based and shiga toxin based IL-2 fusion proteins will provide synergistic effects.

In short, a variety of fusion proteins in which the native receptor binding domain of either DT or PE has been genetically replaced with either a polypeptide cytokine, hormone or other targeting molecule have been reported. In all instances, the chimeric toxins selectively intoxicate receptor bearing target cells *in vitro*. Moreover, cell lines which are devoid of the targeted receptor protein(s) have been found to be resistant to the action of these fusion proteins. Substitution of the toxin receptor binding domain with ligands that bind to receptors that are limited in their cellular distribution offers the potential for a new class of biological response modifiers whose action is based on the selective elimination of target cells.

In Vivo *Effects of Cytokine Fusion Toxins*

For example, both human IL-2 DT[3–5] and human IL-2 PE[6] recombinant fusion proteins have been expressed, purified and studied for immunosuppressive effects (FIG. 2). At low concentrations *in vitro,* IL-2 DT selectively intoxicates activated T cells bearing high affinity IL-2 receptors.[5,7] *In vivo,* the DAB_{486}-IL-2 DT chimeric proteins totally block the delayed type hypersensitivity (DTH) reaction by selectively destroying antigen-activated IL-2 receptor-positive T cells[8] (TABLE 1). IL-2 DT destroys both $CD4^+$ $CD25^+$ and $CD8^+$ $CD25^+$ T cells in the lymph node draining the DTH reaction but not $CD25^-$ T cells. Both IL-2 DT and IL-2 PE produce tolerance in a mouse heart transplant model employing H-2 incompatible donors[9,10] (TABLE 2). Just 10 daily doses of either of the IL-2 toxins produces permanent engraftment. IL-2 PE and IL-2 DT are active in several murine models of autoimmunity. In the rat adjuvant arthritis model treatment during the induction period with either IL-2 PE[11] or IL-2 DT (manuscript in preparation) blocks bone destruction. Delayed therapy administered during the established phase of disease with IL-2 DT inhibits bone erosion[10] (manuscript in preparation). We have found that IL-2 DT blocks diabetogenic autoimmunity (manuscript in preparation) in a virulent model in which autoimmune T cells are passively transferred from diabetic NOD mice into young prediabetic NODs.[12] In untreated NOD mice 50% become diabetic within 1 mo following the cell transfer from older diabetic mice while onset of diabetes is delayed in the majority of IL-2 DT-treated NOD mice for an additional 2 months.

In contrast to conventional immunosuppressive drugs, pan-T cell or anti-CD4 mAbs, the IL-2 toxin selectively targets antigen-activated T cells and spares resting portions of the immune system.[13] The specificity of IL-2 DT for antigen reactive T cell clones was proven in a DTH-model system. Mice were immunized with an i.p. innoculation of TNBS—a chemical hapten—and these were chal-

TABLE 1. IL-2 Toxin Destroys Activated IL-2R+Cells during a DTH Response[a]

Lymph Node	IL-2R+%	
	CD4+	CD8+
Non-immunized	3	2
Immunized	14	18
Immunized IL-2 toxin	5	3

[a] Analysis of 0.5×10^4 cells/sample.

lenged later with TNBS in the foot pad. Both treatment with either anti-CD3 mAb or IL-2DT for seven days beginning on the day of immunization totally blocked the DTH response to the chemical hapten TNBS. Following a rest period anti-CD3-treated or IL-2 DT-treated mice were rechallenged with TNBS or DNFB, a chemically unrelated hapten. No treatment was administered during this rest phase of the experimental protocol. Following the rest period mice were challenged with either TNBS or DNFB. IL-2DT animals failed to respond to TNBS but mounted a normal response to the unrelated hapten (DNFB), thereby proving the specificity of IL-2DT for antigen-activated T cells. Resting T cells are spared. When the rest period was extended to one month, the response to TNBS after IL-2 DT treatment was no longer suppressed unless the NOD mice were thymectomized. This suggests that there is a repopulation of T cell clones from the thymus capable of being sensitized to TNBS. In addition, based on these studies and the results in delaying diabetes in NOD mice, we would predict that newly generated T cell clones must be periodically zapped to maintain a disease-specific suppressive state. In contrast, anti-CD3-treated hosts are broadly and nonselectively immunosuppressed, since they do not mount a response to many haptens and unresponsiveness persists for a protracted period of time.

Recent experiments also demonstrate that IL-2DT powerfully inhibits antigen

TABLE 2. IL-2 Toxin Prolongs Cardiac Allograft Survival

Treatment[a]	Graft Survival Days
IL-2 toxin 1.0 mg	20, >50, >50, >50, >50
IL-2 toxin 0.5 mg	12, 16, 19, 41, >50
CRM45[b] 0.66 mg	11, 12, 12, 13, 19
None	10, 14, 15, 18, 20

[a] i.p. qd for 10 days; $p < 0.01$; mice = B10.BR into C57B1/10.
[b] CRM45: diphtheria toxin lacking the receptor binding domain.

specific (tetanus toxoid) IgG responses *in vitro*. Insofar as production of anti-toxoid IgG-antibodies is a T cell-dependent process, it was important to determine whether IL-2 DT exerted its effects via intoxication of activated T cells or activated B cells. By separately treating highly purified T cells or B cells, it was determined that IL-2 DT targeted upon both activated T cells and activated B cells. Treatment of either B or T cells resulted in significant inhibition of antigen-specific IgG formation.[14] Thus, IL-2 DT inhibits both T and B cell responses.

IL-2 DT is being tested for efficacy in treating patients with a wide variety of drug and radiation resistant, IL-2 receptor positive leukemas or lymphomas. It is evident from these preliminary clinical studies that human IL-2 receptor positive cells can be selectively intoxicated following i.v. administration of IL-2 DT without causing serious side effects. Moreover, treatment with IL-2 DT kills tumor cells in individuals harboring anti-diphtheria toxoid antibodies. Following a short 7-day course of treatment most patients have shown evidence of a tumorcidal effect. In these studies, this short course of phase I study of bolus infusions of the Il-2 toxin has produced enduring remissions in about 15% of the patients. Because toxicity has been mild, phase II studies using longer infusions of the Il-2 toxin have now been initiated. The IL-2 toxin has also been administered by bolus infusion to 5 patients with cyclosporine- and/or methotrexate-resistant rheumatoid arthritis. All other medications were discontinued. Three weeks following cessation of drug therapy, IL-2 DT was infused. Each of the 5 patients evidenced amelioration of the disease. Improvement has been sustained during the very brief follow-up time that has elapsed.

A variety of other cytokine fusion proteins have been expressed including IL-4 DT, IL-4 PE, IL-6 DT and IL-6 PE, and these proteins are undergoing pre-clinical testing. Preliminary results indicate that the murine IL-4 Dt molecule is also a powerful immunosuppressive agent in mice. IL-4 DT blocks DTH responses. The treated mice remain healthy during and following therapy. Since the Il-4 receptor is expressed upon certain resting cells, we initially feared that the IL-4 toxin would create unwanted severe side effects. To our relief, we have determined that a critical number of IL-4 receptors must be expressed to render a cell sensitive to the IL-4 toxin. As a consequence, activated, but not resting macrophages, T or B cells, are sensitive to the Il-4 toxin.[15] It seems clear that the IL-4 toxin will afford an interesting means to assess the role of cells bearing high copy numbers of IL-4 receptors in various immune responses and disease states.

In short, advances in the knowledge of the structure/function relationship of toxins as well as genetic engineering techniques have facilitated development of a large number of antibody and cytokine toxin hybrids. A new generation of chimeric "magic bullets" has been created by deleting or inactivating the domain of the holotoxin responsible for receptor site binding so that the chemically linked or genetically fused targeting element (antibody or cytokine) can dictate the population of cells to be targeted for intoxication. Several hybrid molecules being tested in the clinic show considerable promise.

Nearly one century after Paul Ehlich's remarkably lucid concept of magic bullet therapeutic ligands, several laboratories have succeeded in producing cell-specific hybrid toxins. Antibody or cytokines can be used to direct the therapeutic ligand to the desired target cell. Through the use of new protein engineering and molecular biologic techniques increasingly sophisticated magic bullets are being created, and some of these agents are now being deployed in the clinic.

SUMMARY

Paul Ehrlich first suggested the simple and elegant concept of creating specific cell toxins or "magic bullets" through the fusion of cell-specific antibodies and toxins. In practice it has proven difficult to create safe and effective "magic bullets." In the past several years, several immunotoxins have been applied to clinical testing. These immunotoxins have been created by the biochemical coupling of cell- or lineage-specific monoclonal antibodies to plant toxins or fragments thereof. These immunotoxins have been used to treat bone marrow transplant recipients and patients with autoimmune disorders.

In recent years, another strategy has also been pursued to create hybrid toxins. Rather than use antibodies as the targeting moiety, cytokines have been used to target a select population of cells bearing a high copy number of receptors for the specific cytokine. Rather than biochemically couple a cytokine to the toxin, the cytokine and toxin are fused by a peptide bond established via genetic engineering. A prototype IL-2 diphtheria toxin-related fusion protein is now being tested in the clinic for treatment of hematopoietic malignancies and autoimmune disorders.

REFERENCES

1. PASTAN, I., M. C. WILLINGHAM & D. S. P. FITZGERALD. 1986. Immunotoxins. Cell **47:** 641–648.
2. OLSNES, S., K. SANDRIG, O. W. PETERSEN & B. VANDEWS. 1989. Immunotoxins—entry into cells and mechanisms of action. Immunol. Today **10:** 291–295.
3. MURPHY, J. R., W. BISHAI, A. BOROWSKI, A. MIYANOHARA, J. BOYD & S. NAGLE. 1986. Genetic construction, expression, and melanoma-selective cytotoxicity of a diphtheria toxin-related alpha-melanocyte-stimulating hormone fusion protein. Proc. Natl. Acad. Sci. USA **83:** 8258–8262.
4. WILLIAMS, D. P., K. PARKER, P. BACHA, W. BISHAI, M. BOROWSKI, F. GENBAUFFE, T. B. STROM & J. R. MURPHY. 1987. Diphtheria toxin receptor binding domain substitution with interleukin-2: genetic construction and properties of a diphtheria toxin-related interleukin-2 fusion protein. Protein Eng. **1:** 493–498.
5. BACHA, P., D. P. WILLIAMS, C. WATERS, J. M. WILLIAMS, J. R. MURPHY & T. B. STROM. 1988. Interleukin-2 receptor targeted cytotoxicity: interleukin-2 receptor mediated action of a diphtheria toxin-related interleukin-2 fusion protein. J. Exp. Med. **167:** 612–622.
6. LORBERBOUM-GALSKI, H., D. FITZGERALD, V. CHAUDHARY, S. ADHYA & I. PASTAN. 1988. Cytotoxic activity of an interleukin-2-*Pseudomonas* exotoxin chimeric protein produced in *Escherichia coli*. Proc. Natl. Acad. Sci. USA **85:** 1922–1926.
7. WATERS, C. A., P. SCHIMKE, C. E. SNIDER, K. ITOH, K. A. SMITH, J. C. NICHOLS, T. B. STROM & J. R. MURPHY. 1990. Interleukin-2 binding requirements for entry of a diphtheria toxin related interleukin-2 fusion protein into cells. Eur. J. Immunol. **20:** 785–791.
8. V. E. KELLEY, P. BACHA, O. PANKEWYCZ, J. C. NICHOLS, J. R. MURPHY & T. B. STROM. 1988. Interleukin-2 diphtheria toxin fusion protein can abolish cell-mediated immunity *in vivo*. Proc. Natl. Acad. Sci. USA **85:** 3980–3984.
9. KIRKMAN, R. L., P. BACHA, L. V. BARRETT, S. FORTE, J. R. MURPHY & T. B. STROM. 1989. Prolongation of cardiac allograft survival in murine recipients treated with a diphtheria toxin-related interleukin-2 fusion protein. Transplantation **47:** 327–330.
10. LORBERBOUM-GALSKI, H., L. V. BARRETT, R. L. KIRKMAN, M. OGATA, M. C. WILLINGHAM, D. J. FITZGERALD & I. PASTAN. 1989. Cardiac allograft survival in mice treated with IL-2-PE40. Proc. Natl. Acad. Sci. USA **86:** 1008–1012.
11. CASE, J. P., H. LORBERBOUM-GALSKI, R. LAFFATIS, D. FITZGERALD, R. L. WILDER & I. PASTAN. 1989. Chimeric cytotoxin IL-2-PE40 delays and mitigates adjuvant-induced arthritis in rats. Proc. Natl. Acad. Sci. USA **85:** 287–291.
12. KELLEY, V. K., T. B. STROM & J. R. MURPHY. Manuscript in preparation.
13. BASTOS, M., O. PANKEWYCZ, J. R. MURPHY, V. E. RUBIN-KELLEY & T. B. STROM. 1990. Concomitant administration of hapten and IL-2 toxin (DAB_{486} IL-2) results in specific deletion of antigen activated T-cell clones. J. Immunol. **145:** 3535–3539.
14. GRAILER, A. P., J. C. NICHOLS, T. B. STROM, H. W. SOLLINGER & W. J. BURLINGHAM. Inhibition of human splenic B-cell IgG response to tetanus toxoid by a diphtheria-toxin related interleukin-2 fusion protein. Cell. Immunol. In press.
15. LAKKIS, F., A. STEELE, T. B. STROM & J. R. MURPHY. Interleukin-4 receptor targeted cytotoxicity: genetic construction and properties of diphtheria toxin-related interleukin-4 fusion toxins. Submitted for publication.
16. CHAUDHARY, V. K., D. J. FITZGERALD, S. ADHYA & I. PASTAN. 1987. Activity of a recombinant fusion protein between transforming growth factor type alpha and *Pseudomonas* toxin. Proc. Natl. Acad. Sci. USA **84:** 4538–4542.
17. CHAUDHARY, V. K., T. MIZUKAMI, T. R. FUERST, D. J. FITZGERALD, B. MOSS, I. PASTAN & E. A. BERGER. 1988. Activity of a recombinant fusion protein between transforming growth factor type alpha and *Pseudomonas* toxin. Nature (London) **335:** 369–372.
18. SIEGALL, C. B., V. K. CHAUDHARY, D. J. FITZGERALD & I. PASTAN. 1988. Cytotoxic activity of an interleukin-6 *Pseudomonas* exotoxin fusion protein on human myeloma cells. Proc. Natl. Acad. Sci. USA **85:** 9738–9742.

19. WILLIAMS, D. P., D. REGIER, D. AKIYOSHI, F. GENBAUFFE & J. R. MURPHY. 1988. Design, synthesis and expression of a human interleukin-2 gene incorporating the codon usage bias found in highly expressed *Escherichia coli* genes. Nucleic Acids Res. **16:** 10453–10467.

20. WILLIAMS, D. P., C. E. SNIDER, T. B. STROM & J. R. MURPHY. 1990. Structure/function analysis of interleukin-2 toxin (DAB$_{486}$ IL-2). Fragment B sequences required for the delivery of fragment A to the cytosol of target cells. J. Biol. Chem. **265:** 11885–11889.

21. WILLIAMS, D. P., Z. WEN, R. S. WATSON, T. B. STROM & J. R. MURPHY. 1990. Cellular processing of the interleukin-2 fusion toxin DAB$_{486}$ IL-2 and efficient delivery of diphtheria fragment A to the cytosol of target cells requires Arg194. J. Biol. Chem. **265:** 20673–20677.

22. PAPPENHEIMER, A. M., JR. 1977. Diphtheria toxin. Annu. Rev. Biochem. **46:** 69–94.

23. KACZOREK, M., F. DELPEYROUX, N. CHENCINER, R. E. STREECK, J. R. MURPHY, P. BOQUET & P. TIOLLAIS. 1983. Nucleotide sequence and expression of the diphtheria tox228 gene in *Escherichia coli*. Science **221:** 855–858.

24. GREENFIELD, L., M. BJORN, G. HORN, D. FONG, G. A. BUCK, R. J. COLLIER & D. A. KAPLAN. 1983. Nucleotide sequence of the structural gene for diphtheria toxin carried by corynebacteriophage beta. Proc. Natl. Acad. Sci. USA **80:** 6853–6857.

25. RATTI, G., R. RAPPUOLI & G. GIANNINI. 1983. The complete nucleotide sequence of the gene coding for diphtheria toxin in the corynephage omega (tox+) genome. Nucleic Acids Res. **11:** 6589–6595.

26. GILL, D. M., & A. M. PAPPENHEIMER, JR. 1971. Structure activity relationships in diphtheria toxin. J. Biol. Chem. **246:** 1492–1495.

27. COLLIER, R. J. & J. KANDEL. 1971. Structure and activity of diphtheria toxin. I. Thiol-dependent dissociation of a fraction of toxin into enzymically active and inactive fragments. J. Biol Chem. **246:** 1496–1503.

28. UCHIDA, T., D. M. GILL & A. M. PAPPENHEIMER, JR. 1971. Mutation of the structural gene for diphtheria toxin carried by temperate phage. Nature (New Biol.) **233:** 8–11.

29. BOQUET, P., M. S. SILVERMAN, A. M. PAPPENHEIMER, JR. & W. B. VERNON. 1976. Binding of triton X-100 to diphtheria toxin, crossreacting material 45, and their fragments. Proc. Natl. Acad. Sci. USA **73:** 4449–4453.

30. GREENFIELD, L., V. JOHNSON & R. J. YOULE, 1987. Mutations in diphtheria toxin separate binding from entry and amplify immunotoxin selectivity. Science **238:** 536–539.

31. ROLF, J. M., H. M. GAUDIN & L. EIDELS. 1990. Localization of the diphtheria toxin receptor-binding domain to the carboxyl-terminal Mr approximately 6000 region of the toxin. J. Biol. Chem. In press.

32. MIDDLEBROOK, J. L., R. B. DORLAND & S. LEPPLA. 1978. Association of diphtheria toxin with Vero cells. Demonstration of a receptor. J. Biol. Chem. **253:** 7325–7330.

33. MOYA, M., A. DAUTRY-VERSAT, B. GOUD, D. LOUVARD & P. BOQUET. 1985. Inhibition of coated pit formation in Hep2 cells blocks the cytotoxicity of diphtheria toxin but not that of ricin toxin. J. Cell Biol. **101:** 548–559.

34. SANDVIG, K., T. I. TONNESSEN, O. SAND & S. OLSNES. 1986. Requirement of a transmembrane pH gradient for the entry of diphtheria toxin into cells at low pH. J. Biol. Chem. **261:** 11639–11645.

35. DONOVAN, J. J., M. I. SIMON, R. K. DRAPER & M. MONTAL. 1981. Diphtheria toxin forms transmembrane channels in planar lipid bilayers. Proc. Natl. Acad. Sci. USA **78:** 172–176.

36. KAGAN, B. L., A. FINKELSTEIN & M. COLOMBINI. 1981. Diphtheria toxin fragment forms large pores in phospholipid bilayer membranes. Proc. Natl. Acad. Sci. USA **78:** 4950–4954.

37. YAMAIZUMI, M., E. MEKADA, T. UCHIDA & Y. OKADA. 1978. One molecule of diphtheria toxin fragment A introduced into a cell can kill the cell. Cell **15:** 245–250.

38. WALZ, G., B. ZANKER, K. BRAND, C. WATERS, F. GENBAUFFE, J. B. ZELDIS, J. R. MURPHY & T. B. STROM. 1989. Sequential effects of interleukin-2 diphtheria toxin fusion protein on T-cell activation. Proc. Natl. Acad. Sci. USA **86:** 9485–9488.

39. SHARON, M., R. D. KLAUSNER, B. R. CULLEN, R. CHIZZONITE & W. L. LEONARD. 1986. Novel interleukin-2 receptor subunit detected by cross-linking under high-affinity conditions. Science **234:** 859–863.
40. TSUDO, M., R. W. KOZAK, C. K. GOLDMAN & T. A. WALDMANN. 1987. Contribution of a p75 interleukin-2 binding peptide to a high-affinity interleukin-2 receptor complex. Proc. Natl. Acad. Sci. USA **84:** 4215–4218.
41. TESHIGAWARA, K., H. M. WANG, K. KATO & K. A. SMITH. 1987. Interleukin-2 high-affinity receptor expression requires two distinct binding proteins. J. Exp. Med. **165:** 223–238.
42. DUKOVICH, M., Y. WANO, L. T. BICH-THUY, P. KATZ, D. CULLEN, J. H. KEHRL & W. C. GREENE. 1987. A second human IL-2 binding protein that may be a component of high-affinity IL-2 receptors. Nature (London) **327:** 518–522.
43. ROBB, R. J., C. M. RUSK, J. YODOI & W. C. GREENE. 1987. Interleukin-2 binding molecule distinct from the Tac protein: analysis of its role in formation of high-affinity receptors. Proc. Natl. Acad. Sci. USA **84:** 2001–2006.
44. TANAKA, T., O. SAIKI, S. DOI, M. FUJI, K. SUGAMURA, H. HARA, S. NEGORO & S. KISHIMOTO. 1988. Novel receptor-mediated internalization of interleukin-2 in B cells. J. Immunol. **140:** 866–870.
45. WEISSMAN, A. M., J. B. HARFORD, P. B. SVETLIK, W. L. LEONARD, J. M. DEPPER, T. A. WALDMANN, W. C. GREENE & R. D. KLAUSNER. 1986. Only high-affinity receptors for interleukin-2 mediate internalization of ligand. Proc. Natl. Acad. Sci. USA **83:** 1463–1466.
46. FUJII, M., K. SUGAMURA, K. SANO, K. SAGITA & Y. HINUMA. 1986. High affinity receptor mediated internalization and degradation of interleukin-2 in human T-cells. J. Exp. Med. **163:** 550–562.
47. ROBB, R. J. & W. C. GREENE 1987. Internalization of interleukin-2 is mediated by the beta chain of the high-affinity interleukin-2 receptor. J. Exp. Med. **165:** 1201–1206.
48. WANG, H. M. & K. A. SMITH. 1987. The interleukin-2 receptor. Functional consequences of its bimolecular structure. J. Exp. Med. **166:** 1055–1069.
49. LOWENTHAL, J. L. & W. C. GREENE. 1987. Contrasting interleukin-2 binding properties of the alpha (p55) and beta (p70) protein subunits of the human high-affinity interleukin-2 receptor. J. Exp. Med. **166:** 1156–1161.

The Potential of Restricted T Cell Recognition of Myelin Basic Protein Epitopes in the Therapy of Multiple Sclerosis

DAVID A. HAFLER,[a] MAKOTO MATSUI,
KAI W. WUCHERPFENNIG, KOHEI OTA, AND
HOWARD L. WEINER

Center for Neurologic Diseases
Division of Neurology
Department of Medicine
Brigham and Women's Hospital
and
Harvard Medical School
Boston, Massachusetts, 02115

INTRODUCTION

Multiple sclerosis (MS) is a chronic inflammatory disease of the central nervous system (CNS) characterized by prominent T cell and macrophage infiltrates associated with demyelination. The pathogenesis of MS is thought to arise from autoreactive T cells specific for myelin protein(s) that initiate the inflammatory process.[1,2] Myelin basic protein (MBP) has been studied as a potential autoantigen in the disease because of its role as an encephalitogen in experimental autoimmune encephalomyelitis (EAE)[3] and post-viral encephalomyelitis,[4] and because *in vivo*-activated T cells reactive to MBP are present in the blood of MS patients.[5] Immune involvement in MS has been further suggested by the association with a major histocompatability complex (MHC) class II phenotype DR2, DQw1.[6-8] Although nonspecific immunosuppression can alter the course of severe progressive MS,[9] such therapies are associated with toxic side effects preventing their use in early disease.

Innoculation of attenuated T cell clones recognizing the inciting autoantigen can specifically prevent the induction of experimental autoimmune disease models including experimental autoimmune encephalomyelitis (EAE)[10] and adjuvant arthritis.[11] It has been shown that the mechanism for this protection involves both anti-activated T cell responses[12] which are short-lived and anti-clonotypic responses[13,14] which are long-lived; thus the term T cell vaccination. A major goal in the understanding the treatment of autoimmune disease is to develop antigen-specific, nontoxic forms of immunotherapy. The eventual usage of this type of therapy in autoimmune disease requires the definition of immunodominant epitopes of potential autoantigens in conjunction with the definition of autoreactive T cell receptor usage and MHC restriction. To clarify the T cell fine specificity toward MBP, more than 15,000 short-term T cell lines were established from MS

[a] Address correspondence to: Dr. D. A. Hafler, Center for Neurologic Diseases, Brigham and Women's Hospital, 221 Longwood Ave., Boston, MA 02115.

patients, subjects with other neurologic diseases, and normal controls. We have found a higher frequency of T cells reactive with a DR2-associated region of MBP between residues 84 and 102 in patients with MS, as compared to controls.[15] A second region identified between residues 143 and 168 was recognized equally in MS patients and controls, and was associated with a DRw11 phenotype.[15] The T cell receptor usage for recognition of these immunodominant MBP regions was restricted, particularly among T cells isolated from the same individual.[16] These results suggest the potential utility of antigen-specific immunomodulation in the treatment of MS.

MATERIALS AND METHODS

Patients

Twenty-three early MS patients of definite, relapsing-remitting type were examined. Randomly selected 10 subjects with other neurological diseases who have CNS damage and 6 normal subjects, age- and sex-matched to the MS patients, were also included in the study (TABLE 1).

Antigen-Specific Clones

MBP reactive lines were established from peripheral blood mononuclear cells (MNC) by the method previously published.[15] In brief, for each patient, 288 wells were plated with 2×10^5 blood MNC in 96-well, round-bottom plates. MNC were cultured with MBP (10 μg/ml) in media consisting of RPMI 1640, 10% pooled human serum, 1% hepes buffer, 1% penicillin/streptomycin and 2% glutamine for 13 days. On day 3 and then every 3–4 days, 5% IL-2 (ABI, Columbia, MD) and 2 U/ml of rIL-4 (Genezyme, Boston, MA) were added to the culture. As IL-4 increases the growth rate of T cell clones,[17] between 2.5 and 5.0×10^5 T line cells were generated from every well. On day 13, an aliquot of each T cell line was analyzed for reactivity to MBP by placing 10,000 cells from each T cell line with the same number of MBP-pulsed or nonpulsed irradiated autologous MNC as antigen presenting cells (APC) in duplicate for 72 hrs. Cell proliferation was measured by incorporation of ^{3}H-thymidine pulsed during the last 18 hrs of culture (0.65 μCi/well). Lines positive for proliferation to MBP were retested 72 hrs later for reactivity to 13 different peptides encompassing the human MBP sequence. MBP was extracted from human brain tissue and purified on a CM-52 column.[18] MBP peptides were synthesized by Biosearch Lab Inc, (San Rafael, CA) using the solid phase method and were purified by high pressure liquid chromatography. MBP peptide sequences are as follows (single letter code for amino acid):

```
  1–20:ASQKRPSQRHGSKYLATAST
 11–30:GSKYLATASTMDHARHGFLP
 21–40:MDHARHGFLPRHRDTGILDS
 31–50:RHRDTGILDSIGRFFGGDRG
 41–60:IGRFFGGDRGAPKRGSGKDS
 51–70:APKRGSGKDSHHPARTAHYG
 61–82:HHPARTAHYGSLPQKSHGRT
 71–92:SLPQKSHGRTQDENPVVHFF
 84–102:DENPVVHFFKNIVTPRTPP
```

TABLE 1. Subject Characteristics and Frequency Analysis of MBP- and PLP-Reactive Lines[a]

	Age	Sex (%) (M/F)	MHC (%)				# Ag-Reactive Lines/Total # Lines		Mean Frequency of Ag-Reactive Lines (%)	
			DR2	DR4	DRw11	DQw1	MBP	PLP	MBP	PLP
Multiple sclerosis ($n = 23$)	34.2 ± 1.4	35/65	60.9	26.1	13.0	78.2	554/7746	20/432	7.18 ± 2.38	3.34 ± 1.56
Other neurologic disease ($n = 10$)	38.7 ± 3.2	43/57	14.3	0.0	42.9	85.7	118/2880	3/384	4.10 ± 1.04	0.90 ± 0.62
Normal ($n = 6$)	30.3 ± 1.5	50/50	16.7	0.0	50.0	66.6	73/1742	ND	4.70 ± 1.58	ND
DR2+ controls ($n = 6$)	32.0 ± 2.9	50/50	100	16.7	0.0	100	53/1728	ND	3.08 ± 2.06	ND

[a] Patients with MS were caucasian and had well characterized early relapsing remitting disease with minimal disability with at least two exacerbations within the previous 24 months and positive lesions on magnetic resonance imaging at the time of blood drawing. The total number of lines reactive with either MBP or PLP and the total number of T cell lines generated are shown. In addition, the frequencies of MBP- and PLP-reactive lines were calculated separately for each subject by dividing the number of MBP reactive lines by the total number of lines generated and the mean value ± SEM are given. ND, not determined. (From Ota *et al*.[15] Reprinted by permission from *Nature*.)

93–112:KNIVTPRTPPPSQGKGRGLS
113–132:LSRFSWGAEGQRPGFGYGGR
124–142:RPGFGYGGRASDYKSAHKG
143–168:FKGVDAQGTLSKIFKLGGRD

In pilot experiments, it was found that plating 2×10^5 mononuclear cells per well gave frequencies of between 1 and 20% MBP reactive lines. Thus, according to Poisson probability distribution, most MBP reactive T cell lines represent a single MBP reactive T cell.[15] As 2×10^5 MNC were plated for each of 288 wells per subject, the actual frequency of MBP reactive T cells in total MNC in the blood can be calculated by dividing the percentage (ratio) of MBP reactive wells by 2×10^5. The frequency of specific MBP peptide-reactive T cells was calculated by multiplying the frequency of MBP reactive T cells for each subject by the proportion of lines reactive with each peptide on the second analysis for that same subject. Specifically,

the frequency of circulating T cells reactive with synthetic peptide
$$= \text{frequency of MBP reactive T cells}$$
$$\times \frac{\text{\# T cell lines reactive with synthetic peptide)}}{\text{(total \# MBP reactive lines on 2nd analysis)}}$$

In a subgroup of patients, the frequency of T cells recognizing proteolipid apoprotein (PLP), another major encephalitogenic CNS myelin antigen,[19,20] was investigated preliminarily.

T Cell Receptor Determination

Cells were stimulated twice with MBP and then tested for their peptide specificity by use of a panel of thirteen overlapping synthetic MBP peptides, as described above. Following a third stimulation with the specific MBP peptide, RNA was extracted from cell culture pellets (20,000 to 50,000 cells) by extraction with guanidium-isothiocyanate/phenol-chloroform and isopropanol precipitation in the presence of carrier tRNA. Single-stranded complementary DNAs (cDNAs) were synthesized using oligo-dT and AMV-reverse transcriptase. Polymerase chain reaction (PCR) amplification was done, as previously reported,[16] with a panel of 19 oligonucleotides corresponding to the CDR2 region of the TCR β chain and a C_β primer.[21-25] The sequences of the primers were as follows:

$V_\beta 1$ 5' AAGAGAGAGCAAAAGGAAACATTCTTGAAC 3'
$V_\beta 2$ 5' GCTCCAAGGCCACATACGAGCAAGGCGTCG 3'
$V_\beta 3$ 5' AAAATGAAAGAAAAAGGAGATATTCCTGAG 3'
$V_\beta 4$ 5' CTGAGGCCACATATGAGAGTGGATTTGTCA 3'
$V_\beta 5$ 5' CAGAGAAACAAAGGAAACTTCCCTGGTCGA 3'
$V_\beta 6$ 5' GGGTGCGGCAGATGACTCAGGGCTGCCCAA 3'
$V_\beta 7$ 5' ATAAATGAAAGTGTGCCAAGTCGCTTCTCA 3'
$V_\beta 8$ 5' AACGTTCCGATAGATGATTCAGGGATGCCC 3'
$V_\beta 9$ 5' CATTATAAATGAAACAGTTCCAAATCGCTT 3'
$V_\beta 10$ 5' CTTATTCAGAAAGCAGAAATAATCAATGAG 3'
$V_\beta 11$ 5' TCCACAGAGAAGGGAGATCTTTCCTCTGAG 3'
$V_\beta 12$ 5' GATACTGACAAAGGAGAAGTCTCAGATGGC 3'

$V_\beta14$ 5' GTGACTGATAAGGGAGATGTTCCTGAAGGG 3'
$V_\beta15$ 5' GATATAAACAAAGGAGAGATCTCTGATGGA 3'
$V_\beta16$ 5' CATGATAATCTTTATCGACGTGTTATGGGA 3'
$V_\beta17$ 5' TTTCAGAAAGGAGATATAGCTGAAGGGTAC 3'
$V_\beta18$ 5' GATGAGTCAGGAATGCCAAAGGAACGATTT 3'
$V_\beta19$ 5' CAAGAAACGGAGATGCACAAGAAGCGATTC 3'
$V_\beta20$ 5' ACCGACAGGCTGCAGGCAGGGGCCTCCAGC 3'
C_β 5' GGCAGACAGGACCCCTTGCTGGTAGGACAC 3'
C-probe 5' TTCTGATGGCTCAAACACAGCGACCTCGGG 3'
$V_\beta17$-Leader 5' AGCAACCAGGTGCTCTGCAGTGTGGTCCTT 3'
$J_\beta2.1$ 5' CCCTGGCCCGAAGAACTGCTCATTGTAGGA 3'

Amplifications were done for thirty cycles (94°C 1 min., 55°C 2 min., 72°C 3 min.) with 1 μg of each primer in 50 μl reactions. Amplified products were separated in 1% agarose gels, transferred to nitrocellulose and hybridized with an internal oligonucleotide probe. Probes were endlabeled with $\gamma-^{32}$P ATP and T4 polynucleotide kinase to a specific activity of 10^8 cpm/μg and hybridized. Blots were washed at a final stringency of $6 \times$ SSC/70°C and autoradiographed for 2 to 18 hours. Particular care was taken to prevent contamination of samples. Amplified and nonamplified samples were handled separately, reagents were aliquoted and tested for the presence of amplified material and negative controls were included for different experimental steps, *i.e.*, RNA isolation, cDNA synthesis and PCR amplification.

The validity of this approach was examined by the following experiments. First, all primers except for $V_\beta20$ were confirmed to be able to amplify cDNA from peripheral blood T cells. Second, the specificity of PCR amplification was tested by analysis of V_β gene usage in 69 independent T cell clones previously established from a normal subject and an MS patient[26] by single cell cloning with a combination of phytohemagglutinin (PHA) and interleukin-2.[27] Because of the high cloning efficiencies, these clones provide a representative pattern of V_β gene usage by peripheral blood T cells. TCR V_β gene usage could be determined for 65 of 69 (94.2%) of these T cell clones, indicating that a large proportion of the TCR V_β repertoire was recognized by our V_β primers.[16] Eighty-four percent of these clones were positive for a single V_β, while 7 clones (10.1%) were double-positive.[10] The double positivity could be due to the presence of two rearranged and expressed TCR genes or to the presence of two cell populations in the sample. Therefore, T cell lines found to be positive for more than two V_β segments were excluded from analysis because they were not considered to be derived from a single MBP- or MBP peptide-reactive T cell.

T Cell Receptor Sequencing

For sequencing, amplification was performed, as described elsewhere,[16] with a $V_\beta17$ primer specific for the leader segment containing an internal Pst I restriction site. Amplified DNA was treated with proteinase K, phenol/chloroform extracted, ethanol precipitated, and digested with restriction endonucleases Bgl II and Pst I. Gel-purified DNA was ligated into M13 mp19 and single stranded DNA sequenced by the dideoxy method. Negative controls were included during the procedure to test for possible contamination of RNA samples or reagents used for cDNA synthesis and amplification.

RESULTS

Recognition of Immunodominant Regions of MBP and Association with Class II MHC

A total of 15,824 short-term T cell lines were generated. As shown in TABLE 1,[15] the frequency of MBP reactive cells as well as PLP reactive cells was slightly higher in subjects with MS when compared with the other subjects. However, this was not statistically different. Of a total of 302 lines from patients with MS that could be expanded and confirmed to react with MBP on repeated analysis, 140 (46.4%) reacted with MBP residues 84–102. By contrast, only 11 of a total of 100 MBP-reactive T cell lines (11.0%) derived from control subjects recognized this region of MBP.[15] The actual frequency of T cells reactive with a panel of overlapping MBP peptides was determined for individual subjects, and the mean frequencies for all peptide-reactive T cells evaluated among 23 patients with MS and 16 control subjects are shown in FIGURE 1.[15] The results for peptide-specific T cells from normal subjects and other neurologic disease controls were virtually identical and thus combined for analysis. The mean frequency of peptide 84–102-reactive T cells from subjects with MS was higher than that of controls, while both MS and control subjects showed equally high frequencies of T cells reactive with MBP residues 143–168.[15]

The DR2,DQw1 phenotype was very infrequent in the control subjects and more common in patients with MS (TABLE 1), which was in accordance with previous reports.[6–8] A significant association was observed between the DR2 phenotype and the proportion or the frequency of T cells reactive to MBP residues 84–102 (FIG. 2).[15] To determine whether T cell reactivity to MBP residues 84–102 was associated with DR2,DQw1 expression in non-MS subjects, an additional 6 normal subjects with this MHC phenotype were investigated. A DR2 expression was also associated with the proportion of peptide 84–102 reactive T cell lines among the total MBP reactive lines generated from DR2,DQw1 controls (DR2[+] controls, 31.0 ± 10.8% vs. DR2[−], 10.1 ± 0.4%).[15] However, the actual frequency of T cells reactive with this region of MBP in DR2[+] controls was less than that in DR2[+] MS patients (FIG. 2). Though DQw1 is known to be in linkage disequilibrium with DR2, no particular peptide reactivity was associated with DQw1 pheno-

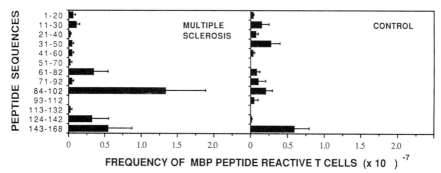

FIGURE 1. Mean frequency of peripheral blood T cells recognizing overlapping synthetic peptides of human MBP in 23 MS patients and 16 randomly selected controls. Sixteen controls consist of 10 subjects with other neurological diseases of the central nervous system and 6 normal controls. (From Ota *et al.*[15] Reprinted by permission from *Nature.*)

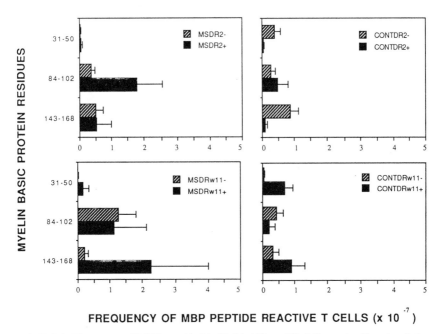

FIGURE 2. Frequency of MBP peptide 31–50, 84–102, or 143–168 reactive lines in relation to class II MHC expression in patients with MS and in controls. Six more DR2-positive normal controls were studied in addition to the original 16 control subjects, and compared with the 23 MS patients. Subjects with the DR2 phenotype had a higher proportion ($p = 0.003$) and frequency ($p = 0.045$) of T cells reactive to MBP residues 84–102. Subjects with the DRw11 phenotype had a higher frequency ($p = 0.006$) of T cells recognizing MBP 143–168 (unpaired t test). (From Ota *et al.*[15] Reprinted by permission from *Nature*.)

type expression. In contrast to the predominance of DR2 phenotype expression in MS, the DRw11 phenotype was more common in controls than in subjects with MS (TABLE 1), and DRw11 expression was positively associated with the frequency of T cells reactive to MBP residues 142–168 both in patients with MS and controls (FIG. 2).[15] Reactivity to MBP residues 31–50, which was predominantly observed in control subjects, was also associated with DRw11.[15] Other MHC associations with the recognition of a particular region of MBP were not found in this analysis.

Fine MHC Restriction for Recognition of DR2-Associated Immunodominant MBP (84–102)

To further investigate the MHC restriction of the T cell lines reactive with the immunodominant MBP epitopes, monoclonal antibody (mAb) blocking studies for five T cell lines reactive with MBP residues 84–102 were performed (TABLE 2).[15] Among clones blocked by anti-DR mAb (TABLE 2b), clone 2E11 proliferated in response to MBP residues 84–102 with the panel of DR2+ antigen-presenting cells (APC) while 2C9 and 2H9 proliferated only with autologous APC (TABLE 2a). The recognition of peptide 84–102 by clones 1A8 and 3A10, which were

TABLE 2a. MHC Restriction of MBP 84–102-Reactive T Cell Lines[a]

^{3}H Thymidine Incorporation (ΔCPM) of T Cell Lines

MHC Phenotype of APC		Hy.1A8			Hy.2C9			Hy.2E11			Hy.2H9			Hy.3A10		
DR	DQw	APC	MBP	Peptide 84–102	APC	MBP	Peptide 84–102	APC	MBP	Peptide 84–102	APC	MBP	Peptide 84–102	APC	MBP	Peptide 84–102
2,7	1,3	32	21,192	10,747	83	3,263	14,991	148	18,593	30,368	169	2,797	10,444	139	6,887	24,411
2	1	83	56	32	82	78	112	217	52,939	49,399	636	327	658	23	28	26
4,7	2,3	32	26	53	45	55	142	37	167	81	226	258	263	306	719	915
3	2	46	32	52	43	44	110	101	98	349	769	402	1,973	23	31	100
3,10	1,2	35	30,737	49,144	158	25	80	36	58	42	49	54	46	42	22,823	31,121
2,7	1,2	38	40	47	43	39	43	78	53,441	32,357	261	190	289	33	19	36
7,w11	2,7	44	39	54	57	124	259	34	25	33	51	58	97	967	1,214	2,744

[a] Five T cell lines reactive to MBP residues 84–102 from subject Hy were expanded by repeated cycles of stimulation with autologous irradiated MNC pulsed with synthetic MBP peptide 84–102 and examined for recognition of this region of MBP and human MBP. The average counts per minute (CPM) values for triplicate wells are shown. DR and DQw haplotypes are given and haplotypes common with the patient (top line), who was DR2, DR7, DQw1, DQw3, are underlined. (From Ota et al.[15] Reprinted by permission from Nature.)

partially blocked by anti-DQ mAbs, was restricted to APC from the responder and one of two APC donor subjects expressing DQw1. These results suggest that in patient Hy both DR and DQ molecules are restricting elements for recognition of this MBP peptide 84–102.

T Cell Receptor Gene Usage in Immunodominant MBP Peptide-Reactive T Cell Clones

TCR V_β gene usage was defined in MBP peptide 84–102-reactive T cell lines established from five patients with MS.[16] Thirty-one MBP-reactive T cell lines from patient Hy were specific for the MBP residues 84–102, of which the $V_\beta 17$ segment was used in 24 (77.4%) T cell lines, other cell lines using either $V_\beta 4$, $V_\beta 7$

TABLE 2b. Blocking Studies for Line Cell Proliferation by Monoclonal Antibodies with Different Specificities for Class II MHC[a]

	[3]H Thymidine Incorporation (ΔCPM) of T Cell Lines				
Monoclonal Abs	Hy.1A8	Hy.2C9	Hy.2E11	Hy.2H9	Hy.3A10
mAb specificity					
APC alone	32	83	39	50	139
none	10,747	14,991	3,325	8,659	24,411
Control mAb	11,375	15,322	4,131	8,156	27,363
Anti-DR					
PL8	11,051	41	31	142	25,016
L243	16,792	586	22	36	21,148
6SP4.1	19,119	405	46	92	26,412
Anti-DQ					
1A3	4,851	11,444	2,102	5,446	15,714
Tu22	1,189	13,442	1,073	7,661	13,488
Leu10	1,128	14,924	2,255	7,678	13,090
Anti-DP					
B7121	7,917	15,922	2,337	6,689	23,452
Anti-DR+DP					
Tu35	13,606	75	21	42	27,104

[a] The panels of five T cell lines reactive with MBP residues 84–102 were plated with autologous APC MNC, as above, in the presence of mAbs (final concentration of 1:100) recognizing different MHC class II gene products. The nomenclature of the antibodies from the Tenth International Histocompatibility Workshop with their specificity are given. (From Ota *et al.*[15] Reprinted by permission from *Nature*.)

or $V_\beta 14$ (patient 1, TABLE 3a). $V_\beta 17$ usage was also found in T cell lines from all of the four remaining patients examined (patients 2–5, TABLE 3a). $V_\beta 12$ was another element used frequently especially among patients 3–5, and this segment is homologous to the mouse $V_\beta 8.2$[28] which is predominantly used among encephalitogenic T cells in mice and rats.[29–32] To determine if there is a restricted usage of TCR genes for recognizing MBP residues 84–102 in healthy subjects, T cell lines reactive with this peptide were examined in five healthy individuals (control 1–5, TABLE 3a). All five cell lines from DR2$^+$ subject Rt were $V_\beta 17^+$. $V_\beta 17$, $V_\beta 6$, $V_\beta 8$, and $V_\beta 12$ were frequently used among MBP 84–102-reactive T cell lines from other healthy subjects. Thus, for each individual, a restricted set of TCR V_β genes appears to be involved in the recognition of the immunodominant MBP 84–102 region. In addition, we had an opportunity to compare TCR V_β usage between

TABLE 3a. MBP Residues 84–102-Reactive Lines from MS and Controls[a]

Cell Line	TCR V_β	Cell Line	TCR V_β	Cell Line	TCR V_β
Multiple sclerosis					
Patient 1 (DR2, DR7)		Patient 1 (cont.)		Patient 3 (DR2, DRw11)	
Hy.1B12	$V_\beta17$	Hy.2C12	$V_\beta17,V_\beta1$	Cy.2C2	$V_\beta12$
Hy.1G9	$V_\beta17$	Hy.2E2	$V_\beta17,V_\beta1$	Cy.3F6	$V_\beta12$
Hy.1H7	$V_\beta17$	Hy.2E11	$V_\beta17,V_\beta2$	Cy.4C1	$V_\beta12$
Hy.2C9	$V_\beta17$	Hy.3A11	$V_\beta17,V_\beta2$	Cy.2G5	$V_\beta17$
Hy.2E4	$V_\beta17$	Hy.2C8	$V_\beta17,V_\beta11$	Cy.2H11	$V_\beta1,V_\beta7$
Hy.2E6	$V_\beta17$	Hy.3A8	$V_\beta17,V_\beta11$	Cy.3D2	$V_\beta1,V_\beta7$
Hy.2F10	$V_\beta17$	Hy.3C3	$V_\beta4$	Cy.2C6	$V_\beta2$
Hy.2G5	$V_\beta17$	Hy.3C6	$V_\beta4$	Patient 4(DR2, DR4)	
Hy.2G11	$V_\beta17$	Hy.3B7	$V_\beta4$	Ns.1G11	$V_\beta12,V_\beta17$
Hy.2H9	$V_\beta17$	Hy.2F11	$V_\beta7$	Ns.2E2	$V_\beta12,V_\beta17$
Hy.3A10	$V_\beta17$	Hy.3B12	$V_\beta7$	Ns.2A5	$V_\beta1$
Hy.3B9	$V_\beta17$	Hy.1H3	$V_\beta14$	Ns.2C10	$V_\beta3,V_\beta14$
Hy.3C7	$V_\beta17$	Hy.2B2	$V_\beta14$	Ns.2D11	$V_\beta5,V_\beta7$
Hy.3G10	$V_\beta17$	Patient 2 (DR2, DR7)		Patient 5 (DR3, Dr4)	
Hy.3F6	$V_\beta17$	Fn.1G6	$V_\beta17$	Tw.B11	$V_\beta12$
Hy.3F7	$V_\beta17$	Fn.1M7	$V_\beta4$	Tw.2F3	$V_\beta12,V_\beta17$
Hy.3F10	$V_\beta17$	Fn.3E17	$V_\beta3,V_\beta5$	Tw.E10	$V_\beta17$
Hy.1A8	$V_\beta17$	Fn.1E6	$V_\beta6,V_\beta8$	Tw.2E2	$V_\beta14$
Controls					
Control 1 (DR2)		Control 2 (Dr2)		Control 4 (DR7, DRw11)	
Rt.1A9	$V_\beta17$	Hr.1B7	$V_\beta12$	An.3E1	$V_\beta8,V_\beta1$
Rt.3C1	$V_\beta17$	Hr.1C9	$V_\beta5$	An.3H3	$V_\beta8$
Rt.3G11	$V_\beta17$	Control 3 (Dr2)		An.3C12	$V_\beta2$
Rt.3A3	$V_\beta17,V_\beta14$	Md.2A4	$V_\beta8,V_\beta6$	Control 5 (Dr1, DR9)	
Rt.3F1	$V_\beta17,V_\beta14$	Md.2F1	$V_\beta8,V_\beta18$	Cr.1B12	$V_\beta17,V_\beta12$

[a] V_β gene usage was determined by PCR amplification of cDNAs derived from MBP-reactive cell lines and Southern blotting. PCR primers covered all published V_β families ($V_\beta1$–20). (From Wucherpfennig *et al.*[16] Reprinted with some modification by permission from *Science*.)

TABLE 3b. Patient Cy Lines Reactive with MBP Residues 143–168

Cell Line	TCR V_β
Patient 3 (DR2, DRw11)	
Cy.1E6	$V_\beta14$
Cy.2B12	$V_\beta14$
Cy.2E2	$V_\beta14$
Cy.3G10	$V_\beta14$
Cy.3H10	$V_\beta14,V_\beta8$
Cy.4C10	$V_\beta14,V_\beta17$
Cy.1C12	$V_\beta12$
Cy.1E9	$V_\beta7$
Cy.3F9	$V_\beta1$

T cell lines reactive with DR2-associated MBP residues 84–102[15] and those specific for DRw11-associated MBP residues 143–168[15] in patient Cy expressing both of these antigens. Six of nine (66.7%) T cell lines recognizing MBP peptide 143–168 used $V_\beta14$ (TABLE 3b), whereas 4 of the seven (57.1%) MBP 84–102-reactive lines used $V_\beta12$ or $V_\beta17$ (TABLE 3a).[16]

To prove the single TCR V_β gene was used for recognition of specific MBP peptide by the line cells established after three cycles of antigen stimulation, two $V_\beta 17^+$ MBP 84–102-reactive T cell lines (Hy.2H9 and Hy.2G5) were cloned by limiting dilution. All 11 individual clones derived from these two cell lines, which were still reactive with both MBP and MBP residues 84–102, were found to be $V_\beta 17^+$.[16] Three of these clones were further analyzed with the complete panel of V_β primers and were all confirmed to be negative for the other V_β segments.

Sequence of $V_\beta 17$ Segment Used by MBP 84–102-Reactive T Cell Clones

T cell receptor $V_\beta 17^+$ PCR products were cloned and sequenced by the dideoxy method from both MS (Hy, Fn and Ns) and control (Rt and Cr) subjects (TABLE 4).[16] The V_β sequences of all 10 lines were homologous to the published $V_\beta 17.1$ sequency[25] except for some nucleotide substitutions at the VD junction observed in four lines, confirming that specific V_β segments were amplified using this approach. Analysis of the V_β junctional sequence indicated that all six T cell lines generated from patient Hy and one line from subject Rt used the $J_\beta 2.1$ segment while three T cell lines from subjects Fn, Ns and Cr used different J_β segments. To further determine how frequently the $J_\beta 2.1$ gene segment was used by other $V_\beta 17^+$ T cells, cDNAs from twenty MBP 84–102-reactive cell lines of patient Hy were amplified using the $V_\beta 17$ primer in combination with a C_β primer or a $J_\beta 2.1$ primer. All of these lines were positive for $V_\beta 17$ as well as $J_\beta 2.1$ gene segments, whereas the negative controls (RNA extracted from all cell lines and not converted to cDNA, and reagents used for cDNA synthesis and amplification) were negative by PCR and Southern blotting. This indicates that $V_\beta 17$-$J_\beta 2.1$ are the major TCR elements used for recognition of MBP residues 84–102 in patient Hy. Comparison of the VDJ sequences of the six T cell lines from subject Hy demonstrated that the line cells used only two types of V_β sequences, though each line was originally derived from separate cultures. These shared sequences could be due to selection of particular TCR structures by stimulation with MBP residues 84–102 *in vitro* or due to oligoclonal expansion of MBP-reactive T cells following *in vivo* antigen exposure.

DISCUSSION

The goal for treatment of autoimmune diseases is to develop antigen-specific immunotherapy that will alter the disease course. This will likely require a basic understanding of T cell receptor and MHC usage in recognition of peptide autoantigens postulated to be involved with inciting the disease. In the present study, we demonstrate that there are MHC-associated immunodominant regions of autoantigen myelin basic protein in humans associated with a restricted T cell recognition of these immunodominant MBP epitopes among T cell clones isolated from each patient.

In EAE, a single immunodominant region of MBP which is presumably influenced by class II MHC has been observed in different mouse and rat strains,[33-36] and these immunodominant peptides are the major encephalitigen if the animal

TABLE 4. Sequence Analysis of TCR V_β Chains of MBP 84–102-Reactive T Cell Lines[a]

	V_β	D_β	J_β	
MS Patients				
Hy.1A8	TyrLeuCysAlaSerSer tatctctgtgccagtagt	ThrAspTrpSer actgactggagc	SerTyrAsnGluGlnPhe tcctacaatgagcagttc	V_β17.1–J_β2.1
Hy.2C9	TyrLeuCysAlaSerSer tatctctgtgccagtagt	ThrAspTrpSer actgactggagc	SerTyrAsnGluGlnPhe tcctacaatgagcagttc	V_β17.1–J_β2.1
Hy.3A10	TyrLeuCysAlaSerSer tatctctgtgccagtagt	ThrAspTrpSer actgactggagc	SerTyrAsnGluGlnPhe tcctacaatgagcagttc	V_β17.1–J_β2.1
Hy.2C8	TyrLeuCysAlaSerArg tatctctgtgccagtagg	ThrSerGly actagcggc	SerTyrAsnGluGlnPhe tcctacaacgagcagttc	V_β17.1–J_β2.1
Hy.2H9	TyrLeuCysAlaSerArg tatctctgtgccagtagg	ThrSerGly actagcggc	SerTyrAsnGluGlnPhe tcctacaacgagcagttc	V_β17.1–J_β2.1
Hy.2G5	TyrLeuCysAlaSerArg tatctctgtgccagtagg	ThrSerGly actagcggc	SerTyrAsnGluGlnPhe tcctacaacgagcagttc	V_β17.1–J_β2.1
Fn.1G6	TyrLeuCysAlaSerSer tatctctgtgccagtagt	IleProPro atccctcca	SerTyrGluGlnTyrPhe tcctacgagcagtacttc	V_β17.1–J_β2.7
Ns.1G11	TyrLeuCysAlaSerSer tatctctgtgccagtagt	AlaAspArg gcggacagg	AspGlnProGlnHisPhe gatcagccccagcatttt	V_β17.1–J_β1.5
Controls				
Rt.1A9	TyrLeuCysAlaSerSer tatctctgtgccagtagt	ThrGlyGlyGlyLeuAsp acgggtcaggggttggat	GluGlnPhe gagcagttc	V_β17.1–J_β2.1
Cr.1B12	TyrLeuCysAlaSerGly tatctctgtgccagtggg	AspAsnGlyGlyGlu gacaatggtggggag	GlnTyrPheGlyProGly cagtacttcgggccgggc	V_β17.1–J_β2.5

[a] Complementary DNAs were amplified with PCR primers for the V_β17-leader segment and the TCR C_β region. Amplified DNA was cloned into M13 and sequenced by the dideoxy method (three M13 plaques/T cell line). All T cell lines use the V_β17.1 gene segment and the sequences are homologous to the published sequence.[25] All TCR V_β chains were found to have an inframe rearrangement. Shared TCR sequences are *underlined*. (From Wucherpfennig et al.[16] Reprinted by permission from *Science*.)

strain is susceptible to EAE. H-2^u mice such as PL/J and B10.PL show selective reactivity to N-terminal MBP peptide 1–9,[29,30,33] while H-2^s mice SJL/J show predominant reactivity to MBP residues 89–101.[34] These strains of mice develop EAE when they are immunized with immunodominant peptides. The majority of T cells recognizing MBP residues 1–9 in H-2^u mice show limited usage of TCR genes, that is V$_\beta$8.2 in combination with V$_\alpha$2 or V$_\alpha$4.[29,30] Lewis rats have also been found to selectively use TCR segments homologous to the mouse V$_\beta$8.2 and V$_\alpha$2 genes for recognition of immunodominant MBP region 68–88.[31,32] Administration of monoclonal antibody against the commonly used TCR gene V$_\beta$8 is effective in prevention or reversal of mice EAE,[29,30] and immunization with V$_\beta$8-specific synthetic peptide protects Lewis rats against EAE.[37,38] Another type of immune intervention that can prevent the development of EAE is T cell vaccination, in which attenuated MBP-reactive T cell clones are innoculated to an animal before active challenge with MBP.[10] It has been shown that the mechanism for this protection involves both anti-activated T cell responses[12] and anti-clonotypic T cell responses.[13,14]

In MS, genetic studies have shown a linkage of disease susceptibility to MHC DR2 allele[6,8] as well as the T cell receptor V$_\beta$ locus.[39] In the present study, we have demonstrated that DR2 phenotype expression is associated with immunodominant regions of the autoantigen myelin basic protein recognized by T cells using limited T cell receptor V$_\beta$ gene.[15,16] Shared TCR V$_\beta$ gene usage is observed among both MS and control subjects, and this finding was most prominent among T cell clones derived from an individual MS patient.[16] It is noteworthy that in EAE experimental animals may not have to be immunized with MBP in determining the relationship between immunodominant regions of MBP and class II MHC because unprimed Lewis rat lymph node cells selectively react with immunodominant MBP residues 48–88 and the T cell clones established are encephalitogenic.[40] Therefore, our findings in humans defining immunodominant region of MBP 84–102 that is linked to MS-associated DR2 phenotype may be analogous to those defined in the encephalitogenic T cells in EAE.

To demonstrate that MS is a cell-mediated autoimmune disease analogous to EAE, a number of criteria can be proposed including: 1. an association between an immunodominant region of the presumed autoantigen- and disease-associated class II MHC haplotypes; 2. an increase in frequency of T cells that react with this immunodominant epitope; and 3. alteration of the disease course by elimination of autoreactive T cells or by inducing tolerance to the autoantigen identified in the first two criteria. The last criterion implies that *in vitro* experiments cannot prove the association of an autoantigen with a disease but that instead such clinical trials of antigen-specific immunotherapy will be required. In this regard, determination of T cell receptor V-gene usage for individual patients may provide a specific target for therapeutic intervention, as has been shown in EAE.[29–32] A potential obstacle to designing TCR V segment-based therapies is the genetic heterogeneity of individuals, in particular at the MHC locus. This type of approach, however, may be of therapeutic value, since DR2-positive MS population corresponding to the majority of MS patients[8] share some degree of antigen reactivity and TCR V$_\beta$ gene usage.

There is strong evidence for T-cell regulation of the immune responses. The presence of T cells reactive with MBP residues 84–102 in DR2$^+$ normal subjects (FIG. 2) suggests that if those T cells possess pathogenic role in MS, other immune mechanisms must exist to prevent the activation of circulating autoreactive T cells. Indeed, although MBP-reactive T cells could be generated by *in vitro* culture from controls to about the same degree as patients with MS (TABLE 1), recent work indicates that MBP-reactive T cells are *in vivo* activated in patients with MS.[5] While altered immunoregulation such as decreased levels in antigennonspecific suppressor mechanisms[41,42] and autologous mixed lymphocyte reaction[43] exists in MS, it may be possible to effectively treat the disease by selectively modulating the immune response to an autoantigen. In this regard, experimental evidence in EAE[10] and adjuvant arthritis[11] has indicated that T cell vaccination can generate an immune response that is capable of further downregulating the generation of new autoreactive T cells sharing the same antigen specificity.[44] This type of clinical trial may be possible by defining the target autoantigen(s) in MS and then isolating autologous autoantigen-reactive T cell lines. In addition, antigen-driven peripheral tolerance following oral administration of autoantigens has been found to be effective in preventing the experimental autoimmune diseases such as EAE with myelin antigens,[45,46] experimental autoimmune uveoretinitis with S antigen,[47] and adjuvant arthritis with type II collagen.[48]

REFERENCES

1. McFarlin, D. E. & H. F. McFarland. 1981. N. Engl. J. Med. **307:** 1193–1197, 1246–1251.
2. Hafler, D. A. & H. L. Weiner. 1989. Immunol. Today **10:** 104–107.
3. Paterson, P. Y. 1977. Autoimmune neurological disease: experimental animal systems and implications for multiple sclerosis. *In* Autoimmunity: Genetic, Immunologic, Virologic, and Clinical Aspects. N. Talal, Ed. 1st edit.: 643–692. Academic Press. New York, NY.
4. Hafler, D. A., D. S. Benjamin, J. Burks & H. L. Weiner. 1987. J. Immunol. **139:** 68–72.
5. Allegretta, M., J. A. Nicklas, S. Sriram & R. J. Albertini. 1990. Science **247:** 718–721.
6. Spielman, R. S. & N. Nathanson. 1982. Epidemiol. Rev. **4:** 45–65.
7. Francis, D. A., J. R. Batchelor, W. I. McDonald, J. E. C. Hern & A. W. Downie. 1986. Lancet **1:** 211.
8. Olerup, O., J. Hillert, S. Fredrikson, T. Olsson, S. Kam-Hansen, E. Moller, B. Carlsson & J. Wallin. 1989. Proc. Natl. Acad. Sci. USA **86:** 7113–7117.
9. Hauser, S. L., D. M. Dawson, J. R. Lehrich, M. Flint Beal, S. V. Kevy, R. D. Propper, J. A. Mills & H. L. Weiner. 1983. N. Engl. J. Med. **308:** 173–180.
10. Ben-Nun, A., H. Wekerle & I. R. Cohen. 1981. Nature **292:** 60–61.
11. Holoshitz, J., Y. Naparstek, A. Ben-Nun & I. R. Cohen. 1983. Science **219:** 56–58.
12. Lohse, A. W., F. Mor, N. Karin & I. R. Cohen. 1989. Science **244:** 820–822.
13. Lider, O., T. Reshef, E. Beraud, A. Ben-Nun & I. R. Cohen. 1988. Science **239:** 181–183.
14. Sun, D., Y. Qin, J. Chluba, J. T. Epplen & H. Wekerle. 1988. Nature **332:** 843–845.
15. Ota, K., M. Matsui, E. L. Milford, G. A. Mackin, H. L. Weiner & D. A. Hafler. 1990. Nature **346:** 183–187.
16. Wucherpfennig, K. W., K. Ota, N. Endo, J. G. Seidman, A. Rosenzweig, H. L. Weiner & D. A. Hafler. 1990. Science **248:** 1016–1019.
17. Brod, S. A., M. Purvee, D. Benjamin & D. A. Hafler. 1990. Cell. Immunol. **125:** 426–436.
18. Chou, F. C.-H., C.-H. Jen Chou, R. Shapira & R. F. Kibler. 1976. J. Biol. Chem. **251:** 2671–2679.
19. Waksman, B. H., H. Porter, M. D. Lees, R. D. Adams & J. Folch. 1954. J. Exp. Med. **100:** 451–471.
20. Yoshimura, T., T. Kunishita, K. Sakai, M. Endoh, T. Namikawa & T. Tabira. 1985. J. Neurol. Sci. **69:** 47–58.

21. TILLINGHAST, J. P., M. A BEHLKE & D. Y. LOH. 1986. Science **233**: 879–883.
22. KIMURA, N., B. TOYONAGA, Y. YOSHIKAI, F. TRIEBEL, P. DEBRE, M. D. MINDEN & T. W. MAK. 1986. J. Exp. Med. **164**: 739–750.
23. TOYONAGA, B., Y. YOSHIKAI, V. VADASZ, B. CHIN & T. W. MAK. 1985. Proc. Natl. Acad. Sci. USA **82**: 8624–8628.
24. CONCANNON, P., L. A. PICKERING, P. KUNG & L. HOOD. 1986. Proc. Natl. Acad. Sci. USA **83**: 6598–6602.
25. KIMURA, N., B. TOYONAGA, Y. YOSHIKAI, R.-P. DU & T. W. MAK. 1987. Eur. J. Immunol. **17**: 375–383.
26. HAFLER, D. A., A. DUBY, S. J. LEE, D. BENJAMIN, J. G. SEIDMAN & H. L. WEINER. 1988. J. Exp. Med. **167**: 1313–1322.
27. MORETTA, A., G. PANTALEO, L. MORETTA, J.-C. CEROTTINI & M. C. MINGARI. 1983. J. Exp. Med. **157**: 743–754.
28. LAI, E., P. CONCANNON & L. HOOD. 1988. Nature **331**: 543–546.
29. ACHA-ORBEA, H., D. J. MITCHELL, L. TIMMERMANN, D. C. WRAITH, G. S. TAUSCH, M. K. WALDOR, S. S. ZAMVIL, H. O. McDEVITT & L. STEINMAN. 1988. Cell **54**: 263–273.
30. URBAN, J. L., V. KUMAR, D. H. KONO, C. GOMEZ, S. J. HORVATH, J. CLAYTON, D. G. ANDO, E. E. SERCARZ & L. HOOD. 1988. Cell **54**: 577–592.
31. BURNS, F. R., X. LI, N. SHEN, H. OFFNER, Y. K. CHOU, A. A. VANDENBARK & E. HEBER-KATZ. 1989. J. Exp. Med. **169**: 27–39.
32. CLUBA, J., C. STEEG, A. BECKER, H. WEKERLE & J. T. EPPLEN. 1989. Eur. J. Immunol. **19**: 279–284.
33. ZAMVIL, S. S., D. J. MITCHELL, A. C. MOORE, K. KITAMURA, L. STEINMAN & J. B. ROTHBARD. 1986. Nature **324**: 258–260.
34. SAKAI, K., S. S. ZAMVIL, D. J. MITCHELL, M. LIM, J. B. ROTHBARD & L. STEINMAN. 1988. J. Neuroimmunol. **19**: 21–32.
35. VANDENBARK, A. A., H. OFFNER, T. RESHEF, R. FRITZ, C.-H. JEN CHOU & I. R. COHEN. 1985. J. Immunol. **135**: 229–233.
36. OFFNER, H., G. A. HASHIM, B. CELNIK, A. GALANG, X. LI, F. R. BURNS, N. SHEN, E. HEBER-KATZ & A. A. VANDENBARK. 1989. J. Exp. Med. **170**: 355–367.
37. VANDENBARK, A. A., G. HASHIM & H. OFFNER. 1989. Nature **341**: 541–544.
38. HOWELL, M. D., S. T. WINTERS, T. OLEE, H. C. POWELL, D. J. CARLO & S. W. BROSTOFF. 1989. Science **246**: 668–670.
39. SEBOUN, E., M. A. ROBINSON, T. H. DOOLITTLE, T. A. CIULLA, T. J. KINDT & S. L. HAUSER. 1989. Cell **57**: 1095–1100.
40. SCHLUESENER, H. L. & H. WEKERLE. 1985. J. Immunol. **135**: 3128–3133.
41. ANTEL, J. P., B. G. W. ARNASON & M. E. MEDOF. 1979. Ann. Neurol. **5**: 338–342.
42. CHOFFLON, M., H. L. WEINER, C. MORIMOTO & D. A. HAFLER. 1988. Ann. Neurol. **24**: 185–191.
43. HAFLER, D. A., M. BUCHSBAUM & H. L. WEINER. 1985. J. Neuroimmunol. **9**: 339–347.
44. LIDER, O., M. SHINITZKY & I. R. COHEN. 1986. Ann. N.Y. Acad. Sci. **475**: 267–273.
45. HIGGINS, P. J. & H. L. WEINER. 1988. J. Immunol. **140**: 440–445.
46. LIDER, O., L. M. B. SANTOS, C. S. Y. LEE, P. J. HIGGINS & H. L. WEINER. J. Immunol. **142**: 748–752.
47. NUSSENBLATT, R. B., R. R. CASPI, R. MAHDI, C.-C. CHAN, F. ROBERGE, O. LIDER & H. L. WEINER. 1990. J. Immunol. **144**: 1689–1695.
48. ZHANG, Z. J., C. S. Y. LEE, O. LIDER & H. L. WEINER. 1990. J. Immunol. **145**: 2489–2493.

Autoregulation of the Immune Response in Autoimmune Disease and Cardiac Transplantation by Photoinactivated Autologous Lymphocytes

CAROLE L. BERGER,[a] RICHARD L. EDELSON,[d]
NILOO EDWARDS,[b] JUAN SANCHEZ,[b] LARRY COPPEY,[b]
XU HE,[b] CHARLES MARBOE,[c] AND ERIC ROSE[b]

[a]Department of Dermatology
[b]Department of Surgery
[c]Department of Pathology
Columbia University
630 W. 168th Street
New York, New York 10032
and
[d]Department of Dermatology
Yale University School of Medicine
500 LCI
P.O. Box 3333
New Haven, Connecticut 06510-8059

The results achieved in clinical trials of photochemotherapy have indicated that a host response occurs which specifically targets the effector T cells that mediate the dysfunctional immune response.[1] Cutaneous T cell lymphoma (CTCL) patients have both a leukemic and skin localized malignancy of inducer T cells.[1] Treatment of the peripheral blood of these patients results in resolution of skin lesions as well as a reduction in the circulating tumor burden.[1] Delayed type hypersensitivity responses to recall antigens are preserved in some patients.[1] The absence of infectious complications in the treated patients also indicates that other immunologically mediated responses remain intact. The results achieved in these patients exceed expectations based on the experience obtained in treatment of CTCL patients with discard leukapheresis.[2] These studies raise questions about the mechanistic basis for this form of therapy, including: 1. Can animal model systems be constructed to investigate photochemotherapy? 2. Does reinfusion of photoinactivated effector T cells result in autoregulation of immune responses? 3. Does the therapy target T cells? 4. Does the therapy result in specific inhibition of an immune response? 5. Can this approach be extended to other conditions mediated by inappropriate regulation of effector T cells such as autoimmune disease and transplantation? To address these issues, murine and primate model systems of autoimmune disease and tissue transplantation were investigated.

The murine model of systemic lupus erythematosus manifested in the MRL/l mouse system was chosen to study autoimmune disease. The MRL/l mouse model of systemic lupus erythematosus (SLE) provides an experimental system that permits exploration of the effect of T cell-targeted therapies on autoimmune disease. MRL/l mice develop aggressive autoimmune disease which is manifested by lymphoid hyperplasia, B cell hyperactivity, autoantibodies, thymic cortical atrophy, dermatitis, arthritis, and fatal immune complex glomerulonephritis.[3,4] The genome of the MRL/1 mouse contains the autosomal recessive mutation lpr. Homozygotes manifest early onset of autoimmune disease with prominent lymphadenopathy and splenomegaly caused by a proliferation of phenotypically aberrant, functional inducer T cells.[3,4] Initiation of autoimmunity in these mice coincides with the onset of T cell hyperproliferation suggesting that the primary defect in this model relates to an absence of regulation of inducer T cells resulting in polyclonal B cell stimulation.

Therapies that effect T cells can improve some of the features of autoimmune disease that are invariably developed, in an age-related fashion, in untreated MRL/1 mice.[3,4] Neonatal thymectomy,[5] injection of monoclonal antibodies directed against the pan T cell marker, Thyl,[6] or the inducer T cell marker, L3T4,[7] and total lymphoid irradiation[8] of MRL/1 mice prevented the development of autoimmune disease, increased survival and depressed T cell proliferation.

If photochemotherapy invokes a host response which regulates abnormal inducer T cell expansions, this approach could be tested in the MRL/1 mouse model where a phenotypically aberrant, benign helper T cell hyperproliferation promotes the development of autoimmune disease. To test whether reinfusion of photomodified lymphocytes can alter the course of a fulminant autoimmune process, recipient mice were exposed to syngeneic autoimmune splenocytes prior to the onset of overt disease when a relatively intact immune system was present.[9] Treated mice were monitored by evaluation of reliable indicators of disease progression including: lymphoid organomegaly, survival, lymphocyte phenotype and anti-DNA antibody production. Control groups were untreated or received injections of unmodified autoimmune cells or lysed phototreated cells to determine if the therapy was contingent on the presence of intact effector cells of the autoimmune process. In addition, the effect of reinfusion of phototreated autoimmune effector cells in actively diseased mice was studied by treating mice at a time when the disease process is normally initiated.[10]

To investigate whether photochemotherapy can inhibit the effector cells of graft rejection, a primate transplantation model was developed. Previous studies in murine models of skin allograft transplantation had demonstrated that injection of naive mice with cells obtained from syngeneic mice rejecting a skin transplant resulted in inhibition of *in vitro* and *in vivo* correlates of allograft rejection.[11] These results were extended to a xenograft model of primate cardiac transplantation where the donor was a cynomolgus monkey separated by centuries of evolution from the recipient a baboon.

The failure of cyclosporine-based immunosuppression to prevent rejection episodes, in xenograft models, suggests that the primary mechanism of this rejection may be humoral in origin. Formation of these antibodies probably reflects the escape from immunoregulation of T cell clones that promote B cell antibody production or the inability to inhibit T cell-independent B cell antibody synthesis. Once antibody formation is established cyclosporine does little to control its continued production.[12] A humoral response as a mechanism of rejection in the presence of cyclosporine A therapy also has been noted in studies of human cardiac allografts where the incidence of anti-donor antibody formation correlated with graft rejection.[12]

A protocol was designed to determine whether treatment of xenografted baboons with photochemotherapy in addition to conventional immunosuppression prolonged the survival of the graft and inhibited the cellular and humoral immune response to xenoantigens. Animals were treated with cyclosporine and steroids alone or with these modalities and photochemotherapy. The baboons were evaluated for the cellular response to donor and unrelated xeno- and alloantigens in mixed leukocyte culture and the humoral response to donor lymphocytes in a lymphocytotoxicity assay. The graft was biopsied weekly and monitored by palpation. Since the primate model was an autologous system the results could be directly extended to the human situation.[13,14]

MATERIALS AND METHODS

Mice

Male MRL/MpJ-lpr/lpr mice were obtained from Jackson Laboratories (Bar Harbor, ME) at 4–6 wk and used as recipients of photoinactivated autoimmune splenocytes or age-matched untreated controls. Donor male MRL/1 mice were retired breeders aged 17–21 wk. BALB/c mice (6–7 wk of age) served as normal controls.

Cells

Splenocytes were obtained by macerating the spleens in a sterile petri dish with forceps. The cells were washed in Hanks buffered salt solution (HBSS, Gibco Laboratories, Grand Island, NY) and red blood cells were lysed with ammonium chloride (0.83%, in water) at 4°C for 10 min. After washing, the cells were resuspended in RPMI 1640 (Gibco) containing 5% fetal calf serum (FCS) for culture or phosphate buffered saline (PBS, Gibco) for treatment with 8 methoxypsoralen (8 MOP) and ultraviolet A (UVA) light. Retroperitoneal lymph nodes were prepared in a similar fashion.

8 MOP-UVA Protocol

The optimal concentration of 8 MOP (Elder, Bryan, OH) and the dose of UVA for inhibition of lymphocyte proliferation was predetermined by a dose response curve (data not presented).

A drug level of 100 ng/ml and a light dose of 1 joule (j)/cm^2 of UVA energy were used for photoinactivation.

The autoimmune status of the donor MRL/1 mice was established by demonstration of anti-DNA antibody or overt lymphoid organomegaly. Splenocytes (20–50 × 10^6/ml) were incubated with 100 ng/ml of 8 MOP in PBS at 23°C, for 20 min and subsequently irradiated with 1 j/cm^2 UVA. The light source was four black lights (FL40, Sylvania GTE Products, Danvers, MA) emitting broad spectrum UVA energy (320–400 nm), filtered through a pane of window glass to remove UVB emission. The light dose was measured with a spectrophotometer (IL700A, International Light, Newburyport, MA.).

After irradiation, the cells were washed to remove excess 8 MOP, and resuspended in PBS at 20–50 × 10^6 splenocytes/100 ul. The cells were injected into the tail vein of recipient MRL/1 mice. The viability of the phototreated cells was 90% or greater by trypan blue exclusion. Mice received their first injection at 6 wk of age, a time point which is prior to the initiation of most of the features of the autoimmune process.[4] The mice were treated at 2-wk intervals until the conclusion of the experiment.

In some protocols, groups of mice were treated with autoimmune splenocytes without 8 MOP-UVA inactivation, or with 8 MOP-UVA-treated autoimmune cells that had been rapidly frozen and thawed to induce lysis. These mice received the equivalent number of whole or lysed splenocytes as the 8 MOP-UVA experimental group.

Active Autoimmune Disease Protocol

To determine whether active autoimmune disease can be inhibited, treatment of a group of MRL/l mice at 9 wk, a time when active disease commences (4) was performed. These mice received photoinactivated splenocytes weekly and were monitored in parallel with untreated controls to assess survival, lymphoid hyperproliferation, anti-DNA antibody titers, and proliferative response to the mitogens lipopolysaccharide and concanavalin A.

Radioimmunoassay for Anti-Double Stranded DNA Antibodies

A solid phase radioimmunoassay (RIA) was performed using calf thymus DNA (Sigma, Chemical Co., St. Louis, MO) at a concentration of 1 mg/ml in PBS. DNA was sonicated for 30 min to obtain small fragments and aliquoted (100 ul/well) into the wells of a round bottom microtiter plate (Flow Laboratories, Rockville, MD). The wells were coated with the DNA solution by rotation on a plate shaker (Dynatech Laboratories, Alexandria, VA) for 1 hr at 23°C. The plate was air dried overnight in a laminar flow hood. The details of the RIA assay have been previously described.[9] Alternatively, an ELISA assay was used to monitor anti-DNA antibodies.

Phenotypic Analysis

Monoclonal antibody binding was used to determine the phenotype of splenocytes in treated mice and controls. Spleen cells were resuspended in RPMI 1640 containing 0.3% bovine serum albumin (BSA). The anti-T cell monoclonal antibodies used were anti-LYT 1.2, 2.1, 3.2, Thy 1.2, Ia^k, and IJ^k (Cedarlane Laboratories, Ontario, Canada). These monoclonal reagents were produced in mice and use of a fluorescein-conjugated rabbit anti-mouse IgG or IgM secondary reagent required preliminary lysis of surface immunoglobulin-positive B cells. To lyse the B cells, splenocytes were incubated (10×10^6 cells/ml) with a 1:20 dilution of the rabbit anti-mouse IgG or as a control nonspecific mouse ascites fluid in RPMI/3% BSA for 30 min at 4°C. The cells were resuspended in 2 ml of a 1:20 dilution of rabbit complement (Cedarlane Laboratories), and incubated at 37°C for 60 min. The cells were washed twice and resuspended in RPMI/3% BSA for assessment of viability by trypan blue exclusion. Indirect immunofluorescence analysis was performed as previously described.[9]

Mitogen Assays

Splenocytes were adjusted to 5×10^6 cells/ml in RPMI 1640 containing 5% FCS. The cells were aliquoted at 100 ul/well in 5 replicate wells of a flat-bottom microtiter plate (Flow Laboratories). Background cultures received 100 ul of RPMI 1640/5% FCS. Stimulated cells received 100 ul of a 4 ug/ml solution of concanavalin A (Con A, Sigma). Splenocytes stimulated with lipopolysaccharide (LPS, Difco Laboratories, Detroit, MI) received 100 ul of a 100 ug/ml solution. Cultures were incubated for 3 days at 37°C under a 5% CO_2 atmosphere. The cultures were pulsed with 1 uCi/well of ^{3}H-thymidine (Amersham, Arlington Heights, IL)) and harvested 12–18 hr later with a Mash II automated harvestor (Whittaker M. A. Bioproducts, Walkersville, MD). The samples were counted in a liquid scintillation Beta counter (Amersham).

Statistics

The weight, size and cellularity of organs obtained from the groups of mice were analyzed for statistical significance by the standard Student t test. Survival data was analyzed using a z statistic to reject the null hypothesis at the $a = 0.01$ level of significance.

Transplantation Model-Animals

Outbred *Papio anubis* baboons (12–16 kg) were heterotopically transplanted with hearts from cynomolgus monkey (*Macaca fascicularis*) donors (4–5 kg). Donor-recipient pairs were matched according to ABO blood groups.

Photochemotherapy and Control Group Protocol

Controls received daily intramuscular injections of cyclosporine A (15 mg/kg) dissolved in cremaphor and ethanol, and subcutaneous steroids (0.8 mg/kg Depomedrol). Photochemotherapy animals received daily cyclosporine A and steroids in parallel with the control group. In addition, starting at 3 days post-transplantation these animals underwent twice weekly photochemotherapy. The baboons were sedated with ketamine (10 mg/kg) during leukapheresis. The lymphocyte enriched buffy coat was incubated with autologous plasma containing 100 ng/ml 8-methoxypsoralen prior to exposure to ultraviolet A light for 1 hr (¯2 j/ml). After irradiation, the cells were reinfused. Lymphocyte and serum samples were obtained for mixed lymphocyte culture and cytotoxicity assays prior to addition of the psoralen.

Monitoring

Graft survival was assessed by daily palpation and weekly percutaneous biopsy. Graft rejection was defined as cessation of a palpable heart beat. Rejection was evaluated by removal of the heart and pathologic examination.

Mixed Lymphocyte Culture Assay

MLC assays were performed with thawed, gamma-irradiated donor lymphocytes, frozen at the time of donor sacrifice. Parallel assays used stimulators obtained from unrelated baboons or monkeys. Irradiated donor lymphocytes (5 × 10^6 cells/ml) were added to the fresh responder lymphocytes (5 × 10^6 cells/ml) and cultured in RPMI 1640 containing a final concentration of 15% unrelated heat-inactivated baboon serum. Samples were adjusted to 100% viability using trypan blue exclusion. As an internal control, parallel assays were performed using lymphocytes from a naive baboon as responder cells.

Cytotoxic Antibody

Donor lymphocytes were labeled with ^{51}chromium and washed prior to incubation with heat-inactivated recipient serum (1 hr, 37°C) and rabbit complement in microtiter plates. The plates were centrifuged and the supernatant radioactivity measured in a gamma counter. Percent cytotoxicity was calculated by the formula:

$$\text{Percent cytotoxicity} = \frac{\text{E-Bg}}{100\% \text{ lysis-Bg}} \times 100$$

TABLE 1. Prophylactic Therapy of Autoimmune Disease[a]

Therapy Splenocyte Tx	50% Survival	Weight		Antibody Anti-DNA	Phenotype		Mitogen	
		LN	SP		THY1	LYT1	Con A	LPS
8 MOP-UVA	3 wk inc	55% dec	29% dec	87% dec	93% dec	86% dec	inc	dec
None	3 wk dec	47% dec	29% dec	ND	71% dec	84% dec	dec	dec
8 MOP-UVA lysed cells	7 wk dec	ND	ND	ND	ND	ND	ND	ND

[a] Results are compared to nontreated control group. Abbreviations: LN; lymph node, SP; spleen, Con A; concanavalin A, LPS; lipopolysaccharide, Tx; treatment, inc; increase, dec; decrease, ND; not done.

E = experimental; Bg = background obtained using media plus complement without antibody; 100% lysis = anti-thymocyte globulin plus complement or detergent lysis.

RESULTS

Prophylactic Model of Autoimmune Disease

TABLE 1 presents the results obtained in the 3 experimental groups of mice in comparison to the nontreated age-matched controls.

Survival

Twice as many of the recipients of photoinactivated autoimmune splenocytes were alive at 23 wk of age. The increased survival demonstrated in the recipients of phototreated splenocytes was statistically significant in comparison to the controls ($a = 0.01$) and maintained from 23 through 29 wk the time point when all of the untreated control mice had died. The 50% mortality level was reached in untreated control mice at 23 wk of age. This rate of control mortality is similar to that reported in other studies.[5-8] In addition, the survival of the phototreated splenocyte group was significantly ($a = 0.01$) prolonged in comparison with the recipients of unmodified cells at 23 and 26 wk. Unmodified cell recipients demonstrated 50% mortality by 20 wk of age. An additional group of mice were recipients of photoinactivated autoimmune cells that had been lysed by freezing and thawing prior to injection. These mice exhibited rapid onset of organomegaly (16–20 wk) and died at an early age (60% mortality by 16 wk of age). The rapid death rate in this group precluded additional studies; however, the massive increase in organ size visible at autopsy indicated that fulminant autoimmune disease was present.

In the group of 46 mice that received photoinactivated autoimmune cells, only 4 mice (9%) were judged to be treatment failures based on early onset of lymphoid organomegaly. In contrast, 20% of the mice tested in the group receiving cells without inactivation were judged to be treatment failures.

Reduced Lymphoid Organomegaly in Treatment MRL/l Mice

The weight of retroperitoneal lymph nodes obtained from mice treated with photoinactivated autoimmune splenocytes was significantly ($p < 0.001$) reduced in comparison with untreated controls, at every age studied. Spleens obtained from the recipients of photoinactivated autoimmune splenocytes showed a significant reduction in weight when compared to controls. MRL/l mice treated with unmodified autoimmune cells also demonstrated decreased lymph node and spleen weights.

Effect of Reinfused Photomodified Splenocytes on Anti-DNA Antibody

The development of autoantibodies to double-stranded DNA was followed over time in MRL/l mice that received photoinactivated autoimmune splenocytes in comparison to untreated controls. Untreated control MRL/l mice had high levels of anti-DNA antibody at 13 and 17 wk of age. Mice that were recipients of photoinactivated splenocytes had low serum levels of anti-DNA antibody at 13 wk. At 19 wk of age, the antibody level in mice that were recipients of photoinactivated autoimmune splenocytes was in the background range found in normal strains of mice.

Phenotype of Splenocytes from Mice Receiving Injections of Autoimmune Splenocytes

The absolute number of Thy1.2^+ T cells was significantly reduced ($p < 0.001$) in the photoinactivated cell-treated group. The recipients of unmodified autoimmune splenocytes also had a profound reduction in the absolute number of splenic T cells but not to the extent demonstrated in the spleens of mice treated with photomodified autoimmune cells ($p < 0.001$). The LY1^+ splenocyte population was reduced in the spleens of mice receiving photomodified ($p < 0.025$) or untreated autoimmune splenocytes.

Response to LPS and Con A

Although the absolute number of T cells was significantly reduced in the group of mice receiving photoinactivated splenocytes, the residual T cells responded better to Con A stimulation ($p < 0.025$) than T cells from the recipients of untreated autoimmune cells or controls. The splenic B cells from the photoinactivated autoimmune cell-treated mice were slightly less responsive to LPS stimulation than controls. The recipients of unmodified autoimmune cells had an equivalent number of B cells when compared to controls but these cells responded poorly to LPS in comparison to B cells obtained from control MRL/1 and the recipients of photoinactivated cells.

Therapeutic Model of Autoimmune Disease

TABLE 2 presents the results of treatment of actively diseased mice with photoinactivated autoimmune splenocytes.

Survival

No improvement in survival was noted when the treated mice were compared with the untreated controls. This inability to improve survival probably reflects an incapacity to reverse established kidney disease which is the major cause of mortality in this mouse model.

Lymphoid Organomegaly

A significant reduction in lymph node weight was achieved in the recipients of photoinactivated autoimmune splenocytes demonstrating inhibition of the T cell hyperproliferation which causes organomegaly in this model. Spleen weight was only modestly decreased perhaps relecting an inability to effect B cell hyperproliferation once T cell dependency is lost.

Anti-DNA Antibody Production

A substantial decrease in the production of anti-DNA antibody production was achieved in the group of mice receiving photoinactivated autoimmune splenocytes. Apparently, even though established disease is present a reduction in autoantibody production can be achieved in actively autoimmune mice.

Response to Mitogens

Lymph node cells from treated mice retained the capacity to respond to the mitogens con A and LPS. These results probably reflect a retention of normal

TABLE 2. Treatment of Active Autoimmune Disease with Photochemotherapy[a]

Therapy Splenocyte Tx	50% Survival	Weight		Antibody Anti-DNA	Mitogen	
		LN	SP		Con A	LPS
8 MOP-UVA	no change	55% dec	14% dec	62% dec	inc	inc

[a] Results are compared to nontreated control group. Abbreviations as in TABLE 1.

lymphoid populations in the lymph nodes of the mice treated with photoinactivated autoimmune splenocytes.

Taken as a whole, the results of reinfusion of photoinactivated autoimmune splenocytes in actively autoimmune mice demonstrate that this approach is less effective than prophylactic therapy but can decrease T cell hyperproliferation and thereby decrease reduce lymphadenopathy and autoantibody production.

Primate Transplantation Model

This protocol was designed to determine whether treatment of xenografted baboons with photochemotherapy in addition to conventional immunosuppression prolonged the survival of the graft and inhibited the cellular and humoral immune response to xenoantigens. Animals were treated with cyclosporine and steroids alone or with these modalities and photochemotherapy. An overview of the results obtained in this model is presented in TABLE 3.

Survival

Control xenograft survival averaged 36 ± 31 days. Control grafts developed progressive cellular infiltrates, myocyte necrosis and edema. Graft survival in the photochemotherapy group was $X = 49 \pm 32$ days. Reversal of cellular rejection episodes was documented by pathology in 2 animals. These results were not statistically significant due to the small numbers of animals in each group ($N = 6$, 8 MOP-UVA; $N = 7$, controls).

TABLE 3. Reinfusion of Photoinactivated Autologous Leukocytes in Cardiac Xenograft Recipients[a]

Therapy	Survival	MLC	Antibody	AMLR
8 MOP-UVA cyclo & steroids	49 ± 32	donor-specific inhibition	83% dec	pres 50%
Cyclo & steroids	36 ± 31	nonspecific inhibition	inc	pres 14%

[a] Abbreviations: MLC; mixed leukocyte culture, AMLR; autologous mixed lymphocyte reaction, Cyclo; cyclosporine A, Pres; present.

Mixed Leukocyte Culture

The mixed leukocyte culture (MLC) response to the donor was suppressed at intervals in all control animals, but the response to unrelated baboons and xenoantigens was also inhibited at these time points. The average suppression in the control group to the specific donor lymphocytes was $49 \pm 28\%$ while $39 \pm 25\%$ of the response to unrelated allogeneic stimulators, and $64 \pm 30\%$ of the response to unrelated xenogeneic animals was also inhibited. Photochemotherapy animals developed enhanced specific suppression of the MLC response to the donor with relative preservation of the response to unrelated allogeneic and xenogeneic stimulators. Average suppression of the mixed lymphocyte response to the specific xenogeneic donor in photochemotherapy animals was $50 \pm 29\%$. The response to unrelated xenogeneic ($X = 14 \pm 13\%$) and allogeneic stimulators ($X = 19 \pm 27\%$) was relatively spared. The specificity of the suppression against the donor in the photochemotherapy group was significantly increased ($p < 0.01$) when compared to the control group.

Cytotoxic Anti-Donor Antibodies

Two of five control animals developed increasing levels of cytotoxic antibody that correlated with graft demise. Continued treatment with cyclosporine and steroids did not control the production of anti-donor antibody. Eighty percent of the animals treated with photochemotherapy in addition to cyclosporine and steroids demonstrated a reduction in cytotoxic antibody production.

Autologous Mixed Leukocyte Culture

An enhanced response in autologous mixed lymphocyte (AMLR) culture was observed in 3 of 6 photochemotherapy animals. This response to self was generally evident one week prior to suppression of the MLR. The baseline response to self increased from <600 CPM to >17000 CPM (6–57 $\times$ pretransplantation AMLR). Animals treated with cyclosporine and steroids did not develop an autologous mixed lymphocyte reaction except in one case in which a preexistent enhanced response to self stimulators was noted (pre: 3372 to 13958 CPM). The increased response to self-stimulators may represent induction of an autologous, autoreactive population in the photochemotherapy group. Autoreactive cells might serve to promote inhibition of the MLR response and downregulate the production of cytotoxic antibodies.

DISCUSSION

The results obtained in the murine and primate models have provided insights into the mechanism of photochemotherapy. These studies indicate that this form of therapy may be useful in other conditions besides CTCL. Autoimmune diseases that are mediated by unregulated inducer T cells may be autoregulated by treatment with photochemotherapy if the therapy is initiated at an early time point. Transplantation regimens demonstrate improved donor specificty and decreased anti-donor antibody formation when photochemotherapy is added to con-

ventional immunosuppression. These protocols demonstrate that photochemotherapy can be studied in animal models. The results obtained in these models
have identified the conditions that may be amenable to photochemotherapy and
have helped to determine the most efficacious manner of intervention in these
systems.

Observations in Murine Models of SLE

The MRL/l mouse models demonstrate that photochemotherapy can modify
the course of autoimmune disease, if therapy is initiated prior to disease onset.
The therapy is still effective during active disease; however, established lesions
such as kidney disease cannot be reversed. Since the autoimmune disease in this
model is mediated by inducer T cells, reinfusion of photoinactivated autoimmune
cells must invoke a regulatory response in the recipient that inhibits the proliferation of these T cells. The effect on autoantibody production is secondary to
regulation of the inducer T cells. The reduction in organomegaly, which is more
prominent in the lymph nodes than the spleen, demonstrates that T cell hyperproliferation is inhibited. The improved response to Con A also confirms that abnormal T cells that lose the capacity to respond to T cell mitogens are diminished. In
spite of the fulminant progression of the autoimmune disease in this model, beneficial effects of therapy were achieved and maintained. These results suggest that
comparable therapy in a human situation may provide prolonged amelioration of
the disease process. Though this approach clearly is not curative in this genetically encoded disorder, the capacity to inhibit T cell proliferation approximates
the results achieved with monoclonal antibodies and irradiation.[6-8] The T cell-
targeted effect of photochemotherapy may reflect a host response to the reinfused
T cell receptors of the autoimmune cells. Photoinactivation of the autoimmune
cells may render these cells more immunogenic perhaps through inhibition of
membrane modulation of target antigens, localization of dying effector cells in
lymphoid organs where immune responses occur,[15] or release of lymphokines
from the dying cells. Alteration of the TCR by psoralen and UVA therapy is
possible. However, the immune response engendered in the recipient is specific
for untreated abnormal T cells, as well as phototreated T cells. This specificity
suggests that the host recognizes an unmodified target. The magnitude of the
specific inhibition mediated by photochemotherapy is demonstrated in the primate model where donor specific suppression is maintained despite the presence
of nonspecific immunosuppressive drugs.

Primate Transplantation Model

The cardiac transplantation model is analgous to the human system since the
animals are leukapheresed and autologous lymphocytes are treated and returned.
The only modification is the addition of psoralen to the pheresed blood in place of
in vivo ingestion. The suppression induced in the treated animals is equivalent in
magnitude to that found in the cyclosporine-treated control group. However, the
response to unrelated challenges is retained. Specificity of inhibition has also been
noted in the clinical situation,[1] and the murine transplantation model.[11] These
results support the contention that the therapy targets the TCR of the reinfused
immunoreactive lymphocytes and induces a host response that inhibits the generation and function of these effector cells. The reversal of cytotoxic anti-donor

antibody formation found in the photochemotherapy group probably reflects a secondary effect on B lymphocytes due to inhibition of the inducer T cell population. The absence of infectious complications in this immunosuppressed model also suggests that general immune surveillance is not compromised.

SUMMARY

These studies demonstrate that photochemotherapy can be successfully evaluated in animal models. The therapy mediates specific suppression of immune responses and appears to operate at the level of the effector T cells. Future studies will focus on isolation and characterization of the host response to photochemotherapy. The extention of this form of therapy to conditions mediated by dysfunctional regulation of effector T cells is already in progress in clinical trials of cardiac allograft transplantation and autoimmune disease. The results of these trials will provide more evidence on the role of this form of therapy in autoregulation of the immune response.

REFERENCES

1. EDELSON, R. L., C. L. BERGER, F. GASPARRO *et al.* 1987. Treatment of leukemic cutaneous T cell lymphoma with extracorporeally-photoactivated 8-methoxypsoralen, N. Engl. J. Med. **316:** 297–303.
2. EDELSON, R. L., C. L. BERGER & R. ARMSTRONG. 1981. Lymphapheresis in the treatment of the leukemic phase of cutaneous T-cell lymphoma and pemphigus vulgaris. *In* Proceedings of the Workshop on Therapeutic Plasmapheresis and Cytapheresis. G. J. Nemo & H. Taswell, Eds. NIH PUBL. No. 82-1665. 55–71. U.S. Dept. of Health and Human Services. Rochester, NY.
3. MORSE, H. C., III, W. F. DAVIDSON, R. A., YETTER, E. D. MURPHY, J. B. ROTHS & R. L. COFFMAN. 1982. Abnormalities induced by the mutant gene LPR: expansion of a unique lymphocyte subset. J. Immunol. **129:** 2612–2615.
4. THEOFILOPOULOS, A. N. & F. J. DIXON. 1981. Etiopathogenesis of murine SLE. Immunol. Rev. **55:** 179–216.
5. STEINBERG, A. D., J. B. ROTHS, E. D. MURPHY, R. T. STEINBERG & E. S. RAVECHE. 1980. Effects of thymectomy or androgen administration upon the autoimmune disease of MRL/MP-lpr/lpr mice. J. Immunol. **125:** 871–874.
6. WOFSKY, D., J. A. LEDBETTER, P. L. HENDLER & W. E. SEAMAN. 1985. Treatment of murine lupus with monoclonal anti-T cell antibody. J. Immunol. **134:** 852–857.
7. SANTORO, T. J., J. P. PORTANOVA & B. L. KOTZIN. 1988. The contribution of L3T4⁻ T cells to lymphoproliferation and autoantibody production in MRL-lpr/lpr mice. J. Exp. Med. **167:** 1713–1718.
8. THEOFILOPOULOS, A. N., R. BALDERAS, D. L. SHAWLER *et al.* 1980. Inhibition of T cell proliferation and SLE-like syndrome of MRL/l mice by whole body or total lymphoid irradiation. J. Immunol. **125:** 2137–2142.
9. BERGER, C. L., M. PEREZ, L. LAROCHE & R. L. EDELSON. 1990. Inhibition of murine autoimmune disease by reinfusion of syngeneic lymphocytes inactivated with psoralen and ultraviolet A light. J. Invest. Dermatol. **94:** 52–57.
10. BERGER, C., C. DELEON, C. MARBOE & R. L. EDELSON. 1989. Amelioration of active murine lupus by treatment with photoinactivated splenocytes. J. Invest. Dermatol. **92:** 402a.
11. PEREZ, M., R. L. EDELSON, L. LAROCHE & C. L. BERGER. 1989. Specific suppression of anti-allograft immunity by vaccination with syngeneic photoinactivated splenocytes. J. Invest. Dermatol. **92:** 669–676.
12. PETROSSIAN, G. A., A. B. NICHOLS, E. REED *et al.* 1989. The relationship between

survival and the development of coronary artery disease and anti-HLA antibodies following cardiac transplantation. Circulation 80(Suppl. #3): 122–125.

13. PEPINO, P., C. L. BERGER, L. FUZESI *et al.* 1989. Primate cardiac allo- and xenotransplantation: modulation of the immune response with photochemotherapy. Eur. Surg. Res. **960:** 1–8.

14. FUZESI, L., P. PEPINO, C. L. BERGER *et al.* 1989. Immunomanipulation of the response to cardiac allo and xenoreactive leukocytes. Transplant. Proc. **21:** 837–841.

15. CHIANG, Y.-C., C. GURIERREZ, L. LAROCHE, R. L. EDELSON & C. L. BERGER. Homing pattern of photoinactivated antigen-reactive splenocytes. (Submitted.)

Immunopotentiation of Anti-Viral and Anti-Tumor Immune Responses Using Anti-T Cell Receptor Antibodies and Mitogens[a]

KENNETH A. NEWELL,[b] JOSHUA D. I. ELLENHORN,[c]
RAPHAEL HIRSCH,[d] AND JEFFREY A. BLUESTONE[e]

[b]Department of Surgery
Division of Transplantation
University of Chicago Hospitals
Chicago, Illinois 60637

[c]Department of Surgery
University of Cincinnati Hospitals
Cincinnati, Ohio 45208

[d]Experimental Immunology Branch
National Cancer Institute
National Institutes of Health
Bethesda, Maryland 20892

[e]University of Chicago
Ben May Institute
Committee on Immunology
Chicago, Illinois 60637

Rationale for Developing T Cell Receptor-Specific Immunotherapy

Current modalities employed in the treatment of malignant neoplasms and viral infections are of limited efficacy and are associated with significant toxicities. In particular many chemotherapeutic regimens are associated with increased infectious complications resulting from leukopenia and generalized immunosuppression. In addition, impaired hematopoiesis and idiosyncratic toxicities often limit the usefulness of many treatment protocols. Given these limitations, it would be ideal to develop a means of augmenting the host's native anti-tumor or anti-viral immune response. Some groups have attempted to enhance existing, but inadequate, host immune responses by administering exogenous lymphokines systematically or by isolating tumor infiltrating lymphocytes (TIL) which are then expanded *in vitro* and reinfused into the patient.[1,2] Although these strategies may offer an improvement over conventional therapy, the toxicity of systemic lymphokine administration and the inability to isolate TIL from many tumors has limited their application. For these reasons we have attempted to boost immune responses by using T cell receptor (TCR) specific agents to activate T cells *in vivo*. Early studies investigating an anti-murine CD3 monoclonal antibody (mAb) suggested that it may be one such agent. This paper summarizes our observations on

[a] This work was supported by Grants PO1 AI 29531, RO1 CA 49260, and P30 CA 14599. K.A.N. is supported by National Institute of Health Training Grant HL-07665.

279

the T cell activating and immunopotentiating properties of one such anti-CD3 mAb, 145-2C11, and reports our initial studies of the effects of the T cell mitogen *Staphylococcal* enterotoxin B (SEB).

Immunosuppressive Properties of Anti-CD3 Monoclonal Antibodies

Due to the lack of a suitable animal model, initial studies of the *in vivo* properties of anti-CD3 mAbs were performed in humans.[3] These studies demonstrated the profound immunosuppressive effects of OKT3 (an anti-human CD3 mAb). In fact, the principal use of OKT3 remains the prevention and treatment of allograft rejection.[4] The identification of an anti-murine CD3 mAb (145-2C11) in 1986 allowed a more systematic investigation of the effects of anti-CD3 mAbs than was possible in humans.[5] 145-2C11 was similar in most, if not all, respects to its anti-human CD3 counterpart OKT3. Initial studies characterizing the effects of *in vivo* treatment of mice with 145-2C11 showed that it dramatically prolonged survival of allogeneic skin grafts and that T cells obtained from treated mice demonstrated significantly decreased MLR and CTL responses.[6] The observed immunosuppression was shown to be the consequence of multiple factors including T cell depletion, T cell receptor coating and modulation, and an as yet incompletely under-

TABLE 1. Dose-Dependent Effect of T Cell Mitogens on IL-2 Receptor Expression by Lymph Node T Cells

	In Vivo Treatment							
	Anti-CD3[a]				SEB[b]			
	0 μg	4 μg	40 μg	400 μg	0 μg	5 μg	50 μg	250 μg
% IL-2R expression	8	38	55	78	8	49	78	86

[a] IL-2R expression as a percent of total T cells.
[b] IL-2R expression as a percent of $V_\beta 8+$ T cells.

stood prolonged T cell dysfunction that is independent of T cell depletion or receptor blocking.[6]

Anti-CD3 Monoclonal Antibodies Also Result in T Cell Activation

Earlier studies of the effects of anti-CD3 mAbs (both OKT3 and 145-2C11) *in vitro* demonstrated a transient but definite T cell activation as evidenced by proliferation and lymphokine secretion.[5,7,8] In subsequent studies we demonstrated that T cell activation was also a consequence of *in vivo* administration of an anti-CD3 mAb.[9] High doses of mAb (40 to 400 μg administered I.P.) result in a transient activation of T cells followed by marked T cell depletion, TCR modulation, and immunosuppression. The anti-CD3-induced *in vivo* T cell activation was reflected by increased IL-2 receptor (IL-2R) expression (TABLE 1), CSF secretion, extramedullary hematopoiesis, and enhanced proliferation *in vitro* to both exogenous IL-2 and allogeneic cells (FIG. 1).[9,10] In addition, other groups have recently reported the production of IFN-γ, TNFα, IL-2, IL-3 and IL-4 *in vivo* following the administration of anti-CD3 mAb in mice.[11,12] Similarly, IFN-γ, TNFα and IL-2 have been detected in the serum of patients following treatment with OKT3 and

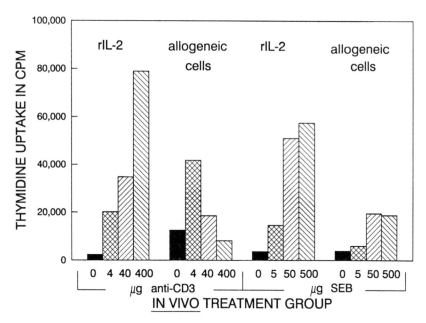

FIGURE 1. *In vitro* proliferative response of lymph node cells to exogenous IL-2 or allogeneic cells.

are thought to play a major role in the nearly uniform side effects seen especially with the first dose of mAb.[13] Further evidence supporting the *in vivo* activation of human T cells following treatment with OKT3 has come from recent studies in which lymph node T cells from allograft recipients were examined before and after treatment with OKT3. These studies showed that the TCR of T cells from treated patients were coated with murine mAb and that they displayed increased IL-2R expression as well as increased proliferation to exogenous IL-2 and allogeneic cells.[14]

Having observed that mAb specific for the CD3 molecule were capable of activating T cells *in vivo*, we next asked whether this property could be exploited to augment the inadequate immune response of mice to a weakly immunogenic, malignant, UV-induced fibrosarcoma (PRO4L). Since the immunosuppressive and activating properties of 145-2C11 are strictly dose dependent, the conditions resulting in maximal activation with minimal suppression were first determined. While high doses (40 to 400 µg) of anti-CD3 mAb resulted in transient activation followed by profound, prolonged immunosuppression, low dose (4 µg) therapy resulted in activation without appreciable suppression.[10] As shown in TABLE 2, intraperitoneal administration of 4 µg of an anti-CD3 mAb to C3H mice at the time

TABLE 2. Mitogen-Induced T Cell Activation Prevents Outgrowth of Malignant Tumors

	Control	Anti-CD3	Control	SEB	SEB + F23.1
Tumor incidence	54/56	17/48	34/46	14/51	9/9
(%)	(96)	(35)	(74)	(27)	(100)

of inoculation with syngeneic tumor fragments significantly decreased the tumor incidence. The mechanism by which anti-CD3 mAb mediates this response was investigated by depleting cell subsets *in vivo*. Early on an increase in non-MHC-restricted cytotoxic cells was noted in the spleen of mice treated with anti-CD3 mAb. In order to evaluate the role of these cells in enhanced tumor rejection, *in vivo* depletions of NK cells were performed using the mAb SH34 (anti-ASGM1) prior to treatment with anti-CD3 mAb. While this treatment abolished NK activity, it did not diminish the anti-tumor effect of 145-2C11.[15] On the other hand, depletion of CD8+ cells at any time (4 days prior to or 8 days following tumor inoculation and treatment with anti-CD3) abolished the anti-tumor effect of 145-2C11.[15] Depletion of CD4+ cells from 4 days prior to tumor inoculation to 4 days after also abolished the protective effect of 145-2C11. However, depletion of CD4+ cells at later time points did not influence the tumor incidence.[15] Furthermore, TIL isolated from mice treated with anti-CD3 mAb demonstrated increased cytolysis of the PRO4L tumor target relative to controls.[15] These cytotoxic T cells were specific for PRO4L and were uniformly of the CD8+ phenotype.[15] These data show that while CD4+ cells are necessary during the initial phase of the response to 145-2C11 and tumor antigen, CD8+ cells are necessary throughout the response. This is compatible with a mechanism by which the anti-CD3 mAb activates CD4+ helper cells which in turn secrete lymphokines that then provide a costimulatory signal for the CD8+ cytotoxic cells which serve as the final effectors.

While the findings obtained using the PRO4L tumor model are consistent with the mechanism suggested above, it is possible that other mechanisms may be operative in different models. It has recently been shown that treatment of mice with low doses of anti-CD3 mAb provides protection against lethal Sendai virus infection and allows the development of long-term, specific anti-viral immunity.[16] Treatment of C57BL/6 mice with 1.0 or 2.0 μg of 145-2C11 18 hours prior to challenge with Sendai virus resulted in 60 and 64% survival respectively (controls 0% survival). Interestingly, mice treated with 8.0 μg of anti-CD3 mAb all died earlier than control mice demonstrating the narrow therapeutic window of anti-CD3 mAbs. Mechanistic studies demonstrated that anti-CD3 mAb treatment did not alter the kinetics of the virus-specific CTL response, antibody response, or T cell proliferation. In addition, anti-CD3 mAb did not increase the Sendai-specific CTL precursor frequency. Anti-CD3 therapy did, however, dramatically increase NK cell activity. Unlike the tumor model, the protective effect of anti-CD3 therapy could be reversed by depletion of NK cells prior to administration of 145-2C11. It was also shown that treatment with anti-CD3 mAb resulted in the production of IL-2 *in vivo* and that administration of exogenous IL-2 could also augment NK activity and protect against Sendai virus infection. Thus, in the Sendai virus model, anti-CD3 mAb therapy appears to act by stimulating IL-2 production which in turn enhances NK activity against virally infected cells. The finding that treated mice do develop long-term, virus-specific immunity is important in that it suggests that the immunosuppressive effects of anti-CD3 mAb therapy do not interfere with the development of a normal memory response.

SEB-Induced T Cell Activation Augments Anti-Tumor Responses

Two properties of anti-CD3 mAbs may eventually limit their clinical application for potentiating host immune responses. First, as has already been addressed, there is very fine balance between the activating and suppressive properties of anti-CD3 mAbs. Though these effects are largely dose dependent, even low "activating" doses of anti-CD3 mAb may be associated with some long-term T cell dysfunction. Secondly, anti-CD3 mAbs act equally on all T cells. It may be advantageous to develop agents capable of acting on only the relevant subset of necessary effector T cells. This might minimize the first dose side effects of anti-CD3 mAbs that result from massive T cell activation and lymphokine release and may minimize the percentage of T cells affected by any potential immunosuppressive effects of anti-CD3 mAbs. In addition, since anti-CD3 mAbs activated all T cells, it is difficult to trace the fate and assess the functional roles of these mAb-activated cells. In this regard the identification of more selective agents might improve our understanding of the mechanisms by which mitogen-activated T cells exert their immune-potentiating effects.

Along these lines, we have recently begun the investigation of the T cell mitogenic properties of *Staphylococcal* enterotoxin B (SEB). This *Staphylococcal* protein has been shown to activate both murine and human T cells *in vitro* in a subset-specific manner based solely on their Vβ chain expression.[17] SEB activates T cells expressing the Vβ gene products 7 and 8.1–8.3.[18–20] *In vitro* SEB-induced T cell activation is reflected by increased IL-2R expression, lymphokine production, and proliferation.[21–27] This activation requires the presence of MHC class II positive accessory cells.[28] It has recently been shown that SEB binds to nonpolymorphic portions of both the MHC class II molecule and the variable portion of the TCR β chain at sites separate from the antigen recognition site.[29,30] It has been hypothesized that SEB thus bound delivers an activation signal to T cells by cross-linking their TCRs.[31]

Since SEB is capable of activating T cells *in vitro* in much the same way as anti-CD3 mAbs (except that it shows Vβ subset specificity), we sought to determine whether or not SEB activated T cell subsets *in vivo*. As shown in TABLE 1, *in vivo* treatment with doses of SEB ranging from 5 to 250 μg (administered intraperitoneally [i.p.] in phosphate-buffered saline) resulted in a dose-dependent increase in IL-2R expression on Vβ8+ cells. This increase in IL-2R expression was not seen on Vβ2+ (non-SEB-reactive) cells. Similarly, CD8 expression was increased on CD8+/Vβ8+ cells following i.p. treatment with SEB.[32] Anti-CD3-mediated T cell activation has previously been shown to result in similar increases in CD8 expression on all CD3+CD8+ cells.[6] Additional evidence supporting SEB-mediated *in vivo* T cell activation comes from the observation that lymph node T cells harvested from mice following treatment with SEB demonstrate enhanced proliferation *in vitro* both with and without exogenous IL-2 (FIG. 1). These same cells also display increased proliferation in MLR assays (FIG. 1). Other findings confirming the ability of SEB to activate T cells *in vivo* include the demonstration that i.p. administration of SEB results in a dose-dependent increase in IFN-γ production in the serum of treated mice as detected by ELISA[32] and the finding that Vβ8+ cells proliferate *in vivo* in treated mice.[32,33] Interestingly, the *in vivo* proliferation of Vβ8+ cells that we observed was confined exclusively to the CD8+ subset of cells (TABLE 3). This is somewhat surprising given the requirement for MHC class II positive APCs and suggests that the class II molecules themselves are not directly involved in the activation of Vβ8+ cells by SEB. In support of this finding, it has recently been reported that SEB causes CD8+ cells to proliferate *in vitro*.[34] Although the cause of this preferential proliferation remains uncertain, it is of note that recent reports have documented that *in vivo* treatment with SEB administered intravenously results in anergy of the CD4+ subset of Vβ8+ cells.[35] Whether the different responses of CD4 and CD8 cells to SEB *in vivo* are the result of different sensitivity to costimulatory signals delivered by accessory cells or are the consequence of as yet undetermined factors, the data suggest that CD4 and CD8 cells respond differently to SEB *in vivo*.

We have also examined the time course of the response of T cells to SEB and have found that maximal T cell activation occurs 18 hours following administration of SEB *in vivo*.[32] Examination of lymph node T cells harvested at 48 and 72 hours after administration of SEB, shows that SEB-induced T cell activation has begun to diminish by 48 hours and has returned to normal by 72 hours as determined by proliferation to exogenous IL-2 or allogeneic cells *in vitro*. This data correlates well with the disappearance of IL-2R from the cell surface as determined by fluorocytometry.[32] Importantly, at no time point did we see suppression of the T cell responses from SEB-treated mice (1 to 14 days). During these studies we observed that the kinetics of the proliferative response of T cells from SEB-treated mice were markedly different from control mice.[32] While the proliferative response of T cells from normal mice to allogeneic stimulator cells continued to increase after 96 hours in culture, the proliferative response of *in vivo* SEB-activated cells peaked after 48 hours in culture. The peak response was quantitatively similar in both groups (control 66347 cpm, SEB-treated 65265) suggesting that SEB-treated animals develop full alloresponses but do it much more rapidly (48 hours vs 96 hours). These kinetics are nearly identical to the proliferative

TABLE 3. *In Vivo* Treatment with SEB Increases the Proportion of CD8+ T Cells

	Control	50 μg SEB	250 μg SEB
% CD8+/Vβ2+	40.2	41.5	41.6
% CD8+/CD3+	31.3	37.5	37.6
% CD8+/Vβ8+	34.6	60.5	65.7

kinetics of primed T cells.[36] This suggests that SEB-induced T cell activation may cause resting (G_0) T cells to differentiate into a memory-like (G_1) or primed state.

If SEB does promote the differentiation of resting T cells into a primed state, treatment with SEB may be capable of potentiating endogenous host immune responses. We therefore examined the effect of SEB-mediated T cell activation on the incidence of tumor development in C3H mice following inoculation with the malignant fibrosarcoma PRO4L. As is shown in TABLE 2, a 50-μg dose of SEB, when administered i.p. following tumor inoculation, significantly decreased the frequency of tumor outgrowth. These data confirm the hypothesis that SEB-mediated T cell activation can be exploited to augment certain immune responses. Whether the potentiation of the anti-tumor response is the result of expansion of anti-tumor effector cells (recall that SEB causes the proliferation of Vβ8+/CD8+ T cells *in vivo*) or converts resting T cells into a primed or activated state such that their requirements for triggering by tumor antigens is decreased, remains to be determined. The data in TABLE 2 also show that the anti-tumor effect of SEB in C3H mice is dependent on the presence of Vβ8+ cells in that the prior depletion of Vβ8 cells totally abolished the anti-tumor effect of SEB. In this regard it is important to note that Vβ8+ T cells are the only SEB-reactive cells present in C3H mice.

SUMMARY

Although the immunosuppressive properties of anti-CD3 mAbs are now widely recognized, we have accumulated data characterizing the T cell activating properties of these antibodies. While in some situations these activating properties may be viewed as unwanted side-effects (for instance OKT3-mediated T cell activation may be responsible for some of the first dose toxicity seen with patients receiving OKT3 for suppression of allograft rejection), we have shown that anti-CD3 mAb therapy can augment host immune responses and provide protection against some tumors and viral infections. Importantly, this augmented response allows the development of long term, specific immunity. Because the immunosuppressive and activating properties of anti-CD3 mAbs are so closely overlapping, we have sought to identify other agents that are capable of activating T cell subsets selectively. We have found that SEB activates T cell subsets selectively *in vivo* and that this activation can be exploited to prevent the outgrowth of a malignant murine tumor. Studies currently in progress, including phenotypic and functional analysis of TILs and *in vivo* T cell subset depletions, should result in a more precise understanding of how SEB-induced T cell activation inhibits tumor growth.

ACKNOWLEDGMENT

We thank Dr. David S. Bruce for his helpful discussion of the data and review of the manuscript.

REFERENCES

1. ROSENBERG, S. A., J. J. MULE, P. J. SPIESS, C. M. REICHERT & S. L. SCHWARZ. 1985. Regression of established pulmonary metastases and subcutaneous tumor mediated by the systemic administration of high-dose recombinant interleukin 2. J. Exp. Med. **161**: 1169–1188.

2. TOPALIAN, S. & S. A. ROSENBERG. 1990. Tumor infiltrating lymphocytes. *In* Important Advances in Oncology 1990. V. Devita, S. Hellman & S. Rosenberg, Eds. 19–37. Lippincott. Philadelphia, PA.

3. COSIMI, A. B., R. C. BURTON, R. B. COLVIN *et al.* 1981. Treatment of acute renal allograft rejection with OKT3 monoclonal antibody. Transplantation **32**: 535–539.

4. ORTHO MULTI-CENTER TRANSPLANT STUDY GROUP. 1985. A randomized clinical trial of OKT3 monoclonal antibody for acute rejection of cadaveric renal transplants. N. Engl. J. Med. **313**: 337–341.

5. LEO, O., M. FOO, D. H. SACHS, L. E. SAMELSON & J. A. BLUESTONE. 1987. Identification of a monoclonal antibody specific for a murine T3 polypeptide. Proc. Natl. Acad. Sci. USA **84**: 1374–1378.

6. HIRSCH, R., M. ECKHAUS, H. AUCHINCLOSS, JR., D. H. SACHS & J. A. BLUESTONE. 1988. Effects of *in vivo* administration of anti-T3 monoclonal antibody on T cell function in mice. I. Immunosuppression of transplantation responses. J. Immunol. **140**: 3766–3772.

7. VAN WAUWE, J. P., J. R. DE MEY & J. G. GOOSSENS. 1980. OKT3: a monoclonal anti-human T lymphocyte antibody with potent mitogenic properties. J. Immunol. **124**: 2708–2713.

8. MARUSIC-GALESIC, S., D. PARDOLL, T. SAITO, O. LEO, B. J. FOWLKES, J. COLIGAN, R. N. GERMAIN, R. H. SCHWARTZ & A. M. KRUISBEEK. 1988. Activation properties

of T cell receptor–gamma delta hybridomas expressing diversity in both gamma and delta chains. J. Immunol. **140:** 411–418.

9. HIRSCH, R., R. E. GRESS, D. H. PLUZNIK, M. ECKHAUS & J. A. BLUESTONE. 1989. Effects of *in vivo* administration of anti-CD3 monoclonal antibody on T cell function in mice. II. *In vivo* activation of T cells. J. Immunol. **142:** 737–743.

10. ELLENHORN, J. D. I., R. HIRSCH, H. SCHREIBER & J. A. BLUESTONE. 1988. *In vivo* administration of anti-CD3 prevents malignant progressor tumor growth. Science **242:** 569–571.

11. FERRAN, C., K. SHEEHAN, M. DY, R. SCHREIBER, S. MERITE, P. LANDAIS, L-H. NOEL, G. GRAU, J. A. BLUESTONE, J-F. BACH & L. CHATENOUD. 1990. Cytokine related syndrome following injection of anti-CD3 monoclonal antibody: further evidence for transient *in vivo* T cell activation. Eur. J. Immunol. **20:** 509–515.

12. FLAMAND, V., D. ABRAMOWICZ, M. GOLDMAN, C. BIERNQUX, G. HUEZ, J. URBAIN, M. MOSER & O. LEO. 1990. Anti-CD3 antibodies induce T cells from unprimed animals to secrete IL-4 both *in vitro* and *in vivo*. J. Immunol. **144:** 2875–2882.

13. CHATENOUD, L., C. FERAN, C. LEGENDRE, I. THOUARD, S. MERITE, A. REUTER, Y. GEVAERT, H. KREIS, P. FRANCHIMONT & J. F. BACH. 1990. *In vivo* cell activation following OKT3 administration. Transplantation **49:** 697–702.

14. ELLENHORN, J. D. I., E. S. WOODLE, I. GOBREAL, J. R. THISTLETHWAITE & J. A. BLUESTONE. 1990. Activation of human T cells *in vivo* following treatment of transplant recipients with OKT3. Transplantation **50:** 608–612.

15. ELLENHORN, J. D. I., H. SCHREIBER & J. A. BLUESTONE. 1990. Mechanism of tumor rejection in anti-CD3 monoclonal antibody-treated mice. J. Immunol. **144:** 2840–2846.

16. KAST, W. M., J. A. BLUESTONE, M. H. M. HEEMSKERK, J. SPAARGAREN, A. C. VOORDOUW, J. D. I. ELLENHORN & C. J. M. MELIEF. 1990. Treatment with monoclonal anti-CD3 antibody protects against lethal Sendai virus infection by induction of natural killer cells. J. Immunol. **145:** 2254–2259.

17. MARRACK, P. & J. KAPPLER. 1990. The staphylococcal enterotoxins and their relatives. Science **248:** 705–711.

18. JANEWAY, C. A., JR., J. YAGI, P. J. CONRAD, M. E. KATZ, B. JONES, S. VROEGOP & S. BUXSER. 1989. T-cell responses to Mls and to bacterial proteins that mimic its behavior. Immunol. Rev. **107:** 61–88.

19. WHITE, J., A. HERMAN, A. M. PULLEN, R. KUBO, J. W. KAPPLER & P. MARRACK. 1989. The Vβ-specific superantigen staphylococcal enterotoxin B: stimulation of mature T cells and clonal deletion in neonatal mice. Cell **56:** 27–35.

20. CALLAHAN, J. E., A. HERMAN, J. W. KAPPLER & P. MARRACK. 1990. Stimulation of B10.BR T cells with superantigenic staphylococcal toxins. J. Immunol. **144:** 2473–2479.

21. PEAVY, D. L., W. H. ADLER & R. T. SMITH. 1970. The mitogenic effects of endotoxin and staphylococcal enterotoxin B on mouse spleen cells and human peripheral lymphocytes. J. Immunol. **105:** 1453–1458.

22. SMITH, B. G. & H. M. JOHNSON. 1975. The effect of staphylococcal enterotoxins on the primary *in vitro* immune response. J. Immunol. **115:** 575–578.

23. WARREN, J. R., D. I. LEATHERMAN & J. F. METZGER. 1975. Evidence for cell-receptor activity in lymphocyte stimulation by staphylococcal enterotoxins. J. Immunol. **115:** 49–53.

24. LANGFORD, M. P., G. J. STANTON & H. M. JOHNSON. 1978. Biological Effects of staphylococcal enterotoxin A on human peripheral lymphocytes. Infect. Immun. **22:** 62–68.

25. JOHNSON, H. M. 1985. Mechanism of gamma interferon production and assessment of immunoregulatory properties. Lymphokines **11:** 33–46.

26. BUXSER, S. & S. VROEGOP. 1988. Staphylococcal enterotoxin B stimulation of BALB/c lymphocyte mitogenesis and potential relationship to the Mls response. J. Immunogenet. **15:** 153–159.

27. CARLSSON, R. & H. O. SJOGREN. 1985. Kinetics of IL-2 and interferon-gamma production, expression of IL-2 receptors, and cell proliferation in human mononuclear cells exposed to staphylococcal enterotoxin A. Cell. Immunol. **96:** 175–183.

28. FLEISCHER, B., H. SCHREZENMEIER & P. CONRADT. 1989. T lymphocyte activation by staphylococcal enterotoxins: role of class II molecules and T cell surface structures. Cell. Immunol. **120:** 92–101.

29. CHOI, Y., A. HERMAN, D. DIGIUSTO, T. WADE, P. MARRACK & J. KAPPLER. 1990. Residues of the variable region of the T-cell-receptor β-chain that interact with *S. aureus* toxin superantigens. Nature **346:** 471–473.

30. DELLABONA, P., J. PECCOUD, J. KAPPLER, P. MARRACK, C. BENOIST & D. MATHIS. 1990. Superantigens interact with MHC class II molecules outside of the antigen groove. Cell **62:** 1115–1121.

31. FLEISCHER, B. 1989. Bacterial toxins as probes for the T-cell antigen receptor. Immunol. Today. **10:** 262–264.

32. NEWELL, K. A., J. D. I. ELLENHORN, D. S. BRUCE & J. A. BLUESTONE. 1991. *In vivo* T cell activation by staphylococcal enterotoxin B prevents outgrowth of a malignant tumor. Proc. Natl. Acad. Sci. USA **88:** 1074–1078.

33. MARRACK, P., M. BLACKMAN, E. KUSHNIR & J. KAPPLER. 1990. The toxicity of staphylococcal enterotoxin B in mice is mediated by T cells. J. Exp. Med. **171:** 455–464.

34. HERRMANN, T., J. L. MARYANSKI, P. ROMERO, B. FLEISCHER & H. R. MACDONALD. 1990. Activation of MHC class I-restricted CD8+ CTL by microbial T cell mitogens. J. Immunol. **144:** 1181–1186.

35. KAWABE, Y. & A. OCHI. 1990. Selective anergy of Vβ8+, CD4+ T cells in *Staphylococcus* enterotoxin B-primed mice. J. Exp. Med. **172:** 1065–1070.

36. PECK, A. M., L. C. ANDERSSON & H. WIGZELL. 1977. Secondary *in vitro* responses of T lymphocytes to non-H-2 Alloantigens. J. Exp. Med. **145:** 802–818.

Cytokine Release by Peripheral Blood Lymphocytes Targeted with Bispecific Antibodies, and Its Role in Blocking Tumor Growth

DAVID M. SEGAL,[a] JIA-HUA QIAN, SARAH M. ANDREW,
JULIE A. TITUS, DELIA MEZZANZANICA,
MARIA A. GARRIDO, AND JOHN R. WUNDERLICH

Experimental Immunology Branch
National Cancer Institute
National Institutes of Health
Bethesda, Maryland 20892

INTRODUCTION

Cytolytic cells can be induced by bispecific antibodies (BA) to kill cells they normally would not lyse.[1-4] In order to be effective, BAs must bind to both triggering structures on cytotoxic cells and surface antigens on target cells. BAs with these specificities form multicellular conjugates between effector and target cells, and trigger the lytic machinery of the effector cells. A number of types of cells can mediate targeted cytotoxicity, but the number of triggering molecules is limited. The two major types of cytolytic triggers are TcRs and Fc_γRs; TcRs can be triggered through either their Ti or CD3 subcomponents,[5-7] and at least three classes of Fc_γR can serve as cytolytic triggers, depending upon the cell type that expresses them.[8-11] In addition, CD2[12,13] and CD59[14] can also trigger lysis. TcRs and Fc_γRs have the dual functions of specifically binding target cells, and triggering lysis. CD2 is thought to be a nonspecific adhesion molecule, one of whose ligands is LFA-3,[15,16] and the function of CD59 is unknown.

Cytolytic cells can be specifically targeted against tumor cells with an appropriate BA,[2,17,18] and targeted effector cells have therefore been studied in tumor-bearing animals[3,11,19-21] and in man[22] with the ultimate purpose of developing anti-cancer immunotherapies. We have previously found that targeted human peripheral blood T[19] and NK[11] cells mediate a powerful anti-tumor effect against human tumors injected subcutaneously in nude mice. We found, however, that one subset of cells, CD8⁻ T cells, was inactive in a 4-hour cytotoxic assay, but was able to block subcutaneous tumor growth in mice.[19] To explain this discrepancy, we established an *in vitro* assay that measures the ability of targeted T cells to block the growth of human tumor cell lines over a period of 5–7 days. Using this assay, we compared the ability of PBL to block tumor growth with their ability to lyse target cells in the presence of appropriate BAs.

[a] Corresponding author: Dr. David M. Segal, Building 10, Room 4B17, NIH, Bethesda, MD 20892.

FIGURE 1. Tumor growth inhibition assay. LS174T human colon adenocarcinoma cells were incubated with (*squares*) or without (*circles*) PBL from a normal donor. In the presence of PBL and anti-CD3 (Fab) × anti-tumor (Fab) BA (*triangles*) tumor growth was inhibited. The PBL : tumor ratio was 10 : 1, and BA concentration was 1 μg/ml. Tumor growth was measured using an MTT assay, as described,[25,26] and is expressed as absorbance at 570 nm.

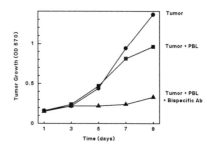

In Vitro *Tumor Growth Inhibition by Targeted PBL*

In order to mimic *in vivo* tumor neutralization by targeted lymphocytes, tumor growth was followed in culture over several days in the presence and absence of targeted PBL from normal donors. An example of data obtained from one experiment is shown in FIGURE 1. In the absence of PBL or in the presence of PBL without bispecific antibody, LS174T tumor cells began growing rapidly at about day 5 and reached high levels by day 9. Most importantly, tumor growth was markedly inhibited by PBL plus anti-CD3 × anti-tumor BA. In other experiments (not shown) we found that the anti-tumor effect was dependent upon the effector : target ratio and that NK cells targeted with anti-CD16 × anti-tumor BA could also block tumor growth. Neither anti-CD16, anti-CD3, anti-tumor nor mixtures of these antibodies blocked tumor growth in the presence of PBL. We next compared lysis *in vitro* with tumor growth inhibition *in vitro* using unfractionated or CD8-depleted PBL to see whether the CD8⁻ cells could block tumor growth *in vitro,* as they do in mice.[19] TABLE 1 shows that in two different experiments, CD8-depleted PBL were unable to mediate targeted lysis in a 4-hour assay, but were able to block tumor growth. Thus the tumor growth inhibition assay better reflects *in vivo* tumor growth inhibition than does the 4-hour cytolytic assay.

TABLE 1. Lysis and Tumor Growth Inhibition Mediated by Targeted T Cell Subsets[a]

Exp.	Cells	% Specific Lysis		% Tumor Growth Inhibition	
		−Ab	+Ab	−Ab	+Ab
1	PBL	2	19	10	91
	CD8⁻	4	5	37	94
	CD4⁻	15	44	30	94
2	PBL	4	35	ND	ND
	CD8⁻	0	6	0	61
	CD4⁻	0	29	13	82

[a] Subsets of PBL were prepared by panning in Exp. 1 or with antibody and C' in Exp. 2. Lysis at an E : T ratio of 30 : 1 or tumor growth inhibition at an E : T of 3 : 1 of LS174T cells was measured in the presence or absence of anti-CD3 (Fab) × anti-tumor (Fab) (+/−Ab). Percent inhibition of tumor growth (P) was calculated using the equation $P = 100[A_{control} - A_{sample}/(A_{control} - A_{bkg})]$, where $A_{control}$ indicates the absorbance at 570 nm arising from tumor cells grown in medium alone, A_{sample} refers to the absorbance of tumor cells grown in the presence of inhibitor (PBL or culture supernatants), and A_{bkg} is the absorbance of wells not containing tumor cells.

Blockage of Growth of Bystander Tumor Cells by Targeted PBL

It has been established in several systems that bystander cells are not lysed by targeted cytotoxic cells in 4-hour ^{51}Cr release assays.[2] For example in FIGURE 2, panel A, activated PBL specifically lysed tumor cells but not H-2^k spleen (bystander) cells in the presence of anti-CD3 (Fab) × anti-tumor (Fab), whereas the reverse was true in the presence of anti-CD3 (Fab) × anti-K^k (Fab). In panel B, PBL were tested for the ability to block bystander tumor growth. In contrast to

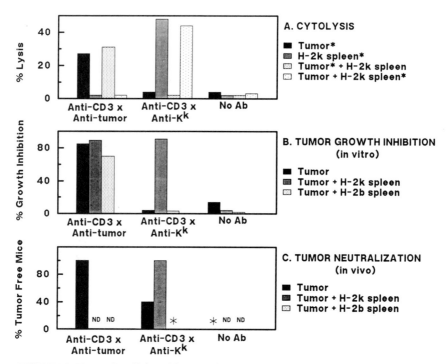

FIGURE 2. Bystander effects with targeted PBL. Panel **A** shows a lack of bystander lysis by targeted PBL. PBL effector cells (3 × 10^5) were incubated with 10^4 radiolabeled target cells or 10^4 radiolabeled cells plus 10^4 unlabeled cells in the presence of the indicated BA or no antibody. Radiolabeled cells are indicated in the legend by "*". The tumor is LS174T, and H-2^k and H-2^b spleen cells are 2-day Con A blasts from C3H and C57BL/6 mice, respectively. Effector cells were PBL from a normal donor, activated for 3 days with immobilized OKT3 and IL-2, followed by 9 days with IL-2 alone. Panel **B** shows inhibition of bystander tumor cell growth *in vitro* using aliquots of the same cells used in panel **A**. All wells contained 2 × 10^3 tumor cells, 4 × 10^4 PBL, and where indicated, 5 × 10^4 spleen cells. Percent inhibition of tumor growth (relative to tumor in the absence of PBL or antibody) was measured on day 8. Panel **C** shows that targeted PBL block subcutaneous tumor growth in nude mice. Mice in each group, 5 mice/group, received 4 × 10^6 LS174T tumor cells on day 0. PBL from a normal donor were coated with bispecific antibodies, washed, and added to tumor cells prior to injection, at a PBL : tumor ratio of 5 : 1. Some mice also received 5 × 10^7 irradiated C3H (H-2^k) or C57BL/6 (H-2^b) spleen cells added to the tumor/PBL mixture prior to injection. Mice were evaluated for tumor growth on day 30. ND, not done. "*" indicates 0 tumor-free mice.

FIGURE 3. Generation of tumor growth inhibitory activity in antibody coated microtiter wells. PBL were incubated with 10^3 LS174T cells at a 30 : 1 effector : target ratio for 7 days. Samples contained either soluble anti-CD3 (Fab) × anti-tumor (Fab) BA, the indicated mAbs adsorbed to the microtiter wells, or no antibody.

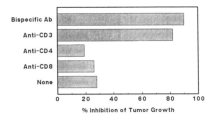

% Inhibition of Tumor Growth

the lytic experiments, bystander tumor growth was inhibited by PBL in the presence of anti-CD3 (Fab) × anti-K^k (Fab) and H-2^k, but not H-2^b, spleen cells. Thus targeted PBL block the growth of bystander tumor cells, but do not lyse bystander cells, suggesting that lysis and tumor growth inhibition are different processes.

Next, we asked whether targeted T cells could block the growth of bystander cells *in vivo* in tumor neutralization assays. Panel C of FIGURE 2 shows that in the presence of anti-CD3 (Fab) × anti-K^k (Fab), the subcutaneous growth of the LS174T tumor cells in nude mice is blocked when H-2^k, but not H-2^b, spleen cells are also present. Thus, targeted human T cells can block the growth of bystander tumor cells *in vivo*.

Because tumor growth inhibition did not require a direct linkage between PBL and tumor cells, experiments were carried out to determine whether anti-CD3 alone would induce PBL to block tumor growth. Several monoclonal antibodies against cell surface components on PBL were adsorbed to the bottoms of plastic tissue culture flasks, and PBL and LS174T tumor cells were added. Anti-CD3 × anti-tumor was used as a positive control. FIGURE 3 shows that immobilized anti-CD3 was as effective at blocking tumor growth as the bispecific antibody. Immobilized anti-CD4, CD8, or CD16 were unable to consistently elicit strong anti-tumor responses.

Tumor Growth Inhibition Is Mediated by Factors Secreted by Targeted PBL

The above data suggest that TcR crosslinking induces peripheral T cells to secrete factors into the medium that block tumor growth. To test this hypothesis, PBL were cultured in anti-CD3-coated flasks or in flasks coated with no antibody. At various times, supernatants were removed and tested for the ability to block tumor growth. FIGURE 4 shows that supernatants of PBL grown on CD3-coated flasks blocked tumor growth at high dilutions, whereas supernatants from cells

FIGURE 4. Inhibition of tumor growth by supernatants from PBL. PBL were incubated in flasks coated with anti-CD3 (*squares*) or with no antibody (*triangles*). At the indicated times supernatants were removed, centrifuged, and frozen. At the end of the experiment all supernatants were thawed, diluted, and added to LS174T cells to test for tumor growth inhibition. The final dilution of factors was 1 : 54. Factors from this donor were particularly effective at inhibiting tumor growth.

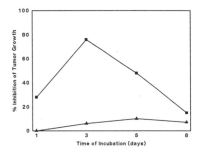

Time of Incubation (days)

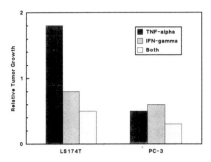

FIGURE 5. Blockage of tumor growth by added cytokines. Indicated tumor cells were incubated in either 4×10^3 units/ml IFN-γ, 10^3 units/ml TNF-α, or a mixture of both cytokines at these concentrations. On day 9, tumor growth was measured and expressed relative to tumor growth in the absence of added cytokine. LS174T and PC-3 are human colon and prostate tumor lines, respectively.

grown in the absence of antibody were much less effective. The maximum amount of inhibitory factor was obtained at day 3. The decrease in activity after 3 days suggests that the factor is not stable or is consumed in culture. Culture supernatants from targeted PBL have also been tested for growth inhibitory activity against a number of other tumor lines, in addition to LS174T. Cell growth of PC-3 (human prostate adenocarcinoma), OVCAR3 (human ovarian carcinoma), B16 (murine melanoma), and K562 (human myelogenous leukemia), but not RBL5 (murine leukemia) or F2B (human B cell line) was blocked by the supernatants produced by PBL grown on CD3 coated flasks (data not shown).

To identify the substances responsible for blocking tumor growth we first cultured tumor cells in the presence of various cytokines. FIGURE 5 shows that the growth of both LS174T and PC-3 was blocked by mixtures of IFN-γ and TNF-α. With PC-3 either TNF-α or INF-γ alone partially inhibited tumor growth, while with LS174T, TNF-α reproducibly enhanced tumor growth when added alone, but had the opposite effect in the presence of IFN-γ. We next tested the ability of antibodies against TNF-α and IFN-γ to reverse the anti-tumor effects of targeted lymphocytes. FIGURE 6 shows that antibodies to TNF ($\alpha + \beta$) and IFN-γ do in fact block the anti-tumor activity of PBL incubated with tumor cells in anti-CD3-coated microtiter wells. With both PC-3 and LS174T, the blockage of tumor growth could be reversed by mixtures of anti-INF-γ and anti-TNF($\alpha + \beta$) antibodies, suggesting that TNF and IFN-γ are necessary components of bystander anti-tumor activity. Similar studies (not shown) indicated that these same antibodies could reverse tumor growth inhibition of LS174T cells mediated by PBL in the presence of anti-CD3 $\times$ antitumor bispecific antibody even though they had no effect upon lysis in a 4-hour ^{51}Cr release assay. These data show that cytokines

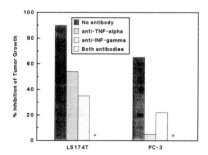

FIGURE 6. Reversal of tumor growth inhibition by antigen-cytokine antibodies. PBL were incubated in anti-CD3-coated microtiter wells with either LS174T or PC-3 tumor cells at a 20:1 effector target ratio. Also included were either anti-IFN-γ anti-serum (5 units/ml), anti-TNF ($\alpha + \beta$) mAb (10 μg/ml), both antibodies together at these concentrations, or no antibody. The inhibition of tumor growth relative to tumor alone, was measured on day 7. "*" indicates no inhibition of tumor growth.

are unimportant in cytolysis as measured by ^{51}Cr release, but do play an essential role in inhibiting tumor growth over a longer term.

CONCLUSIONS

Targeted cytotoxicity holds great promise as a means for treating tumors or virally infected cells in patients. Many investigators have assumed that the results of short term cytolysis experiments *in vitro* would lay the groundwork for clinical uses of targeted cells. However, as we report here, the ability of targeted human lymphocytes to block tumor growth in culture or in nude mice correlates poorly with their ability to mediate lysis, mainly because targeted tumor growth inhibition and targeted cytolysis result from two different activities. Targeted cytolysis as measured by ^{51}Cr release occurs rapidly, usually within 4–6 hours, and does not involve bystander cell lysis. Tumor growth inhibition, by contrast, is mediated by secreted factors that block the growth of both target and bystander cells.

Cytolysis and tumor growth inhibition are initiated by the crosslinking of triggering molecules on the effector cells. However, targeted lysis occurs only when target cells are bound directly to effector cells (*e.g.*, with BAs), while targeted tumor growth inhibition is induced by receptor crosslinking *per se*, for example, in T cells by anti-CD3 antibody adsorbed to the bottoms of culture flasks. For therapeutic use bispecific antibodies with anti-tumor cell specificity would have an advantage over other forms of TcR crosslinking because they would result in a local release of inhibitory cytokines at the tumor site. Such factors could act upon all cells within a tumor, killing even those cells that were sterically inaccessible to targeted PBL or that had lost antigen expression. Localized release of tumoristatic cytokines could circumvent problems of toxicity frequently observed when cytokines are given systemically. For example, cytotoxic T cells, LAK, and NK cells all require IL-2 for the maintenance of cytotoxic activity. Therefore immunotherapeutic protocols which use cytotoxic cells to treat tumors also require that the patients be given high doses of IL-2.[23] Because IL-2 is toxic at high doses, such therapies are greatly limited. Likewise, TNF-α is often able to block tumor growth *in vitro*, but is highly toxic when given *in vivo*.[24] Targeted PBL might be able to release cytokines at tumor sites that would act locally to eradicate the tumor, without producing toxic, life-threatening reactions in patients.

REFERENCES

1. SEGAL, D. M. & J. R. WUNDERLICH. 1988. Targeting of cytotoxic cells with hetero-crosslinked antibodies. Cancer Invest. **6:** 83–92.
2. SEGAL, D. M. & D. P. SNIDER. 1989. Targeting and activation of cytotoxic lymphocytes. Chem. Immunol. **47:** 179–213.
3. STAERZ, U. D. & M. J. BEVAN. 1986. Use of anti-receptor antibodies to focus T cell activity. Immunol. Today **7:** 241–245.
4. FANGER, M. W., R. F. GRAZIANO, L. SHEN & P. M. GUYRE. 1989. FcγR cytotoxicity exerted by mononuclear cells. Chem. Immunol. **47:** 214–253.
5. STAERZ, U. D., O. KANAGAWA & M. J. BEVAN. 1985. Hybrid antibodies can target sites for attack by T cells. Nature **314:** 628–631.
6. PEREZ, P., R. W. HOFFMAN, S. SHAW, J. A. BLUESTONE & D. M. SEGAL. 1985. Specific targeting of cytotoxic T cells by anti-T3 linked to anti-target cell antibody. Nature **316:** 354–356.

7. Liu, M. A., D. M. Kranz, J. T. Kurnick, L. A. Boyle, R. Levy & H. N. Eisen. 1985. Heteroantibody duplexes target cells for lysis by cytotoxic T lymphocytes. Proc. Natl. Acad. Sci. USA **82:** 8648–8652.

8. Karpovsky, B., J. A. Titus, D. A. Stephany & D. M. Segal. 1984. Production of target-specific effector cells using hetero-cross-linked aggregates containing anti-target cell and anti-Fcγ receptor antibodies. J. Exp. Med. **160:** 1686–1701.

9. Shen, L., P. M. Guyre, C. L. Anderson & M. W. Fanger. 1986. Heteroantibody-mediated cytotoxicity: antibody to the high affinity Fc receptor for IgG mediates cytotoxicity by human monocytes that is enhanced by interferon-γ and is not blocked by human IgG. J. Immunol. **137:** 3378–3382.

10. Graziano, R. F. & M. W. Fanger. 1987. FcγRI and FcγRII on monocytes and granulocytes are cytotoxic trigger molecules for tumor cells. J. Immunol. **139:** 3536–3541.

11. Titus, J. A., P. Perez, A. Kaubisch, M. A. Garrido & D. M. Segal. 1987. Human K/NK cells targeted with heterocrosslinked antibodies specifically lyse tumor cells *in vitro* and prevent tumor growth *in vivo*. J. Immunol. **139:** 3153–3158.

12. Siliciano, R. F., J. C. Pratt, R. E. Schmidt, J. Ritz & E. L. Reinherz. 1985. Activation of cytotoxic T lymphocyte and natural killer cell function through the T11 sheep erythrocyte binding protein. Nature **317:** 428–429.

13. Scott, C. F., Jr., J. M. Lambert, R. S. Kalish, C. Morimoto & S. F. Schlossman. 1988. Human T cells can be directed to lyse tumor targets through the alternative activation/T11-E rosette receptor pathway. J. Immunol. **140:** 8–14.

14. Leo, O., M. Foo, D. M. Segal, E. Shevach & J. A. Bluestone. 1987. Activation of murine T lymphocytes with monoclonal antibodies: detection on Lyt2+ cells of an antigen not associated with the T cell receptor complex but involved in T cell activation. J. Immunol. **139:** 1214–1222.

15. Shaw, S., G. E. G. Luce, R. Quinones, R. E. Gress, T. A. Springer & M. E. Sanders. 1986. Two antigen-independent adhesion pathways used by human cytotoxic T-cell clones. Nature **323:** 262–264.

16. Dustin, M. L., M. E. Sanders, S. Shaw & T. A. Springer. 1987. Purified lymphocyte function-associated antigen 3 binds to CD2 and mediates T lymphocyte adhesion. J. Exp. Med. **165:** 677–692.

17. Perez, P., J. A. Titus, M. T. Lotze *et al.* 1986. Specific lysis of human tumor cells by T cells coated with anti-T3 cross-linked to anti-tumor antibody. J. Immunol. **137:** 2069–2072.

18. Jung, G., C. J. Honsik, R. A. Reisfeld & H. J. Muller-Eberhard. 1986. Activation of human peripheral blood mononuclear cells by anti-T3: killing of tumor target cells coated with anti-target-anti-T3 conjugates. Proc. Natl. Acad. Sci. USA **83:** 4479–4483.

19. Titus, J. A., M. A. Garrido, T. T. Hecht, D. F. Winkler, J. R. Wunderlich & D. M. Segal. 1987. Human T cells targeted with anti-T3 crosslinked to anti-tumor antibody prevent tumor growth in nude mice. J. Immunol. **138:** 4018–4022.

20. Barr, I. G., S. Miescher, V. von Fliedner *et al.* 1989. *In vivo* localization of a bispecific antibody which targets human T lymphocytes to lyse human colon cancer cells. Int. J. Cancer **43:** 501–507.

21. Garrido, M. A., M. J. Valdayo, D. F. Winkler *et al.* 1990. Targeting human T lymphocytes with bispecific antibodies to react against human ovarian carcinoma cells in nu/nu mice. Cancer Res. **50:** 4227–4232.

22. Nitta, T., K. Sato, H. Yagita, K. Okumura & S. Ishii. 1990. Preliminary trial of specific targeting therapy against malignant glioma. Lancet **335:** 368–371.

23. Rosenberg, S. A. 1988. Immunotherapy of patients with advanced cancer using interleukin-2 alone or in combination with lymphokine activated killer cells. Important Adv. Oncol. **4:** 217–257.

24. Old, L. J. 1985. Tumor necrosis factor (TNF). Science **230:** 630–632.

25. Mosmann, T. R. 1983. A rapid colorimetric assay for cellular growth and survival: application to proliferation and cytotoxic assays. J. Immunol. Methods **65:** 55–63.

26. Tada, H., O. Shiho, K. Kuroshima, M. Koyama & K. Tsukamoto. 1986. An improved colorimetric assay for interluekin 2. J. Immunol. Methods. **93:** 157–165.

Antigen-Induced Tolerance to Organ Allografts[a]

PETER J. MORRIS, KATHRYN J. WOOD, AND
MARGARET J. DALLMAN

Nuffield Department of Surgery
University of Oxford
John Radcliffe Hospital
Oxford, OX3 9DU, United Kingdom

INTRODUCTION

The induction of neonatal tolerance to a skin allograft in the mouse by antigen pretreatment at the time of birth was first demonstrated almost 40 years ago.[1] Since that time there has been a continuing effort directed at inducing tolerance to an allograft in the adult animal, with the expectation that such a phenomenon might ultimately be applicable to clinical organ transplantation. Pretreatment of rodents with alloantigen either as whole cells or crude antigen extracts has been shown to produce prolongation of skin allograft survival by a few days at most (*e.g.*, REF. 2). However in the late 1960's it was reported, contrary to expectation, that patients who had received large numbers of transfusions before renal transplantation did not show poorer graft survival than those who had received relatively few. This led to the suggestion that some degree of specific immunodepression or partial tolerance might be produced in patients by prior blood transfusions.[3] An experimental model of a vascularised organ graft was needed to test this hypothesis and about that time the technique of renal transplantation in the rat was described, which allowed the phenomenon of antigen pretreatment to be explored in a vascularised organ allograft model.[4]

Early experiments showed that pretreatment of the recipient with whole blood led to the prolonged survival, and in many instances indefinite survival, of a renal allograft across major and minor histocompatibility barriers.[5] The phenomenon was found to be dependent on dose of antigen used, the intravenous route of administration, the timing relative to transplantation, and the strain combination investigated.[5,6] The importance of these experimental findings was given further impetus by the observation in clinical renal transplantation that recipients who had received no blood transfusions before transplantation had very poor graft survival,[7] and this lead to the uniform adoption of a deliberate blood transfusion policy in nontransfused patients awaiting renal transplantation. Even more persuasive was the demonstration that the transfusion of blood from the potential donor of one haplotype disparate recipients of a living related renal transplant led to a much improved graft survival in those recipients who did not become sensitised by the blood pretreatment.[8]

These observations in the clinic have led to renewed interest in the phenomenon of antigen-induced tolerance in adult recipients. Over the past few years in our laboratory we have continued to explore the requirements for induction of

[a] This work was supported by grants from the Medical Research Council, the National Kidney Research Fund, and the British Heart Foundation.

295

tolerance to vascularised organ allograft and the mechanisms of induction and maintenance of this tolerant state using two experimental models, renal allografts in the rat and cardiac allografts in the mouse. Some aspects of this work will be reviewed in this paper.

METHODS AND MATERIALS

Animals

C3H (H-2k), C57BL/10 (H-2b) and Balb/C (H-2d) male mice were purchased from Harlan Olac Ltd (Bicester, UK), and were between 8 and 14 weeks old when used. LEW-RT1l, DA-RT1a and PVG-RT1c male rats were purchased from Harlan Olac Ltd or bred in the Biomedical Services Unit of the John Radcliffe Hospital, Oxford, UK.

Organ Transplantation

Renal allografts in the rat were performed essentially as previously described[4] with removal of the contralateral kidney delayed until seven days after transplantation. Function was assessed by monitoring the blood urea. Fully vascularised heterotopic cardiac allografts in the mouse were performed as described,[9] rejection being defined as loss of palpable cardiac contractions or the cessation of all electrical activity on electrocardiogram.[10]

Transfected L Cells

L cells derived from C3H (H-2K) were transfected with the H-2D^b, H-2K^b, and H-2IA^b α and β genes and cloned by flow cytometry as previously described.[11] Expression of H-2 antigens was evaluated by staining with a panel of polymorphic monoclonal antibodies specific for K^b, D^b, and IA^b molecules.[11]

Preparation of Infiltrating Cells from Graft

Viable cell suspensions were prepared from rejecting and nonrejecting kidneys by collagenase digestion.[12,13] Cells were used immediately after isolation in *in vitro* cytotoxicity assays (Cr release) and assessed for IL-2 responsiveness and IL-2 production as previously described.[14]

Anti-CD4 Monoclonal Antibody

The anti-CD4 (rat anti-mouse IgG2b) mab, YTS191.1, was generously provided by Dr. Herman Waldmann.[15] The antibody was purified from ascites by NH$_4$SO$_4$ precipitation and DEAE sephagel chromatography. Purity was assessed by PAGE and the antibody concentration quantitated.

Adoptive Transfer of Splenocytes in the Rat

Spleen cells were prepared by passing the spleen through a stainless steel mesh and the T cells were enriched by passage over a nylon column. CD4$^+$ and CD8$^+$ T cells were prepared by negative selection using anti-CD8 (MRC OX8) and anti-CD4 (W3/25) monoclonal antibodies respectively as previously described.[16] Syngeneic DA recipients were given 200 rads irradiation (day -2) followed the next day by the adoptive transfer of splenocytes from DA rats bearing long surviving LEW kidney grafts (day -1). A fresh LEW kidney was transplanted 24 hours after the adoptive cell transfer (day 0) and graft survival monitored.

RESULTS

Requirements for Induction of Antigen-Induced Tolerance to a Vascularised Allograft

As previously demonstrated in our laboratories on many occasions, pretreatment of a DA recipient with 0.5–1.0 ml of LEW blood 7 or 14 days before transplantation of a LEW kidney leads to indefinite survival of that kidney[5,17] (TABLE 1). The phenomenon is donor specific in that a kidney from a third party strain, *e.g.*, PVG, is rejected. Furthermore we have shown previously, both in a rat model and mouse model, that the sharing of an MHC haplotype (class I and class II) between the blood donor and the organ donor or even the sharing of class II antigen alone (class I alone not tested) can produce prolonged survival of a subsequent renal allograft.[18,19] We have also explored the role of different components of blood in the rat model and shown that pretreatment with affinity-purified erythrocytes or purified hepatocytes, expressing donor class I MHC antigen only, can also produce prolonged renal allograft survival[17,20] (TABLE 1). However, as pretreatment with B lymphocytes, expressing both class I and class II MHC antigen, can produce prolonged graft survival,[21] these experiments did not unequivocally confirm that pretreatment with cells expressing only class I MHC antigen could induce tolerance to a subsequent allograft. To allow this question to be addressed very precisely a mouse model was developed in which recipients of a heterotopic cardiac allograft were pretreated with syngeneic cells transfected with donor MHC class I or class II genes.[11]

C3H (H-2k)-derived fibroblasts (L cells) were transfected with H-2D, H-2K, or H-2IA α and β genes from C57BL/10 (H-2b) mice and cloned by flow cytometry. Expression of the transfected H-2b gene product was confirmed by monoclonal antibody binding, virus-specific killing by H-2K^b- or H-2D^b-restricted T cell clones and activation of H-2IA^b-restricted T cells.[11] The number of antigenic sites per cell in each transfected clone was determined by antibody saturation analysis, and the results are shown in TABLE 2.

C3H recipients treated with 0.25–0.5 ml of C57BL/10 whole blood IV 14 days before transplantation of a C57 heart showed prolonged survival of the cardiac allograft (mean survival = 34.2 days).[11] Pretreatment with L cells alone or transfected with an irrelevant gene(s), *e.g.*, influenza haemagglutinin or IA^k α and β, did not prolong graft survival. In contrast, pretreatment with the optimal dose of L cells expressing a single H-2b gene product all showed prolonged survival (TABLE 3). Prolongation of graft survival in both situations was dose related in

TABLE 1. Pretreatment of DA or LEW Rates with LEW or DA Whole Blood (0.5 ml) or Affinity-Purified Erythrocytes (1300 Leukocytes per 8×10^9 Erythrocytes) Given 7 Days before Transplantation of a LEW, DA, or BN Kidney

Donor-to-Recipient	Blood Donor	Blood (B) or Erythrocytes (E)	Mean Survial (Days)
LEW to DA	LEW	B	>100
	BN	B	10
	DA	B	10
	LEW	E	>100
	BN	E	10
	DA	E	10
DA to LEW	DA	B	56
	BN	B	10
	LEW	B	11
	DA	E	>100
	BN	E	11
	LEW	E	10

that larger doses of whole blood, or larger and smaller doses of the transfected L cells produced a less marked or no effect[11] (data not shown). The unresponsive state induced by blood transfusion or treatment with transfected cells was donor specific, as BALB/c hearts were rejected within 10 days.[11]

Thus in this model pretreatment with donor MHC class I products specifically prolonged cardiac allograft survival in the absence of donor class II or minor histocompatibility antigens. Similarly pretreatment with donor class II MHC antigen alone was effective. The degree of unresponsiveness induced appeared to be related to the antigen load presented to the recipient. At equivalent class I antigen loads the H-2K locus appeared immunodominant over the H-2D locus and, furthermore, lower doses of L-IA^b cells, which have a greater antigen density per cell than the above, were required to prolong survival (TABLES 2 and 3).

Mechanisms for the Induction of Tolerance by Alloantigen Pretreatment

The immune status of recipients after antigen pretreatment but before transplantation was explored. CD4$^+$ suppressor T cells could be demonstrated transiently, 3 and 4 days after a blood transfusion, in the spleen and then by day 7, in the thoracic duct lymph (but not in the spleen), both *in vitro* and *in vivo*.[16,22,23] *In vitro* suppression of both donor-specific proliferation and the generation of cytotoxic T cells by this CD4$^+$ T cell suppressor population has been demonstrated.[22] *In vivo* adoptive transfer of CD4$^+$ T cells, but not CD8$^+$ T cells, from the thoracic duct lymph of the transfused recipients into lightly irradiated (200 rads) syngeneic

TABLE 2. Expression of H-2b Antigenic Sites per Cell in L Cell Clones Transfected with H-2b Genes

L-D^6 clone R-1	$1.0 \pm 0.1 \times 10^5$ (mean $\pm$ SD)
L-K^b clone G	$2.2 \pm 0.3 \times 10^5$
L-IA^b clone 1-C	$7.7 \pm 1.8 \times 10^5$

TABLE 3. Survival of C57BL/10 (H-2b) Hearts Transplanted into C3H (H-2k) Recipients after Pretreatment of Recipient with Donor-Specific Whole Blood (0.25 ml) or Transfected L Cells 14 Days Before Transplantation[a]

Antigen Pretreatment	N	Mean Survival Days (Range)
Nil	6	9.2 (8–10)
C57 blood	14	34.2 (13–72)
10^7 L cells	7	9.8 (9–11)
10^7 L-D^b cells	6	14.3 (9–18)
5×10^6 L-K^b cells	12	45.2 (9– >100)
10^6 L-IA^b cells	13	19.6 (10–44)

[a] The results for the optimal doses of antigen are given.

recipients prolonged the survival of a renal allograft from the same strain as the blood donor[16] (TABLE 4).

After transplantation of a renal allograft to the transfused recipient there is a significant cellular infiltration demonstrable in the transplanted kidney, comparable with that in an untreated recipient, but despite this, rejection does not occur and these grafts survive indefinitely.[13,25] However, cells extracted from the graft by collagenase digestion produce donor-specific lysis of lymph node con A blasts.[13] The absence of rejection in spite of the presence of these donor specific cytotoxic cells was shown not to be due to the lack of expression of target, MHC antigens in the transplanted organ, as the nonrejecting kidneys in the transfused recipients expressed increased amounts of class I and II MHC antigens, at least as much as that expressed in rejecting kidneys implanted in untreated rats.[24]

To explore this observation further we have investigated the role of the IL-2 pathway. The results from these experiments may be summarised as follows:[14,44]

a) The cell surface expression of high affinity IL-2 receptors was reduced in the infiltrating cells isolated from the graft of the tolerant animals.

b) Cells retrieved from the tolerated grafts responded poorly to recombinant IL-2 *in vitro*, and were not able to produce biologically active IL-2 when stimulated with donor alloantigen.

c) Administration of recombinant IL-2 to transfused animals *in vivo* immediately following transplantation-abrogated tolerance allowing rejection of the renal allografts to occur (TABLE 5).

TABLE 4. The Survival of LEW Kidneys in Lightly Irradiated (200 rads) DA Rats following the Adoptive Transfer of Purified Lymphocyte Subpopulations Prepared from Thoracic Duct Lymph (TDL) of DA Rats 7 Days after a Single Transfusion of LEW Blood[a]

Adoptively Transferred TDL Cells	Transferred No. of Cells	N	Median Survival
T cells	4.25×10^7	5	>100
CD4$^+$ T cells	2.5×10^7	5	>100
CD8$^+$ T cells	4.0×10^6	5	13
CD8$^+$ T cells	1.6×10^7	4	12

[a] PVG renal allografts (specificity controls) did not show prolonged survival.

These results suggest that following renal transplantation in a rat which has been rendered tolerant of the allograft by a donor-specific transfusion, there is altered regulation of the IL-2 pathway in the induction phase of the immune response to the graft, such that the aggressor response, responsible for graft destruction seen in the untreated animal, is suppressed.

Mechanism for Maintenance of Tolerance following Antigen Pretreatment

We have shown previously that rats tolerant of a renal allograft following pretreatment with blood appear to have a normal response in the popliteal node GVH assay.[25] Furthermore, in the maintenance phase the tolerant state cannot be abrogated by the injection of syngeneic lymphocytes.[26,27] In general it is not possible to adoptively transfer suppression with serum from the tolerant rats.[25] However, it is possible to transfer unresponsiveness with the IV transfer of splenocytes from tolerant recipients bearing long surviving grafts, to either untreated (mouse model) or lightly irradiated (200 rads) recipients (rat model).[11,25,26]

Antigen Pretreatment under Cover of Anti-CD4 MAB Treatment

Treatment of an allograft recipient with anti-CD4 mab at the time of transplantation results in prolonged survival of skin allografts and indefinite survival of vascularised organ allografts.[28-30] However the immunodepression produced in the first instance, although profound, is immunologically nonspecific.[29,31] In contrast antigen pretreatment produces unresponsiveness that is immunologically specific but it is not a particularly potent form of immunosuppression.[11] B cell tolerance to soluble antigens has been produced in mice by pretreatment with soluble antigen under an umbrella of anti-CD4 mab treatment.[32,33] Based on this protocol we explored the possibility of inducing T cell tolerance to a vascularised organ allograft by pretreatment with donor MHC antigen at the same time as the administration of an anti-CD4 mab.[31,34]

To induce specific unresponsiveness, 2 doses of YTS191.1 (50 g) was given IV to a C3H recipient 27 and 28 days before implantation of a heterotopic C57BL/10 cardiac allograft. The second dose of antibody was combined with a transfusion of 0.25 ml of blood from a C57BL/10 donor. This protocol produced indefinite survival of the cardiac allograft in antigen-specific fashion. Administration of the mab alone or blood transfusion alone 28 days before a cardiac allograft had little or no

TABLE 5. DA Rats Transfused with PVG Blood 7 Days before Transplantation of a PVG Kidney[a]

Daily Dose of rIL-2[b]	N	Survival (Days)
60×10^4	9	10 ($\times$ 4), 11 ($\times$ 3), 34, >100
30×10^4	8	11 ($\times$ 3), 12 ($\times$ 5)
15×10^4	8	14, >100 ($\times$ 7)
7.5×10^4	8	12, 13 ($\times$ 4), 16, >100 ($\times$ 2)
Buffer	6	>100 ($\times$ 6)

[a] On the day of transplantation and for the following 5 days the recipients were given intraperitoneal injections of recombinant IL-2 generously donated by Cetus Corporation.
[b] International units.

TABLE 6. Induction of Tolerance by Treatment with a Combination of Anti-CD4 MAB (50 μg) and C57BL/10 Donor-Specific Blood Transfusion (0.25 ml) 27 and 28 Days before Transplantation of a C57BL/10 Heart into a C3H Recipient[a]

Pretreatment (Days −28 & −27)	N	Median Survival	(Range)
Nil	4	10	(8–12)
C57BL/10 blood	6	16	(7–71)
YTS191.1	7	13	(8– >100)
C57BL/10 blood + YTS191.1	5	100	(>100– >100)

[a] Pretreatment with blood or mab alone did not result in tolerance.

effect on graft survival (TABLE 6). The dose of mab was important in that lower (10 g) and higher (150 g) doses were much less effective (data not shown). Animals tolerant of C57BL/10 cardiac allografts accepted C57BL/10 skin allografts while promptly rejecting Balb/c allografts and were thus truly tolerant.[34]

Analysis of the lymphoid compartments of mice treated with anti-CD4 mab showed that by 28 days after treatment CD4[+] cells were at least 50% restored.[34] Thus complete elimination of the CD4[+] T cells is not necessary for the induction of tolerance. Furthermore recipients were immunocompetent despite partial depletion of the CD4[+] population; heart grafts transplanted at least 28 days after mab treatment alone were rejected.[31,34]

DISCUSSION

The studies briefly reviewed in this paper confirm that tolerance to a vascularised organ allograft can be produced by pretreatment with antigen, in a variety of forms, in adult rodents.[5,11,17,19–24,35–37] It is of interest that antigen pretreatment in a form that produces long-lasting survival of a vascularised organ allograft will only produce a modest prolongation of survival of a skin allograft. This difference in the behaviour of two different types of allograft, one vascularised and one not, remains unexplained but presumably is related to the different route of presentation of antigen by the graft itself.

Not only does pretreatment with whole blood produce tolerance to a renal allograft in the rat, but also pretreatment with erythrocytes, lymphocytes and platelets will also all produce specific suppression and tolerance.[5,17,36,37] As pretreatment with whole blood in clinical practice does present the risk of sensitisation which could preclude a subsequent renal transplant, attention has been directed at pretreatment with class I MHC antigen only, which in general will not produce sensitisation and may induce specific immunodepression. This was shown to be the case some time ago with platelet pretreatment in the rat model[38] and has been confirmed in our own studies by the use of both platelets and highly purified erythrocytes in which contamination with lymphocytes was minimal.[17,37] Furthermore, we were able to show that pretreatment with either hepatocytes, which again express only class I MHC antigen, or purified membrane class I antigen in the form of protein micelles, would also produce tolerance to a subsequent renal allograft.[20,35] These studies investigating the requirements for antigen-induced tolerance were further extended in the murine experiments in which the recipient was pretreated with syngeneic cells transfected with donor MHC class I or class II antigens. The data obtained showed that a single MHC class I or class II gene product would produce specific immunodepression and prolonged survival of a subsequent cardiac allograft.[11] How a single gene product can produce specific immunodepression of the response to a subsequent cardiac allograft which is incompatible for the whole MHC and multiple minor histocompatibility antigens remains unexplained, but these experiments do provide a rational explanation for the clinical observation that a few random blood transfusions before transplantation does improve graft survival.

Examination of the immunological status of the rodent pretreated with blood, at least in the strain combinations used in our studies, revealed the presence, both *in vitro* and *in vivo*, of a CD4$^+$ T suppressor cell population which appeared transiently within the spleen on day 3, but thereafter was found only in the thoracic duct lymph.[16,22,23]

Following transplantation of a kidney in these rats there is a cellular infiltration and a marked induction of both MHC class I and class II expression in the renal parenchyma of the graft (suggesting that there must be a considerable release of some cytokines, especially interferon-gamma).[13,24] If lymphocytes are extracted from the kidney, a level of donor-specific cytotoxicity can be demonstrated which is similar to, or in some strain combinations greater than, that seen in lymphocytes extracted from rejecting grafts.[13] Thus, tolerance exists despite the presence of cells reactive with the donor alloantigen.

Investigation of the IL-2 pathway in these graft-infiltrating leucocytes has shown that these cells proliferate poorly in response to IL-2, do not produce functional IL-2 when stimulated with donor antigen and have lower expression of high affinity IL-2 receptors on the cell surface.[14,44] All of this suggests an altered regulation of the IL-2 pathway in the first few days after transplantation. Final confirmation of this is provided by the demonstration that the administration of recombinant IL-2 on the day of transplantation and daily thereafter for 5 days will result in a reversal of tolerance as demonstrated by the rejection of a renal allograft in animals pretreated with whole blood.[14,44] These results are certainly not compatible with a mechanism of clonal deletion, but would be consistent with the induction of clonal anergy in antigen-pretreated recipients in the induction phase of the response immediately following transplantation. Of relevance in this context is the recent demonstration that tolerance to antigens expressed outside the thymus seems to be due to anergy within the autoreactive population also possibly related to altered regulation of the IL-2 pathway.[39,40]

The maintenance of this tolerant state in recipients with long-surviving grafts also does not appear to be due either to clonal deletion, for transfer of syngeneic lymphocytes does not break the tolerant state and the lymphocytes of these long surviving animals have a normal popliteal node GVH response.[25,27] Furthermore, failure to transfer suppression with serum from these animals tends to exclude the presence of blocking factors including anti-idiotypic antibodies.[25] However, as it is possible to transfer tolerance by the adoptive transfer of splenocytes from these long surviving mice or rats bearing cardiac or renal allografts, an active regulatory mechanism involving suppressor cells is suggested.[25,26] The anxiety about using adoptive transfer experiments to demonstrate suppressor T cells is that a modified recipient, *e.g.,* one treated with 200 rads irradiation, is usually needed to demonstrate a strong effect of the transferred T cells.[26] Nevertheless, in our cardiac allograft model in the mouse transfer of splenocytes into naive untreated syngeneic mice will result in marked prolongation of survival of a cardiac allograft.[41]

Thus we have demonstrated in two different experimental models that antigen pretreatment in the form of whole blood, or with cells expressing a single MHC gene product, may produce tolerance to a subsequent organ allograft. In rats which have received a single donor-specific transfusion we have demonstrated the presence of a CD4[+] T cell population present in the thoracic duct lymph immediately before transplantation which is capable of transferring unresponsiveness,[22] while immediately after transplantation there appears to be an altered regulation of the IL-2 pathway within the leucocytes infiltrating the grafts of the tolerant recipients.[14,44] Finally, the maintenance phase of the response, 50–100 days after transplantation, appears to be associated with an active form of suppression, and suppressor T cells (generally of the CD8[+] phenotype) adoptively transfer the suppression into syngeneic recipients.[25,26]

However, as yet we have no further information about the interaction of the 3 phases of antigen-induced tolerance to a vascularised organ allograft that we have described in adult recipients. There is no doubt that the phenomenon of suppressor T cells can be demonstrated in these allograft models, but scepticism quite rightly exists because no separate T suppressor cell population has been detected, and T suppressor cells have not yet been cloned. It would seem unlikely that there is a separate cell population that gives rise to suppressor T cells, but a plausible explanation for these findings is that T cells given certain signals in the right environment might behave as suppressor cells when explored in adoptive transfer models. At the moment, until the signals which trigger this event can be characterised this explanation remains purely speculative. But the demonstration of an altered regulation of the IL-2 pathway indicates that at least one signal needed for proliferation of the graft infiltrating leucocytes and production of an aggressor response responsible for the destruction of the allograft is missing. No doubt other signals may be suppressed or enhanced as a result of antigen pretreatment and transplantation and these combined with the altered regulation of the IL-2 pathway result in the inhibition of the whole cascade of the allograft response and, as a result, indefinite graft survival.

Finally, the confirmation that T cell tolerance, which appears to be highly specific, can be produced by pretreatment with anti-CD4 monoclonal antibody together with antigen some weeks before transplantation of a cardiac allograft in mice, points the way towards the development of protocols which might have clinical application in the future. That antigen-induced tolerance to a vascularised organ allograft can be produced in the adult by treatment before transplantation and with different protocols explored elsewhere, *e.g.*, post-transplant treatment with ALG and bone marrow,[42,43] encourages one to feel that this phenomenon can be reproduced clinically once the mechanisms by which tolerance is induced and maintained are better understood.

REFERENCES

1. BILLINGHAM, R. E., L. BRENT & P. B. MEDAWAR. 1953. Actively acquired tolerance of foreign cells. Nature **172:** 603–606.
2. BRENT, L., J. HANSEN, P. KILSHAW & A. THOMAS. 1973. Specific unresponsiveness to skin allografts in mice. 1. Properties of tissue extracts and their synergistic effects with anti-lymphocyte serum. Transplantation **15:** 160–171.
3. MORRIS, P. J., A. TING & J. STOCKER. 1968. Leucocyte antigens in renal transplantation. The paradox of blood transfusion in renal transplantation. Med. J. Aust. **2:** 1088–1090.
4. FABRE, J., S. LIM & P. J. MORRIS. 1971. Renal transplantation in the rat: details of a technique. Aust. N.Z. J. Sur. **41:** 69–75.

5. FABRE, J. W. & P. J. MORRIS. 1972. The effect of donor strain blood pretreatment on renal allograft rejection in rats. Transplantation 14: 608–617.
6. FABRE, J. 1982. Specific immunosuppression. In Tissue Transplantation. P. J. Morris, Ed. Churchill Livingstone. Edinburgh.
7. OPELZ, G. & P. I. TERASAKI. 1974. Poor kidney transplant survival in recipients with frozen-blood transfusions or no transfusions. Lancet 2: 696–698.
8. SALVATIERRA, O., F. VINCENTI & W. AMEND. 1983. Four year experience with donor-specific blood transfusions. Transplant. Proc. 15: 924–931.
9. CORRY, R. J., H. J. WINN & P. S. RUSSELL. 1973. Primarily vascularized allografts of hearts in mice: the role of H-2D, H-2k, and non H-2 antigens in rejection. Transplantation 16: 343–350.
10. SUPERINA, R. A., W. N. PEUGH, K. J. WOOD & P. J. MORRIS. 1985. Assessment of primarily vascularised cardiac allografts in mice. Transplantation 42: 226–227.
11. MADSEN, J. C., R. A. SUPERINA, K. J. WOOD & P. J. MORRIS. 1988. Immunological unresponsiveness induced by recipient cells transfected with donor MHC genes. Nature 332: 161–164.
12. MASON, D. & P. J. MORRIS. 1984. Inhibition of the accumulation in rat kidney allografts of specific but not non-specific cytotoxic cells by cyclosporine. Transplantation 37: 46–51.
13. DALLMAN, M. J., K. J. WOOD & P. J. MORRIS. 1987. Specific cytotoxic T cells are not found in the non-rejected kidneys of blood transfused rats. J. Exp. Med. 165: 566–571.
14. DALLMAN, M. J., K. J. WOOD & P. J. MORRIS. 1989. Recombinant interleukin-2 (IL-2) can reverse the blood transfusion effect. Transplant. Proc. 21: 1165–1167.
15. COBBOLD, S. P., A. JAYASURIYA, A. NASH, T. D. PROSPERO & H. WALDMANN. 1984. Therapy with monoclonal antibodies by elimination of T cell subsets in vivo. Nature 312: 548–551.
16. QUIGLEY, R. L., K. J. WOOD & P. J. MORRIS. 1989. Mediation of antigen-induced suppression of renal allograft rejection by a CD4 (W3/25+) T cell. Transplantation 47: 684–688.
17. WOOD, K. J., J. EVINS & P. J. MORRIS. 1985. Suppression of renal allograft rejection in the rat by class I antigen on purified erythrocytes. Transplantation 39: 56–62.
18. HUTCHINSON, I. V. & P. J. MORRIS. 1986. The role of major and minor histocompatibility antigens in active enhancement of rat kidney allograft survival by blood transfusion. Transplantation 41: 166–170.
19. PEUGH, W. N., K. J. WOOD & P. J. MORRIS. 1987. The importance of sharing major histocompatibility complex and minor antigens between blood and graft donors in the blood transfusion effect. Transplant. Proc. 19: 744–745.
20. FOSTER, S., D. CRANSTON, K. J. WOOD & P. J. MORRIS. 1987. Pretreatment with viable and non-viable haptocytes or liver membrane extracts produces indefinite renal allograft survival in the rat. Transplantation 45: 228–231.
21. CRANSTON, D., K. J. WOOD, N. CARTER & P. J. MORRIS. 1986. Pretreatment with lymphocyte subpopulations and renal allograft survival in the rat. Transplantation 43: 809–813.
22. QUIGLEY, R. L., K. J. WOOD & P. J. MORRIS. 1989. Transfusion induces blood-donor specific suppressor cells. J. Immunol. 142: 463–470.
23. QUIGLEY, R. L., K. J. WOOD & P. J. MORRIS. 1989. Mediation of the induction of immunologic unresponsiveness following antigen pretreatment by a CD4 (W3/25+) T cell appearing transiently in the splenic compartment and subsequently in the TDL. Transplantation 47: 689–697.
24. WOOD, K. J., A. HOPLEY, M. DALLMAN & P. J. MORRIS. 1987. Donor major histocompatibility antigens are induced on non-rejected renal allografts in transfused rats. Transplantation 42: 759–767.
25. FABRE, J. W. & P. J. MORRIS. 1972. The mechanism of specific immunosuppression of renal allograft rejection by donor strain blood. Transplantation 14: 634–640.
26. HUTCHINSON, I. V. 1986. Suppressor T cells in allogeneic models. Transplantation 41: 547–555.

27. BOWEN, J. E., J. R. BATCHELOR, M. E. FRENCH, H. BURGESS & J. W. FABRE. 1974. Failure of adoptive immunization or parabiosis with hyperimmune syngeneic partners to abrogate long-term enhancement of rat kidney allografts. Transplantation **18:** 322–327.

28. COBBOLD, S. & H. WALDMANN. 1986. Skin allograft rejection by L3T4+ and LYT-2+ T cell subsets. Transplantation **41:** 634–639.

29. MADSEN, J. C., W. N. PEUGH, K. J. WOOD & P. J. MORRIS. 1987. The effect of anti-L3T4 monoclonal antibody on first-set rejection of murine cardiac allografts. Transplantation **44:** 849–852.

30. MOTTRAM, P. L., J. WHEELAHAN, I. F. C. MCKENZIE & G. J. A. CLUNIE. 1987. Murine cardiac allograft survival following treatment of recipients with monoclonal anti-L3T4 or LY-2 antibodies. Transplant. Proc. **19**(2): 2898–2901.

31. PEARSON, T. C., J. C. MADSEN, P. J. MORRIS & K. J. WOOD. 1990. The induction of transplantation tolerance using donor antigen and anti-CD4 monoclonal antibody. Transplant. Proc. **22:** 1955–1956.

32. WOFSY, D., D. C. MAYES, J. WOODCOCK & W. E. SEAMAN. 1985. Inhibition of humoral immunity *in vivo* by monoclonal antibody to L3T4: studies with soluble antigens in intact mice. J. Immunol. **135:** 1698–1701.

33. BENJAMIN, R. J. & H. WALDMANN. 1986. Induction of tolerance by monoclonal antibody therapy. Nature **320:** 449–451.

34. PEARSON, T., J. MADSEN, P. J. MORRIS & K. J. WOOD. 1991. The induction of transplantation tolerance using donor antigen and anti-CD4 monoclonal antibody. Transplant. Proc. **23:** 565–566.

35. FOSTER, S., K. J. WOOD & P. J. MORRIS. 1989. Comparison of the effect of protein micelles containing purified class I MHC antigen and a cytostolic preparation containing water soluble class I molecules on rat renal allograft survival. Transplant. Proc. **21:** 375–376.

36. HIBBERD, A. & L. SCOTT. 1983. Allogeneic platelets increase survival of rat renal allografts. Transplantation **35:** 622–624.

37. WOOD, K. J. & P. J. MORRIS. 1985. The blood transfusion effect: suppression of renal allograft rejection in the rat using purified blood components. Transplant. Proc. **17:** 2419–2420.

38. WELSH, K., H. BURGOS & J. BATCHELOR. 1977. The immune response to allogeneic rat platelets (Ag-B) antigens in matrix form lacking Ia. Eur. J. Immunol. **7:** 267–272.

39. RAMMENSEE, H. G., R. KROSCHEWSKI & B. FRANGOULIS. 1989. Clonal anergy induced in mature $V\beta6^+$ T lymphocytes on immunizing M1S-1^b mice with M1S-1^a expressing cells. Nature **339:** 541–544.

40. MORAHAN, G., J. ALLISON & J. F. A. P. MILLER. 1989. Tolerance of class I histocompatibility antigens expressed extra thymically. Nature **339:** 622–624.

41. SUPERINA, R. A., K. J. WOOD & P. J. MORRIS. 1987. Class I antigen pretreatment prolongs allograft survival in mice by induction of suppressor cells. Transplant. Proc. **19:** 3459–3460.

42. WOOD, M. L. & A. P. MONACO. 1984. Induction of unresponsiveness to skin allografts in adult mice disparate at defined regions of the H-2 complex. II. Effect of donor-specific bone marrow in ALS-treated mice. Transplantation **37:** 35–39.

43. BARBER, W. H. 1990. Induction of tolerance to human renal allografts with bone marrow and antilymphocyte globulin. Transplant. Rev. **4:** 68–78.

44. DALLMAN, M. J., O. SHIHO, T. H. PAGE, K. J. WOOD & P. J. MORRIS. 1991. Peripheral tolerance to alloantigen results from altered regulation of the interleukin 2 pathway. J. Exp. Med. **173:** 79–87.

Antigen-Specific Immunoregulation and Autoimmune Thyroiditis[a]

NOEL R. ROSE AND EYAL TALOR

The Johns Hopkins School of Hygiene and Public Health
Department of Immunology and Infectious Diseases
615 North Wolfe Street
Baltimore, Maryland 21205

INTRODUCTION

It is still problematical to explain the basis for unresponsiveness to self-antigens.[1] Recent evidence directly supports Burnet's original concept of clonal deletion.[2] T cells capable of reacting with prominent self-antigens, such as Mls and I-E, are eliminated almost entirely in the thymus.[3] Such deletional mechanisms, however, do not affect self-antigens that do not occur in the thymus.[4] By definition organ-specific antigens are restricted to a particular organ. They may not circulate at all or may be present in the blood stream in small amounts only.[5] Autoimmune responses to organ-specific antigens can be induced relatively easily by experimental immunization.[6] Indeed, many of the most prevalent autoimmune diseases result from autoimmune responses to organ-specific antigens.[7]

Experimental thyroiditis offers an ideal model for the study of organ-specific autoimmunity.[8–10] With the appropriate adjuvant, it can be instigated in a variety of animals by immunization with thyroglobulin (Tg). It occurs spontaneously in genetically selected strains such as the OS chicken and BUF rat.[11,12] The counterpart human disease, chronic thyroiditis, is associated with an autoimmune response to Tg.[13,14]

A decade ago, one of us reviewed the evidence that T cell regulation is critical in the induction of autoimmune thyroiditis in animals.[15] A triad of T-cell-based regulatory activities was defined at that time. Helper T cells are required for the initiation of autoimmune thyroiditis in both spontaneous and experimental forms of the disease. Tg recognition is regulated by a class II MHC immune response gene, Ir-Tg, located at I-A. Finally, suppressor T cells may occur naturally or may be stimulated by raised levels of native, nonaggregated Tg.[15] In addition, effector T cells, associated with class I MHC control, determine the severity of thyroid lesions in the presence of good responder Ir-Tg genes. It was suggested that self-tolerance to Tg is based not on elimination of Tg-specific T cells, but rather on the balance of helper and suppressor T-cell responses in given situations. This concept, referred to as clonal balance, emphasizes the importance of the ratio among the T-cell populations that promote the autoimmune response and those that control it.[16]

Neonatal thymectomy of OS chickens and BUF rats increases the severity of spontaneous thyroiditis, suggesting that the thymus is a source of cells that can dampen the autoimmune response.[17] It was found later that the injection of soluble, nonaggregated mouse Tg (MTg) without adjuvant into mice prevents the

[a] This study was supported by Public Health Service–National Institutes of Health research grant #AR31632.

induction of experimental thyroiditis.[18] The timing and dosage of antigen used in these experiments are critical, but under proper conditions, unresponsiveness could be maintained for at least 30 days. The effect was antigen-specific. Furthermore, the unresponsive state could be transferred to syngeneic recipients using thymus or spleen cells of the nonresponsive mice.[19] These findings suggested that an antigen-specific regulatory T-cell population was activated by treatment with soluble antigen.

Since previous investigations pointed to an important role for the thymus in regulating both spontaneous and induced forms of thyroiditis, it was decided to examine the thymus for evidence of regulatory T cells.[20] In order to simplify the experiments and permit quantitation of the effects, an *in vitro* system was used for measuring the actions of regulatory T-cell populations.[21] The test depends upon the ability of the T cells of immunized mice to inhibit secretion of Tg-specific autoantibody by syngeneic B cells. The method is based on the procedure developed by Richter and Talor for the study of antibody formation in rabbits.[22–24]

MATERIALS AND METHODS

All the animal experiments described here adhered to or exceeded good laboratory practice standards.

Preparation of Mouse Thyroglobulin

Swiss mice (Jackson Laboratories, Bar Harbor, ME) were killed by ether overdose and cervical dislocation. The trachea and larynx were exposed for removal of the thyroid gland. The thyroid was immersed in cold borate-buffered saline, pH 8.2, homogenized and filtered through sterile gauze. The filtrate was centrifuged at 3,000 g for 30 minutes at 4°C and the pellet was discarded. The supernatant was further centrifuged at 100,000 g for 60 minutes at 4°C. The supernatant collected was separated on a sizing column (Sepharose CL/4B200, Sigma, St. Louis, MO); the fractions containing MTg were collected and dialyzed overnight against physiological saline solution. The MTg was stored in aliquots at −80°C until used.

Preparation of Antibody-Secreting Cells

Antibody-secreting cells were produced by immunizing CBA/J mice with intravenous injections of 40 µg MTg plus 20 µg *Salmonella* lipopolysaccharide (LPS, Difco Laboratories, Detroit, MI). At five days the mice were killed and the spleen removed. A mononuclear splenic cell suspension was then prepared. Control mice were immunized with stromal antigens of sheep red blood cells, SSSF (10^8 SRBC equivalents). In some experiments different inbred strains of mice were tested for the induction of antibody-secreting cells.

Preparation of Regulatory Cells

CBA/J mice were injected intravenously with 40 µg or 100 µg MTg without adjuvant or with SSSF (10^9 SRBC equivalents). In some experiments different inbred strains of mice were tested for the induction of regulatory cells. The animals were killed at various times after injection as indicated in the individual protocols and mononuclear cell suspensions prepared from the thymus and spleen. The mononuclear cells were then tested for their ability to suppress the antibody production by the antibody-secreting syngeneic spleen cells. For that purpose, target B cells were incubated with either splenocyte or thymocyte suspensions at various ratios for 4 hours at 37°C in 5% CO_2 and air, prior to their incorporation into the ELISA plaque assay.

ELISA Plaque Assay for the Detection of MTg Antibody-Secreting Cells

Multiwell plates (COSTAR 3524 24 well, Cambridge, MA) were coated with 5 μg MTg per well in a bicarbonate/carbonate buffer, pH 9.6, and kept overnight at 2–4°C in a dark humid chamber. The wells were washed three times with phosphate-buffered saline-Tween 20 (PBS-T), and twice with PBS alone. The coating and washing of the wells were repeated three times. Five tenths ml of the mononuclear cell suspension, 5×10^5 cells per well, were pipetted into the MTg-coated and washed wells, and incubated for one hour at 37°C, 5% CO_2 in air, to allow secretion and binding of antibodies to the antigen. The plates were then drained and washed three times with PBS-T, followed by washing twice with PBS alone. Affinity-purified goat anti-mouse IgG or IgM (Sigma) in a 1 : 500 dilution in PBS-T with 1% bovine serum albumin (BSA) was added to each well (0.5 ml). The plates were then incubated in the dark for 1.5 hours at 37°C or for 18–24 hours at room temperature. The plates were washed as above and 0.5 ml of the chromogen (5 bromo- 4 chloro-3 indolyl-phosphate, Sigma) in a 2 amino- 2-methyl- 1-propionyl-(AMP) buffer solution (Sigma), pH 8.25 in a 36°C gelling agarose (Type I, Sigma), 0.6% final concentration was added to each well. The plates were left at room temperature for 10 minutes for the agarose to gel. They were then incubated at 37°C for 2 hours to allow the development of the dark blue spots that indicate the presence of antibody-secreting cells. The plaques were counted under an inverted microscope at 150X and expressed as the number of antibody-secreting cells per 10^6 splenic mononuclear cells.

Specific Immunoabsorption

Thymic mononuclear cells were obtained from mice injected intravenously with MTg or SSSF 10 days previously or from normal, uninjected, mice. The thymocytes were first panned on uncoated 6-well plastic plates (Nunc, Microbiological Associates, Gaithersburg, MD) to clear them of nonspecific adherent cells. They were then collected and plated on 6-well plastic plates previously coated with 10 μg MTg per well. The adherent cell population was collected by treating the plates with 1% lidocaine solution in RPMI-1640. The cells were then washed three times with RPMI-1640 and panned again on uncoated 12-well plastic plates (Nunc) to clear the suspension of any residual nonspecific adherent cells. The cells in the supernatant were collected and resuspended to the desired concentration in RPMI-1640.

In some experiments, to further ensure the absence of B cells or macrophages, the MTg adherent thymus cell suspension was treated with monoclonal antibodies Mac-1 and Mac-3 plus complement (guinea pig serum). The suspensions were incubated for 18 hours at 37°C in 5% CO_2 to allow the development of phagocytic cells. As an additional precaution, the suspensions were treated with carbonyl iron and the phagocytic cells discarded. B cells were removed by treatment with anti-Ig in the presence of guinea pig complement. In some experiments, the residual T cells were further treated with anti-L3T4 and anti-Lyt-1 and complement to clear them of T-helper cells.

Antibodies for T-Cell Phenotyping

Nine different affinity-purified monoclonal antibodies were obtained commercially. They included antibodies to Thy 1.2, Lyt-1 Lyt-2, L3T4 (Becton Dickinson, Mt. View, CA), Mac-1, Mac-3, Ia, Ig, (Boehringer Mannheim Biochemicals), and asialo-GM-1 (Wako Pure Chemical Industries, Ltd. Osaka, Japan). Antimurine CD3 was kindly provided by Dr. Drew Pardol, Johns Hopkins University, Baltimore, Maryland. The conjugates used for immunofluorescence were goat anti-rat or goat anti-mouse FITC (Cappel-Organon Technika), and goat anti-hamster phycoerythrin (Dr. Pardol).

Flow Cytometric Analysis

Flow cytometric analysis was performed by staining the cells with fluorescein-conjugated affinity-purified monoclonal antibodies and by passing them through an argon-excited laser (Becton-Dickinson, CA). The cells were analyzed for size by forward angle light scatter as well as for fluorescent activity. All measurements were gaited to adjust for autofluorescence and dead cells. The results presented in the text represent triple experiments.

RESULTS

Induction and Specificity of Regulatory T Cells

In order to demonstrate the presence of immunoregulatory cells in the thymus, groups of 5 CBA/J mice were injected intravenously with an aqueous solution of MTg (without adjuvant) at either of two dose levels, 100 μg or 40 μg, or with MTg in combination with LPS or with LPS alone. The mice were killed 10 days later and their thymus cell suspensions tested for their ability to inhibit antibody secretion by syngeneic spleen cells from mice immunized 5 days previously with MTg plus LPS. The results are summarized in FIGURE 1.

A marked inhibition of MTg antibody secretion by syngeneic spleen cells occurred when these cells were incubated with thymocytes from mice injected intravenously with MTg alone at either dose level. In contrast, mice injected with control LPS showed only a weak ability to inhibit antibody secretion. Interestingly, mice injected with MTg plus LPS showed marginal inhibition, suggesting that LPS interferes with the generation of the regulatory T cells. Other control experiments (not shown) indicated that antibody-secreting cells were not found in the thymus of any of the mice at the times indicated.

The next series of experiments was carried out to determine the point of time at which regulatory T cells appear in the thymus after injection of 40 μg of soluble MTg. The results of three such experiments have been combined and are pre-

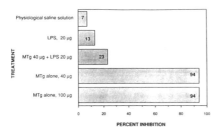

FIGURE 1. Inhibition of thyroglobulin autoantibody production by thymus cells. CBA/J mice were immunized intravenously with 40 µg MTg + 20 µg LPS and killed five days later. The spleen was removed and the cells mixed with thymus cells from CBA/J mice treated nine days previously as described. The inhibition by thymic cells compared with medium alone is based on three separate experiments.

sented in FIGURE 2. As the figure illustrates, significant suppression of MTg antibody is produced by thymus cells 9–16 days after administration of antigen. By days 18–21, loss of inhibitory ability occurs.

To examine the specificity of suppression, CBA/J mice were injected intravenously with either MTg (40 µg) or SSSF (10^9 SRBC equivalents) and tested with spleen cells from mice immunized with MTg plus LPS or with SSSF. The results are shown in FIGURE 3. The thymus cells from mice injected with soluble MTg markedly inhibited the secretion of MTg antibody. In contrast, little or no inhibition was produced by thymus cells from mice given SSSF. In the opposite experiment, thymus cells from SSSF-injected mice were able to inhibit the production of antibody to SSSF, whereas thymus cells from MTg-injected mice produced no such inhibition.

A further time course experiment was carried out to compare the presence of regulatory cells in the thymus and the spleen. The results are given in FIGURE 4. As noted previously, the maximum inhibitory activity was found when thymus cell suspensions were taken 9–16 days after injection of the soluble MTg. Less marked inhibitory activity was found earlier (days 5–7) and later (days 18–21). On the other hand, when spleen cell suspensions were used, inhibitory activity was first found on days 14–16 and was greatest on days 18–21 after injection. No significant inhibition was found with spleen cells taken 36 days after injection. These findings imply, but do not prove, that the regulatory T cells are generated first in the thymus and then migrate to the spleen. More direct evidence supporting this hypothesis has been reported by Richter and associates who used a similar experimental method in the rabbit.[25]

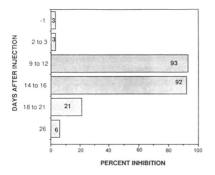

FIGURE 2. Time course of regulatory cells in thymus after injection of 40 µg MTg alone. Methods are the same as described in FIGURE 1.

FIGURE 3. Antigenic specificity of thymus-derived regulatory cells. Thymus cells were taken from mice injected 9–12 days previously with 40 μg MTg or SSSF (10⁹ SRBC equivalents) and treated with spleen cells from mice immunized with MTg-LPS or SRBC.

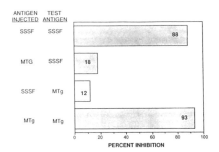

Special note should be taken of the results obtained with spleen cells on days 2 and 3. A marginal level of inhibition (34%) was obtained at this time using syngeneic target cells from animals injected with MTg plus LPS. Similar inhibition was found, however, with target cells from mice immunized with SSSF, indicating that the short-lived suppression detected at this time was not antigen specific.

Separation and Phenotypic Properties of Regulatory T Cells

In view of the antigen specificity of the thymus-derived regulatory T cells, experiments were undertaken to separate them by positive selection. For this purpose, plastic plates were coated with MTg or with SSSF and the thymus cell suspensions allowed to attach to the antigen-coated plates. The nonadherent cells in the supernatant were removed while the adherent cells were released by lidocaine treatment. The two fractions were then tested separately for their ability to suppress the production of antibody to MTg or to SSSF. The results are given in TABLE 1. The thymus cells adhering to the MTg-coated plastic plates strongly inhibited production of antibody to MTg, but failed to inhibit production of anti-

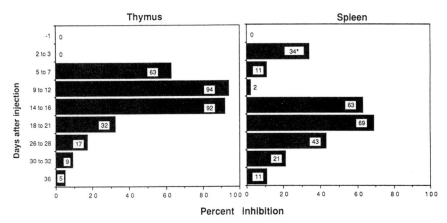

FIGURE 4. Appearance of regulatory cells in the thymus and in the spleen. Methods are the same as described in FIGURE 1. *Non-antigen-specific suppression.

TABLE 1. Adherence of Regulatory Cells to Antigen-Coated Plates

	Percent Inhibition	
Treatment	Anti-MTg	Anti-SSSF
Panned on plastic		
adherent fraction	4	2
supernatant fraction	75	76
Panned on MTg		
adherent fraction	93	10
supernatant fraction	10	88
Panned on SSSF		
adherent fraction	8	97
supernatant fraction	75	4

SSSF. In contrast, thymus cells that adhered to SSSF-coated plates inhibited antibody to SSSF, but not antibody to MTg. This experiment reveals a striking property of the regulatory T cells, namely, their ability to bind to cognate antigen on a plastic surface. These data clearly illustrate the specificity of this binding. The finding permitted us to separate physically the regulatory T cells on the basis of their antigen-binding properties.

The experiments carried out subsequently were undertaken to characterize the T cells responsible for the inhibitory activity observed. The immunoadherent thymus cell population was treated with a panel of antibodies to well-characterized surface markers. As shown in FIGURE 5 anti-Thy-1.2 and anti-Lyt-2 reagents markedly reduced the ability of the thymus cell suspensions to inhibit antibody secretion by spleen cells. No reduction in suppressor activity was evident with antisera to Lyt-1, L3T4, Mac-1 and Mac-3. In addition, anti-Ia antiserum had no effect, suggesting that the T cells did not express this conventional activation marker. Anti-Ig treatment (not shown in the figure) had no ability to reduce the inhibitory effect. Thus, suppression may be attributed to a population of Thy-1$^+$, CD4$^-$, CD8$^+$ T cells.

As another approach to determining the phenotype of the regulatory T-cell population obtained from the thymus of mice injected with soluble MTg, indirect immunofluorescence was carried out with standard typing area. The results are given in TABLE 2. The immunoabsorbed population is clearly depleted of Lyt-1, L3T4, and Asialo-Gm-1$^+$ cells, suggesting the absence of helper T cells and of NK cells. These results reinforce the conclusion that CD8$^+$ cells are the active suppressors.

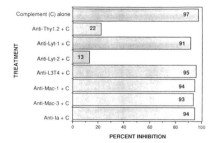

FIGURE 5. Abrogation of inhibitory activity by selected antisera. Methods are the same as described in FIGURE 1.

TABLE 2. Phenotypic Characteristics of Immunoabsorbed Cells

Reagent	Untreated	Immunoabsorbed
Thy1.2	87	90
CD3	53	58
Lyt-1	ND	<1
Lyt-2	45	78
L3T4	29	<1
Asialo GM1	6	<1

Following the assumption that the immunoabsorption procedure described above produces an enrichment in antigen-specific regulatory cells, quantitative experiments were undertaken to measure the proportion of suppressor to target cells required for significant inhibition. The results are given in TABLE 3.

Unseparated thymus cell suspensions produce marked inhibition of antibody synthesis only in a suppressor-to-target ratio of 8:1. In contrast, the adherent thymic cell population inhibits antibody secretion even at a 1:1 ratio. These results then suggest that there is at least an eight-fold enrichment in the regulatory T-cell component of the population.

Additional properties of the thymus-derived regulatory T-cell population were revealed by flow-cytometric analysis (FIG. 6). Ten days after injection of soluble MTg a population of large $Lyt-2^+$ cells appeared in the thymus. Few cells of this type were found in the spleen at that time. On the other hand, on day 26 a similar large Lyt-2 population was seen in the spleen, but not in the thymus. The appearance of this cell population in our experiments corresponds with the presence of an inhibitory cell population in the respective organ. Following this lead, preparative experiments were carried out with the aid of the cell sorter. All of the inhibitory activity of the thymus cell suspension on day 10 after injection was found in the gaited cells, corresponding to the large $Lyt-2^+$ cells illustrated in FIGURE 6. On day 26 the inhibitory activity of the spleen was also found in the large cells in the gaited population. These findings support the view that the regulatory T cells in the thymus and in the spleen are large $Lyt-2^+$ lymphocytes.

Genetic Restriction

Information on the genetic restriction of the thymus-derived regulatory T-cell population using the response to SRBC have been published previously.[26] Experiments were undertaken to determine if these findings apply equally to the MTg-specific regulatory T cells. As TABLE 4 shows, the presence of regulatory T cells differs among various strains, but without any apparent relationship to H-2 haplo-

TABLE 3. Titration of Regulatory Cells before and after Immunoabsorption

Ratio of Suppressors : Targets	Percent Inhibition	
	Untreated	Immunoabsorbed
8:1	92	94
4:1	41	90
2:1	11	84
1:1	4	67

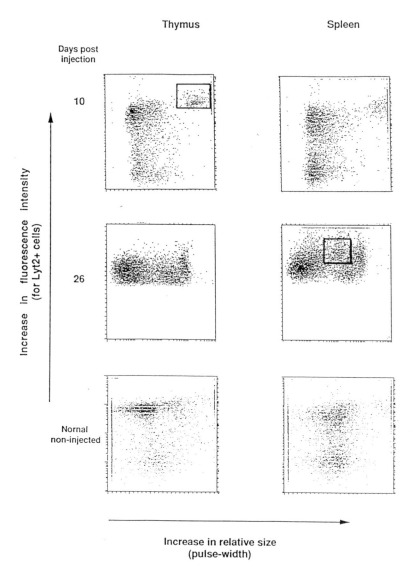

FIGURE 6. FACStar pulse-width dot plot analysis of thymocytes and splenocytes for Lyt2+ cells from mice injected intravenously with MTg thyroglobulin in saline in the absence of adjuvant.

type. A striking finding is the virtual absence of these regulatory cells from the thymus of SJL mice at the time they were studied. This observation correlates with previous reports that this strain of mice is deficient in suppressor cell production.[26,27]

To determine the MHC restriction in the interaction of regulatory T cells with their B-cell targets, checkerboard experiments, such as the one shown in TABLE

TABLE 4. Strain Difference in Thymus-Derived Suppressor Cells

Strain	H-2	Percent Inhibition
CBA/J	k	95
BALB/C	d	90
A/J	a	92
C3H/He	k	87
SJL	s	2

5, were carried out. Surprisingly, complete suppression was observed only when cells of the same inbred strain were mixed. Even mice that were matched at the H-2 region, such as C57BL/10A and CBA/J, were unable to inhibit allogeneic B cells. The results indicate that the cellular interactions necessary for inhibition of antibody secretion depend upon non-H-2 as well as on H-2 congruence.

DISCUSSION

A number of years ago, we emphasized in these *Annals* the important role played by the thymus in the regulation of autoimmune responses.[28] At first, the concept was based on the often cited clinical evidence of thymic abnormality in a number of human autoimmune diseases including myasthenia gravis, Hashimoto's thyroiditis, and systemic lupus erythematosus.[29,30] Experimentally, we showed that neonatal thymectomy leads to a significant increase of thyroid infiltration in two models of spontaneous thyroiditis, the OS chicken and BUF rat.[31,32] Moreover, Kojima[33] and colleagues have clearly shown that thyroiditis can be produced in mice by carefully timed neonatal thymectomy. Penhale and colleagues[34] have induced thyroiditis in rats by a combination of thymectomy and irradiation. The implication of all of these experiments is that the thymus plays a critical role in the prevention of autoimmune disease. It has not, however, been possible to define a particular population of thymus-derived cells that carry out this function. We have now developed a straightforward and quantitative method to assess the ability of thymus-derived cells to regulate autoantibody production. More work is needed to demonstrate whether this population is able to modify the course of autoimmune disease *in vivo*.

The T cells described in this investigation differ from previously reported suppressor cells[35–42] in a number of important aspects. They are, first of all, induced by injection of soluble self-antigen in the absence of adjuvant. When mice are given the same preparation of MTg accompanied by LPS, the inhibitory activity of thymus cell suspensions is markedly reduced. It may be that LPS alters

TABLE 5. Strain Specificity and H-2 Restriction of Suppression

Thymus Cells	Antibody-Secreting Cells Percent Inhibition		
	C57BL/10A(H^k)	C57BL/6(H^b)	CBA/J(H^k)
C57BL/10A	95	22	35
C57BL/6	20	90	9
CBA/J	30	14	98

the mode of antigen presentation, so that the T-cell response differs when antigen is given with adjuvant. In other experiments, we have found that administering MTg with complete Freund's adjuvant, intraperitoneally or subcutaneously, also reduces the production of the regulatory T cells. Perhaps one of the important functions of adjuvant in inducing experimental autoimmune disease is to change the balance of helper and suppressor T cells by altering antigen presentation.

Although the regulatory T cells arise first in the thymus, they appear to migrate to the spleen within 7–10 days. Regulatory activity is never as prominent in the spleen as in the thymus, perhaps because the regulatory T cells are more dilute in peripheral lymphoid organs. It is, however, surprising that inhibition can be demonstrated for as long as 26–28 days after a single intravenous injection of soluble antigen. This finding may indicate that antigen persists in the thymus or that there may be considerable proliferation of the regulatory T-cell population. Support for the notion of antigen persistence may be found in work by Dintzis and colleagues[43] demonstrating the ability of antigen to persist both within cells and on cell surfaces for a prolonged period of time. The antigen specificity of the suppressive effect implies that the T cells are capable of recognizing antigenic determinants by means of an antigen-specific receptor. On that assumption, we initiated experiments to separate the regulatory cells on the basis of their ability to adhere to antigen. To our great surprise the cells were able to bind cognate antigen on plastic surface. We recognize that antigen-presenting cells may be present in the thymic suspensions. Thymic cell suspensions were first incubated on plastic plates to rid them of nonspecific adherent cells followed by incubation on MTg-coated plastic plates. The MTg-adherent cells were removed and treated with anti-Mac-1 anti-Mac-3 and complement as well as anti-Ig and complement. In some experiments, CD4$^+$ T cells were also eliminated by treatment with anti-Lyt-1 and anti-L3T4 and complement. Furthermore, phagocytic cells were removed by treatment with carbonyl iron. Flow cytometric analysis of the thymus cell suspension after each treatment failed to detect cells with surface markers which correspond to the depleted cells (results not shown). The treatment did not reduce the number of Lyt2$^+$ T cells within the limitation of the detecting apparatus (FACScan, Becton-Dickinson). Moreover, the time available for antigen processing and presentation, approximately 1 hour, is limited. Still, we were able to demonstrate binding to cognate antigen on plastic surface. We cannot exclude the possibility that other cells in the thymic suspension, including T cells themselves, might serve as antigen-presenting cells. However, due to treatment, in some experiments of the thymic cell suspensions with anti-Lyt-1 and anti-L3T4, we are forced at this time to conclude that if indeed thymus cells present antigen then they must be either CD4$^-$, CD8$^+$ T cells or CD4$^-$, CD8$^-$ T cells. Moreover, spreading the antigen on a plastic surface may be essential for antigen binding. Studies by Dintzis and colleagues[44] and others[45] have shown that binding of antigen to plastic plates or other surfaces alters the three-dimensional configuration of the antigen, allowing the exposure of antigenic determinants which are sequestered in the native state. It should be noted that these thymus-derived regulatory T cells are induced *in vivo* where optimal conditions for antigen processing, presentation and cellular induction prevail. Thus, it may not be so surprising that the T-cell receptor may recognize an antigenic determinant *in vitro*, to which it has been educated *in vivo*, even in the absence of the appropriate MHC determinant. The antigen binding required for panning is restricted to attachment only and does not involve T-cell activation. No Ia markers were expressed on this adherent regulating cell population. The regulatory T-cell suspensions were tested with monoclonal antibody to the invariant portion of the beta chain of the T-cell receptor. The positive reaction obtained suggested that the T cells express the α-β receptor (results not shown). We conclude inter alia that the ability of the regulatory T cells to adhere to cognate antigen provides an important new opportunity to separate these regulatory cells from other T-cell populations.

In experiments not reported here, we have used successive panning to separate the regulatory T cells and culture them in enriched media. These cells have proliferated for at least 70 days and have been cloned once by limiting dilution. A clone with suppressor activity has been isolated along with a second clone which was unable to suppress. We are now in the process of characterizing these two clones. To determine if suppression can be produced *in vivo*, we have repopulated eight-week-old Balb/c SCID mice with antibody-secreting B cells and regulatory T cells from the thymus of syngeneic donors injected with soluble MTg. Marked suppression of antibody production in the SCID recipients was found, compared with SCID mice that were given the antibody-secreting B cells alone. We concluded that autoantibody production can be suppressed *in vivo* as well as *in vitro*.

At this time, we are unable to determine the mechanism by which these regulatory T cells prevent antibody secretion. The strict syngeneic restriction between regulatory T cell and antibody-secreting B cell suggests that direct cell-cell interaction is required, since not only MHC but other, non-MHC cell determinants limit suppression. This finding makes it less likely that soluble factor(s) secreted by the regulatory T cells are responsible for suppression. We have, in fact, tested the supernatant medium in which the regulatory cells have grown, and have been unable to demonstrate any inhibitory activity. Factors acting at short range or with a short half-life remain a possibility.

The fact that the regulatory cells are CD4$^-$ CD8$^+$ T cells may mean that they are cytotoxic T cells. If so, the target of their cytotoxic activity may be the antibody-producing B cell itself. The antigenic specificity of the regulatory T cells excludes the possibility that they may react with the idiotypic determinant on the B cell. An interesting possibility is that the regulatory cells would recognize antigen or antigen fragments attached to the surface of the B cell as has been demonstrated in other systems.[46,47] We have, however, not yet been able to find any evidence for this possibility in our experiments.

In recent years, the very concept of suppressor T cells has been strongly challenged.[48] The basis of this dispute is the inability to clone a population of T cells with unique phenotypic markers. Some investigators[49] have even suggested that all the so-called suppressor phenomena are attributable to carry-over of antigen. In our experiments we have carried out a number of controls to exclude this possibility. We have shown, for example, that thymus and spleen suspensions suppress only at certain times after antigen injection and that some strains of mice are deficient in suppressor cell production even if they are given 10 times the amount of antigen usually required to induce regulatory T cells in responder strains.

Other investigators[50] have suggested that the same cells that produce suppression under one set of operational conditions may have stimulatory effect under other circumstances. Different subsets of murine T helper cells, for example, are known to produce different mixtures of lymphokines following antigen stimulation. As stated above, we do not feel at this time that the suppression we have observed is due to release of soluble factors, although further investigation is necessary to solidify this point. Others[51] have suggested that suppression is due to anti-idiotypic cytotoxic T cells. Here, again, our data do not support this viewpoint.

Given all of these uncertainties, it is clear that a great deal can still be learned from careful studies of antigen-specific immunoregulation.

SUMMARY

1. Large Thy1$^+$, CD8$^+$ immunoregulatory cells were found in the thymus of mice 9–16 days after injection of soluble mouse thyroglobulin (without adjuvant).
2. Similar immunoregulatory cells appeared in the spleen 14–21 days after antigen administration suggesting that they were generated in the thymus and later migrated to the spleen.
3. The immunoregulatory cells were antigen-specific and attached to cognate antigen.
4. The degree of inhibition by the immunoregulatory cells differed among various inbred strains of mice and were virtually absent from SJL mice.
5. The regulatory function of the cells was strain specific *in vitro* and *in vivo*, and was restricted by both H-2 and non-H-2 haplotype.
6. By panning on antigen-coated plates, immunoregulatory cells were isolated and cell lines and clones with inhibitory function established.

REFERENCES

1. ROSE, N. R. 1988. 1970. Current concepts of autoimmune disease. Transplant Proc. **20:** 3–10.
2. BURNET, F. M. 1957. A modification of Jenne's theory of antibody production using the concept of clonal selection. Aust. J. Sci. **20:** 67.
3. BRONDZ, B. D., I. F. ABRONIVA, M. B. XAICOVA, A. V. FILATOVE & A. V. CHERVONSKY. 1984. Specific suppressor T-cells immune to antigens of the H-2 complex: receptors, clonal structure, genetic restriction an antigen markers. Immunol. Rev. **80:** 29–76.
4. PARASKEVAS, F. 1984. Pathways of T cell suppression. Crit. Rev. Immunol. 5(2): 95–148.
5. ROSE, N. R. 1975. The role of the thymus in spontaneous autoimmune thyroiditis. Ann. N. Y. Acad. Sci. **249:** 116.
6. WITEBSKY, E., N. R. ROSE, K. TERPLAN, J. R. PAINE & R. W. EGAN. 1957. Chronic thyroiditis and autoimmunization. J. Am. Med. Assoc. **164:** 1439–1447.
7. ROSE, N. R. & E. WITEBSKY. 1956. Studies on organ specificity. V. Changes in the thyroid glands of rabbits following active immunization with rabbit thyroid extracts. J. Immunol. **76:** 417–427.
8. BIGAZZI, P. E. & N. R. ROSE. 1975. Spontaneous autoimmune thyroiditis in animals as a model of human disease. Prog. Allergy **19:** 245–274.
9. LIVEZEY, M., R. SUNDICK & N. R. ROSE. 1981. Spontaneous autoimmune thyroiditis in chickens II. Evidence for autoresponsive thymocytes. J. Immunol. **127**(4): 1469–1471.
10. TRUDEN, J. L., R. S. SUNDICK, S. LEVINE & N. R. ROSE. 1983. The decreased growth rate of obese strain chicken thyroid cells provides *in vitro* evidence for a primary target organ abnormality in chickens susceptible to autoimmune thyroiditis. Clin. Immunol. Immunopathol. **29:** 294–305.
11. BACON, L. D., C. R. POLLEY, R. K. COLE & N. R. ROSE. 1981. Genetic influences on spontaneous autoimmune thyroiditis in (CSxOS)F$_2$ chickens. Immunogenetics **12:** 339–349.

12. FARR, A. G., S. K. ANDERSON, P. MARRACH & J. W. KAPPLER. 1985. Expression of antigen-specific, major histocompatibility complex-restricted receptors by cortical and medullary thymocytes in situ. Cell **43**: 543–550.

13. VOLPE, R., P. V. CLARKE & V. V. ROW. 1973. Relationship of age-specific incidence rates to immunological aspects of Hashimoto's thyroiditis. Can. Med. Assoc. J. **109**: 898–901.

14. BANKHURST, A. D., G. TORRIGINA & A. C. ALLISON. 1973. Lymphocytes binding human thyroglobulin in healthy people and its relevance to tolerance for autoantigens. Lancet **1**: 226–230.

15. ROSE, N. R., Y. M. KONG, I. OKAYASU, A. A. GIRALDO, K. BEISEL & R. S. SUNDICK. 1981. T-cell regulation in autoimmune thyroiditis. Immunol. Rev. **55**: 299–314.

16. KONG, Y. M., I. OKAYSU, A. A. GIRALDO, K. W. BEISEL, R. S. SUNDICK, N. R. ROSE, C. S. DAVID, F. AUDIBERT & L. CHEDID. 1982. Tolerance to thyroglobulin by activating suppressor mechanisms. Ann. N. Y. Acad. Sci. **392**: 191–209.

17. WELCH, P., N. R. ROSE & J. H. KITE, JR. 1973. Neonatal thymectomy increases spontaneous autoimmune thyroiditis. J. Immunol. **110**: 575–577.

18. OKAYASU, I., Y. M. KONG, C. S. DAVID & N. R. ROSE. 1981. *In vitro* T-lymphocyte proliferative response to mouse thyroglobulin in experimental autoimmune thyroiditis. Cell. Immunol. **61**: 32–39.

19. CREEMERS, P., A. A. GIRALDO, N. R. ROSE & Y. M. KONG. 1984. T-cell subsets in the thyroids of mice developing autoimmune thyroiditis. Cell. Immunol. **87**: 692–697.

20. CREEMERS, P., N. R. ROSE & Y. M. KONG. 1983. Experimental autoimmune thyroiditis: *in vitro* cytotoxic effects of T lymphocytes on thyroid monolayers. J. Exp. Med. **157**: 559–571.

21. TALOR, E. & N. R. ROSE. 1989. Antigen-specific thymus-derived suppressor cells from mice injected with mouse thyroglobulin. *In* Cellular Basis of Immune Modulation. J. G. Kaplan, D. R. Green & R. C. Bleackley, Eds. 391–394. Alan R. Liss, Inc. New York.

22. RICHTER, M. & E. TALOR. 1986. Cells involved in the immune response XXXXIV. Suppressor cells in the thymus of the rabbit capable of secreting a factor which can suppress the secretion of antibodies from antibody-forming cells *in vitro*. Clin. Immunol. Immunopathol. **41**: 461.

23. TALOR, E., C. A. JODUIN & M. RICHTER. 1988. Cells involved in the immune response XXXVI. The thymic antigen-specific suppressor cell in the immunized rabbit is a T cell with receptors for F_cG and the antigen and it acts, via a secreted suppressor factor, directly on the immune splenic AFC B cell to inhibit antibody secretion. Immunology **64**: 253.

24. TALOR, E. & M. RICHTER. 1988. Cells involved in the immune response XXXV. The antigen-specific antibody response in the rabbit is suppressed by thymocytes of allogeneic immunized rabbits and by the non-toxic suppressor factor (ITSF) secreted by these thymocytes. Clin. Immunol. Immunopathol. **48**(2): 150.

25. RICHTER, M., I. TRUDEL & E. TALOR. 1990. Cells involved in the immune response. XXXVII. Suppressor cells in the spleen of the outbred rabbit following primary immunization are T cells which emigrate from the thymus. Scand. J. Immunol. **32**: 611.

26. TALOR, E. & N. R. ROSE. 1988. The induction of antigen-specific thymic regulatory cells in the mouse. Cell. Immunol. **116**: 24–34.

27. TOMER, Y. & Y. SHOENFELD. 1989. The significance of T suppressor cells in the development of autoimmunity. J. Autoimmunity **2**: 739–758.

28. KONG, Y., I. OKAYASU, A. GIRALDO, K. BEISEL, R. SUNDICK, N. R. ROSE *et al.* 1984. Tolerance to thyroglobulin by activating suppressor mechanisms. Ann. N. Y. Acad. Sci. **392**: 192–209.

29. BRENIHAN, B. & H. E. JASIN. 1977. Suppressor function of peripheral blood mononuclear cells in normal individuals and in patients with systemic lupus erythematous. J. Clin. Invest. **59**(1): 106–116.

30. HOFFMAN, W. H., P. SAHASRANANAN, S. S. FERANDOS, C. L. BUREK & N. R. ROSE. 1982. Transient thyrotoxicosis in an infant delivered to a long-acting thyroid stimula-

tor (LATS)- and LATS protector-negative, thyroid-stimulating antibody-positive woman with Hashimoto's thyroiditis. J. Clin. Endocrinol. Metab. **54:** 354–356.

31. LIVEZEY, M. D., R. S. SUNDICK & N. R. ROSE. 1981. Spontaneous autoimmune thyroiditis in chickens. II. Evidence for autoresponsive thymocytes. J. Immunol. **127:** 1469–1472.

32. SILVERMAN, D. A. & N. R. ROSE. 1974. Neonatal thymectomy increases the incidence of spontaneous and methylcholanthrene-enhanced thyroiditis in rats. Science **184:** 162–163.

33. KOJIMA, A., Y. TANAKA-KOJIMA, T. SAKAKURA & Y. NISHIZUKA. 1976. Spontaneous development of autoimmune thyroiditis in neonatally thymectomized mice. Lab. Invest. **34:** 550–557.

34. PENHALE, W. J., A. FARMER, R. P. McKANNA & W. J. IRVINE. 1973. Spontaneous thyroiditis in thymectomized and irradiated Wistar rats. Clin. Exp. Immunol. **15:** 225.

35. GERSHON, R. K. 1974. T cell control of antibody production. Contemp. Top. Immunobiol. **3:** 1–40.

36. GERSHON, R. K. 1980. Immunoregulation circa 1980: some comments on the state of the art. J. Allergy Clin. Immunol. **66**(1): 18–24.

37. AUNE, T. M. 1987. Role and function of antigen nonspecific suppressor factors. Crit. Rev. Immunol. **7**(2): 93–130.

38. DORF, M. E. & B. BENACERRAF. 1984. Suppressor cells and immunoregulation. Ann. Rev. Immunol. **2:** 127–158.

39. KELLER, R. H. & N. J. CALVANICO. 1984. Suppressor macromolecules. Crit. Rev. Immunol. **5**(2): 149–199.

40. TALOR, E. & M. RICHTER. 1991. Suppressor cells and suppressor factors in the regulation of humoral immunity. *In* Contemporary Clinical Immunology. M. R. Escobar & H. Friedman, Eds. Plenum Press. New York. In press.

41. ZUNIGA-PFLUCHER, J. C., D. L. LONG & A. M. KRÛISBEEK. 1989. Positive selection of CD⁻ CD8⁺ T cells in the thymus of normal mice. Nature **338:** 76–78.

42. MacDONALD, R. H. 1989. Mechanisms of immunological tolerance. Science **246:** 82.

43. DINTZIS, R. Z., M. H. MIDDLETON & H. M. DINTZIS. 1988. Tolerogen-mediated suppression of the immune response. Scand. J. Immunol. **28:** 747.

44. DINTZIS, R. Z., M. OKAJIMA, M. H. MIDDLETON, G. GREEN & H. M. DINTZIS. 1989. The immunogenicity of soluble haptenated polymers is determined by molecular mass and hapten valence. J. Immunol. **143:** 1239.

45. McMASTER, P. R. B., J. D. OWNS & W. E. VANNIER. 1977. The preparation and characterization of a thymic independent antigen: E-dinitrophenyl-lysine-ficoll. Immunochemistry **14:** 189.

46. DINTZIS, H. M., R. Z. DINTZIS & B. VOGELSTON. 1976. Molecular determinants of immunogenicity: the immunon model of immune response. Proc. Natl. Acad. Sci. USA **73:** 3671.

47. TEW, J. G., R. P. PHIPPS & T. E. MANDEL. 1980. The maintenance and regulation of the humoral immune response: persisting antigen and the role of follicular antigen-binding dendritic cells as accessory cells. Immunol. Rev. **53:** 175.

48. MÖLLER, G. 1988. Do suppressor cells exist? Scand. J. Immunol. **27:** 247.

49. DINTZIS, R. X., M. H. MIDDLETON & H. M. DINTZIS. 1983. Studies on the immunogenicity and tolerogenicity of T-independent antigens. J. Immunol. **131:** 2196.

50. MÖLLER, G. 1985. Con A activated lymphocytes suppress immune response *in vitro* but are helper cells *in vivo*. Scand. J. Immunol. **21:** 31.

51. COOKE, A., P. M. LYDYARD & I. M. ROITT. 1983. Mechanisms of autoimmunity: a role for cross-reactive idiotypes. Immunol. Today **4**(6): 170.

Viral-Specific Immunization in AIDS-Related Complex by Photopheresis

EMIL BISACCIA,[a,b,d,f] CAROLE BERGER,[b,c]
FRANCIS X. DiSPALTRO,[d] STEVEN ARMUS,[d]
CAROL CAHILL,[d] AND ALBERT KLAINER[a,e]

Departments of [a]Medicine, [b]Dermatology, and [c]Pathology
Columbia University
College of Physicians and Surgeons
630 West 168th Street
New York, New York 10032
and
[d]Photopheresis Unit
[e]Department of Internal Medicine
Morristown Memorial Hospital
Morristown, New Jersey 07962-1956

Human immunodeficiency virus (HIV) is a pathogenic retrovirus and the causative agent of acquired immunodeficiency syndrome (AIDS) and related disorders. In HIV infection the immunoprotective factors induced by initial infection seem to persist in those who remain healthy but are lost in those who develop full-blown AIDS, an event which may occur over a period of several years. The primary target for human immunodeficiency virus (HIV) infection is the CD4 lymphocyte cell population. Additional susceptible cell types include those of the macrophage/monocyte lineage. The mechanism underlying the CD4 cell depletion that occurs *in vivo* in HIV infection may involve indirect and undefined cytopathic processes, cell fusion and possibly an autoimmune mechanism.[1]

The potential therapeutic value of photopheresis was evaluated in 7 patients with AIDS-related complex (ARC). The rationale for the study was based on: 1. the demonstration that psoralen and UVA could inactivate virus[2] and specifically HIV *in vitro*[3] and possibly *in vivo;*[4] 2. CD4 cells are the primary target population affected by HIV and by photopheresis;[5] and 3. reinfusion of inactivated virus and cell-associated virus might serve to engender a specific immune response. The current study represents an extension of the initial preliminary trial[4] to include two additional patients.

PATIENTS AND METHODS

Patients

Seven patients with AIDS-related complex were selected from the eight patients who volunteered for the study. The patient who was not selected was disqualified because he was enrolled in another drug trial. All seven patients had enlarged lymph nodes (1 cm or more) at two or more sites; and unexplained systemic symptoms, including intermittent or continuous fever for more than 1

---

[f] Address for correspondence: 182 South Street, Morristown, NJ 07960.

321

month, repeated night sweats, a debilitating, persistent weight loss of at least 5%, and a decreased percentage of CD4-positive cells. The study was done according to the provisions for the treatment of human subjects of the Institutional Review Board at Morristown Memorial Hospital, Morristown, New Jersey. On the basis of the Walter Reed (WR) staging classification,[6] patients ranged from WR4 to WR5.

Laboratory Studies

Pretreatment studies included an enzyme-linked immunosorbent assay (ELISA) for HIV and a confirmatory Western blot,[7] antibody tests (HIVAGEN-SKF,[8] SmithKline Beecham, West Norriton, Pennsylvania), HIV isolation by p24 antigen capture[7] (Metpath, Teterboro, New Jersey), peripheral blood phenotyping,[9] hepatitis profile, VDRL, antinuclear antibody, chest roentgenogram, and electrocardiogram. Pretreatment and monthly posttreatment studies included a complete blood count, platelet count, erythrocyte sedimentation rate, reticulocyte count, a 20-parameter automated analysis, urinalysis, determinations of cytomegalovirus[10] and Epstein-Barr virus titers,[11] immunoglobulin electropheresis, assessments of beta2-microglobulin,[12] neopterin,[13] BE2[14] and p24 antigen levels.[7] Isolation of HIV[15] was repeated every 3 months. Skin testing to the recall antigens of tuberculin, mumps, Candida, and Trichophyton was done before treatment and at the completion of approximately 6 months of therapy. Photopheresis was done at monthly intervals as previously described.[4] Clinical evaluation included history and physical exam including monthly weight and calibration of lymph nodes as previously described.[4]

RESULTS

Initially 5 patients were entered into the clinical trial. Due to the absence of deleterious side effects and the demonstration of preliminary favorable responses, an additional 2 patients were added to the study. All of the patients were HIV-positive by either Western blot analysis, antibody titers and/or culture at the initiation of the study. One patient withdrew from the study after 5 months of treatment, and 2 other patients withdrew after 7 and 11 treatments. These patients were followed at intermittent intervals off therapy. Withdrawal from the study was based on patients' personal factors, and 2 of the 3 patients were considered clinically stable or improved during therapy.

All patients demonstrated resolution of lymphadenopathy. Skin test reactivity to recall antigens returned in 6 of the 7 patients. Weight remained stable or increased in 5 of the 7 patients. In addition, subjective measurements of well-being and fitness suggested that all patients tolerated the therapy well; 6 of 7 remained in good health and felt that their quality of life was improved. None of the opportunistic infections associated with transition to AIDS were observed in these patients during the initial trial period and all were able to manage common respiratory tract infections without difficulty. Except for normal variations, laboratory parameters including hemoglobin, hematocrit, reticulocyte count and platelet count remained stable. Chemistry values were unchanged except for slight elevations in aspartate aminotrasferase and alanine aminotransferase. Initial viral studies on the 7 patients demonstrated HIV antibody and positive virus cultures in all cases. Four of the seven (57%) of the patients had negative viral cultures after 5–19 treatments. In two of the four cases, repeated cultures remained negative. Antibody titers to core protein p24, envelope protein gp120, along with gp41, gp55, gp66/31 rose in all patients (TABLE 1). During the course of the study p24 antigen was negative in 4 of the 7 patients (57%). Levels of p24 fell in 2 patients and rose in one patient after 12 treatments. In spite of the rise in p24

TABLE 1. HIV Antibody Titers

	P24[a]	GP41	GP55	GP66/31	GP120[b]
Patient 1					
Pre	2.52	2.42	2.34	2.38	0.01
6 mos.	2.76	2.65	2.71	2.49	1.68
15 mos.	2.78	2.736	2.883	2.907	2.898
18 mos.	2.92	2.935	3.044	2.898	2.956
Patient 2					
Pre	0.12	1.41	0.87	0.45	0.08
6 mos.	0.74	2.54	2.25	1.89	0.14
15 mos.	0.79	2.80	2.53	1.24	2.59
18 mos.	0.72	2.61	2.61	1.97	2.66
Patient 3					
Pre	0.72	2.59	2.16	1.89	1.04
6 mos.	1.69	2.61	2.32	2.28	2.07
15 mos.	1.97	2.69	2.82	2.65	2.82
Patient 4					
Pre	0.62	1.36	1.40	0.93	0.21
6 mos.	1.76	2.59	2.41	2.00	1.25
15 mos.	2.54	2.66	2.66	1.81	2.82
18 mos.	2.51	2.72	2.43	1.90	2.74
Patient 5					
Pre	1.41	1.49	1.83	1.72	0.46
6 mos.	2.80	2.80	2.90	2.80	1.95
13 mos.	2.70	2.70	2.80	1.95	2.80
Patient 6					
Pre	2.68	2.71	2.77	2.73	2.48
6 mos.	2.60	2.63	2.81	2.70	2.70
13 mos.	2.70	2.70	2.80	2.80	2.75
Patient 7					
Pre	0.87	2.44	1.35	1.69	0.76
6 mos.	2.40	2.691	1.37	2.56	2.92
13 mos.	0.80	2.54	0.70	1.50	2.70

[a] Standard deviation for p24 antibody: ± 13%.
[b] Standard deviation for gp120 antibody: ± 20%.

in this patient, his viral cultures became negative and no other signs of progression were noted. The percentages and absolute numbers of CD4 and CD8 at several measured endpoints are presented for all 7 patients in TABLE 2. If the percentage of CD4+ lymphocytes is graphed over the treatment course and a best fit trend line drawn, the data reveals that 2 of 7 (29%) patients had a slight decline

TABLE 2. Clinical Characteristics and Laboratory Results

	Patient 1	Patient 2	Patient 3	Patient 4	Patient 5	Patient 6	Patient 7
Sex, age	M, 38	M, 30	M, 27	M, 42	F, 27	M, 38	M, 30
Predisposing factor	homosexuality	homosexuality	homosexuality	IVDA	IVDA	het.	het.
Walter Reed staging classification	4	5	5	4	5	4	4
Known duration of HIV antibody positivity (yrs)	3	2	4	2	1	2	3
Weight (kg)							
Before treatment	71.3	64.5	63.6	109	61.0	79.3	62
6 mos.[a]	70.5	66.0	64.7	108	57.7	75.9	64.5
15 mos.	71.0	68.7	64.5	110	56.0	71.4[b]	64.4
Absolute lymphocyte count/mm							
Before treatment	2600	1824	1617	1024	1936	1357	858
6 mos.	1768	1533	893	2067	522	1188	1056
15 mos.	1620	1554	546	2176	594	1593[b]	1380
Present	3150	1630	1148	2430	200		1220
CD4-percent positive cells/mm (%)							
Before treatment	4	29	34	11	12	45	30
6 mos.	34	31	40	33	13	37	43
15 mos.	25	29	52	27	7	36[b]	25
CD-percent positive cells/mm (%)							
Before treatment	26	30	33	14	46	42	46
6 mos.	52	45	53	40	42	41	50
15 mos.	50	46	40	32	48	42[b]	45
Beta2-microglobulin, mg/L							
Before treatment	NA[c]	NA	3.6	NA	3.9	2.6	3.21
6 mos.	7.6	2.8	3.6	4.3	4.3	2.6	3.3
15 mos.	6.2	2.6	3.6	3.1	NA	1.9[b]	3.5
p24 antigen, pg/mL							
Before treatment	NA	NA	NA	NA	NA	—	77
6 mos.	—	495	—	135	—	—	175
15 mos.	—	258	—	54	—	—	243

[a] After 6 months of therapy except in patient 3 who received only 5 months of therapy (see text).
[b] After 9 months.
[c] Not available.

in CD4 percentage, 2 of 7 patients (29%) maintained a stable percentage of CD4+ cells, 2 of 7 patients had an increase in their CD4 percentage (29%) and 1 patient (patient # 5) (14%) demonstrated a sharp decline in CD4-positive cells. Patient #5 also manifested a declining white count, weight loss and persistence of skin test anergy. No infectious complications were noted in this patient, and she withdrew from the study for personal reasons after 11 treatments. The remaining 6 patients did not develop a rapid decline in CD4 percentage and had no signs of progression to AIDS. Three of the seven patients had CD4 percentages of <25% and only 1 of these patients (#5) had signs of progression, while one patient demonstrated a trend towards a minimal decline in CD4 percentage over time and the other patient manifested an increase. Therefore, in the three patients most at risk for progression, no frank cases of AIDS were seen during the 1 year to 18 month monitoring period.

When the CD8+ percentages were compared and a trend line drawn, all patients demonstrated a substantial increase in CD8+ cells over the treatment course. In addition, when the absolute number of CD4 and CD8 lymphocytes were evaluated, 3 of the 7 (43%) patients had an increase in the absolute number of CD4 cells at the latest time point available. Two patients (29%) manifested a minimal decrease in the absolute number of CD4 cells and two patients demonstrated a marked decline in the absolute number of CD4+ cells. The absolute number of CD8+ lymphocytes decreased in the two patients that had a fall in the absolute number of CD4+ cells. The remaining patients had marked increases in CD8+ cells ranging from 1.2 to 6.1 times their initial level. This increase in CD8 cells correlates in 5 patients with the rising percentage of CD8+ cells seen in all patients.

Levels of beta2-microglobulin were followed in the 7 patients during their treatment with photochemotherapy. Beta2-microglobulin fell in 6 patients and increased slightly in 1 patient. High levels of beta2-microglobulin (>3 mg/L) are another predictive indicator of progression to AIDS. Five of the seven patients began the study with levels of beta2-microglobulin in this range. The level declined in 3 of the 5 patients but remained in the elevated range. Two patients had levels of beta2-microglobulin that were considered moderate (2–2.9 mg/L). These levels fell with one patient (patient #6) attaining a normal level (1.9 mg/L).

DISCUSSION

Immunosuppressed individuals do not usually respond properly to antigen stimulation. HIV-seropositive men have shown multiple immunologic abnormalities, including a reduction in CD4 cells and a decreased CD4 : CD8 ratio. Antibody titers to EBV and CMV in HIV infection have been shown to be negatively correlated with CD4 depletion and CD4 : CD8 ratio.[16] Patients with ARC/AIDS typically show a decline in antibody titers to HIV over time. McDougal and colleagues showed a correlation between HIV antibody titer and the severity of immunodeficiency regardless of clinical status. Decreasing levels of antibody to p24 and gp120 are predictive of disease progression while increasing levels are indicative of nonprogression. This association is independent of the levels of CD4-positive cells.[17]

The present study provides evidence of elevation of HIV-specific antibodies to p24, gp120, gp66/31, gp55, gp41, while antibody titers to EBV and CMV remained essentially unchanged. The increase in antibody titers was not an isolated event, but was accompanied by: the maintenance of relatively stable percentages and absolute numbers of CD4-positive cells; a stabilization of or decline in the activation markers beta2-microglobulin and neopterin; resolution of clinical symptoms and lymphadenopathy in 6 of 7 patients and a failure to culture virus in 4 patients. If these results are an immune response to the virus, one might expect the suppression of viral replication to be directly or indirectly related to psoralen ultraviolet A therapy. The direct response may be due to the irradiation of virus with long wavelength ultra-violet (UVA) in the presence of psoralen which results in cross-linking of the base-pair regions of nucleic acids[2] with the formation of covalent monoadducts. This treatment can destroy the infectivity of DNA and RNA viruses,[18] including HIV.[3] The indirect response is suggested by *in vitro* studies which have shown that a specific cellular immune response can be engendered by exposing herpes virus to psoralen and UVA. Redfield and colleagues[19] have shown that *in vitro* exposure of virus infected cells causes the loss of infectivity in both the intact virus and virus-infected cells. Viral antigenicity was not affected by the treatment and the infected cells induced a specific lymphocyte proliferation *in vitro*.[19]

The humoral response to HIV infection is initially vigorous, reflecting the influence of an intact immune system at the time of infection. Antibodies produced against HIV have been implicated in a variety of humoral and cell-mediated immune responses, the most significant of which is blocking of viral cytopathic effects by neutralizing antibodies. The present study has demonstrated elevations in antibody titers to the main HIV antigens. The major viral antigens targeted by these antibodies are the glycoproteins 120, 41, 55/66/31 and the core protein p24. Antibodies to HIV antigens have been identified that are able to neutralize the infectivity of all HIV substrains and thus are cross-reactive.[20] This is important given the genomic diversity in the viral envelope gene and the propensity of the virus to mutate even during the infection of a single patient. However, the transmission of HIV from cell to cell without "free" virus makes destruction difficult by neutralizing antibodies alone. Consequently, appropriate therapeutic intervention would be required to include a cytotoxic cell-mediated response that is virus specific. This response may involve cytotoxic T lymphocytes, antibody-dependent cell-mediated cytotoxicity and "null" killer cells. Our study demonstrates a dramatic increase in the CD8 cell population in the context of a stable CD4 T lymphocytes and a stable clinical status. The possibility exists that the observed increase in CD8 cells in the majority of treated patients represents a virus-specific response. It has been suggested that CD8 T cells are the major defense mechanism by which the body eliminates virus-infected lymphocytes. Murine models of retroviral infection indicate a positive relationship between stable clinical status and the presence of HIV-specific cytotoxic T lymphocytes (CTL).[21] Furthermore, Walker and colleagues have shown that a subset of CD8 T lymphocytes is capable of producing the suppression of HIV replication[22] as determined by the culture of the peripheral blood mononuclear cells.

However, in other studies increased numbers of CD8-positive cells may reflect the generation of CTL which recognize gp120 and can cross react with other viral and possibly self antigens might result in destruction of self. Indirectly, CTL may also mediate the observed CD4 cell depletion by specific lysis of virus-negative CD4 by cells due to recognition of antigens released from HIV-infected cells in association with HLA Class I. This mechanism of lysis has been demonstrated using noninfected CD4 T lymphocytes coated with gp120.[23] In addition, there is sequence homology between HLA Class II antigens and HIV gp41 envelope protein. Beretta *et al.* demonstrated that monoclonal antibody directed against this antigen recognizes the HLA marker in macrophases.[24] This suggests that although a strong capacity to mount a specific CTL response exists in the HIV patient, this same response may account for the killing of noninfected gp120 coated or noncoated CD4 lymphocytes bearing cross-reactive antigens. However, we have not seen the indication of autoimmune disease in our study and the percent CD4-positive cells have remained relatively stable. It seems clear that any therapeutic intervention should elicit both a specific and protective CTL along with the appropriate humoral response which overcomes the problem of viral type and strain variation. A method of immunization previously employed to deal with this problem has been to include both type-specific and strain-specific variants along with the use of a potent immunologic adjuvant to induce durable immunity to a broad spectrum of variants.[25,26] The functional adjuvant in our study may be the treated virus, viral antigens, peptides, infected cells, along with the release of lymphokines and/or other factors after the photopheresis therapy. The use of an appropriate adjuvant could heighten, prolong and possibly broaden the specificity of the immune response. The immunopathological consequences of the adjuvant used is of interest since it may reveal the different effects of an immunogen either in the induction of an immunopathologic disease or its prevention. An example of this is seen in experimental allergic encephalomyelitis (EAE). EAE is a disease induced in rodents by injecting myelin basic protein (MBP) in complete Freunds' adjuvant.[27] EAE induced in this fashion can be prevented by the administration of MBP in incomplete Freunds' adjuvant (which does not contain mycobacterial). This "vaccination" occurs if the immunogen in incomplete adjuvant are given early enough after the administration of the MBP in the complete adjuvant. As a result of our observations in HIV, we feel that a unique advantage of photoche- motherapy might be its ability to "vaccinate" an individual post-exposure to HIV. The strategy of post-exposure "vaccination" or immunization has been previously practiced in rabies and has been suggested as an approach in HIV. This strategy attempts to immunize a person early enough in the infection so as to boost existing immunoprotective factors, *i.e.*, at minimum to maintain, but prefer- ably potentiate, the immunologic response that may prevent the progression of the viral infection to AIDS. However, previous studies have found that HIV- infected individuals often have impaired antibody responses and that the humoral response to viral "vaccination" is T cell dependent.[27] Therefore, subjects with ARC or AIDS might be significantly more impaired with respect to mounting an antibody or cellular response to vaccination reflecting the severity of these immu- nologic impairments. What then is the relationship of photopheresis to engender- ing the elevated levels of HIV antibodies and the quantitative and functional (return of skin test reactivity) cellular response in light of the severity of the immunodeficiency and clinical status? Unlike antiviral drugs, extracorporeal pho- topheresis spares the tissue-fixed elements of the immune system from exposure to the therapy, thereby minimizing damage to the antigen processing system. It has been demonstrated that the magnitude of the response of antigen-specific T lymphocytes to a viral antigen depends largely on the conformation of the antigen molecule and an intact processing system. For example, hepatitis B viral surface antigen (HBsAG) has been denatured by various methods (*e.g.*, formic acid) and its capacity to stimulate an immune response has been enhanced.[28] As a conse- quence of these studies a denatured antigen has been shown to stimulate the response of T cells with significantly higher efficiency that the native antigen.[29] Photopheresis may inactivate and possibly physically alter free HIV, soluble antigen and/or cells both associated with or without virus to unmask and/or to photomodify antigen to induce an enhanced immunologic response.

The operative mechanism of photopheresis in ARC patients is presently under intensive study. The present results suggest that this therapy is at a minimum well-tolerated and stabilizing and perhaps results in an improved immunocompetence in some patients. These results and the expanded Phase II trial which is underway, will help determine the ultimate role of photopheresis in the treatment of people with HIV infection.

SUMMARY

The potential for therapeutic intervention in 7 patients with AIDS-related complex (ARC) was evaluated through the use of photopheresis. The rationale for the study was based on: 1. the demonstration that psoralen and UVA could inactivate HIV/virus in $vitro$; 2. CD4 cells are the primary target population effected by HIV and photopheresis; and 3. reinfusion of inactivated virus and cell-associated virus might serve to engender an immune response. Preliminary results in 7 patients with ARC over 6 to 18 months revealed a virus-specific response with an elevation of HIV antibodies, while EBV and CMV titers remained unchanged. The immunologic results revealed an increase in the CD8 lymphocyte population, stable activation markers (B2 microglobulin neopterin), a decrease in p24 antigen titers and inability to culture HIV virus in 3 patients. All of these results were in the context of a stable or increasing CD4+ percent. Six patients did not reveal a generalized inhibition of other immune responses as demonstrated by recovery of DTH. In addition, the resolution of lymphadenopathy, night sweats, fever and weight loss, paralleled the immunologic response.

REFERENCES

1. GALLO, R. C. 1988. HIV-the cause of AIDS: an overview of its biology, mechanisms of disease induction and out attempts to control it. J. Acquire Immune Defic. Syndr. **1:** 521–535.
2. MASAJO, L., G. RODIGHLER, J. COLOMBO, V. TERTONE & F. DALLACQUA. 1965. Photosensitizing furocoumarines: interactions with DNA and photoinactivation of DNA containing viruses. Experientia **21:** 22–24.
3. QUINNAN, G. V., M. A. WELLS, A. E. WITTEK et al. 1986. Inactivation of human T-cell virus, type III by heat, chemicals and irradiation. Transfusion **26:** 481–483.
4. BISACCIA, E., C. BERGER & A. KLAINER. 1990. Extracorporeal photopheresis in the acquired immunodeficiency syndrome (AIDS)-related complex: a pilot study. Ann. Intern. Med. **113:** 270–275.
5. EDELSON, R., C. BERGER, F. GASPARRO et al. 1987. Treatment of cutaneous T-cell lymphoma by extracorporeal photochemotherapy. Preliminary results. N. Engl. J. Med. **316:** 297–303.
6. REDFIELD, R. R., D. C. WRIGHT & E. C. TRAMONT. 1986. The Watler Reed staging classification for HTLV-III/LAV infection. N. Engl. J. Med. **314:** 131–132.
7. JACKSON, G. G., D. A. PAUL, L. A. FALK et al. 1988. Human immunodeficiency virus (HIV) antigenemia (p24) in acquired immune deficiency syndrome (AIDS) and the effect of treatment with zidovudine (AZT). Ann. Intern. Med. **108:** 175–180.
8. VALERIE, L. N. G. et al. 1989. Reliable confirmation of antibodies to human immunodeficiency virus type I (HIV-I) with an enzyme-linked immunoassay using recombinant antigens derived from HIV-I gag, pol, and env Genes. J. Clin. Microbiol. **27:** 977–982.
9. KUNG, P. C., C. BERGER, G. GOLDSTEIN, P. LoGERFO & R. L. EDELSON. 1981. Cutaneous T-cell lymphoma: characterization by monoclonal antibodies. Blood **57:** 261–266.

10. HENLE, W., G. HENLE & C. A. HOROWITZ. 1979. Infectious mononucleosis and Esptein-Barr virus associated malignancies. *In* E. H. Lennett, N. J. Schmidt, Eds. Diagnostic procedures for viral, rickettsial, and chlamydia infections. 5th edit. 441–475. American Public Health Association. Washington, DC.

11. BRODY, J. P., J. H. BINKLEY & S. A. HARDING. 1979. Evaluation and comparison of two assays for detection of immunity to rubella infection. J. Clin. Microbiol. **10:** 708–711.

12. LACEY, J. N., M. A. FORBES, M. A. WAUGH, E. H. COOPER & M. H. HAMBLING. 1987. Serum beta-microglobulin and human immunodeficiency virus infection. AIDS **1:** 123–127.

13. FAHEY, J. L., J. M. TAYLOR, R. DETEKS *et al.* 1990. The prognostic value of cellular and serologic markers in infection with human immunodeficiency virus, type 1. N. Engl. J. Med. **322:** 166–172.

14. BERGER, C. L., D. MORRISON, A. CHU, J. PATTERSON, A. ESTABROOK, S. TAKEZAKI, J. SHARON, D. WARBURTON, G. IRGOYINO & R. L. EDELSON. 1982. Diagnosis of cutaneous T-cell lymphoma by use of monoclonal antibody reacted with tumor associated antigen. J Clin. Invest. **70:** 1205–1215.

15. VELLECA, W. N., D. F. PALMER, R. W. FEORNO, D. T. WARFIELD, J. CREBS, R. FORRESTA & L. PHILLIP. 1986. Training Manual of the Centers for Disease Control: Isolation Culture and Identification of Human T-Cell Lymphotrophic Virus III. Lymphadenopathy Associated Virus. Atlanta, Georgia. Centers for Disease Control.

16. DETELS, R., B. R. VISSHER, J. L. FAHEY, K. SCHWARTZ, R. S. GREENE, D. L. MADDEN, J. L. SEVER & M. S. GOTTLIEB. 1984. The relation of cyto-megalovirus and Epstein-Barr virus antibodies to T-cell subsets in homosexually active men. J. Am. Med. Assoc. **251:** 1719–1722.

17. MCDOUGAL, J. S., M. S. KENNEDY, J. K. NICHOLSON *et al.* 1987. Antibody response to human immunodeficiency virus in homosexual men. Relation of antibody specificity, titer, and isotype to clinical status: severity of immunodeficiency, and disease progression. J. Clin. Invest. **80:** 316–324.

18. NAKASHIMA, K. & A. J. SHATKIN. 1978. Photochemical cross-linking of retrovirus genome RNA in situ and inactivation of viral transcriptase. J. Biol. Chem. **253:** 8680–8682.

19. REDFIELD, D. C., D. D. RICHMAN, M. N. OXMAN & L. H. KRONENBERG. 1981. Psoralen inactivation of influenza and herpes simplex viruses and of virus-infected cells. Infect. Immun. **32:** 1216–1226.

20. HAHN, B. H., G. M. SHAW, M. E. TAYLOR *et al.* 1986. Genetic variation in HTLV-III/LAV over time in patients with AIDS or at risk for Aids. Science **232:** 1548–1553.

21. PLATA, F., P. LANGLADE-DEMOYEN, J. P. ABASTADO, T. BERBAR & P. KOURILSKY. 1987. Retrovirus antigens recognized by cytolytic T lymphocytes activate tumor rejection. Cell **48:** 231–240.

22. WALKER, B. D., S. CHAKRABARTI, B. MOSS, T. J. PARADIS, T. FLYNN, A. G. DURNO, R. S. BLUMBERG, J. C. KAPLAN, M. S. HIRSCH & R. T. SCHOOLEY. 1987. HIV-specific cytotoxic T lymphocytes in seropositive individuals. Nature (London). **328:** 345–348.

23. LANZAVECCHIA, A., E. ROOSNEK, T. GREGORY, P. BERMAN & S. ABRIGNANI. 1988. T cells can present antigens such as HIV gp120 targeted to their own surface molecules. Nature **334:** 530–532.

24. BERETTA, A., F. GRASSI, M. PELAGI, A. CLIVIO, C. PARRAVICINI, G. GIOVINAZZO, F. ANDRONICO, L. LOPALCO, P. VERANI, S. BUTTO, P. TITTI, G. G. ROSSI, G. VIALE, E. GINELLI & A. G. SICCARDI. 1987. HIV env glycoprotein shares a crossreacting epitope with a surface protein present on activated human monocytes and involved in antigen presentation. Eur. J. Immunol. **17:** 1793–1798.

25. SALK, J., M. CONTAKOS, A. M. LAURENT *et al.* 1963. Use of adjuvants in studies on influenza immunization: degree of persistence of antibody in human subjects two years after vaccination. J. Am. Med. Assoc. **151:** 1169–1175.

26. MEIKLEJOHN, G. 1962. Adjuvant influenza adenovirus vaccine. J. Am. Med. Assoc. **79:** 594–597.

27. SALK, J. 1987. Prospects for the control of AIDS through immunization of seropositive individuals. Nature **327:** 473–476.
28. CELIS, E. & T. W. CHANG. 1984. HBsAg-serum protein complexes stimulate immune T lymphocyte more efficiently than do pure HBsAG. Hepatology **4:** 1116–1123.
29. CELIS, E., I. KATO, R. W. MILLER & J. W. CHANG. 1985. Regulation of the human immune response to HBsAG: effects of antibodies and antigens conformation in the stimulation of helper T cells by HbsAG. Hepatology **5:** 744–751.

Protein Engineering of DAB-IL-2 Fusion Toxins to Increase Biologic Potency[a]

TETSUYUKI KIYOKAWA,[b] DIANE P. WILLIAMS,
CATHERINE E. SNIDER, CORY A. WATERS,
JEAN C. NICHOLS,[c] TERRY B. STROM,[d] AND
JOHN R. MURPHY[b]

[b]Evans Department of Clinical Research
and
Department of Medicine
The University Hospital
Boston University Medical Center
Boston, Massachusetts 02118
[c]Seragen, Inc.
97 South Street
Hopkinton, Massachusetts 01748
[d]The Charles A. Dana Research Laboratory
Harvard Thorndike Laboratory
of the Beth Isreal Hospital
Boston, Massachusetts 02215

INTRODUCTION

The genetic replacement of either the native diphtheria toxin or *Pseudomonas* exotoxin A receptor binding domain with eukaryotic cell receptor-specific polypeptide hormones or growth factor sequences has resulted in the development of a new class of biological response modifier—the fusion toxin.[1–6] The first of these fusion toxins, DAB_{486}-IL-2, is currently in human Phase I clinical trials and the early results clearly demonstrate that this molecule is safe, well-tolerated, and biologically active in the elimination of high-affinity IL-2 receptor-positive leukemia and lymphoma cells without adverse side effect (LeMaistre, personal communication). DAB_{486}-IL-2 is a bipartite fusion protein composed of diphtheria toxin fragment A and fragment B sequences to Ala^{486} linked to Pro^2 through Thr^{133} of human interleukin-2 (IL-2).[2] This chimeric protein is the product of a genetic fusion between a truncated gene encoding fragment A and the membrane-associating domains of fragment B of diphtheria toxin and a synthetic gene encoding human IL-2.[7] DAB_{486}-IL-2 has been shown to selectively bind to high-affinity IL-2 receptors, be internalized by receptor-mediated endocytosis, and facilitate the delivery of diphtheria toxin fragment A to the cytosol of target cells.[8,9] Recent studies have defined the minimal size of fragment B that is required to deliver fragment A across the endocytic vesicle membrane in target cells, and defined the site of proteolytic processing involved in the release of fragment A from the intact fusion toxin molecule.[10,11]

[a] Preparation of this review was supported in part by Public Health Service Grants R01 CA-41746 and U01 CA-48626 (J.R.M.) from the National Cancer Institute, and R01 AI-22882 (T.B.S.) from the National Institute of Allergy and Infectious Diseases.

331

While the application of protein engineering to the development of new biologicals is in its infancy, it is now clear that one can design and genetically construct a wide variety of fusion toxins that are extraordinarily selective and potent in the elimination of receptor-bearing target cells. Indeed, the early results from human Phase I/II clinical trials of DAB_{486}-IL-2 suggest that the fusion toxin technology will play an important role in the development of new biological agents for the treatment of specific human malignancies.

Diphtheria Toxin

Biochemical and genetic analyses of diphtheria toxin has clearly shown that the toxin molecule is composed of at least three functional domains: (i) the enzymatically active fragment A, (ii) the membrane-associating domains and (iii) the receptor-binding domain of fragment B. Moreover, each domain of diphtheria toxin has been shown to play an essential role in the intoxication of intact sensitive eukaryotic cells.[12] In mature form, diphtheria toxin is a single polypeptide chain 585 amino acids in length, and contains four cysteine residues which form two disulfide bridges: Cys^{186}-Cys^{201} and Cys^{461}-Cys^{471}.[13-15] The fourteen amino acid loop subtended by the first disulfide bridge contains three arginine residues (Arg^{190}. Arg^{192}, and Arg^{193}) and is extremely sensitive to proteolytic attack by serine proteases. Upon trypsin "nicking" and reduction of the first disulfide bridge, diphtheria toxin can be separated under denaturing conditions into two polypeptide fragments.[16,17] Fragment A, the N-terminal 21.1-kDa polypeptide, carries the catalytic centers for the nicotinamide adenine dinucleotide (NAD+)-dependent adenosine diphosphoribosylation (ADPR) of eukaryotic elongation factor 2 (EF-2).[18] The B fragment of diphtheria toxin, the 37.1-kDa polypeptide, carries at least two functional domains: the hydrophobic membrane-associating domains which are responsible for the translocation of fragment A through the cell membrane and into the cytosol,[19] and the native diphtheria toxin receptor-binding domain.[18] The toxin receptor-binding domain has been recently located at the extreme C-terminal end of the toxin molecule.[20,21]

Interactions between diphtheria toxin and toxin-sensitive eukaryotic cells involve (i) the binding of intact toxin to the cell surface receptor,[22] (ii) internalization of bound toxin by receptor-mediated endocytosis into acidification competent vesicles,[23] and upon "nicking" of the toxin in this acidic environment [pH 5.3–5.1],[22,24] (iii) insertion of the hydrophobic domain(s) into the vesicle membrane,[25,26] thereby facilitating the (iv) delivery of fragment A to the cytosol. Once delivered to the cytosol, fragment A catalyzed ADP-ribosylation of EF-2 abolishes cellular protein synthesis and as a result leads to the death of the cell. Yamaizumi et al.[27] have demonstrated that a *single* molecule of fragment A delivered to the cytosol of a cell is sufficient to be lethal for that cell.

IL-2-Toxin (DAB₄₈₆-IL-2)

Williams et al.[2] described the genetic construction and properties of a fusion toxin that was assembled from a truncated form of diphtheria toxin and human interleukin-2 (IL-2), DAB_{486}-IL-2. In this construct, the 3'-end of the *tox* structural gene encoding the C-terminal receptor binding domain of diphtheria toxin was removed and replaced by a synthetic gene encoding amion acids 2 through 133 of mature human IL-2. Since the native diphtheria toxin receptor binding domain was replaced with IL-2 sequences, the resulting fusion toxin is directed towards cells bearing the IL-2 receptor. Importantly, cells which lacked the IL-2 receptor were found to be resistant to the inhibitor action of DAB_{486}-IL-2. Bacha *et al.*[8] have confirmed and extended these initial observations and have shown that the cytotoxic action of this fusion toxin is mediated through the IL-2 receptor and can be blocked by excess free recombiant IL-2, as well as by antibodies that bind to the p55 subunit (Tac antigen) of the IL-2 receptor. Moreover, since lysozomatrophic agents (*e.g.*, chloroquine) also block the cytotoxic action of DAB_{486}-IL-2, it is apparent that the fusion toxin must pass through an acidic compartment in order to deliver its ADP-ribosyltransferase to the cytosol of target cells. Bacha *et al.*[8] also demonstrated that inhibition of protein synthesis in target cells was, in fact, due to the specific ADP-ribosylation of elongation factor 2 in the target cell cytosol. Thus the cytotoxic action of DAB_{486}-IL-2 (i) is directed through the IL-2 receptor, (ii) requires passage through an acidic compartment in a manner analogous to native diphtheria toxin, and (iii) catalyzes the ADP-ribosylation of elongation factor 2 in a manner indistinguishable from that of native diphtheria toxin fragment A.

It is well known that the high-affinity form of the IL-2 receptor is composed of at least two subunits: a low-affinity 55-kDa glycoprotein (p55, Tac antigen) and an intermediate-infinity 75-kDa glycoprotein (p75, Tic antigen).[29-34] Moreover, it is known that both the high-affinity (p55 + p75) and intermediate-affinity receptor, but not the low-affinity receptor, undergo accelerated internalization after binding native IL-2.[33-36] Based on these observations, Waters *et al.*[9] have examined the receptor binding requirements of DAB_{486}-IL-2 for the efficient intoxication of target cells. As can be seen in FIGURE 1, dose response analysis of high-, intermediate-, and low-affinity IL-2 receptor-bearing cells demonstrates that only cell lines which bear the high-affinity form of the IL-2 receptor are sensitive to the cytotoxic action of DAB_{486}-IL-2 ($IC_{50} \leq 1 \times 10^{-10}$ M). In marked contrast, cell lines which bear either isolated p55 chains or p75 chains are resistant to the action of the fusion toxin and require exposure to ca. 1,000-fold higher concentrations ($IC_{50} \geq 1 \times 10^{-7}$ M) of DAB_{486}-IL-2.

Weissman *et al.*[35] have shown that the p55 subunit of the IL-2 receptor does not mediate efficient internalization of bound [^{125}I]-labeled IL-2. By comparison, native IL-2 bound to the p75 subunit of the receptor is known to be internalized as rapidly as the high-affinity receptor ($t\frac{1}{2}$ = 15 min).[37] Since p75-only-bearing cell lines were resistant to the action of DAB_{486}-IL-2, we reasoned that this resistance was due to altered binding of the fusion toxin to this subunit of the receptor. Waters *et al.*[9] have also determined the receptor binding properties of DAB_{486}-IL-2 by competitive displacement experiments using [^{125}I]-labeled IL-2. Approximately 200-fold higher concentrations of DAB_{486}-IL-2 are required to displace radiolabeled IL-2 from the high-affinity (p55 + p75) receptor. It is of interest to note that only 18-fold higher concentrations of DAB_{486}-IL-2 than native IL-2 are required to displace radiolabeled ligand from the p55 subunit; whereas, 120-fold higher concentrations are required for the p75 subunit.

The receptor-binding experiments described above strongly suggest that the relative resistance of p75-only-bearing cells to the cytotoxic action of DAB_{486}-IL-2 is due to altered binding to the p75 subunit of the receptor. Although both the p75 and the high-affinity heterodimer share the common property of rapidly internalizing bound ligand, p75 binding is characterized by slow kinetics of association/dissociation. In contrast, the high-affinity receptor displays the fast "on" rate of p55 and the slow "off" rate of p75.[38,39] Thus, an alteration in DAB_{486}-IL-2 binding to the p75 subunit may more dramatically influence the kinetics of this fusion toxin's binding to the intermediate vis-a-vis high-affinity receptor. Clearly, the results of the competitive displacement studies described by Waters et al.[9] are consistent with this interpretation. As determined by the concentration of fusion toxin required to inhibit radiolabeled IL-2 binding, it is evident that DAB_{486}-IL-2 displays altered binding to *both* subunits of the IL-2 receptor; however, binding to the p75 subunit appears to be more significantly affected than binding to the p55 subunit.

DAB_{389}-IL-2

Williams et al.[10] have demonstrated that the inframe deletion of 97 amino acids from Thr^{387} to His^{485} of DAB_{486}-IL-2 increases both the potency ($IC_{50} \approx 2$–5×10^{-11} M) and the apparent dissociation constant (K_d) of the resulting DAB_{389}-IL-2

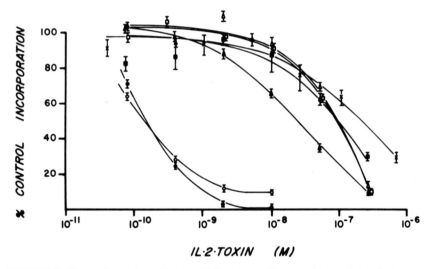

FIGURE 1. Comparison of sensitivity of high-, intermediate-, and low-affinity IL-2 receptor-bearing cell lines to DAB_{486}-IL-2. High-affinity receptor-bearing cell lines, HUT 102/6TG (○), C91/PL (●); intermediate-affinity receptor-bearing cell lines, YT2C2 (□), SKW6.4 (△), MLA-144 (▲); low-affinity receptor-bearing cell line, MT-1 (■). (Adapted from Waters et al.[9]

for high affinity IL-2-receptor-bearing T cells. In marked contrast, the deletion of an additional 94 amino acids (Asp^{291} to Gly^{483}) results in a greater than 1,000-fold loss of cytotoxic potency in the fusion toxin DAB_{295}-IL-2. It should be noted that the structural regions between Asp^{291} and Gly^{483} include the hydrophobic putative membrane spanning helical regions of fragment B that have been postulated to facilitate the delivery of fragment A across the endocytic vesicle membrane.[19] The results of experiments described by Williams et al.[10] strongly suggested that the putative membrane spanning helices of fragment B are essential in the intoxication process.

In addition, Williams et al.[10] have shown that the amphipathic membrane surface binding region of fragment B contained between Asn^{204} and Ile^{290} is also

TABLE 1. Bacterial Strains and Plasmids

Strain	*tox* Product	Reference
E. coli JM101	—	Yanisch-Perron *et al.*, 1985
E. coli (pDW24)	DAB_{486}-IL-2	2
E. coli (pDW27)	DAB_{389}-IL-2	45
E. coli (pDTK98)	DAB_{389}-(Glu^{408})IL-2	45
E. coli (pDTK99)	DAB_{389}-(1–10)$_2$IL-2	45
E. coli (pDTK100)	DAB_{389}-(1–10)$_3$IL-2	45
E. coli (pDTK101)	DAB_{389}-(1–10)$_4$IL-2	45

essential to the cytotoxicity of the DAB-IL-2 fusion toxins. It is important to note that the genetic deletion of this region of fragment B in both DAB (205–289)$_{486}$-IL-2 and DAB (205–289)$_{389}$-IL-2 also decreases biologic activity of the fusion toxin by ca. 1,000-fold. Most interestingly, these in-frame internal deletion mutations also effect the apparent K_d of the fusion toxin for the high-affinity IL-2 receptor. Since the region that has been deleted carries an amphipathic domain(s),[40] it is reasonable to postulate that this region of fragment B associates with the T cell membrane surface forming a nonspecific secondary binding event and appears to stabilize the interaction of the fusion toxin with the target cell surface.

DAB$_{389}$-IL-2 with Flexible Linkers (TABLE 1)

We have analyzed the primary amino acid sequence of DAB_{486}-IL-2 and DAB_{389}-IL-2 fusion toxins for predicted secondary structure using the PC GENE software (Intelligenetics, Mountain View, CA). In particular, the FLEXPRO program of Karplus and Schulz[41] was used to predict the flexibility of the DAB-IL-2 fusion toxins at each point of their sequence. This program calculates the theoretical flexibility of the peptide chain at each amino acid and is measured from the average value of the atomic temperature factor (B value) of the alpha carbon atom, as affected by the adjacent amino acids. The "neighbor-correlated" average normalized B values for each amino was found from a set of proteins whose three dimensional structural was known. The predicted flexibility at an amino acid is the weighted sum of the normalized B values (taking account of neighbors) of the seven amino acids closest to that point in the sequences.

It is of particular interest to note that this analysis of the DAB-IL-2 toxins has revealed a common predicted "most" flexible region— amino acids 1 through 10 of human IL-2 (TABLE 2). Since this region was also found to be unordered in the 5.5 Å crystal structure of IL-2,[42] we postulated that the apparent flexibility of this region of the fusion toxin might allow for some degree of mobility of the IL-2 component with respect to the diphtheria toxin-related sequences. Were this the case, amplification of the flexible region might result in a fusion toxin with in-

TABLE 2. Position and Amino Acid Sequence of the Predicted Most Flexible Segments of DAB_{486}-IL-2 and DAB_{389}-IL-2

Fusion Toxin	from	to	B[Norm]	Sequence
DAB_{486}-IL-2	487	493	1.135	Pro-Thr-Ser-Ser-Ser-Thr-Lys
DAB_{389}-IL-2	390	396	1.135	Pro-Thr-Ser-Ser-Ser-Thr-Lys

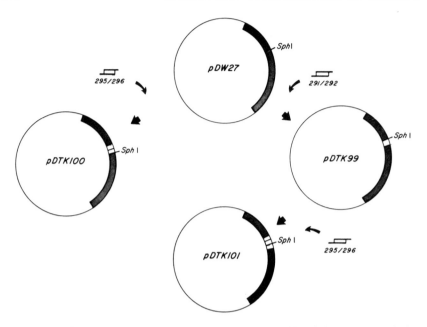

FIGURE 2. Plasmid DNA constructions used in the assembly of the DAB-IL-2 fusion toxins used in this study.

creased receptor binding affinity and potency. In order to amplify amino acids 1 through 10 of IL-2 sequences, two sets of oligonucleotides were designed and synthesized. It should be noted that in order to insure genetic stability of the oligonucleotide linkers codon usage was varied. The 291/292 oligonucleotide encodes the first ten amino acids of IL-2; whereas, the 295/296 oligonucleotide encodes two tandem repeats of IL-2 amino acids 1 through 10. As shown in FIGURE 2, pDW27 was digested by *Sph* I and either 291/292 or 295/296 oligonucleotides were ligated into place to form pTK99 and pTK100, respectively. In a similar fashion, pDTK101 was constructed from pDTK99 with insertion of the 427/428 oligonucleotides. pDTK101 has the putative flexible portions of IL-2 quadruplicated.

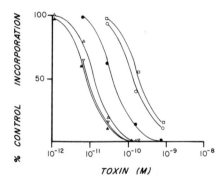

FIGURE 3. Dose-response analysis of DAB-IL-2 fusion toxins on high-affinity IL-2 receptor-bearing HUT 102/6TG cells. DAB_{486}-IL-2 (○); DAB_{389}-IL-2 (●); DAB_{389}-(Glu^{408})IL-2 (□); DAB_{389}-$(1-10)_2$IL-2 (▲); DAB_{389}-$(1-10)_3$IL-2 (▽); DAB_{389}-$(1-10)_4$IL-2 (△). Results are plotted as percent control [^{14}C]-leucine incorporation.

TABLE 3. Comparison of Dose-Response Analysis and Competitive Displacement of [^{125}I]-rIL-2 on Intermediate-Affinity IL-2 Receptor-Bearing YT2C2 Cells

Protein	IC$_{50}$ × 10^{-9} M	50% displacement × 10^{-9} M
IL-2	—	2
DAB$_{486}$-IL-2	70	120
DAB$_{389}$-IL-2	11	110
DAB$_{389}$-(Asp^{408}→Glu)IL-2	110	720
DAB$_{389}$-(1–10)$_2$IL-2	2	30
DAB$_{389}$-(1–10)$_3$IL-2	2	28
DAB$_{389}$-(1–10)$_4$IL-2	2	32

We have characterized the cytotoxic activity of DAB-IL-2 fusion toxins by dose-response analysis using cell lines which bear either the high, intermediate, or low affinity forms of the IL-2 receptor. Dose-response analysis using the high affinity receptor bearing HUT102 cell line shows that exposure to DAB$_{389}$-IL-2 at a concentration of 3.5 × 10^{-11} M for 18 hours results in 50% inhibition of protein synthesis (IC$_{50}$) FIGURE 3. It is of particular interest to note that all three of the insertion mutant variant forms of the fusion toxin were found to be more potent than DAB$_{389}$-IL-2. The IC$_{50}$ of DAB$_{389}$(1–10)^2-IL-2 and DAB$_{389}$(1–10)^3-IL-2 are almost identical (IC$_{50}$ = 7 × 10^{-12} M). DAB$_{389}$(1–10)^4-IL-2 was found to be slightly less potent than other insertion mutants (IC$_{50}$ = 1.3 × 10^{-11} M).

Moreover, relative to DAB$_{389}$-IL-2 the insertion mutants are also more potent against the YT$_{2c2}$ cell line which expresses only the intermediate-affinity form of the IL-2-receptor. However, as shown in TABLE 3, the concentrations of the insertion mutant forms of the DAB-IL-2 fusion toxin required to achieve an IC$_{50}$ are approximately 5-fold lower than DAB$_{389}$-IL-2.

In order to determine whether the relative cytotoxic potency binding affinity of the DAB-IL-2 fusion toxins was directly related to their binding affinity of IL-2 receptor, we conducted a series of competitive displacement experiments using [^{125}I]-labeled rIL-2. FIGURE 4 shows the results obtained with the high-affinity IL-2 receptor bearing HUT102/6TG cell line, both DAB$_{389}$-IL-2 (K$_d$ = 1.3 × 10^{-9} M vs K$_d$ = 2.9 × 10^{-9} M).

As shown in TABLE 3, a similar pattern of results was obtained using the intermediate-affinity YT$_{2c2}$ cells. The insertion mutant forms of the fusion toxin consistently showed a higher binding affinity than DAB$_{389}$-IL-2. In the case displacement of [^{125}I]-rIL-2 from the low-affinity form of the IL-2 receptor, similar concentrations of DAB$_{389}$-IL-2 and the mutant fusion toxins were required to achieve a 50% displacement of label (data not shown).

FIGURE 4. Competitive displacement of [^{125}I]-rIL-2 from the high-affinity IL-2 receptor by unlabeled rIL-2 ($\diamond$); DAB$_{486}$-IL-2 ($\bigcirc$); DAB$_{389}$-IL-2 ($\bullet$); DAB$_{389}$-(Glu^{408}IL-2 ($\square$); DAB$_{389}$-(1–10)$_2$IL-2 ($\blacktriangle$); DAB$_{389}$-(1–10)$_3$IL-2 ($\triangle$); DAB$_{389}$-(1–10)$_4$IL-2 ($\triangledown$).

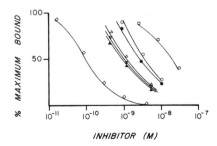

These studies clearly demonstrate that the application of protein engineering methodologies towards the development of second generation DAB-IL-2 fusion toxins will result in variants with increased biologic potency.

REFERENCES

1. MURPHY, J. R., W. BISHAI, M. BOROWSKI, A. MIYANOHARA, J. BOYD & S. NAGLE. 1986. Proc. Natl. Acad. Sci. USA 83: 8258–8262.
2. WILLIAMS, D. P., K. PARKER, P. BACHA, W. BISHAI, M. BOROWSKI, F. GENBAUFFE, T. B. STROM & J. R. MURPHY. 1987. Protein Eng. 1: 493–498.
3. CHAUDHARY, V. K., D. J. FITZGERALD, S. ADHYA & I. PASTAN. 1987. Proc. Natl. Acad. Sci. USA 84: 4538–4542.
4. LORBERBOUM-GALSKI, H., D. J. FITZGERALD, V. CHAUDHARY, S. ADHAYA & I. PASTAN. 1988. Proc. Natl. Acad. Sci. USA 85: 1922–1926.
5. CHAUDHARY, V. K., T. MIZUKAMI, T. R. FUERST, D. J. FITZGERALD, B. MOSS, I. PASTAN & E. A. BERGER. 1988. Nature (London) 335: 369–372.
6. SIEGALL, C. B., V. K. CHAUDHARY, D. J. FITZGERALD & I. PASTAN. 1988. Proc. Natl. Acad. Sci. USA 85: 9738–9742.
7. WILLIAMS, D. P., D. REGIER, D. AKIYOSHI, F. GENBAUFFE & J. R. MURPHY. 1988. Nucleic Acids Res., 16: 10453–10467.
8. BACHA, P., D. P. WILLIAMS, C. WATERS, J. M. WILLIAMS, J. R. MURPHY & T. B. STROM. 1988. J. Exp. Med. 167: 612–622.
9. WATERS, C. A., P. SCHIMKE, C. E. SNIDER, K. ITOH, K. A. SMITH, J. C. NICHOLS, T. B. STROM & J. R. MURPHY. 1990. Eur. J. Immunol. 20: 785–791.
10. WILLIAMS, D. P., C. E. SNIDER, T. B. STROM & J. R. MURPHY. 1990. J. Biol. Chem. 265: 11885–11890.
11. WILLIAMS, D. P., Z. WEN, R. S. WATSON, T. B. STROM & J. R. MURPHY. 1990. J. Biol. Chem. In press.
12. PAPPENHEIMER, A. M., JR. 1977. Ann. Rev. Biochem. 46: 69–94.
13. KAZCOREK, M., F. DELPEYROUX, N. CHENCINER, R. E. STREECK, J. R. MURPHY, P. BOQUET & P. TIOLLAIS. 1983. Science 221: 855–858.
14. GREENFIELD, L., M. BJORN, G. HORN, D. FONG, G. A. BUCK, R. J. COLLIER & D. A. KAPLAN. 1983. Proc. Natl. Acad Sci. USA 80: 6853–6857.
15. RATTI, G., R. RAPPUOLI & G. GIANNINI. 1983. Nucleic Acids Res. 11: 6589–6595.
16. GILL, D. M. & A. M. PAPPENHEIMER, JR. 1971. J. Biol. Chem. 246: 1492–1495.
17. COLLIER, R. J. & J. KANDEL. 1971. J. Biol. Chem. 246: 1496–1503.
18. UCHIDA, T., D. M. GILL & A. M. PAPPENHEIMER, JR. 1971. Nature (New Biol.) 233: 8–11.
19. BOQUET, P., M. S. SILVERMAN, A. M. PAPPENHEIMER, JR. & W. B. VERNON. 1976. Proc. Natl. Acad. Sci. USA 73: 4449–4453.
20. GREENFIELD, L., V. JOHNSON & R. J. YOULE. 1987. Science 238: 536–539.
21. ROLF, J. M., H. M. GAUDIN & L. EIDELS. 1990. J. Biol. Chem. In press.
22. MIDDELBROOK, J. L., R. B. DORLAND & S. LEPPLA. 1978. J. Biol. Chem. 253: 7325–7330.
23. MOYA, M., A. DAUTRY-VERSAT, B. GOUD, D. LOUVARD & P. BOQUET. 1985. J. Cell Biol. 101: 548–559.
24. SANDVIG, K., T. I. TONNESSEN, O. SAND & S. OLSNES. 1986. J. Biol. Chem. 261: 11639–11645.
25. DONOVAN, J. J., M. I. SIMON, R. K. DRAPER & M. MONTAL. 1981. Proc. Natl. Acad. Sci. USA 78: 172–176.
26. KAGAN, B. L., A. FINKELSTEIN & M. COLOMBINI. 1981. Proc. Natl. Acad. Sci. USA 78: 4950–4954.
27. YAMAIZUMI, M., E. MEKADA, T. UCHIDA & Y. OKADA. 1978. Cell 15: 245–250.
28. WALZ, G., B. ZANKER, K. BRAND, C. WATERS, F. GENBAUFFE, J. B. ZELDIS, J. R. MURPHY & J. R. MURPHY. 1989. Proc. Natl. Acad. Sci. USA 86: 9485–9488.

29. SHARON, M., R. D. KLAUSNER, B. R. CELLEN, R. CHIZZONITE & W. L. LEONARD. 1986. Science **234:** 859–863.
30. TSUDO, M. R., W. KOZAK, C. K. GOLDMAN & T. A. WALDMANN. 1986. Proc. Natl. Acad. Sci. USA **83:** 9694–9698.
31. TESHIGAWARA, K., H. M. WANG, K. KATO & K. A. SMITH. 1987. J. Exp. Med. **165:** 223–238.
32. DUKOVICH, M., Y. WANO, L. T. BICH-THUY, P. KATZ, D. CELLEN, J. H. KEHRL & W. C. GREENE. 1987. Nature (London) **237:** 518–522.
33. ROBB, R. J., C. M. RISK, J. YODOI & W. C. GREENE. 1987. Proc. Natl. Acad. Sci. USA **84:** 2001–2006.
34. TANAKA, T., O. SAIKI, S. DOI, M. FUJI, K. SUGAMURA, H. HARA, S. NEGORO & S. KISHIMOTO. 1988. J. Immunol. **140:** 866–870.
35. WEISSMAN, A. M., J. B. HARFORD, P. B. SVETLIK, W. L. LEONARD, J. M. DEPPER, T. A. WALDMANN, W. C. GREENE & R. D. KLAUSNER. 1986. Proc. Natl. Acad. Sci. USA **83:** 1463–1466.
36. FUJII, M., K. SUGAMURA, K. SANO, K. SAGITA & Y. HINUMA. 1986. J. Exp. Med. **163:** 550–562.
37. ROBB, R. J. & W. C. GREENE. 1987. J. Exp. Med. **165:** 1201–1206.
38. WANG, H. M. & K. A. SMITH. 1987. J. Exp. Med. **166:** 1055–1069.
39. LOWENTHAL, J. L. & W. C. GREENE. 1987. J. Exp. Med. **166:** 1156–1161.
40. LAMBOTTE, P., P. FALMAGNE, C. CAPIAU, J. ZANEN, J. M. RUYSSCHAERT & J. DIRKX. 1980. J. Cell Biol. **87:** 837–840.
41. KARPLUS, P. & G. E. SHULTZ. 1986. Naturwissenschaften **72:** 212–213.
42. BRANDHUBER, B. J., T. BOONE, W.C. KENNEY & D. B. MCKAY. 1987. Science **238:** 1707–1709.
43. KIYOKAWA, T., D. P. WILLIAMS, C. E. SNIDER, T. B. STROM & J. R. MURPHY. 1990. Protein Eng. Submitted for publication.

Photopheresis for the Treatment of Lupus Erythematosus

Preliminary Observations

ROBERT M. KNOBLER,[a] WINFRIED GRANINGER,[b]
ANDREAS LINDMAIER,[a] AND FRANZ TRAUTINGER[a]

[a]Department of Dermatology II
[b]Department of Internal Medicine II
University of Vienna General Hospital
Alserstrasse 4
A-1090 Vienna, Austria

INTRODUCTION

A highly specific therapy for systemic lupus erythematosus (SLE) is up to the present not available;[1-3] in this sense, nonspecific immunosuppressive therapy, such as corticosteroids and/or cytotoxic agents, is often necessary to control the disease. These drugs, however, are known to lead to serious side effects and complications.[4,5] Recently, extracorporeal phototreatment (EP) of circulating blood leucocytes was described as an effective way of immunomodulation.[13-21] This method employs extracorporeal low-energy ultraviolet A (UVA) irradiation of leucocytes after ingestion of a photoactivatable drug, 8-methoxypsoralen (8-MOP). Reinfusion of such photomodified leucocytes is thought to cause a modulation of the immune system. Exploratory experiments in a murine model of SLE have shown that administration of photoinactivated syngeneic splenocytes lead to inhibition of abnormal T cell proliferation and diminution of production of high titer anti-DNA antibodies.[13] Similarly, it has been demonstrated that experimental arthritis in rats can be prevented by the injection of modified autologous pathogenic T lymphocytes.[22-24] Although the exact mechanisms underlying the clinical responses documented with photopheresis have not been elucidated, beneficial clinical effects with EP have been documented in the treatment of human cutaneous T cell lymphoma, pemphigus vulgaris,[15,16,19] progressive systemic sclerosis,[20] and AIDS-related complex.[21]

In a two-year open clinical trial we investigated the clinical and laboratory effect of this new treatment modality in 10 patients diagnosed as having lupus erythematosus.

PATIENTS AND METHODS

Patients

Using the American Rheumatism Association (ARA) criteria[26] for lupus erythematosus we entered ten patients into the study. Of these, two were diagnosed as having subacute cutaneous LE (SCLE) with widespread cutaneous involvement. Patients were eligible for the study if they presented:

1. mild-to-moderate disease activity adequately controlled with conventional treatment including nonsteroidal antiinflammatory drugs (NSAIDs), low-dose steroids, chloroquin, oral azathioprine and/or oral cyclophosphamide; and
2. flare of disease activity upon attempted reduction and/or elimination of these drugs within three months prior to inclusion.

Furthermore, patients had to have serum-creatinine <2.5 mg/dl, leucocyte count >2.500 leukocytes/mm³, platelet count >75.000 platelets/mm³, hematocrit >25% and no involvement of the central nervous system. Patients were also excluded if they were under 18 years of age or had chronic or acute infections, or if their cardiopulmonary status did not permit the temporary blood volume changes associated with photopheresis. Female patients of child-bearing age were required to practice an accepted form of contraception. Disease activity was evaluated by using the SLE activity index scoring system (SIS) as previously described.[27] This score has been validated in other studies and against other indices such as SLAM, SLEDAI and BILAG.[28–32]

All patients gave written informed consent. The treatment protocol was approved by the Ethical Review Committee of the University of Vienna. Some characteristics of the patients who entered the study are summarized in TABLE 1.

Photopheresis Procedure

Photopheresis was performed as previously described:[15] one-half hour after ingestion of 0.6 mg/kg of 8-MOP patients were connected to the photopheresis device via a venous canula placed in the antecubital vein. The instrument used (UVAR II, Therakos, King of Prussia, PA) performs a combined parallel plasma and leukapheresis step with subsequent exposure of leukocytes and plasma to ultraviolet A light in a single unit. A continuous heparin dose of 500 IU/h was used for extracorporeal anticoagulation during EP. A plasmapheresis/leukapheresis was performed for a total volume of 540 ml (300 ml plasma + 240 ml buffy coat). The red blood cells were reinfused in 250 ml of saline. In this fashion approximately 10% of the circulating lymphocyte pool is collected, radiated and returned to the patient. The original 270-minute exposure to ultraviolet A was considerably shortened due to a more efficient light source (increased exposure surface per unit time), and an earlier start of radiation, namely immediately after collection of the first of the six fractions of 40 ml buffy coat. The final percentage of red blood cells in the exposate was 3.98 ± 0.79 percent (mean ± SD). Exposure of leucocytes to UVA light (334–346 nm range) was set so as to obtain a final energy delivery of photo energy of 2 J/cm² to the white blood cell DNA.[15] After exposure to UVA light the entire leukocyte-enriched plasma volume was reinfused within a period of 30 minutes.

Treatment Protocol

In all patients entering the study a sham-photopheresis (*i.e.*, no reinfusion of the treated plasma/buffy coat fraction) was performed before the actual treatment period. The leukocyte concentrate and 300 ml plasma which had been irradiated with UVA were used to obtain data on cell viability, proliferation assays, other cellular studies, as well as optimal effective psoralen levels.

TABLE 1. Clinical Characteristics of Patients Entered in the Study Protocol

Patient No.	Onset of Disease (Age)	Duration of Disease Before EP	LE Criteria[a]	Previous Treatment[b]	Anti-DNA (n <50 IU/ml)	ANA (n <1:10)
1	42	3 yrs	MR,PS,OU,A,IM,ANA,Sm, Ro,nRNP,My,Ry,AR	100 mg diclofenac/day azathioprine (AZA) 100 mg/day prednisone 20/10 mg/day	57.5	ANA 1:40
2	68	4 yrs	MR,DR,S.H,IM,ANA,Ro, AR,My,Ry	100 mg diclofenac/day prednisone 5/10 mg/day chloroquine 100 mg/day	59	ANA 1:3200
3	39	3 yrs	MR,OU,A,S,IM,ANA,Ro	150 mg diclofenac/day prednisone 20 mg/day AZA 250 mg/day	215	ANA 1:800
4	20	4 yrs	MR,PS,A,S(SC),H,IM, ANA,NE,Ro,La	chloroquine 100 mg/day 200 mg indomethacin AZA 100 mg/day	266	ANA 1:800
5	20	9 yrs	AR,My,Ry,MR,PS,A,IM, ANA,nRNP,AR	prednisone 40 mg/day 100 mg diclofenac/day chloroquine 100 mg/day prednisone 8/4 mg/day	197	ANA 1:1600
6	31	6 yrs	MR,DR,PS,A,S,H,IM,ANA	prednisone 20/10 mg/day 0.5 g aspirin/day	120	ANA 1:320
7	26	9 yrs	MR,PS,A,RE,NE,IM, ANA,AR,GN	prednisone 16/8 mg/day chloroquine 100 mg/day	640	ANA 1:800
8	58	6 yrs	A,SP,RE,HL,IM,ANA,Ro, La,AR,Ry	AZA 100 mg/day prednisone 20 mg/day	68.5	ANA 1:2560
9	27	21 yrs	DR,PS,IM,ANA	chloroquine 100 mg/day	0	ANA 1:20
10	20	4 yrs	MR,DR,PS,ANA	chloroquine 100 mg/day prednisone 40 mg/day	0	ANA 1:100

a ARA revised criteria for the classification of SLE (1–11) (1982):[25]

1. Malar rash (MR)
2. Discoid rash (DR)
3. Photosensitivity (PS)
4. Oral ulcers (OU)
5. Arthritis (A)
6. Serositis (S)
   a) Pleuritis or (SP)
   b) Pericarditis (SC)
7. Renal disorder (RE)
8. Neurologic disorder (NE)

b Since diagnosis of disease.

9. Hematologic disorder (H)
   a) Hemolytic anemia or (HA)
   b) Leucopenia or (HL)
   c) Thrombocytopenie (HT)
10. Immunoglioc disorder (IM)
    a) Positive LE preparation or
    b) Anti-DNA or
    c) Anti-Sm or
    d) False-positive serologic test for syphilis

11. Antinuclear antibody (ANA)

Other:

12. Myalgia (My)
    (normal SCPK and EMG)
13. Raynauds (Ry)
    (confirmed by rheography)
14. Arthralgias (AR)
15. Glomerulonephritis (GN)
16. Sm, Ro(SSA), La(SSB), nRNP

TABLE 2. Medication Use before and after Photopheresis

Patient	Beginning of EP	End of EP
1	a) 100 mg diclofenac/day b) prednisone alt. 20/10 mg/day c) azathioprine 100 mg/day	none
2	a) 100 mg diclofenac/day b) prednisone alt. 5/10 mg/day	none
3	a) 150 mg diclofenac/day b) azathioprine 150 mg/day c) chloroquine 100 mg/day	none
4	a) 200 mg indomethacin b) prednisone 80 mg/day c) azathioprine 100 mg/day	a) none b) prednisone alt. 5/10 mg/day c) none
5	a) 100 mg diclofenac/day b) prednisone alt. 8/4 mg/day c) chloroquine 100 mg/day	a) none b) prednisone alt. 6/2 mg/day c) none
6	prednisone alt. 20/10 mg/day	none
7[a]	a) 0.5 g aspirin/day b) prednisone 16/8 mg/day alt.	a) NC[b] b) NC
8[a]	a) azathioprine 100 mg/day b) prednisone 20 mg	a) NC b) NC
9	chloroquine 100 mg/day	none
10	prednisone 40 mg/day	none

[a] Did not complete study.

[b] NC = no change during period of observation.

Two months after the sham treatment and continuation of the previously established treatment (TABLE 2), patients entered the actual therapeutic trial with monthly EP on two consecutive days for 6 months followed by EP every 3 months. Conventional therapy was maintained upon initiation of EP and modified subsequently as a function of the patient's response to treatment.

Patients were evaluated at monthly intervals for a minimum period of 1 year after their last photopheresis treatment.

Laboratory and Clinical Scores

Based on the mentioned activity index scoring system all patients evaluated had, upon entering the study, a total score of at least 7 (mean ± SD: 11.1 ± 2.7).

TABLE 3. Score Changes[a] in 8 LE Patients Treated by Extracorporeal Photochemotherapy[b]

Variable	Base Line	Final	p Value	Follow-up[c]	p Value
Clinical score	7.25 ± 1.48	1.81 ± 1.64	<0.001	1.2 ± 1.25	<0.001
Laboratory score	3.8 ± 1.8	3.4 ± 2.06	NS	3.6 ± 1.94	NS
Total score	11.12 ± 2.69	5.18 ± 2.61	<0.001	4.8 ± 1.15	<0.001
Medication score	4 ± 0	0.25 ± 0.46	<0.001	0.4 ± 0.89	<0.0001

[a] Laboratory score and clinical score were assigned to each patient based on the SLE activity index scoring system (SIS).

[b] Plus-minus values are mean ± SD; NS denotes not significant.

[c] At least 12 months after last EP.

For the laboratory parameters, significant response to therapy was defined as a sustained improvement of >25% in the laboratory parameters of the activity scoring system.[27] Where applicable a score of the extent of dermatological involvement was adapted from Edelson *et al.*[15] Evaluation of arthritic symptoms and response to treatment was performed as previously described.[33] A medication necessity score[15] was calculated as follows: the total daily dose of steroid, nonsteroidal antiinflammatory drugs (NSAIDs), and/or cytotoxic therapy before EP treatment was taken as baseline (100%). The prescribed dosage of each of these drugs was then evaluated in monthly intervals. A reduction of the dosage prescribed by >25% of the initial value was assigned a one-point reduction of a four-point score (TABLE 3). Parameters were recorded before and at the end of the treatment period and 12 months thereafter (TABLE 4).

TABLE 4. Photpheresis in SLE Arthritis: Clinical Results

Patient No.	Joint No. (Score)[a]		Pain Score[b]
1	beginning	4	3
	end	1	1
	control (12 mo)	0	1
3	beginning	5	3
	end	0	0
	control (12 mo)	0	1
4	beginning	4	2
	end	1	1
	control (12 mo)	0	1
5	beginning	5	3
	end	1	2
	control (12 mo)	2	1
6	beginning	3	2
	end	0	0
	control (12 mo)	0	0
Mean ± SD	beginning	4.2 ± 0.84	2.6 ± 0.55
	end	0.6 ± 0.55[c]	0.8 ± 0.84[c]
	control (12 mo)	0.4 ± 0.89[c]	0.8 ± 0.45[c]

[a] Joint no: number of joints with swelling and pain.
[b] Pain score: 0 = absent, 1 = slight, 2 = moderate, 3 = severe.
[c] $p < 0.001$ vs beginning.

Cellular Studies

Mitogen Stimulation

DNA synthesis of irradiated and nonirradiated peripheral blood mononuclear cells (PBMC) was investigated by mitogen stimulation. Cell count was adjusted to 5×10^6 cells/ml in complete culture medium (CM): RPMI 1640 medium with 25 mM Hepes buffer with L-glutamine (Gibco, Ltd., UK) and 5% heat-inactivated fetal calf serum (Gibco, Ltd., UK).[34]

The cells were aliquoted at 100 μl/well in five replicate wells into a 96-well flat-bottom microtiter plate (Flow Laboratories) and incubated with and without phytohemagglutinin (PHA, Sigma, St. Louis, MO) at a final concentration of 2 μg/

ml.[35] After culture for 72 hours at 37°C under a 5% CO_2 atmosphere, the cultures were pulsed with 1 μl/well of ^{3}H-thymidine (Amersham, Arlington Heights, IL) and harvested 12 hours later with a Mash II automated harvester (Whittaker M.A. Bioproducts, Walkersville, MD). The samples were counted in a liquid scintillation counter (Amersham).

Viability of Mononuclear Cells

The radiated PBMCs were isolated by ficoll gradient density centrifugation.[15] The viability of mononuclear cells before and after EP was evaluated by trypan blue exclusion before incubation and after a 72-hour incubation at 37°C in CM.

Serum Levels of Methoxsalen

8-methoxypsoralen was administered in a liquid formulation (Oxsoralen, Gerot, Vienna, Austria), with better bioavailability than the previously used crystalline formulation.[15] Thirty minutes after ingestion peak blood levels were determined according to the newly developed method of Gasparro et al.[34] which detects amounts of 8-MOP as low as 10 ng/ml in a 1-ml serum sample.[36,37] To analyse 8-MOP serum levels high pressure liquid chromatography (HPLC) was performed after plasma extraction by solid phase affinity cartridges.[36,37] Additional plasma samples were obtained during every treatment from the collection bags after the collecting cycles had been terminated. Oral psoralen dosage was adjusted by 10 mg increments in order to maintain a minimum of 50 ng/ml 8-MOP in the radiated fraction of blood cells.

Laboratory Parameters

Standard chemical parameters (analyzed in a Technicon parallel analyzer), complement levels (C2,C3,C4, detected by nephelometry), ANA (detected by indirect imunofluorescence on rat liver sections), anti-DNA (Amersham RIA) and ANA subsets (double immunodiffusion) were determined routinely at baseline during the treatment period and for follow up in all patients. In addition, circulating soluble interleukin-2 receptor levels (sIL-2R) were determined in sera from seven SLE patients before and after EP, and in 20 healthy controls. For this purpose we used an enzyme-linked immunosorbent assay (ELISA; T Cell Sciences, Cambridge, MA), according to the modified method of Rubin et al.[38,39]

Statistical Analysis

Statistical significance was performed using the paired t test. A p value of less than 0.05 was considered significant.

RESULTS

Clinical Response

Of the ten patients initially entered into the study, eight were able to complete this experimental clinical investigation. Patient No. 8 refused further treatment due to personal reasons after her fourth EP. A second patient (patient No. 7) died six months after the initiation of the EP program. Autopsy did not demonstrate pulmonary embolism or occluded arteries. Although this patient's death occurred 10 days post EP, a relationship to EP treatment cannot be ruled out. A significant clinical improvement could be documented in 7 of the 8 patients evaluable for response (TABLE 3, FIGS. 1 and 2). One patient (No. 5) has remained stable without significant reduction in medication (TABLE 2). Patients 3, 5, 9, 10 showed improvement of symptoms after 3 to 5 months of treatment. In none of the patients could disease activation due to EP be documented. During the observa-

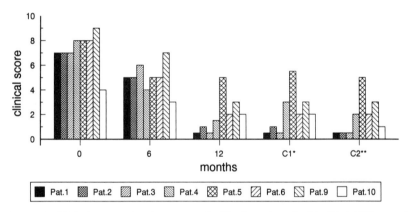

FIGURE 1. Clinical score of patients treated with photopheresis. Modified NIH score.[26] *Control #1, 6 months after last treatment; **control #2, 12 months after last treatment.

tion period the laboratory score of the SLE index remained unchanged in all patients (baseline of 3.8 ± 1.8 to a final value of 3.4 ± 2.1) (TABLE 4, FIG. 3). Based on independent clinical judgement of disease activity, the dosage of steroids and immunosuppressive agents as well as NSAIDs could be reduced progressively in 8 patients. In 6 patients steroids and/or cytotoxic medication were ommitted completely (TABLE 2). Patients presenting cutaneous lesions (8 patients) continuously improved as a function of the number of treatments increased, particularly patients 2, 3, 4, 6, 9 and 10. First signs of improvement were noted 4 to 6 months into the treatment. In contrast to the diagnostic skin biopsies in patients 3, 5, 6 and 7, repeat biopsies after treatment in patients 3 and 6 were negative by histology and immunofluorescence, in affected as well as normal skin. The response of cutaneous lesions to natural UVA/UVB-light exposure was not affected, implying that strict avoidance of sun exposure had to be maintained during as well as after treatment. Among the clinical symptoms that appear to respond consistently to EP were arthritis, arthralgias and myalgias. Four of five patients who initially presented with swollen and tender joints (patients 1, 3, 4, 5, 6; TABLE 4 and FIG. 2) showed an improvement with cessation of symptoms and no recurrence; in those patients, NSAIDS and steroids could be reduced or withdrawn and did not have to be reinstated (patients 1, 3, 5, 6; TABLE 2).

Review of Patients

In patient No. 1 fatigue diminished substantially as well as arthralgia, arthritis, myalgia and muscle weakness so that she was able to resume her household and

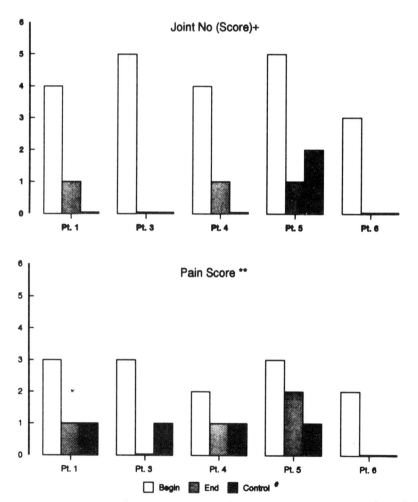

FIGURE 2. Response of SLE arthritis, joint no., and pain score to photopheresis treatment. +Joint no: number of joints with swelling and pain. **Pain score: 0 = absent, 1 = slight, 2 = moderate, 3 = severe. #12 months after last treatment. *p <0.001 vs begin.

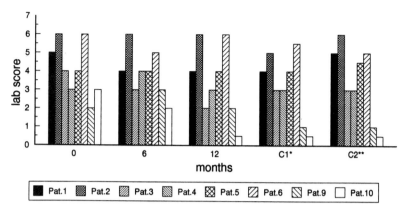

FIGURE 3. Laboratory score of patients treated with photopheresis. Modified NHI score.[26] *Control #1, 6 months after last treatment; **control #2, 12 months after last treatment.

work chores. Joint swelling has not recurred. Sensitivity to UV light remains unchanged. On rare occasions the patient uses 50 mg/day of the NSAID diclofenac for arthralgia. Twelve months after her last treatment the patient remains well with no signs of disease progression.

Skin lesions showed continuous improvement in patient No. 2. Fatigue and muscle pain have improved significantly. UV sensitivity, though diminished, persists. At 12 months after her last treatment a major short-lived rise in serological parameters was observed (ANA rose from 1:800 to 1:12.800, anti-DNA from 1:50 to 535 IU/ml), but neither organ involvement nor concomitant clinical symptoms could be identified.

Patient No. 3 also experienced significant clinical improvement: symptoms attributed to Raynaud's phenomenon as well as migraine-like headaches have ceased. Recurrent fever and solitary skin lesions disappeared; diclofenac 25 mg/day is sufficient to control occassional arthralgia. Twelve months after her last treatment the patient maintains her clinical improvement.

In patient No. 4 (who had been diagnosed as having SLE after severe pericardial effusion of 2000 ml two years before start of EP) pericardial effusion has remained minimal as confirmed by echocardiography (5–10 ml). Mitigated bouts of joint pain can be controlled by use of 50–100 mg/day of diclofenac. Ten months after her last treatment she reports continuing subjective improvement regarding fatigue and organic brain syndrome. Patient No. 5 has shown subjective improvement of her arthralgias. At the last treatment (9th treatment series) the systemic prednisone intake could be reduced from 8/4 mg to alternate 6/0 mg per day. Chloroquin has been discontinued. The extensive skin involvement of patient No. 6 has shown slow but constant resolution of lesions. Fatigue is not present anymore, arthritis swelling has resolved with no further significant clinical joint pain. Except for occasional use of 1% hydrocortisone cream on unresolved cutaneous lesions all medication has been stopped. Slight increase of perilesional cutaneous inflammatory infiltrates can be observed during menstruation with resolution thereafter.

Patients 9 and 10, both of whom have SCLE, have shown a slow but definite resolution of cutaneous lesions with no new lesions. Systemic therapy (see TABLE

2) has not been resumed and bouts have not recurred since EP treatment was implemented.

Patient No. 9 was treated for 12 months. She has maintained a clear skin status with no signs of exacerbation for 11 months. Alopecia regions on scalp have shown areas of hair regrowth.

Laboratory Parameters during and after Treatment

In the course of EP we were not able to find any marked changes in specific routine laboratory parameters (TABLES 3, 6; FIG. 3). All parameters of SLE activity including sIL2r remained essentially unaffected. The soluble sIL2r levels (TABLE 5, last line) before and after treatment phases showed a clear correlation

TABLE 5. Laboratory Changes in 8 LE Patients Treated by Extracorporeal Photochemotherapy[a]

Variable	Base Line	Final	p Value	% Change
Complement C_3 (mg/liter) n: 80–180	83.9 ± 19.7	84 ± 28.9	NS	+0.12
Complement C_4 (mg/liter) n: 20–60	13.1 ± 2.75	15.1 ± 5.51	NS	+15.20
Total complement (CH_{50} units) n: 150–250	117 ± 53	115 ± 62	NS	−1.71
Immunoglobulin A (mg/liter) n: 700–3500 mg/l	328 ± 217	363 ± 193	NS	+10.60
Immunoglobulin G (mg/liter) n: 6500–22,000 mg/l	1747 ± 558	2045 ± 529	p < 0.01	+17.05
Immunoglobulin M (mg/liter) n: 500–3500 mg/l	128 ± 63	168 ± 74	p < 0.05	+31.25
Anti-DNA (U/ml) n <50	256 ± 220	227 ± 198	NS	−11.33
CD3 (%)	72.33 ± 19.19	67 ± 7.64	NS	−7.34
CD4 (%)	42.33 ± 11.96	40.66 ± 9.87	NS	−3.95
CD8 (%)	25.83 ± 10.45	26.5 ± 9.52	NS	+2.69
CD4/CD8	1.97 ± 1.07	1.75 ± 0.78	NS	−11.16
s-IL2 (n = 8)	1093 ± 366	1035 ± 369	NS	−5.60

[a] Plus-minus values are mean 5 SD; NS denotes not significant.

with laboratory disease activity (score manifestation) but not with the clinical score. This is in accordance with previous reports.[39] Evaluation of T cell subsets (TABLE 5) showed no significant changes throughout the study.

Complications

During the course of treatment the following clinical abnormalities were observed. Hypovolemic hypotension with slight nausea was documented in one patient during EP procedure. Three patients were found to develop nausea after ingestion of the 8-MOP capsules. One patient presented with an urticarial rash after two treatments; it was found to be due to sunlight sensitivity and psoralen could still be detected in the patient's serum. The patient had not been compliant with recommended UV light protection measures. A later repeat exposure of the

TABLE 6A. Viability of PBMC after Extracorporeal Photochemotherapy[a]

	Exposure	
Days of Incubation after Exposure	8-MOP Leukapheresis (Mean ± SD)	8-MOP Leukapheresis Ultraviolet A (Mean ± SD)
0	98 ± 1.6	98 ± 2.0 NS[b]
1	96 ± 1.8	69 ± 16.1[c]
2	91 ± 4.6	24 ± 6.0[c]
3	90 ± 4.1	10 ± 4.9[c]

[a] Viability was determined using the trypan blue exclusion method.[32] All readings were done in triplicate. PBMC were isolated from the collection compartment by ficoll density centrifugation. Incubation was performed at 37°C in 5% heat inactivated fetal calf serum in RPMI 1640 medium with 25 mm buffer hepes buffer with L-glutamine (complete medium[32]).
[b] NS = not significant.
[c] p <0.005.

patient, after treatment, to natural UV light under controlled conditions (8-MOP serum level at time of exposure: 65 ng/ml) reproduced the observed urticarial reaction. None of the unwanted effects led to interruption or cessation of photopheresis cycles.

Viability and Mitogen Stimulation Studies

Our results confirm the effects of photopheresis on the viability of peripheral blood mononuclear cells (PBMC):[15] the viability of unirradiated cells remained >90% in the 3-day incubation period, while the viability of the UVA-treated fraction dropped to 10% of the simultaneous control (TABLE 6A). Mitogen stimulation showed that complete photopheresis led to a mean 96.4% inhibition when compared to the cells treated in an analogous manner but without UVA irradiation (TABLE 6B).

Treatment Time and Psoralen Levels

Treatment time for every photopheresis procedure averaged 182.9 ± 4.74 minutes (mean ± SD). Concentrations of plasma 8-MOP before and after radiation

TABLE 6B. Inhibition of PHA[a]-Stimulated DNA Synthesis of Mononuclear Cells of 6 Patients before and after Extracorporeal UV-A Exposure (after 72 Hours in Culture)

8-MOP + UV-A Exposure (Joules/cm²)	CPM[b] × 10³	Stimulation Index[c]	% Inhibition
0	33.6 ± 12.0[c]	86.5	0
2	1.2 ± 3[c]	3.0	96.4
Control	38.9 ± 14.1[c]		

[a] Phytohemagglutinin.
[b] Counts per minute.
[c] Mean ± SD (same patients before 8-MOP + UV-A).

were found to be unchanged by UVA exposure in all cases. The mean ± SD of 8-MOP levels in the irradiated plasma fraction were 125 ± 68.99 ng/ml. In one treatment a maximum concentration of 382 ng/ml after oral intake of 60 mg 8-MOP was observed.

DISCUSSION

In the present preliminary study we have evaluated the effects of extracorporeal photochemotherapy in the treatment of lupus erythematosus. The eight patients who remained in the study experienced clinical improvement. In five patients these changes were maintained during a one-year follow-up period after the end of the EP treatment. Among the symptoms that showed objective improvement were skin lesions and arthritis. The subjective amelioration of complaints like fatigue and arthralgia was reported in almost all patients. The use of immunosuppressive drugs, steroids and NSAIDs could be reduced significantly. However, since this was not a double blind study, an "in-study" effect during the treatment phase cannot be excluded. A control group using 8-MOP alone was not included due to ethical considerations.

Laboratory parameters were not significantly affected by EP: they did not appear to correspond to the clinical improvement. This is in contrast to the results of the animal model where ANA titers dropped significantly under EP,[13] as well as in SLE patients with renal involvement where levels of anti-ds-DNA antibodies appear to correlate with disease activity.[40-42]

It is another important observation of this study that extracorporeal irradiation of blood with UVA followed by reinfusion did not induce exacerbation of SLE symptoms, regardless of whether the patients were UV sensitive or not. This is in contrast to previous experience in exposing patients directly to UVA light with or without the use of psoralen; moreover, recent reports have described the induction of connective tissue disease including subacute cutaneous lupus erythematosus in association with PUVA treatment for psoriasis.[38-42] The clinical effects of photopheresis appear to be induced by the synergistic effects of 8-MOP and UVA.[13-21] In treatments where 8-MOP levels were below 50 ng/ml response appeared to be less pronounced.[13-24] In this sense the major difficulty encountered was the great variability in obtaining appropriate serum psoralen levels. Studies on the intravenous or extracorporeal application of 8-MOP directly into the buffy coat/plasma collecting bag should help obtain constant predictable levels in the future and eliminate this source of error. Although the mechanisms responsible for the clinical improvement are currently unclear it is conceivable that a modulation of the immune system is achieved by the reinfusion of physicochemically altered lymphocytes. This is supported by the observation of Lider et al.[24] that reinfusion of physically altered autologous effector T lymphocytes prevented the development of adjuvant arthritis, as well as by the successful elimination by EP of autologous (malignant) T cell clones in CTCL patients.[15] A hypothetical generation of anti-clonotypic T cells is further supported by studies in the MRL/1 mice: re-infusion of methoxsalen photoinactivated mononuclear cells suppressed the development of the SLE-like syndrome as well as lymphoid hyperplasia;[13] moreover, the modification of an autoimmune-directed T cell deregulation has been shown in experimental allergic encephalitis (EAE) by the injection of modified autoantigen specific T cell lines.[22] The results obtained in using the 8-MOP-UVA procedure to prepare T cell vaccines for trial in adjuvant arthritis and EAE have been reported to be similar to those obtained by the same group using glutaraldehyde or formaldehyde treatment of activated, autoimmune T cell clones.[48] Similar effects have been recently described in related autoimmune disorders.[52-55]

Despite all this experimental support of possible clonotypic changes, nonspecific immunosuppression could also be additionally responsible for the observed clinical improvement in our patients as in the transplant animal model, where it is considered to be instrumental in the control of allograft skin rejection.[14]

The well-known "cytostatic" effects on nucleated cell replication and viability attributed to the effect of 8-MOP plus UVA cannot account for the observed effects since only a small fraction of lymphocytes (10–20%) are treated during photopheresis. Though unlikely, the effect of heparinoids on T cell trafficking mechanisms as reported by Y. Naporstek[53] seems to indicate that this important factor in EP will need further investigation. Although functional and investigative laboratory changes are not sufficient for a full explanation of EP effects yet, our study shows the feasibility and safety of this experimental approach and gives encouraging results with respect to clinical improvement. Our observations show that extracorporeally activated drugs such as 8-methoxypsoralen do not induce exacerbations in patients with proven photosensitivity and LE. In future studies, a more extended, controlled clinical trial will have to be performed. Moreover, detailed studies of immunoregulation[54-59] and clonal function will be necessary to pinpoint the precise mechanism by which clinical improvements are induced by photopheresis.

REFERENCES

1. BLAESE, R. M., J. GRAYSON & A. D. STEINBERG. 1980. Increased immunoglobulinsecreting cells in the blood of patients with systemic lupus erythematosus. Am. J. Med. **69:** 345–350.
2. KOFFLER, D., P. SCHUR & H. KUNKEL. 1967. Immunohistochemical studies on the nephritis of lupus erythematosus. J. Exp. Med. **126:** 617–619.
3. BALOW, J. E. & G. C. TSOKOS. 1984. T and B lymphocyte function in patients with lupus nephritis: correlation with renal pathology. Clin. Nephrol. **21:** 93–97.
4. EISENBERG, D., Y. SCHÖNFELD & R. S. SCHWARTZ. 1987. The importance of the study of monoclonal antibodies. *In* Systemic Lupus Erythematosus, Clinical and Experimental Aspects. J. S. Smolen & C. C. Zielinski, Eds. 88–104. Springer Verlag. Berlin.
5. MORROW, W. J. W., P. YOUNION, D. A. ISENBERG & M. L. SMITH. 1983. Systemic lupus erythematosus: 25 years of treatment related to immunopathology. Lancet **2:** 206–211.
6. STROBER, S., E. FIELD, R. T. HOPPE *et al.* 1985. Treatment of intractable lupus nephritis with total lymphoid irradiation. Ann. Intern. Med. **102:** 450–458.
7. BRAHN, E., S. M. HELFGOTT, J. A. BELLI *et al.* 1984. Total lymphoid irradiation therapy in refractory rheumatoid arthritis. Arthritis Rheum. **27:** 481–488.
8. TRENTHAN, D. E., J. A. BELLI, R. J. ANDERSON *et al.* 1981. Clinical and immunologic effects of fractionated total lymphoid irradiation in refractory rheumatoid arthritis. N. Engl. J. Med. **305:** 976–982.
9. DWOSH, I. L., A. R. GILES, P. M. FORD *et al.* 1983. Plasmapheresis therapy in rheumatoid arthritis. N. Engl. J. Med. **308:** 1124–1129.
10. TENENBAUM, J., M. B. UROWITZ, E. C. KEYSTONE *et al.* 1979. Leucapheresis in severe rheumatoid arthritis. Ann. Rheum. Dis. **38:** 40–44.
11. WALLACE, D., D. GOLDFINGER, C. LOWE *et al.* 1982. A double-blind, controlled study of lymphoplasmapheresis versus sham apheresis in rheumatoid arthritis. N. Engl. J. Med. **306:** 1406–1410.

12. STROBER, S., M. DHILLON, M. SCHUBERT et al. 1989. Acquired immune tolerance to cadaveric renal allografts: a study of three patients treated with total lymphoid irradiation. N. Engl. J. Med. **321:** 28–33.
13. BERGER, C. L., M. PEREZ, L. LAROCHE & R. EDELSON. 1990. Inhibition of autoimmune disease in a murine model of systemic lupus erythematosis induced by exposure to syngeneic photoinactivated lymphocytes. J. Invest. Dermatol. **94:** 52–57.
14. PEREZ, M., R. EDELSON, L. LAROCHE & C. BERGER. 1989. Inhibition of antiskin allograft immunity by infusions with syngeneic photoinactivated effector lymphocytes. J. Invest. Dermatol. **92:** 669–676.
15. EDELSON, R., C. BERGER, F. GASPARRO et al. 1987. Treatment of cutaneous T-cell-lymphoma by extracorporeal photochemotherapy. N. Engl. J. Med. **316:** 297–303.
16. HEALD, P. W. & R. EDELSON. 1988. Photopheresis for T cell mediated diseases. Adv. Dermatol. **3:** 25–40.
17. KNOBLER, R. M. 1987. Photopheresis—extracorporeal irradiation of 8-MOP containing blood—a new therapeutic modality. Blut **54:** 247–250.
18. KNOBLER, R. M. & R. L. EDELSON. 1986. Cutaneous T cell lymphoma. Med. Clin. North Am. **70:** 109–138.
19. ROOK, H. L., B. V. JEGASOTHY, P. HEALD, G. T. NAHASS, C. DITRE, W. K. WITMER, G. S. LAZARUS & R. L. EDELSON. 1990. Extracorporeal photochemotherapy for drug-resistant pemphigus vulgaris. Ann. Intern. Med. **112:** 303–305.
20. ROOK, A. H., B. FREUNDLICH, G. T. NAHASS, R. WASHKO, B. MACELIS, M. SKOLNICKI, P. BROMLEY, W. K. WITMER & B. V. JEGASOTHY. 1989. Treatment of autoimmune disease with extracorporeal photochemotherapy: progressive systemic sclerosis. Yale J. Biol. Med. **62**(6): 639–646.
21. BISSACIA, E., C. BERGER & A. S. KLAINER. 1990. Extracorporeal photopheresis in the treatment of AIDS-related complex: a pilot study. Ann. Intern. Med. **113:** 270–275.
22. COHEN, I. R. 1985. The study and manipulation of experimental autoimmune disease using T lymphocyte lines. J. Invest. Dermatol. **85:** 34S–38S.
23. HOLOSHITZ, J., Y. NAPARSTEK, A. BEN-NUN & I. R. COHEN. 1983. Lines of T lymphocytes induce or vaccinate against autoimmune arthritis. Science **219:** 56–58.
24. LIDER, O., K. NORTHAN, M. SHINITZKY & I. R. COHEN. 1987. Therapeutic vaccination against adjuvant arthritis using autoimmune T cells treated with hydrostatic pressure. Immunology **84:** 4577–4580.
25. BEN-NUN, A., H. WEKERLE & I. R. COHEN. 1981. Vaccination against autoimmune encephalomyelitis with T lymphocyte cell lines reactive against myelin basic protein. Nature **292:** 60–61.
26. TAN, E. M., A. S. COHEN, J. FRIES et al. 1982. The 1982 revised criteria for the classification of systemic lupus erythematosus. Arthritis Rheum. **25:** 1271–1277.
27. SMOLEN J. S. 1987. Clinical and serological features—incidence and diagnostic approach. In Systemic Lupus Erythematosus—Clinical and Experimental Aspects. J. S. Smolen & C. C. Zielinski, Eds. 170–196. Springer-Verlag. New York–Heidelberg.
28. LIANG, M. H., S. STERN & J. M. ESDAILE. 1988. Towards an operational definition of SLE activity for research. Rheum. Dis. Clin. **14:** 57–66.
29. BILAG: BRITISH ISLES LUPUS ASSESSMENT GROUP. 1986. A comparison of disease activity scores in SLE. Br. J. Rheumatol. **25:** 16.
30. French Cooperative Study Group. 1985. Activity criteria count. A randomized trial of plasma exchange in severe acute SLE. Plasma Ther. Trans. Tech. **6:** 535–539.
31. UROWITZ, M. B., D. D. GLADMAN & E. C. S. TOZMAN. 1984. The lupus activity criteria count LACC. J. Rheumatol. **11:** 783–787.
32. LIANG, M. H., S. A. SCOHER, M. G. LARSON & P. H. SCHUR. 1989. Reliability and validity of six systems for the clinical assessment of disease activity of systemic lupus erythematosus. Arthritis Rheum. **32**(9): 1107–1118.
33. WILFERT, H., H. HÖNIGSMANN, G. STEINER, J. SMOLEN & K. WOLFF. 1990. Treatment of psoriatic arthritis by extracorporeal photochemotherapy. Br. J. Dermatol. **122:** 225–232.

34. EISINGER, M. 1985. Cultivation of normal human epidermal keratinocytes and melanocytes. *In* Methods in Skin Research. D. Skerrow & C. J. Skerrow, Eds. 195. John Wiley. New York.

35. BERGER, C. L., C. CANTOR, J. WELSH *et al.* 1985. Comparison of synthetic psoralen derivatives and 8-MOP in the inhibition of lymphocyte proliferation. Ann. N.Y. Acad. Sci. **453:** 80–90.

36. GASPARRO, F. P., J. BATTISTA, J. SONG & R. L. EDELSON. 1988. Rapid and sensitive analysis of 8-methoxypsoralen in plasma. J. Invest. Dermatol. **90:** 234–236.

37. PUGLISI, C. V., A. J. DE SILVA & J. C. MEYER. 1977. Determination of 8-methoxypsoralen, a photoactive compound, in blood by high pressure liquid chromatography. Anal. Lett. **10:** 39–50.

38. RUBIN, L. A., C. C. KURMAN, M. E. FRITZ, W. E. BIDDISON, B. BOUTIN, R. M. YARCHOAN & D. L. NELSON. 1985. Soluble interleukin-2 receptors are released from activated human lymphoid cells *in vitro*. J. Immunol. **135:** 3172–3177.

39. WOLF, R. E. & W. G. BRELSFORD. 1988. Soluble interleukin-2 receptors in systemic lupus erythematosus. Arthritis Rheum. **31**(6): 729–735.

40. MACKWORTH, C. G., J. K. H. CHAN, C. C. BUNN, G. R. V. HUGHES & A. E. GHARAVI. 1986. Complement fixation by anti-dsDNA antibodies in SLE: measurement by radioimmunoassay and relationship with disease activity. Ann. Rheum. Dis. **45:** 314–318.

41. GRIPPENBERG, M. & T. HELVE. 1986. Anti-DNA antibodies of IgA class in patients with systemic lupus erythematosus. Rheumatol. Int. **6:** 53–65.

42. SPERANSKY, A. I., M. J. IVANOVA, T. A. RJAZANTCEVA, V. A. PIVEN & T. D. BULANOVA. 1988. Antinuclear antibodies in lupus erythematosus and Sjögren's syndrome: clinical and immunological investigations. Scand. J. Rheumatol. Suppl. **67:** 39–43.

43. DOWDY, M. J., P. N. THOMAS & W.F. BARTH. 1989. Subacute cutaneous lupus erythematosus during PUVA therapy for psoriasis. Case report and review of the literature. Arthritis Rheum. **32:** 343–346.

44. EYANSON, S., M. C. GREIST, K. D. BRANDT & B. SKINNER. 1979. Systemic lupus erythematosus-association with psoralen-ultraviolet: a treatment of psoriasis. Arch. Dermatol. **115:** 54–56.

45. MILLNS, J. L., F. S. MCDUFFLE, S. A. MULLER & R. E. JORDON. 1978. Development of photosensitivity and an SLE-like syndrome in a patient with psoriasis. Arch. Dermatol. **114:** 1177–1181.

46. BRUZE, M., G. KROOK & B. LJUNGGREN. 1984. Fatal connective tissue disease with antinuclear antibodies following PUVA therapy. Acta Dermato-Venereol. (Stockholm) **64:** 157–160.

47. DOMKE, H. F., D. LUDWISEN & J. THORMANN. 1979. Discoid lupus erythematosus possibly due to photochemotherapy (letter). Arch. Dermatol. **115:** 642.

48. COHEN, I. R. & H. L. WEINER. 1988. T-cell vaccination. Immunol. Today **9:** 332–335.

49. COHEN, I. R., A. BEN-NUN, J. HOLOSHITZ *et al.* 1983. Vaccination against autoimmune disease with lines of autoimmune T lymphocytes. Immunol. Today **4**(8): 227–230.

50. BEN-NUN, A. & I. R. COHEN. 1982. Experimental autoimmune encephalomyelitis (EAE) mediated by T cell lines: process of selection of lines and characterization of the cells. J. Immunol. **129:** 303–308.

51. BEN-NUN, A., H. WEKERLE & I. R. COHEN. 1981. The rapid isolation of clonable antigen-specific T lymphocyte lines capable of mediating autoimmune encephalomyelitis. Eur. J. Immunol. **11:** 195–199.

52. RICO, J. M. & R. P. HALL. 1989. Anti-idiotypic antibodies as vaccine candidates. Arch. Dermatol. **125:** 271–275.

53. NAPARSTEK, Y., I. R. COHEN & Z. FUKS. 1984. Activated T lymphocytes produce a matrix-degrading heparan sulphate endoglycosidase. Nature **310**(19): 241–244.

54. EDELSON, R. L. 1988. Light-activated drugs. Sci. Am. **259:** 68–75.

55. BENNET, R. M., B. L. KOTZIN & M. J. MERRIT. 1987. DNA receptor dysfunction in systemic lupus erythematodes and kindred disorders. J. of Exp. Med. **166:** 850–863.

56. LASKIN, J. D., E. LEE, E. J. YURKOW, D. L. LASKIN & M. A. GALLO. 1985. A possible mechanism of psoralen phototoxicity not involving direct interaction with DNA. Cell Biol. **82:** 6158–6162.

57. LASKIN, J. D., E. LEE, D. L. LASKIN & M. A. GALLO. 1986. Psoralens potentiate ultraviolet light-induced inhibition of epidermal growth factor binding. Cell Biol. **83:** 8211–8215.

58. LASKIN, J. D., E. LEE, D. L. LASKIN & M. A. GALLO. 1986. Psoralens potentiate ultraviolet light-induced inhibition of epidermal growth factor binding. Proc. Natl. Acad. Sci. USA **83:** 8211–8215.

59. TRAUTINGER, F., R. M. KNOBLER, W. GRANNINGER, W. MACHEINER, R. NEUMANN & M. MICKSCHE. 1990. The ability of neutrophils to release oxygen free radicals is reduced by extracorporeal photochemotherapy (photopheresis). J. Invest. Dermatol. **94**(4): 586 (abstract).

Immunophenotypic Marker Analysis of Peripheral Blood Lymphocytes during Extracorporeal Photopheresis

A. AL-KATIB,[a] M. VOLBERGS, C. SHEARER,
L. HEILBRUN, B. READING, AND L. SENSENBRENNER

Division of Hematology and Oncology
Wayne State University
School of Medicine
and
Harper-Grace Hospitals
Detroit, Michigan 48202

Mycosis Fungoides is a primary malignant lymphoma of the skin with T cell phenotype (cutaneous T cell lymphoma, CTCL). The clinical course is usually indolent and characterized by frequent relapses, resistance to treatment and progression of disease to lymph nodes and internal organs with fatal consequences. There are several treatment modalities for this disease that are variably effective.[1] In 1987, Edelson *et al.* reported on the efficacy of extracorporeal photopheresis (ECPP) therapy in CTCL.[2] This treatment modality involves the extracorporeal exposure of a lymphocyte-enriched blood fraction to ultraviolet A light following the oral administration of methoxypsoralen. The lymphocytes will then be returned to the patient. Although the mechanism of the beneficial effect is uncertain, an immune reaction is believed to be involved.

At our institution, we have serially analyzed the peripheral blood lymphocyte marker profile before and after each ECPP treatment on three patients with CTCL. All patients had a histologically confirmed diagnosis of CTCL; patient #1 (TK) had Stage IB (limited plaque), patient #2 (HS) Stage III (generalized erythroderma) and patient #3 (RG) Stage IIA (generalized plaque with clinical adenopathy). All patients had previously treated and recurrent disease. ECPP was performed on two consecutive days every 4 weeks. However, in patients 2 and 3, treatment frequency was increased to every two weeks when there was no evidence of response. Blood samples were obtained either immediately before starting the first day run (pre) or 10 min following the completion of the second day run (post). Lymphocytes were separated by Ficoll-Hypaque density centrifugation, stained with monoclonal antibodies to CD2, CD3, CD4, CD8, CD16, CD19, CD25, Leu 7, CD71, and HLA-DR. Stained cells were analyzed by flow cytometry.

Clinically, patient #1 achieved a complete remission and therapy was discontinued after a total of 14 monthly treatments. This patient, however, relapsed 2 months later in the lung and was treated with systemic chemotherapy. The second patient had 19 treatments in 12 months. There was no evidence of response following the first three monthly treatments, with a skin score of 225. Subsequently, the prednisone therapy was discontinued and the treatment schedule changed to ever two weeks; three months later, he achieved a partial response

[a] Correspondence to: Ayad Al-Katib, M.D., Division of Hematology/Oncology, Wayne State University, P.O. Box 02188, Detroit, MI 48202.

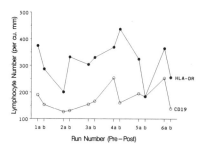

FIGURE 1. Comparison of mean HLA-DR and CD19 levels. Each point on the line represents the mean HLA-DR or CD19 level for 3 patients for pre- and postphotopheresis measures.

with the score of skin disease being 73. Response lasted 6 months before disease progressed and did not respond to continued ECPP. Patient #3 has received 6 treatments and is still on therapy at the time of this writing. He showed evidence of stabilization of disease following the first 3 treatments. Therefore, the treatment schedule was switched to biweekly, together with the addition of interferon-α (3 million u/m^2 BSA S.C—three times per week) as was previously reported;[3] so far the patient has not shown clinical response.

Our analysis showed no apparent effects of ECPP on any of the total WBC or absolute lymphocyte counts. The only consistent finding in the marker analysis is the presence of higher numbers of HLA-DR (+) cells compared with the CD19 (+) B cells (FIG. 1). There were no apparent changes in the proportion of cells expressing any of the markers tested either between the pre- and post-analysis or over the course of the therapy. In patient #2, however, there was an increase in the lymphocyte count following discontinuation of the prednisone therapy with subsequent clinical response (FIG. 2). However, at the same time the schedule of therapy was changed to every two weeks.

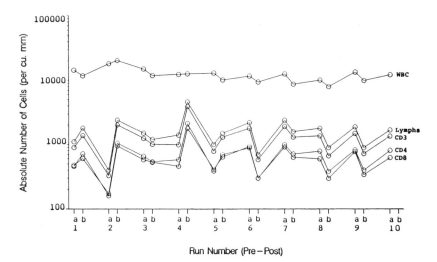

FIGURE 2. Patient #2. Each point on the line represents the absolute cell count (WBC, lymphocytes, CD3, CD4, CD8) for 10 measures taken pre- and postphotopheresis for patient #2.

In conclusion, our results show that there is no consistent change in any of the lymphocyte markers that can predict for clinical response. Considering the limited number of patients, these results are preliminary and we plan to continue our analysis on future patients.

REFERENCES

1. MINNA, J. D., H. H. ROENIGK & E. GLATSTEIN. 1979. Report of the committee on therapy for mycosis fungoides and Sezary syndrome. Cancer Treat. Rep. **63:** 729.
2. EDELSON, R., C. BERGER, F. GASPARRO *et al.* 1987. Treatment of cutaneous T-cell lymphoma by extracorporeal photochemotherapy. N. Engl. J. Med. **316:** 297.
3. SPRINGER, E., S. ROSEN & H. ROENIGK. 1989. Interferon alpha-2a combined with photochemotherapy for cutaneous T-cell lymphomas (abst.). Clin. Res. **37:** 630A.

Regulation of Immune Activation/Retroviral Replication by CD8+ T Cells

JONATHAN D. POWELL,[a] DANIEL P., BEDNARIK,[c]
TAMAR JEHUDA-COHEN,[a] FRANCOIS VILLINGER,[a,b]
THOMAS M. FOLKS,[c] AND A. A. ANSARI[a,b,d]

[a]Department of Pathology
and
[b]Yerkes Regional Primate Research Center
Emory University School of Medicine
Atlanta, Georgia 30322
[c]Retrovirus Disease Branch
Centers for Disease Control
Atlanta, Georgia 30333

CD8+ T cells from humans infected with HIV and monkeys infected with simian immunodeficiency virus (SIV) have the ability to inhibit viral replication *in vitro*.[1,2] The exact mechanism of this inhibition remains to be elucidated. In light of the fact that viral replication is intimately linked to T cell activation, we hypothesized that CD8+ T cells may inhibit viral replication at the level of cellular activation. To test this hypothesis an EBV-transformed cell line from a naturally SIV-infected sooty mangabey monkey was transfected with a human CD4 gene (courtesy of Dr. R. Morgan NHLBI, NIH) and shown to be replication competent for SIV, HIV-1 and HIV-2. Autologous activated lymphocytes from the sooty mangabey monkey from which the cell line was derived were shown to have the ability to inhibit replication of all three of these lentiviruses as measured by reverse transcriptase activity (data not shown). Such findings suggest that the inhibition is not viral-type specific and is directed at a pathway common to all three of these diverse lentiviruses.

Next the EBV-transformed cell line was transiently transfected with the plasmid pU3RIII which contains an LTR-driven CAT reporter gene.[3] As seen in FIGURE 1 (lane a vs b), autologous activated lymphocytes are able to inhibit viral activity as measured by CAT activity. It should be noted that this inhibition does not appear to be secondary to the cytolysis of the transfected cells by the autologous lymphocytes. These data suggest that the inhibition of viral replication can occur at the level of transcription. Experiments utilizing a dual-chamber culture vessel separated by a semipermeable membrane were performed in order to determine whether this effect was mediated by a soluble factor(s). As seen in FIGURE 1 (lane a vs c) even when the lymphocytes are not in direct contact with the transfected cells the inhibition of viral replication as measured by CAT activity is apparent. However, it should be noted that in these experiments and in similar experiments measuring reverse transcriptase activity, the inhibition is quantita-

[d] Address for correspondence: Dr. A. A. Ansari, Emory University School of Medicine, Winship Cancer Center, 5th Floor, 1327 Clifton Road, NE, Atlanta, GA 30322.

tively less than when the effector cells are in direct contact with the transfected or infected targets.

It has been shown that cellularly derived nuclear binding factors have the ability to bind to the NFkB element of the LTR and activate viral replication.[4] It was of interest to determine whether such NFkB binding proteins were responsible for the activation of pU3RIII in our cell line. In an effort to address this issue, a pU3RIII plasmid with mutations in the NFkD binding motifs of the LTR (termed Kb-) was employed.[4] When the CD4 expressing EBV-transformed cell line was

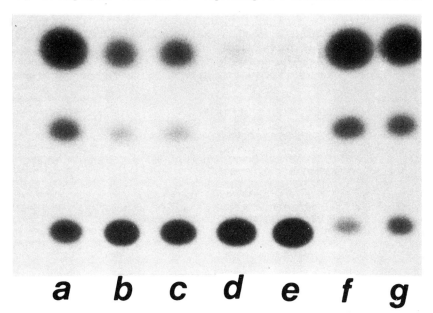

FIGURE 1. The CD4 expressing EBV-transformed cell line was transfected with the plasmid pU3RIII and aliquoted at 2×10^6 cells/well in a 6-well plate. The data represented in lane a show the CAT activity of the cells cultured alone. The data in *lane b* show the activity when 2×10^6 autologous activated lymphocytes were added to the well and *lane c* represents the CAT activity when 2×10^6 autologous activated lymphocytes were added to the well separated from the transfected cells by a semipermeable membrane. *Lanes d and e* represent CAT activity of cells transfected with the Kb- plasmid and cultured either alone (*lane d*) or with autologous activated lymphocytes (*lane e*). *Lanes f and g* represent CAT activity of cells co-transfected with the Kb- plasmid and a plasmid which constitutively expresses TAT. The transfected cells were cultured either alone (*lane f*) or with autologous activated lymphocytes (*lane g*).

transfected with the Kb- plasmid, no significant CAT activity was demonstrable (FIGURE 1, lanes d and e). On the other hand, when the cell line was co-transfected with the Kb- plasmid and a plasmid which constitutively expresses TAT (PIIIextatIII)—which can drive the Kb- plasmid in trans independently of the NFkB binding sites—there is marked CAT activity, thus demonstrating that the lack of activity seen in lanes d and e is not secondary to a defective plasmid. These data suggest that the majority of viral activation, as measured by CAT activity, in this model is dependent upon the binding of cellularly derived nuclear binding proteins to the NFkB elements of the LTR. As such, our data suggest that

CD8+ T cells have the ability to inhibit viral replication at the level of NFkB activation.

The model described herein involves EBV immortalized B cells and may not faithfully mimic HIV infection in T cells and monocytes. However, the mode of action of NFkB binding proteins in a variety of diverse cells is remarkably similar.[5] In T cells NFkB binding proteins have been implicated in the upregulation of the IL-2 receptor as well as the production of IL-2.[5] Since viral replication is so intimately linked to T cell activation, it is unclear as to whether CD8+ T cell inhibition of viral replication is primarily an antiviral or immunosuppressive response. Indeed it has been proposed that the downregulation of the immune response seen early on in HIV infection may represent active immunosuppression which plays a protective role by concomitantly inhibiting viral replication.[6] If such is the case, we hypothesize that this suppression may in fact be mediated by CD8+ T cells and may be directed at NFkB-mediated activation of infected cells.

REFERENCES

1. WALKER, C. M., D. J. MOODY, D. P. STITES & J. A. LEVY. 1986. Science 234: 1563–1566.
2. POWELL, J. D., T. YEHUDA-COHEN, F. VILLINGER, H. M. McCLURE, K. W. SELL & A. A. ANSARI. 1990. J. Med. Primatol. 19: 239–249.
3. ROSEN, C. A., J. G. SODROSKI & W. A. HASELTINE. 1985. Cell 41: 813–823.
4. NABEL, G. & D. BALTIMORE. 1989. Nature 326: 711–713.
5. GREENE, W. C., E. BOHNLEIN & D. W. BALLARD. 1989. Immunol. Today 10: 272–277.
6. VIA, C. S., H. C. MORSE & G. M. SHEARER. 1990. Immunol. Today 11: 250–255.

CD45 Isoforms on T Cells during Ontogeny

CLARA G. BELL

Department of Microbiology and Immunology
M/C 790
University of Illinois at Chicago
Chicago, Illinois 60612

The leukocyte common antigens family of heavily glycosylated glycoproteins designated T200, cluster differentiation marker CD45—encoded by a single, 33 exons gene (that maps to chromosome $1/q^{32}$)—span the membrane of leukocytes of their thymic and marrow precursors, and of early erythroid lineages, as a 22-residue transmembrane segment yielding two domains chimeric in character. Common to the CD45 isoforms is the highly conserved cytoplasmic domain (705 residues with >81% identity among human, rat, and mouse species), which consists of two ~300-residue tandem homologous subdomains that display 33% and 40% sequence identity to a placental major protein tyrosine (PT) phosphate (PTPase) 1B, and function as PTPases. There is accumulating evidence that it actively modulates the transmembrane signal transduction pathway dephosphorylating tyrosyl residues[1] that underlie the T cell (Tc) activation, by interacting with the CD4 or CD8 glycoproteins—which function as coreceptors in antigen (Ag)-specific, Tc receptor (TcR)-mediated signal transduction. Critical in this process is the TcR-coupled lymphocyte (LC) PT kinase (PTK), $p56^{lck}$, association with the cytoplasmic tail of the CD4 or CD8. ($p56^{lck}$ is critical for phosphorylating the ζ chain of the CD3ζ-TcR complex, essential for the Ag-stimulated signaling.) The extracellular NH_2-terminal domain (391–552 residues length, with 40% homology among the three species) is transcribed by the alternate usage of the exons 4, 5, and 6. The isoforms of CD45—produced by the alternative splicing of the mRNA (resulting in a potential for eight different mRNAs)—differ in size (180, 190, 205, and 220 kDa); the NH_2-terminal sequence and antigenicity; in the potential O-linked carbohydrate sites, functioning in cell-cell interactions; and in the posttranscriptional modification pattern of the N- and O-glycosylation.[2,3] They are expressed in cell-type specific pattern on LC lineages. The Tc expression of the CD45 isoforms is developmentally regulated with immature thymocytes—splicing out exons 4 to 6—exhibiting the 180-kDa CD45 variant only, and with the most mature thymocytes exiting the thymus, expressing the highest 220-kDa CD45 variant. Since peripheral blood (PB) matures Tc, uses the multiple transcripts, and exhibits the multiple CD45 isoforms in different patterns during activation—finding when in development each CD45 isoform expression is acquired and the extend to which the CD45-isoform expression is associated with specialization to the functionally distinct Tc subsets, may prove to be pivotal for dissecting the cascade of events that underlie the postthymic Tc maturation and activation.

Using the monoclonal antibodies [mAbs] against the NH_2-terminal variant restricted epitopes CD45R, that dissected the human CD4 Tc into functionally distinct reciprocal subsets:—the high MW isoform expressing subset $CD45R^+$, $CD45RA^{+(2H4+)}$, associated with suppressor/inducer (s/i) effector function, effective in interleukin-2 (IL-2)-related functions; and the low MW isoform expressing

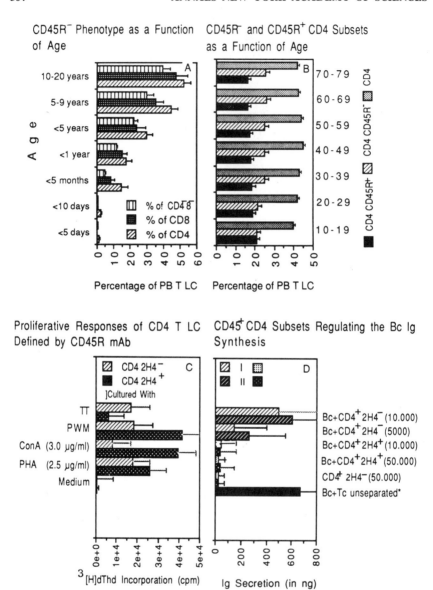

FIGURE 1. Mononuclear cells (MC) were separated from erythrocytes and debris by Ficoll-Hypaque (Pharmacia Fine Chemicals, Piscataway, NJ) density gradient sedimentation of heparinized peripheral blood (PBMC) from healthy humans, and from cord blood, washed, and separated into plastic-adherent and -nonadherent MC by incubation of 2-3- × 10[7] MC/in 10 ml medium (RPMI 1640 [Gibco Laboratories, Grand Island, NY] supplemented with heat inactivated human serum [7.5%] or FCS [10%], L-glutamine [4 mM], Hepes buffer [15 mM], sodium bicarbonate [0.5%], penicillin/streptomycin [1%]) in 90-mm petri dishes, for 2 h at 37°C. Nylon wool enriched nonadherent Tc were fractionated into CD4+, CD8+, and CD4-8- Tc by negative selection. An Epics V cell sorter with two-color fluorescence staining was used for some experiments. Fractionated Tc (showing >96% viability by trypan

subset CD45R⁻, CD45RO$^{+(UCHL1+)}$, responsive to recall Ags, functioning as helper/inducer (h/i) for Tc-dependent B cell (Bc) differentiation—to tag Tc, I report a cytofluorometric ontogenic dissection of human PB and of cord blood Tc, linked with an in-depth analysis of the function of the Tc to show: (i) a decrease, with increasing age, from birth to the 8th decade of life, in the CD45R⁺, CD45RA⁺, CD4⁺ and CD8⁺ Tc subsets expressing predominantly the $\alpha\beta$TcR heterodimer, and in the CD4⁻8⁻ Tc expressing the Vδ1TcR; and (ii) an exponential increase in the reciprocal CD45R⁻, CD45RO⁺ subset in the $\alpha\beta$TcR CD4⁺ and CD8⁺, from the low percentage expressed in the newborn to the ~50% of the circulating Tc PB pool in adults (principally in the CD4⁺ Tc), and in the CD4⁻8⁻ Tc expressing the $\gamma\delta$TcR heterodimer (which comprise 0.5–10% of the PB Tc) (FIG. 1A, 1B). That the upregulation in the expression of the CD45RO⁺ characteristic of the memory phenotype is consistent with postthymic *in vivo* dynamic developmental activation of the CD45RA⁺, and not with a distinct Tc lineage, is indicated by the shift from the CD45RA⁺ to the CD45RO⁺ phenotype delineated

---

blue exclusion) were analyzed by direct immunofluorescence with saturating concentration of phycoerythrin- or fluorescein-conjugated mAbs: anti-CD4 (Leu-3a, IgG1), anti-CD8 (Leu-2a, IgG1), anti-CD3 (Leu-4, IgG1), anti-CD16 (Leu-11b, IgM), and/or anti-CD14 (Leu-M3, IgG2b) from Becton Dickinson (Mountain View, CA). These were subdivided into subsets by further staining (by direct fluorescence) with: conjugated anti-CD25 (anti-IL-2R, p55, IgG1), anti-CD45 (Hle-1, p180-200 kDa, IgG1), and anti-CD45RA, leukocyte common antigen (Leu-18) from Becton Dickinson; and anti-CD45RA (2H4, CD45R, p220 kDa, IgG1, Coulter Immunology, Hialeah, FL);[4,5] or by indirect immunofluorescence using unconjugated, purified mAb anti-CD45RO (UCHL1, p180 kDa, IgG2a, Dako Corp., Santa Barbara, CA),[6] followed by fluorescein-conjugated goat anti-mouse Ig, and characterized phenotypically by two-color flow cytometry with scatter gates set on LC (for volume and light scatter) to exclude contaminating erythrocytes and debris. Nonspecific binding of conjugated mAb to Tc via the Fc receptor was excluded by inhibition of binding assays. Only the unlabelled mAb but not the nonspecific mouse Ig mAb inhibited the binding of the conjugated mAb. Histogram A depicts the exponential increase, from birth to the second decade of life, in the PB CD45R$^{-(CD45RO+)}$ phenotype (characteristic of activated) CD4⁺, CD8⁺, and CD4⁻8⁻ Tc. Histogram B shows that the exponential increase, from the first to the eighth decade of life, in the CD45R$^{-(CD45RO+)}$ subset, is paralleled by a decrease, with age, in the expression of the CD45RA$^{+(CD45RO-)}$ (depicted for the CD4⁺ subset). Histogram C depicts the functional proliferative responses of the CD4⁺CD45R$^{+(2H4+)}$ and CD4⁺CD45R$^{-(2H4-, UCHL1+)}$ PB CD4⁺ subsets cultured in triplicate, 2×10^5 cells/200 μl, round-bottomed microtiter wells with 10^5 adherent (2,000 rad irradiated) MC, and stimulated with mitogens or recall (tetanus toxoid [TT]) Ag. Four- to 5-day cultures were pulsed with 1 μCi [³H]thymidine ([³H]dThd) 16 h before harvesting, and proliferation was assessed by [³H]dThd incorporation measured on a Packard Scintillation Counter. The *bars* depict the CD4⁺CD45RA⁺ Tc mean cpm effective proliferative response to PHA (2.5 μg/ml), ConA (3.0 μg/ml), and PWM (1 : 100 dilution, Gibco Laboratories), of triplicate cultures corrected by subtraction of control medium alone, and the CD4⁺CD45RO⁺ Tc mean cpm effective proliferative response to TT (1 : 300 dilution). The functional significance of the expression of the CD45RA and CD45RO in immunoregulation of Ig synthesis by PWM-stimulated Bc (as measured by an ELISA quantification of the Ig produced in quadruplicate cultures) and in the pathogenesis of autoimmune SLE, RA, and AIT is shown in histogram D, which depicts the regulatory h/i function of the CD4⁺CD45RO$^{+(2H4-)}$ subset, and s/i function of the CD4⁺CD45RA⁺ (2H4⁺) subset, in an Ig synthesizing system, when added to autologous Bc cultured for 7 days with PWM (1 : 100 dilution, Gibco). Note the lack of s/i function within PB Tc derived from an active SLE patient, in the Ig synthesizing system (depicted in the *lower panel* of histogram D [Bc + Tc unseparated*]). Of note is that the s/i function of the normal PB CD45RA⁺ CD4⁺ pretreated with the serum derived from this patient was abrogated.

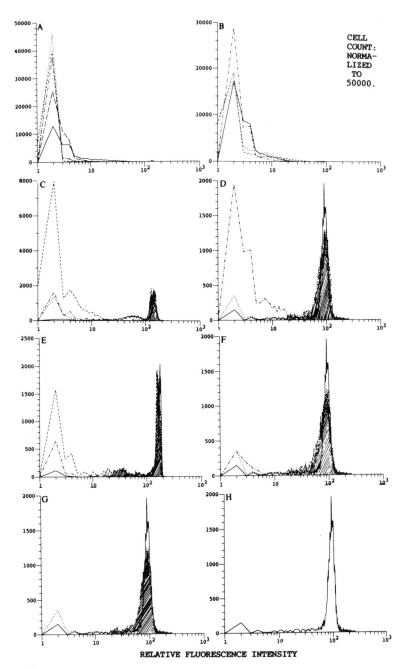

FIGURE 2. Phenotypic characterization of PB Tc. Induction of CD45RO⁺ isoform expression on PB CD45RA⁺ Tc (representative profiles). PBMC were purified and separated into CD45RA⁺ and CD45RA⁻ subsets as described in the legend to FIGURE 1. CD45RA⁺ Tc were

within the CD45 expressing CD4$^+$, when cultured with concanavalin A (ConA), phytohemagglutinin (PHA), or mAbs in limiting dilution/or bulk cultures (FIGS. 1C, 2C–D), as measured by flow cytometry (FIG. 2), and by the functional effectiveness of the latter to proliferate in response to tetanus toxoid (TT), (FIG. 1C), and to help/or suppress the immunoglobulin (Ig) synthesis by pokeweed mitogen (PWM)-stimulated Bc (FIG. 1D). The association of the CD45RA$^+$, of the naive Tc phenotype, with the Vδ1 Tc, and of the CD45RO$^+$, of the activated Tc phenotype, with the Vδ2, suggests that the predominant $\gamma\delta$ Tc subset in PB of normal individuals is *in vivo* activated. The patterns of reactivity depicted within normal PB Tc during ontogeny, suggests that the thymus plays a principal role in the acquisition and exiting of the CD45RA$^+$ to the periphery, and contributes to the peripheral CD45RA$^+$ pool self renewal throughout life. Alterations in the CD45RA$^+$: CD45RO$^+$ ratio, and the higher frequencies of the CD45RO$^+$ activation phenotype CD8$^+$, as a consequence of the lower frequencies of the CD4$^+$ CD45RA$^+$ s/i, delineated in PB and in synovial- and thyroidal-aspirates from rheumatoid arthritis (RA), SLE, and autoimmune thyroiditis (AIT) diseased subjects, characteristic of the compartmentalization of the naive and memory Tc at sites of Agnic stimulation, contribute, with the autoAbs against these, to the basic mechanism underlying the dysfunction of these autoimmune diseases.

ACKNOWLEDGMENTS

I thank Drs. L. Barkan, P. Lydyard, and R. Serenas for generously providing cells, and Dr. K. Hagen and the Flow Cytometry Laboratory of the Research Resources UIC for providing equipment and technical expertise.

---

cultured (as described in legend to FIG. 1) with: medium alone ([A] for 8 h, [B] for 24 h); or with mitogens PHA, ConA (at concentration indicated in legend to FIG. 1) (C, D); or with mAbs (0.2–0.5 μg) ([E, F] for 24 h). Cells resuspended in phosphate buffered saline (PBS) containing FCS (5%) were incubated with saturating concentration of the different conjugated mAb, alone for 30 min at 4°C, and washed in PBS-FCS, or in combinations each for 30 min at 4°C, or with the unconjugated mAb for 30 min followed by the conjugated, second layer, goat anti-mouse Ig mAb (Cappel Laboratories). Graph profiles (transmitted via a VAX-11/750) depict the relative fluorescence intensity vs number of cells ($\sim$5 $\times$ 10^3–2 $\times$ 10^4 analyzed for each indicated population; normalized to 50,000) examined on a EPICS Coulter by gating for the LC. In each panel the smallest *dotted lines* in the left depict cells stained with the control, with unrelated FITC-conjugated mouse mAb or with the second layer mAb only. Binding of conjugated anti-CD45RO to cells was unaffected by the presence of the purified unconjugated mouse Ig isotype (*dashed lines*). The examination (by gating for the LC on log forward and log right angle light scatter parameters) and measuring of two-color immunofluorescence showing the interindividual variations in the CD45RA$^+$: CD45RO$^+$ ratio, and the proportion of CD45RA^{low},CD45RO^{+high} dual positive Tc delineated after the mitogenic stimulation are not depicted in the histograms. An observation of note was that, while within a given healthy control individual, the proportion of the CD45RA$^+$ and CD45RO$^+$ on the CD4$^+$ highly correlated with that on the CD8$^+$, the frequency distribution of the CD45RO$^+$ was significantly higher on CD8$^+$ > CD4$^+$ from RA, SLE, and AIT PB ([D, F, G, H] bold *solid lines*) in relation to that of the age-matched controls. This suggests that the acquisition of immunological memory, in addition to being a function of ontogenic age, is subject to some central immunologic experience and dynamic regulation.

REFERENCES

1. VEILETTE, A. *et al*. 1988. Cell **85:** 8628.
2. LEFRANCOIS, L. 1987. J. Immunol. **139:** 2220–2229.
3. CHARBONNEAU, H. *et al*. 1988. Proc. Natl. Acad. Sci. USA **85:** 7182–7186.
4. COBBOLD, S. *et al*. 1987. *In* Leukocyte Typing III. A. J. McMichael *et al*., Eds. 7896.
5. MORIMOTO, C. *et al*. 1985. J. Immunol. **134:** 1508–1515.
6. MERKENSCHLAGER, M. *et al*. 1988. Eur. J. Immunol. **18:** 1653–1661.

Microbial Stimulus in the
γδ T Cells Localization

CLARA G. BELL

Department of Microbiology & Immunology
M/C 790
University of Illinois at Chicago
Chicago, Illinois 60612

The majority of the mature, peripheral blood (PB) and lymphoid organs, functional helper (CD4$^+$ Th) and cytotoxic (CD8$^+$ Tc) CD3$^+$ T lymphocytes (TLC) responsible for known forms of cell-mediated immunity utilize $\alpha\beta$ T cell receptor (TcR) heterodimers in association with their membrane CD3 polypeptide complex for recognition of foreign antigens (Ags) associated with class II major histocompatibility complex (MHC) molecules (for the CD4$^+$), and with class I MHC molecules (for the CD8$^+$), respectively.[1,2] A small subpopulation (<5%) of the adult CD3$^+$ T LC in PB, characterized as double negative (DN) with respect to the CD4 and CD8 glycoproteins (CD4$^-$8$^-$); a subset of the adult CD3$^+$ thymocytes in the thymus, the DN CD4$^-$8$^-$; and a subset of fetal CD3$^+$, early DN CD4$^-$8$^-$ thymocytes, express a disulphide-linked γδTcR in association with the CD3$^+$ complex. The function of these early, "fetal" CD3$^+$, DN CD4$^-$8$^-$, γδTcR-bearing thymocytes, which appear well prior to the $\alpha\beta$TcR-bearing thymocytes during thymic ontogeny (as early as day [d] 14 of gestation)[3] is undefined. The cells evolve as a dynamic population with selective outgrowth, and proliferative, and export potential, and migrate out of the thymus. Some persist in PB T LC of adults as a minor (<5%) DN CD4$^-$8$^-$, relatively immature subset, with significant developmental potential.[4] Others migrate to distal organs to predominantly and specifically localize within the epithelia (dendritic epidermal cells [DEC]).[5] A role, unrelated to the MHC, in the surveillance of the epithelial integrity was proposed for the γδTcR-bearing murine CD3$^+$, DN CD4$^-$8$^-$ T LC, on the basis of the latter.

I report a study addressing the question of the function, localization, and specificity of the γδTcR-bearing DN CD4$^-$8$^-$ T LC in conventionally-reared (CR) and germ-free (GF), euthymic, and congenitally athymic (nu/nu) BALB/cJ and C57Bl/6J mice, age 4 to 16 wks; and of the γδTcR-bearing DN CD4$^-$8$^-$ splenocyte (SpC) subset of nu/nu mice. I show microscopic differences in the detectable lymph nodes (LN) and Peyer's patches (PP) of the various groups of mice, and differences in the frequency distribution: of the $\alpha\beta$TcR-bearing CD3$^+$ T LC, cytofluorometrically characterized as single positive (SP) CD4$^+$8$^-$/or CD4$^-$8$^+$; and of the γδTcR-bearing CD3$^+$ T LC, cytofluorometrically characterized as DN CD4$^-$8$^-$, indicative of the susceptibility of the $\alpha\beta$TcR- to bacterial Ags, and suggestive of a distinct $\alpha\beta$TcR-bearing T LC potential defensive role against bacterial invasion (FIGS. 1 and 2). Notably, CR, gut associated bacteria (*Enterobacteria cloacae* [*E. cloacae*]) immunized mice, showed selective localization and expansion of the $\alpha\beta$TcR- with no apparent change in the frequency distribution of the γδTcR-bearing T LC. The GF mice showed reduced $\alpha\beta$TcR- SP to a barely detectable level, but increased frequency of the γδTcR-bearing T LC in the 2–8

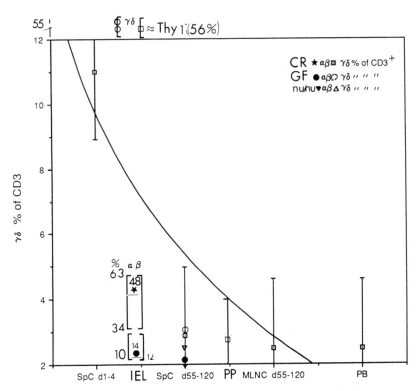

FIGURE 1. Frequency distribution of γδ LC in periphery. Splenocytes (SpC), mesenteric lymph node cells (MLNC), Peyer's patch (PP), peripheral blood (PB) LC, and thymocytes were purified from BALB/c and C57Bl/6 mice ages 1–4 d, 55 d and 120 d by density centrifugation and by panning methods as previously described. The cells from newborn 1–4-day-old mice were pooled. IEL were prepared from 75–100-day-old BALB/c and C57Bl/6 mice's small intestine free of PP, cut longitudinally into 1 cm fragments, shaken and dispersed repeatedly at ~20°C first in Ca- and Mg-free Hank's balanced salt solution (HBSS) only, then for 10 min in Ca- and Mg-free medium containing EDTA (5 mM) and DTT (70 mg/ml). Large debris were sedimented on ice and non adherent cells were collected, washed, purified on Percoll gradients, assessed for viability, and stained, but there was no selection of the LC and IEL population via culturing and *in vitro* stimulation. Cells (10^6) in 200 μl PBS or HBSS containing FCS (5%) were incubated in microtiter plates for 25 min on ice with each of the conjugated or unconjugated mAb, washed as previously described, and single and two-color immunofluorescence analysis for each of the various markers performed. The figure depicts the frequency distribution of γδ cells as percentage of CD3+ calculated (for 10,000 cells counted) from two-color immunofluorescence analysis of γδTcR and CD3 Ags on various LC of mice at different ages. Of note was the high frequency of the γδTcR+ IEL in both conventionally-reared (CR) and germ-free (GF) mice (as shown in the *upper left* of the graph) (numbers tabulate the mean percentages). The percentage of the γδTcR+ among the CD3+ was higher in the newborn GF IEL than in the newborn CR IEL. In contrast the αβTcR+ percentage of CD3+ was lower in GF IEL than in CR IEL (as shown in the *lower left* of the graph) (numbers tabulate the mean and the range percentages). The profile of the thymocytes was essentially similar and is not depicted. Of note was the high frequency of the γδTcR+ T LC among the SpC population of the newborn <5 d, as compared to that of the adult 55–120 d SpC, and the essential low frequency of the γδTcR+ LC among the PP, MLNC, and PB T LC population. The frequency of the αβTcR+ LC in the periphery was

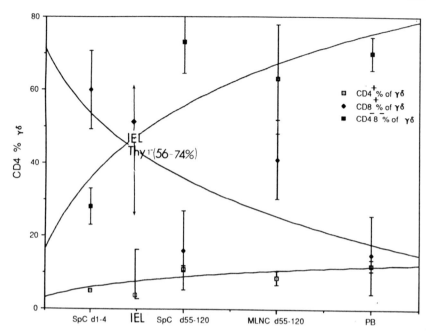

FIGURE 2. Frequency and phenotypic characteristics of the $\gamma\delta$TcR$^+$ cells in periphery. The figure depicts the frequency distribution and membrane phenotype of the $\gamma\delta$TcR$^+$ cells characterized as SP CD4$^+$, SP CD8$^+$, and DN CD4$^-$8$^-$/Thy-1, with respect to the CD4 and CD8 glycoproteins and the Thy-1 Ag. Of note was the higher frequency, among the <5-day-old SpC, of the $\gamma\delta$TcR$^+$ exhibiting the SP CD8$^+$ phenotype, than among the >55-day-old mice SpC (59% mean, 50–70% range; vs 16 mean, 11–28 range), and the relative lower frequency, among the SpC of both age groups, of the $\gamma\delta$TcR$^+$ SpC exhibiting the CD4$^+$ phenotype. The $\gamma\delta$TcR$^+$ SpC exhibiting the DN CD4$^-$8$^-$ were significantly lower in the <5-day-old as compared to the >55-day-old mice (mean 28, range 21–32; vs mean 72, range 62–81). Most $\gamma\delta$TcR$^+$ IELs SP CD8$^+$ were Thy-1$^-$ (see also FIG. 1, *upper*).

wks old, with $\gamma\delta$TcR- CD3$^+$, SP CD4$^-$8$^+$ cells predominant, if not exclusive, localization to the intestinal intraepithelial LC (IEL). That argues that self-Ags autoreactive to MHC and food Ags may play a role in the $\gamma\delta$TcR-bearing cells localization and expansion. The differences, in the various groups of mice, in the localization and frequency distribution of the CD3$^+$ subsets, characterized cytofluorometrically as SP CD4$^+$8$^-$/or CD4$^-$8$^+$ $\alpha\beta$TcR-; and as DN CD4$^-$8$^-$ $\gamma\delta$TcR-bearing T LC, indicate the $\alpha\beta$- and $\gamma\delta$TcR-bearing T LC exhibit distinct homing patterns. In this vein, the nu/nu mice essential lack of $\alpha\beta$TcR- and reduced frequencies of $\gamma\delta$TcR-bearing T LC, may suggest that $\alpha\beta$TcR-bearing T LC play a role in the expansion of the $\gamma\delta$TcR-bearing IEL.[6] Yet the ontogenic study suggests

high in euthymic (minus numbers not tabulated in the Figure) but low in nu/nu peripheral organs. The frequency of the $\alpha\beta$TcR$^+$ T LC was only bearly detectable among the GF SpC and was below the detection level among the nu/nu SpC (depicted for the SpC). Depicted also is the low frequency of the $\gamma\delta$TcR$^+$ T LC among the nu/nu SpC, as compared to the frequency of the $\gamma\delta$cR$^+$ T LC among the CR euthymic SpC, and among the GF SpC.

that while the gut associated bacterial flora Ags+$\alpha\beta$TcR- T LC, may drive the $\gamma\delta$TcR- expansion, the $\gamma\delta$TcR-bearing cells localized independently of foreign Ag stimulation. Expression, by only a proportion (23-<-~44%) of the $\gamma\delta$TcR-bearing IEL, of the murine pan T LC marker Thy-1 (Thy-1$^+$) (which is expressed by most of the mature CD3$^+$, SP CD4$^-$8$^+$ PB T LC) make the thymic origin and the lineage distinction of the $\gamma\delta$TcR-bearing CD3$^+$ CD4$^-$8$^+$ Thy-1$^-$ IEL unclear. Functional effective lysis of M104E (an *E. cloacae*, α(1–3) dex-binding BALB/c plasmacytoma), by (flow cytometry, phenotypically characterized) $\gamma\delta$TcR-bearing CD3$^+$ SP CD4$^-$8$^+$ BALB/c IEL (expressing the CD45 differentiation marker characteristic of the activated T LC,[7] indicates these SP $\gamma\delta$TcR-bearing IEL to be activated. However, whether these IEL function as singularly autoreactive to MHC, or can recognize via the variable-joining (VJ) junction of the $\gamma\delta$ heterodimers (which is equivalent to the CD3 complementarity loop of antibody [Ab] V regions), the foreign α(1–3) dex Ag of *E. cloacae*, or the regulatory idiotype (IdX J558/M104E) associated with the class I MHC-linked CD3$^+$ CD8$^+$ (as do T LC of M104E-bearer BALB/c mice), regards a $\gamma\delta$TcR- vs $\alpha\beta$TcR- T LC recognition to be studied.

ACKNOWLEDGMENTS

Drs. R. A. Good's, F. W. Shen's, E. E. Simpson's, A. J. Edwards', and P. Lalor's generous provision of mice and reagents is gratefully acknowledged.

REFERENCES

1. MARRACK, P. & J. KAPPLER. 1986. Adv. Immunol. **38**: 1–30.
2. SAITO, T., A. WEISS, J. MILLER, M. NORCROSS & R. GERMAIN. 1987. Nature **325**: 125–130.
3. BLUESTONE, J. A., D. PARDOLL, S. O. SHARROW & B. J. FOWLKES. 187. Nature **326**: 82–84.
4. LANIER, L. & A. WEISS. 1986. Nature **324**: 268–270.
5. KONING, F. *et al.* 1987. Science **236**: 834–837.
6. YOSHIKARA, Y., M. D. REIS & T. W. MAK. 1986. Nature **324**: 482–485.
7. BELL, C. 1991. This volume, preceding poster.

Preparation and Combining Site Characterization of Mouse Monoclonal Anti-B Blood Group Substances

HUA-TANG CHEN[a] AND XIAO-QING WANG

Department of Biochemistry
Anhui Medical University
People's Republic of China 230032

We have prepared a group of hybridomas by different immunization procedures using BALB/c mice with B blood group substances, Beach phenol insoluble or Tijll phenol insoluble as antigen. Three of them, 3-3-D9(IgG1), 3-5-D12(IgG1) and 6-1-G11(IgA), which secreted high level and high specific monoclonal anti-B, were studied immunochemically. The agglutination titers of their tissue culture supernatant were 4096, 4096 and 16384 by Takatsy microtitration assays (TABLE 1).

The combining sites and specificities of the monoclonal anti-Bs have been characterized with ELISA quantitative assays and ELISA quantitative oligosaccharide inhibition assays. All of them bind to B blood group substances, but not to A, H, Le^a and Le^b blood substances. It is demonstrated that 3-3-D9 and 3-5-D12 were most complementary to the difucosyl containing B-penta. Galα1→3Galβ1→4Glc; the third monoclonal 6-1-G11 was complementary to

$$\underset{\text{Fuc}\alpha}{\overset{2}{\underset{1}{\uparrow}}} \qquad \underset{\text{Fuc}\alpha}{\overset{3}{\underset{1}{\uparrow}}}$$

monofucosyl containing oligosaccharides, Galα1→3Galβ1→0(CH2)$_8$COOCH3

$$\overset{2}{\underset{1}{\uparrow}}$$
$$\text{Fuc}\alpha$$

(TABLE 2).

We also use these monoclonal anti-Bs in clinical blood typing for over 3700 samples, and no error was produced. They all would be excellent blood grouping reagents.

TABLE 1. Agglutination Titers, Avidies and Clinical Tests of Anti-Bs Monoclonals

			Results of Clinical Test			
Hybridoma	Titer of TCS[a]	Avidies of TCS (Second)	A (1141)	B (1047)	O (1177)	AB (339)
3-3-D9	4096	3	−	+ + + +	−	+ + + +
3-5-D12	4096	3	−	+ + + +	−	+ + + +
6-1-G11	16384	2	−	+ + + +	−	+ + + +

[a] TCS: Tessue culture supernatant.

[a] Address for correspondence: Building 10, Rm, DO3, NIH, Bethesda, MD 20892.

TABLE 2. Oligosaccharides Active in Inhibition Assays by Elisa[a]

Symbol	Oligosaccharide Structure	nMoles for 50% Inhibition		
		3-3-D9	3-5-D12	6-1-G11

B-Tri.	Galα1→3Gal
	   ↑2
	   1
	  Fucα
		28.1%
		(102 nM)
			41.0%
			(102 nM)
				35.2%
				(102 nM)

O2E	Galα1→3Gal-O(CH2)8-COOCH3
	   ↑2
	   1
	  Fucα
		22.7	18.0	34.0

B-Penta	Galα1→3Galβ1→4Glc
	  ↑2 ↑3
	   1 1
	Fucα Fucα
		8.0	9.0	inactive

[a] The following mono- and oligosaccharides give no inhibition with the anti-B monoclonals: D-Gal; D-GalNAc; L-Fuc; Galα1→3Galβ1→3GlcNAc; A-Tri.GalNAcα1→3Gal; 11E.Fucα1→2Galβ1→3Gal; 11E.Fucα1→2GalβO(CH2)8COOCH3.

Increased Gamma/Delta T Cells and Thy-1 Cells in Cutaneous T Cell Lymphoma

DAVID P. FIVENSON,[a] JAMES J. NORDLUND,[b]
MARGARET C. DOUGLASS,[a] AND EDWARD A. KRULL[a]

Departments of Dermatology
[a]Henry Ford Hospital
2799 West Grand Boulevard
Detroit, Michigan 48202-2689
and
[b]University of Cincinnati
Cincinnati, Ohio 45267

The Thy-1 antigen was one of the first T cell markers described. In mice, Thy-1 cells are dendritic antigen presenting epidermal cells which express the γ/δ T cell receptor (TCR).[1,2] Thy-1 expression has been reported in mycosis fungoides.[3] Increased γ/δ T cells have been reported to be present in immunologic diseases such as sarcoidosis[4] and rheumatoid arthritis[5] but only a minority of cases of MF.[6,7]

We have used monoclonal antibodies to study human Thy-1 antigen and TCR heterodimer expression (α/β vs γ/δ) in cutaneous T cell lymphoma (CTCL) and benign dermatoses. Sixteen cases of CTCL (4 patch, 10 plaque, and 2 tumor stage mycosis fungoides), 4 premycotic parapsoriasis, 2 small plaque parapsoriasis, 2 lichen planus, 10 lupus erythematosus, 9 dermatitis, 2 drug eruptions and 9 normal skin specimens were evaluated. Immunoperoxidase studies using the ABC technique on serial frozen sections were performed. Primary antibodies included: anti-human Thy-1, anti-TCR α, anti-TCR β, and anti-TCR δ.

Epidermal lymphocytes were <5% TCR $\gamma/\delta+$ in the inflammatory dermatoses or in normal skin, while the mean number of epidermotropic TCR $\gamma/\delta+$ cells in CTCL was 32%. TCR $\gamma/\delta+$ cells were also increased in the dermis of CTCL patients but TCR $\alpha/\beta+$ cells remained in the majority (FIG. 1).

Thy-1 was expressed by dendritic cells in all CTCL cases in the dermis, while epidermotropic cells remained Thy-1−. Thy-1 was seen perivascularly in normals and patients as previously reported. Normals and benign dermatoses differed from CTCL by the lack of Thy-1 on dermal cells and a relative paucity of TCR $\gamma/\delta+$ cells. Thy-1+ dermal cells appeared TCR $\alpha/\beta+$ and TCR $\gamma/\delta-$ on serial sections.

The role of the Thy-1 expression by dendritic dermal cells in CTCL is unclear, but the shear numbers and characteristic distribution suggests that these cells are involved in the pathogenesis of CTCL. The increased numbers of TCR $\gamma/\delta+$ T cells in the epidermis and dermis may help induce a state of immune tolerance to the transformed lymphocytes in CTCL.

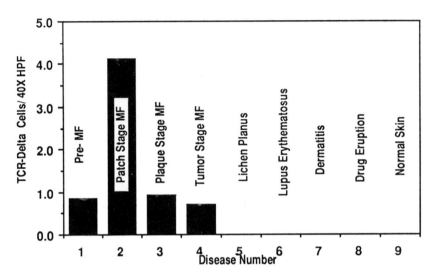

FIGURE 1. Epidermal TCR delta cells in MF and benign dermatoses. The average number of TCR delta positive epidermal lymphocytes was calculated by averaging the number of cells staining with the TCRδ1 antibody in each 40X high power field (HPF) of epidermis. At least 5–10 HPF of epidermis were examined in each specimen; all specimens of each disease were subsequently averaged to form the bar graph.

REFERENCES

1. SULLIVAN, S., P. R. BERGSTRESSER, R. E. TIGELAAR & J. W. STREILEIN. 1986. Induction and regulation of contact hypersensitivity by resident, bone marrow-derived, dendritic epidermal cells: Langerhans cells and Thy-1+ cells. J. Immunol. **137:** 2460–2467.
2. KONING, F., G. STINGL, W. M. YOKOYAMA, H. YAMADA, W. L. MALOY, E. TSCHACHLER, E. M. SHEVACH & J. E. COLIGAN. 1987. Identification of T3 associated γ/δ T cell receptor on Thy-1+ dendritic epidermal cell lines. Science **236:** 834–836.
3. HAYNES, B. F., L. L. HENSLEY & B. V. JEGATHSOTHY. 1982. Differentiation of human T lymphocytes: II. Phenotypic differences in skin and blood malignant T cells in cutaneous T-cell lymphoma. J. Invest. Dermatol. **78:** 323–326.
4. BABLI, B., D. R. MOLLER, M. KIRBY, K. J. HOLROYD & R. G. CRYSTAL. 1990. Increased numbers of T lymphocytes with γ/δ-positive antigen receptors in a subgroup of individuals with pulmonary sarcoidosis. J. Clin. Invest. **85:** 1353–1361.
5. REME, T., M. PORTIER, F. FRAYSSINOUX, B. COMBE, P. MIOSSEC, F. FAVIER & J. SANY. 1990. T cell receptor expression and activation of synovial lymphocyte subsets in patients with rheumatoid arthritis. Phenotyping of multiple synovial sites. Arthritis Rheum. **33:** 485–492.
6. MICHIE, S. A., E. A. ABEL, R. T. HOPPE, R. A. WARNKE & G. S. WOOD. 1989. Expression of T-cell receptor antigens in mycosis fungoides and inflammatory skin lesions. J. Invest. Dermatol. **93:** 116–120.
7. HORN, T. A. & E. R. FARMER. 1990. Distribution of lymphocytes bearing TCR γ/δ in cutaneous lymphocytic infiltrates. J. Cutaneous Pathol. **17:** 165–170.

Role of T Cell Activation in the Pathogenesis of Psoriasis[a]

ALICE B. GOTTLIEB, JAMES G. KRUEGER,
LAKSHMI KHANDKE, RACHEL M. GROSSMAN,
JEFFREY KRANE, AND D. MARTIN CARTER

The Rockefeller University
1230 York Avenue
New York, New York 10021

The increased frequency of certain mixed histocompatibility complex antigens, especially HLA-Cw6, in populations of psoriasis patients provides some of the strongest clinical evidence that immune mechanisms may be important in the pathogenesis of psoriasis.[1] Active psoriatic plaques demonstrate a similar immunologic phenotype as do ongoing cellular immune responses: IL-2 receptor[+] and HLA-DR[+] T cells are found in active psoriatic plaques in significantly higher numbers than are found in uninvolved skin or in treated plaques.[2,3] The epidermal compartment is also dramatically altered. Keratinocytes in active plaques are HLA-DR[+] and gamma-IP-10[+] similar to the detection of these gamma interferon-induced proteins in ongoing cellular immune responses.[2-4] Keratinocytes displayed a growth-activated phenotype similar to that seen in epidermis undergoing regenerative maturation, *i.e.*, increased TGF-alpha, IL-6, EGF-receptor levels and altered keratin expression.[5-7]

Eight severe psoriasis patients were treated with cyclosporine A (CSA) at a dose of 5–7 mg/kg/day for 1 to 3 months. Skin biopsies, obtained before and after treatment, were studied for evidence of immune activation and keratinocyte regenerative maturation using immunoperoxidase techniques (TABLE 1). All patients showed improvement in erythema, thickness and scale as a result of treatment with CSA. The number of IL-2 receptor[+], presumably activated, T cells in plaques after CSA treatment was reduced in all patients (FIG. 1). Decreases in the number of CD3+, CD4+ and CD8+ T cells were noted in 5/8, 4/6 and 6/7 patients, respectively. 5/8 patients showed a decrease in keratinocyte HLA-DR expression and 5/7 showed a decrease in gamma-IP-10 immunoreactivity, suggesting a decline in gamma interferon levels in plaques after CSA therapy. In contrast, increased TGF-alpha, IL-6, and EGF receptor expression were rela-

[a] This work was supported in part by General Clinical Research Center Grant RR-00102 from the National Institutes of Health to the Rockefeller University Hospital; by a training grant (AR07525) from the National Institutes of Health to the Laboratory for Investigative Dermatology; by the Skin Disease Society; by the Dermatology Foundation's 1989 National Psoriasis Foundation Research Grant; by a grant from Squibb/ConvaTec; by a grant from Sandoz Corporation; by a grant from Ms. Susan Weil and with general support from the Pew Trusts.

TABLE 1. Cyclosporine A Treatment Decreases Immune Activation More Than Regenerative Maturation

Marker	Number of Patients Showing Decreased Levels After Cyclosporine A Treatment
IL-2 receptor	8/8
CD3	5/8
CD4	4/6
CD8	6/7
HLA-DR	5/8
IP-10	5/7
TGF-alpha	0/8
EGF receptor	1/6
IL-6	0/7
Hyperproliferative keratin	4/6

tively resistant to CSA treatment. Hyperproliferative keratin expression was diminished by CSA treatment in 4/6 patients. Northern blotting analysis, and radiolabeled-ligand binding studies demonstrated that TGF-alpha levels and EGF-receptor number and binding affinity in cultured normal keratinocytes were not affected by CAS treatment.[8]

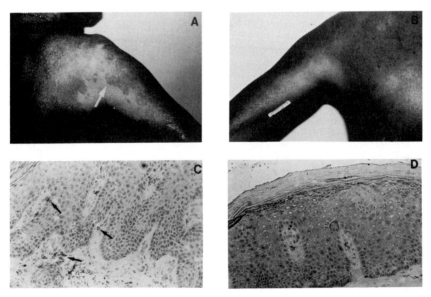

FIGURE 1. Cyclosporine A (CSA) treatment decreases the number of IL-2 receptor+ T lymphocytes in psoriatic plaques. Clinical photographs of patient MS before **(A)** and after **(B)** CSA treatment demonstrate reduced erythema, elevation and scaling of the plaques. *White arrow* indicates a typical large raised, erythematous, scaly plaque in the patient before CSA treatment. The number of IL-2 receptor+ T lymphocytes (*black arrows*) in this pretreatment plaque **(C)** decreased to 0 in this CSA-treated plaque **(D)**.

Diminution of T cell activation in plaques, with resulting decreases in the production of cytokines such as gamma interferon, is a likely mechanism of action of CSA in psoriasis plaques *in vivo*. These studies suggest that immune activation is important in the pathogenesis of psoriasis and that immunomodulating therapies which interfere with T cell activation or inhibit subsequent cytokine secretion will play a major role in the future treatment of psoriasis.

REFERENCES

1. GOTTLIEB, A. B. & J. G. KRUEGER. 1990. Arch. Dermatol. **126:** 1083–1086.
2. GOTTLIEB, A. B., B. LIFSHITZ, S. M. FU, L. STAIANO-COICO, C. Y. WANG & D. M. CARTER. 1986. J. Exp. Med. **164:** 1013–1028.
3. GOTTLIEB, A. B. 1988. J. Am. Acad. Dermatol. **18:** 1376–1380.
4. GOTTLIEB, A. B., A. D. LUSTER, D. N. POSNETT & D. M. CARTER. 1988. J. Exp. Med. **168:** 941–948.
5. GOTTLIEB, A. B., C. K. CHANG, D. N. POSNETT, B. FANELLI & J. P. TAM. 1988. J. Exp. Med. **167:** 670–675.
6. GROSSMAN, R. M., J. KRUEGER, D. YOURISH, A. GRANELLI-PIPERNO, D. P. MURPHY, L. T. MAY, T. S. KUPPER, P. B. SEHGAL & A. B. GOTTLIEB. 1989. Proc. Natl. Acad. Sci. USA **86:** 6367–6371.
7. KRUEGER, J. G., J. F. KRANE, D. M. CARTER & A. B. GOTTLIEB. 1990. J. Invest. Dermatol. **94:** 135S–140S.
8. KHANDKE, L., J. F. KRANE, R. ASHINOFF, L. STAIANO-COICO, A. GRANELLI-PIPERNO, A. D. LUSTER, D. M. CARTER, J. G. KRUEGER & A. B. GOTTLIEB. 1991. Arch. Dermatol. **127:** 1172–1179.

Prevention of *In Vivo* Alloreactions by Adoptive Immunotherapy with Lymphokine-Activated Killer Cells

JOSEPH KAPLAN[a,b,c] AND JOSEPH UBERTI[b]

Departments of [a]Pediatrics and [b]Medicine
Wayne State University School of Medicine
Detroit, Michigan 48201

Veto is a relatively recently discovered mechanism for clone-specific control of T cells. Cells with veto activity have the ability to specifically eliminate the precursors of cytotoxic T cells (CTL) which recognize cell surface antigens expressed by the veto cells themselves. Upon recognizing and binding to veto active cells, the CTL precursors are somehow inactivated or destroyed. Although mature cytotoxic T cells have been shown to have veto activity, most veto cells are non-T lymphoid cells. In the course of investigating the nature of cells with veto activity we found that lymphokine-activated killer (LAK) cells have veto activity.[1] When added at relatively low doses to mixed lymphocyte cultures LAK cells specifically block the generation of allospecific CTL directed against their own MHC antigens. At higher doses they show natural suppressor activity, *i.e.,* they nonspecifically inhibit generation of allo-CTL directed against MHC-unrelated targets. Prompted by these *in vitro* observations we proceeded to test the ability of adoptively transferred LAK cells to block *in vivo* alloreactions. Using murine transplantation model systems, we found that administration of recipient-type LAK cells to lethally irradiated recipients of totally allogeneic spleen cells prevented lethal graft-versus-host disease, and that administration of either recipient or donor-type LAK cells inhibited the resistance of irradiated mice to short term growth of allogeneic hematopoietic stem cells.

Whether veto or natural suppression accounts for the ability of LAK cells to prevent alloreactions *in vivo* remains to be determined. Nevertheless, the findings suggest that adoptive immunotherapy with LAK cells might prove useful as a strategy for controlling transplantation alloreactions in human transplant recipients. With that in mind we have sought to determine whether human LAK cells, like murine LAK cells, have veto and nonspecific suppressor activities. LAK cells were generated by culturing peripheral blood lymphocytes for 4 days with 1500 units/ml human recombinant IL-2. Stimulator, responder, or 3rd party-unrelated-type LAK cells were added to MLC on day 0. After 6 days MLC cultured cells were tested in a 4 hr chromium release assay for specific killing of stimulator-type cells. At LAK/responder cell ratio of 1 : 4 veto-type inhibition was observed (TABLE 1). Stimulator-type LAK cells inhibited generation of allospecific CTL 79% whereas responder or 3rd party-type LAK cells failed to inhibit. At the higher LAK/responder cell ratio of 1 : 1 natural suppressor-type inhibition was oberved since all 3 types of LAK cells were inhibitory. LAK proliferation is

---

[c] Address for correspondence: Children's Hospital of Michigan, 3901 Beaubien Blvd., Detroit, MI 48201.

TABLE 1. Veto and Natural Suppressor Activities of Human LAK Cells

MLC	Source of LAK Cells (LAK : Responder)[a]	% Inhibition Target Cell Lysis[b]
ABX	B(1 : 4)	79
ABX	B(1 : 2)	64
ABx	B(1 : 1)	90
ABx	A(1 : 4)	15
ABx	A(1 : 2)	19
ABx	A(1 : 1)	56
ABx	C(1 : 4)	-12
ABx	C(1 : 2)	15
ABx	C(1 : 1)	52

[a] LAK cells added on day 0 of MLC.

[b] % Inhibition $= 100 \times \dfrac{\text{LU}/10^7 \text{ cells without LAK} - \text{LU}/10^7 \text{ cells with LAK}}{\text{LU}/10^7 \text{ cells without LAK}}$

required for inhibition since exposure to 30 Gy irradiation eliminated LAK inhibitory activity (TABLE 2). This and the fact that stimulator-type LAK cells inhibited generation of CTL when added on day 0 and day +2 of MLC but not when added on day +5 just prior to harvest indicates that the LAK cell veto effect is not simply due to "cold target" inhibition and is directed at an early stage in generation of allo-CTL.

Together with the previous findings in animal models, and the fact that large numbers of human LAK cells can be routinely generated from human peripheral blood by culturing lymphocytes obtained by leukopheresis with recombinant IL-2, the observed veto and natural suppressor activities of human LAK cell preparations suggest that LAK cells might prove useful as an adoptive immunotherapy approach to the prevention of transplant rejection and graft-versus-host disease. Moreover, since conjugation of haptens to cell surface membranes of veto-active cells renders these cells capable of preventing generation of hapten-specific CTL, it may be possible to use adoptive immunotherapy with chemically-modified veto-active LAK cells to prevent or ameliorate T cell-mediated autoimmune disorders.

TABLE 2. LAK Inhibitory Activity but Not Cytolytic Activity is Radiosensitive and Affects an Early Event in MLC Generation

Expt	MLC	B LAK Added to MLC	Lysis of Daudi (LU/10⁷ Cells)	Day Added to MLC	Allospecific CTL (LU/10⁷ Cells)
1	ABx	—	—	—	4.2
	ABX	+	19.8	0	0.09
	ABx	+ (30 Gy)	17.0	0	3.32
2	ABx	—	—	—	3.80
	ABx	+	ND[a]	0	1.77
	ABx	+	ND	+2	1.24
	ABx	+	ND	+5	4.70

[a] Not done.

REFERENCES

1. AZUMA, E. & J. KAPLAN. 1988. Role of lymphokine-activated killer (LAK) cells as mediators of veto and natural suppression. J. Immunol. **141:** 2601–2606.
2. AZUMA, E., H. YAMAMOTO & J. KAPLAN. Use of lymphokine activated killer cells to prevent bone marrow graft rejection and lethal graft-vs-host disease. J. Immunol. **143:** 1524–1529.

Release of Oxygen-Free Radicals by Neutrophils Is Reduced by Photopheresis

F. TRAUTINGER,[a] R. M. KNOBLER,[a,c] W. MACHEINER,[b]
C. GRÜNWALD,[a] AND M. MICKSCHE[b]

[a]Second Department of Dermatology
[b]Institute of Applied and Experimental Oncology
University of Vienna
A-1090 Vienna, Austria

In the present study we investigated the effect of extracorporeal photoche-motherapy (EP) on the respiratory burst activity (RBA) of polymorphonuclear neutrophils (PMN). EP is a new treatment modality that has been shown to be beneficial in the treatment of cutaneous T cell lymphoma (CTCL).[1] Its usefulness in other dermatological/immunological disorders (*i.e.*, lupus erythematosus, systemic scleroderma) is currently under investigation.[2,3] During EP white blood cells are exposed to the photoactivatable drug 8-methoxypsoralen (8-MOP) that is activated extracorporeally by irradiation of the cells with ultraviolet A light (UVA) prior to reinfusion.

Neutrophil respiratory burst activity was evaluated in 8 patients who were treated with EP (TABLE 1). The diagnoses of the patients were systemic lupus erythematosus (n = 3), systemic scleroderma (n = 3) and cutaneous T cell lymphoma (n = 2).

PMN of patients treated with EP were isolated from the buffy coat fraction before and immediately after UVA exposure. Dextran sedimentation, ficoll density gradient centrifugation and hypotonic shock were used to obtain PMN cell fractions with less than 1% contaminating mononuclear cells. PMN of healthy donors were used for *in vitro* experiments. Cells were incubated with different concentrations of 8-MOP and 5-MOP (0 ng/ml, 25 ng/ml, 50 ng/ml, 100 ng/ml) under standard conditions. After 20 min of incubation PMN were exposed to UVA (2 J/cm^2) and immediately used for RBA determination. Sham irradiation was performed as a control. Respiratory burst activity was evaluated by two different methods after stimulation of the cells with phorbol-myristate-acetate (PMA, 40 nM).[4] Luminol-amplified chemiluminescence was used for the determination of myeloperoxidase-dependent toxic oxygen metabolites. An assay based on the O_2 dependent reduction of cytochrom-c was used for the determination of superoxide anion (O_2^-).

EP treatment of PMN induced a significant decrease of RBA determined by luminol-amplified chemiluminescence in all patients ($51.9.0\% \pm 19.1\%$, mean $\pm$ SD). No clear correlation between 8-MOP serum levels and inhibition of RBA could be detected (TABLE 1). However, *in vitro* experiments demonstrated that inhibition of chemiluminescence is directly correlated to the concentration of the photoactivatable drug. No difference between the inhibitory effect of 8-MOP and its analog 5-MOP could be observed (FIG. 1). Neither psoralens alone nor UVA alone had a significant effect on RBA. In contrast to chemoluminescence O_2^-

---

[c] Address for correspondence: Dr. Robert M. Knobler, II. Dept. of Dermatology, University of Vienna, Alserstraße 2, A-1090 Vienna, Austria.

TABLE 1. 8-MOP Serum Levels (2 Hours after Oral Administration) and Inhibition of RBA in Patients Treated with EP

Diagnosis[a]	8-MOP in Serum	Inhibition of RBA
CTCL	146 ng/ml	71.2%
CTCL	62 ng/ml	47.5%
SLE	34 ng/ml	66.4%
SLE	164 ng/ml	24.1%
SLE	79 ng/ml	71.2%
SS	14 ng/ml	65.2%
SS	163 ng/ml	30.1%
SS	142 ng/ml	39.6%

[a] CTCL: cutaneous T cell lymphoma, SLE: systemic lupus erythematosus, SS: systemic scleroderma.

release was not significantly affected by photochemotherapy indicating that photochemotherapy has no direct effect on NADPH-oxidase activity, responsible for the generation of superoxide-anions from molecular oxygen. However, the observed reduction of myeloperoxidase dependent oxygen metabolites by EP suggests that, besides DNA-intercalation, photoactivated psoralens may interact with intracellular enzymes involved in respiratory burst of PMN.

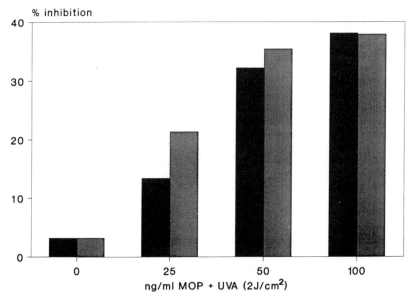

FIGURE 1. Inhibitory effect of photochemotherapy on PMN luminol dependent chemoluminescence. PMN of healthy donors were incubated *in vitro* with different concentrations of 8-MOP (*black bars*) and 5-MOP (*hatched bars*) prior to UVA exposure (2 J/cm^2).

REFERENCES

1. EDELSON, R. L. *et al.* 1987. N. Engl. J. Med. **316:** 297–303.
2. KNOBLER, R. M., *et al.* 1991. Ann. N. Y. Acad. Sci. In press.
3. ROOK, H. L., *et al.* 1989. Yale J. Biol. Med. **62:** 639–646.
4. JOHANSSON, A., *et al.* 1989. J. Leukocyte Biol. **45:** 444–451.

Proto-Oncogene Transcription after Activation of Th-1 and Th-2 Cells[a]

PENELOPE A. MOREL,[b,e] JEFFREY A. WALKER,[c]
ALEXANDRA M. LIVINGSTONE,[d] DAVID J. TWEARDY,[b]
AND J. SCOTT CAIRNS[c]

Departments of [b]Medicine and [c]Pathology
University of Pittsburgh
Pittsburgh Cancer Institute
Pittsburgh, Pennsylvania 15213
and
[d]Basel Institute for Immunology
Grenzacherstrasse, 487
CH-4005 Basel, Switzerland

Murine helper T cells can be divided into two subsets on the basis of the lymphokines they secrete; Th-1 cells secrete IL-2, IFN-γ and lymphotoxin and mediate the delayed hypersensitivity response whereas Th-2 cells secrete IL-4, IL-5, IL-6 and IL-10 and mediate specific B cell help.[1] Recent studies have revealed that there are differences in the responses of these two types of cells to various stimuli. Whereas Th-2 cells can be readily stimulated to proliferate in response to immobilized anti-CD3 or concanavalin A (ConA), Th-1 cells cannot.[2] In addition, Th-1 cells stimulated in either of these ways do not respond well to exogenous IL-2,[3] (FIG. 1). These cells do, however, secrete IL-2 and IL-3 and respond by activation of the known second messenger systems, *i.e.,* an increase in intracellular calcium and activation of protein kinase C.[4]

In order to further dissect this phenomenon we have examined the early molecular events that occur after stimulation of Th-1 and Th-2 clones with various agents. Three T cell clones were examined; one of these is a Th-1 cell (11.3.7) and the 2 others (14.16.12 and Ly1$^+$2$^-$/9) are Th-2 cells. Proliferation assays carried out in the presence or absence of ConA (FIG. 1) demonstrated the induction of unresponsiveness to exogenous IL-2. 11.3.7 (Th-1) proliferated vigorously in response to IL-2, but when the cells were stimulated with ConA this response was abrogated. In contrast 14.16.12 (Th-2) responded to ConA in the absence of IL-2 and the presence of ConA enhanced the response of these cells to IL-2. To study activation-induced proto-oncogene expression the cells were cultured using the following conditions: No treatment, IL-2 alone (5 U/ml), CD3 alone, CD3 + IL-2, immobilized CD3 (XCD3), and XCD3 + IL-2. For the CD3 treatment, cells (30 × 10^6/ml) were incubated for 30 min at 4°C in a 1:1 dilution of culture supernatant containing anti-CD3 antibodies. The cells were washed and placed in culture in 6-well plates (5 × 10^6/ml) that either had or had not been coated with 10 μg/ml anti-hamster Ig. Cells were removed from culture 30 min or 4 hr after stimulation and lysed and RNA was isolated. Northern blot analysis was carried out to

[a] This work was supported by a grant from the Lupus Foundation of America, Inc.

[e] Address for correspondence: The Pittsburgh Cancer Institute, B.S.T., 9th Floor, De Soto at O'Hara Street, Pittsburgh, PA 15213.

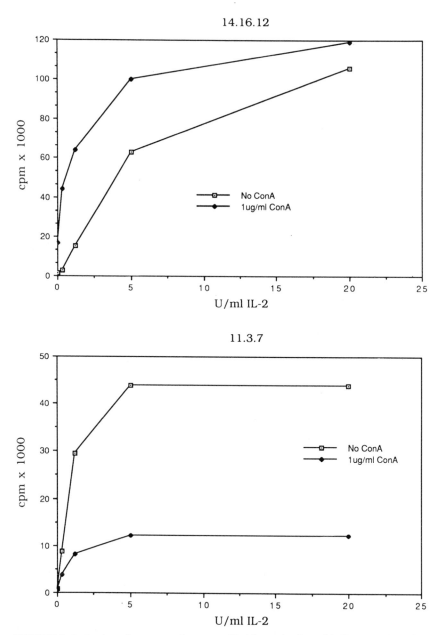

FIGURE 1. Induction of unresponsiveness to IL-2 by activation with ConA. 11.3.7 (Th-1) and 14.16.12 (Th-2) cells were washed and placed in culture in the presence (◆——◆) or absence (□——□) of 1 μg/ml ConA with increasing concentrations of IL-2. Cells were incubated for 48 hr at 37°C after which time the wells were pulsed with 0.5 μCi/well [³H]thymidine. Cells were harvested and counted in a beta scintillation counter, and results are the mean of triplicate wells.

examine the expression of c-fos, c-myc and the proliferation cell nuclear antigen (PCNA).[5]

The results, shown in TABLE 1, demonstrate major differences in the activation requirements of the two cells types. In the case of the Th-1 cell (11.3.7) uncrosslinked CD3 was unable to stimulate expression of c-fos or c-myc. IL-2 provided the strongest stimulus for c-myc in 11.3.7 and XCD3 was the strongest stimulus for c-fos expression. In contrast each stimulus applied to the Th-2 cells was able to upregulate expression of c-myc and c-fos. These data suggest that the requirements for activation of Th-2 cells are less stringent than those required for the activation of Th-1 cells. Thus, whereas both cell types, were induced to express c-myc and c-fos following stimulation with XCD3, only Th-2 cells expressed these proto-oncogenes following stimulation with uncrosslinked CD3.

TABLE 1. Activation Requirements of the Two Th Cell Types

T Cell	Conditions	cpm[a]	c-fos[b]	c-myc[b]	PCNA[b]
11.3.7	unstim	588	−	−	−
(Th-1)	IL-2	30949	+/−	++	+
	CD3	1131	−	−	+
	CD3 + IL-2	30151	+/−	+++	+
	XCD3	812	+++	+	+
	XCD3 + IL-2	4967	+++	++	+
Ly1+2−/9	unstim	245	−	−	−
(Th-2)	IL-2	66177	+	++	+
	CD3	435	+	++	+
	CD3 + IL-2	29645	++	+++	+
	XCD3	1331	++	++	+
	XCD3 + IL-2	31472	++	+++	+
14.16.12	unstim	511	ND	+	−
(Th-2)	CD3	1125	ND	++	+
	XCD3	5107	ND	+++	+

[a] Cells were incubated with anti-CD3 antibodies for 30 min at 4°C. After washing, cells were placed in the presence or absence of 5 U/ml IL-2 and cultured in plates that either had or had not been coated with 10 μg/ml anti-hamster Ig. Aliquots of cells were removed before plating and placed in 96-well plates (2×10^4/well) in the conditions described above. After incubation at 37°C for 48 hr the plates were pulsed for 16 hr with 0.5 μCi/well [^{3}H]thymidine. Cells were harvested and counted on a beta scintillation counter.

[b] Cells were removed from the various culture conditions and lysed 30 min (c-fos) and 4 hr (c-myc and PCNA) after activation.

Interestingly, PCNA, a gene whose expression was previously thought to correlate with proliferation was found to be upregulated in Th-1 and Th-2 cells following any stimulation including those which did not induce substantial levels of [^{3}H-] thymidine incorporation.

Two conclusions are suggested by these data: One is that c-myc and c-fos are independently regulated in Th-1 cells and require different activation signals to be expressed. The second is that, in Th-1 cells, it is possible that the high levels of c-fos expression in response to XCD3 could be responsible for the induction of unresponsiveness to IL-2 observed in these cells. These phenomena could be important in some autoimmune diseases (e.g., systemic lupus erythematosus) that may be associated with an excess of Th-2 cells.

REFERENCES

1. MOSMANN, T. R. & R. L. COFFMAN. 1989. TH1 and TH2 cells: different patterns of lymphokine secretion lead to different functional properties. Ann. Rev. Immunol. **7:** 145–173.
2. JENKINS, M. K., C. CHEN, G. JUNG, D. L. MUELLER & R. H. SCHWARTZ. 1990. Inhibition of antigen-specific proliferation of type 1 murine T cell clones following stimulation with immobilized anti-CD3 monoclonal antibody. J. Immunol. **144:** 16–23.
3. WILLIAMS, M. E., A. H. LICHTMAN & A. K. ABBAS. 1990. Anti-CD3 antibody induces unresponsiveness to IL-2 in Th1 clones but not in Th2 clones. J. Immunol. **144:** 1208–1214.
4. MUELLER, D. L., M. K. JENKINS, L. CHIODETTI & R. H. SCWHARTZ. 1990. An intracellular calcium increase and protein kinase C activation fail to initiate T cell proliferation in the absence of a costimulatory signal. J. Immunol. **144:** 3701–3709.
5. CRABTREE, G. R. 1989. Contingent genetic regulatory events in T lymphocyte activation. Science **243:** 355–361.

Acetylcholine Receptor-Reactive T Cells in Murine Experimental Myasthenia React to All Subunits of the Receptor

ANDREW R. PACHNER, ANDREA ITANO, AND
NANCY RICALTON

Department of Neurology
Georgetown University Hospital
3800 Reservoir Road
Washington, DC 20007

Myasthenia gravis (MG) is an autoimmune disease which spontaneously occurs in humans and is associated with a high titer of autoantibodies to the nicotinic acetylcholine receptor (AChR). Animal models of MG, experimental autoimmune myasthenia gravis (EAMG), exist in which immunization with purified AChR, usually from electric eels or fishes, results in a clinical state mimicking the human disease. As interest in the neurosciences has focused on neural receptor structure and function, the AChR has become an archetypal receptor protein that is important also as an autoantigen.

The immunopathogenesis of MG and role of the T cell in the autoimmune process are unclear. Most theories presume that receptor function is interferred with and AChRs damaged by pathogenic autoantibodies; this theory is supported by the ability of passive transfer to effect disease with either polyclonal antibodies in serum or certain monoclonal anti-AChR antibodies. However, there are some reasons to feel that autoantibodies may not be the only or even the primary pathogenic agent.[1] *E.g.,* many patients with severe MG have no detectable anti-AChR antibodies. In addition, many anti-AChR monoclonal antibodies that bind mouse AChR will not passively transfer disease, and the doses of antibodies needed to cause myasthenia in the passive transfer model are generally quite large. If one, however, assumes that autoantibody is the primary pathogenetic mechanism and that the development of the autoimmune process is T-dependent, then the primary role of pathogenic T cells might be expected to be the recognition of autoantigen and subsequent production of help for B cell clones making anti-AChR antibody.

Our aim for the past few years has been to isolate, grow, and study T cells specific for the AChR. An AChR-specific T cell response can be readily found in the lymph nodes draining the sites of immunization of mice with *Torpedo* AChR. Since whole mouse or human AChR is impossible to obtain at reasonable yields from tissue, synthetic or recombinant peptides of the AChR have been used by many laboratories as antigens in assays of human and animal myasthenic T cells. We have adopted a different approach and are studying the possibility of using native AChR proteins isolated electrophoretically as antigens for AChR-specific T cells. The first question we addressed was the subunit specificity in murine EAMG of T cells specific for *Torpedo* AChR.

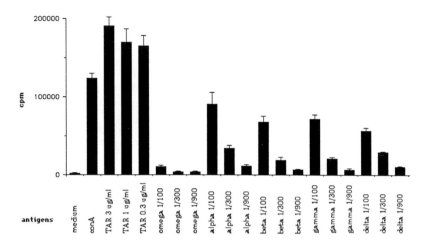

FIGURE 1. AChR and its subunits as antigens for T cells.

MATERIALS AND METHODS

Details of AChR purification, immunizations, ELISA, and *in vitro* culture methodology have been previously described in depth.[2,3]

Torpedo AChR was applied to a polyacrylamide gel, separated into its 4 subunits, the subunits identified at the sides of the gel by amido black staining, and the polyacrylamide cut with a razor along straight lines determined by the subunits. The slabs of polyacrylamide were placed in water and cut into pieces. The proteins were allowed to leach overnight, and the polyacrylamide removed. The proteins were then concentrated, and tested in either SDS-PAGE, ELISA, or lymphocyte proliferation assays.

RESULTS

The separation procedure resulted in electrophoretically pure isolates of AChR subunits (FIG. 1). Use of these subunits as coating proteins in a standard

FIGURE 2.

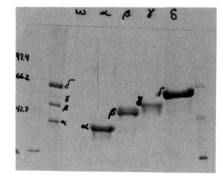

ELISA against serum from mice with EAMG revealed that all four subunits were recognized with very little or no difference in degree of recognition between the four. When the four subunits were used as antigen in proliferation assays using lymph node T cells of mice both singly and multiply immunized with *Torpedo* AChR, excellent proliferation was found to all four subunits (FIG. 2) Proliferation to whole TAR was strong as expected; there was little to no proliferation to polyacrylamide obtained from parts of the gel where none of the subunits was found.

In addition, the separated proteins were used in immunoprecipitation assays using iodinated bungarotoxin and hyperimmune serum. The alpha subunit retained activity in this assay.

DISCUSSION

These investigations answer two questions. The first question is: can receptor subunits be separated electrophoretically and retain antigenic and ligand-binding capacity? and the answer is yes, at least in the case of *Torpedo* AChR. The second question is: is there preferential subunit reactivity of either antibodies or T cells in murine EAMG induced by immunization with *Torpedo* AChR? and the answer is no.

These findings do not rule out the possibility that some peptide sequences may be preferentially identified, to some degree, by T cells for two reasons. First, there are shared stretches of sequences between subunits and, second, the populations of T cells used were polyclonal. In previous studies in which we isolated T cell hybridoma clones were tested for reactivity to synthetic peptides of the alpha subunit, the alpha sequence 146–162 seemed to be a preferential target.

These data also provide confirmation that AChR proteins leached from polyacrylamide can be used as antigens in T cell assays, and raise the possibility that this method of identification of antigenic material may be useful in the study of human myasthenia.

REFERENCES

1. PACHNER, A. R. 1988. Myasthenia gravis, immunology and allergy clinics of North America. **8:** 277–293.
2. PACHNER, A. R. & F. S. KANTOR. 1984. The relationship of clinical disease to antibody titer, proliferative responses, and neurophysiology in murine experimental autoimmune myasthenia gravis. Clin. Exp. Immunol. **56:** 614.
3. PACHNER, A. R. & F. S. KANTOR. 1985. Helper T cell lines specific for the acetylcholine receptor: induction, characterization, and *in vitro* effects. Clin. Immunol. Immunopathol. **35:** 245.
4. PACHNER, A. R., B. MULAC-JERICEVIC, M. Z. ATASSI & F. S. KANTOR. 1989. An immunodominant T cell epitope of the acetylcholine receptor in experimental myasthenia mapped with T cell clones and synthetic peptides. Immunol. Lett. **20:** 199–204.

An Outer Surface Protein Is a Major T Cell Antigen in Experimental Lyme Disease in CB6F1 Mice

ANDREW R. PACHNER, ANDREA ITANO, AND
NANCY RICALTON

Department of Neurology
Georgetown University Hospital
3800 Reservoir Road
Washington, DC 20007

Lyme disease is a protean infectious illness[1] with clinical manifestations primarily in skin,[2] nervous system,[3] joint,[4] and heart. The causative organism is an invasive spirochete, *Borrelia burgdorferi,* which in many ways resembles *Treponema pallidum,* the causative agent of syphilis. Latency of organism in immunocompent humans has been demonstrated by culture of *B. burgdorferi* from skin and CSF months to years after initial infection. The mechanisms the organism uses to establish latency and the reasons for failure of immunosurveillance despite high anti-*B. burgdorferi* antibody titers are unknown. In order to pursue these questions we have established an animal model of Lyme disease by injecting *in vivo* passaged spirochete into susceptible inbred mice.

In infected CB6F1 mice an immune response to the organism develops slowly with an initial IgM response and then an IgG response. Target organs of infection are bladder, spleen, heart, and brain, and spirochetemia is present until significant IgG antibody titers appear. Very little is known about the T cell response to *B. burgdorferi.* In the experiments outlined below we attempted to address the question of whether a significant T cell proliferative response can be measured in the murine model and if so whether any particular protein is preferentially identified by *B. burgdorferi*-specific T cells.

MATERIALS AND METHODS

Growth of *Borrelia burgdorferi* in Kelly's medium, intraperitoneal infection of mice, preparation of *B. burgdorferi* sonicates, and SDS-PAGE of sonicates have been previously described.[5]

Methods for nylon wool column preparation of T cells, and proliferative assay have been previously described with acetylcholine receptor as antigen.[6]

CB6F1 mice were infected with the TLS strain of *B. burgdorferi* (obtained from Julie Rawlings, Dept. of Public Health, Dallas, TX) and immunized into the footpads with 10 micrograms of a sonicate of the spirochete in CFA one month later. Draining lymph node T cells were isolated on nylon wool columns and tested for reactivity by proliferative response to whole TLS sonicate and proteins of the sonicate. Sonicate proteins were separated by SDS-PAGE and transferred to nitrocellulose. The nitrocellulose bands were dissolved in DMSO and particles precipitated with carbonate buffer.

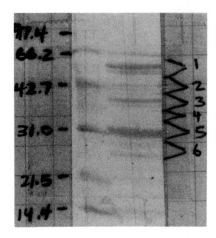

FIGURE 1.

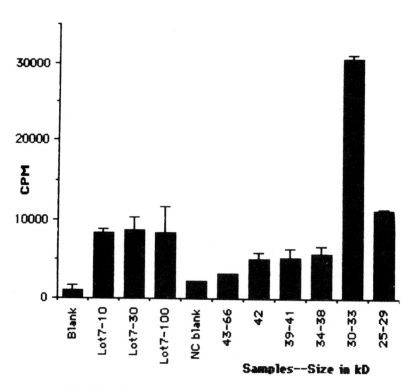

FIGURE 2. Lyme lymph node proliferation—T cell Western.

RESULTS

Separation of *B. burgdorferi* sonicate proteins on SDS-PAGE resulted in multiple bands (FIG. 1) stained on nitrocellose between 20 and 66 kD.

A robust proliferative response was present to 10, 30, and 100 micrograms per ml of sonicate. Although some proliferation could be induced by proteins from each band, the most vigorous response was to proteins of molecular weight 30–33 (FIG. 2), corresponding to the OspA protein.

DISCUSSION

The OspA protein (*outer surface protein A*) is known to be encoded by genes in extrachromosomal DNA, and has been felt to represent a unique protein of *Borrelia burgdorferi* not found in other Borrelia species or other spirochetes. There is generally not a strong antibody response early in the course of infection; proteins of MW 41, 60, 66, and 20 kD are usually major early antigens for the antibody response.

Little is known about T cell responses although it is likely that the T cells are a major regulator of the quantity and quality of the immune response. These experiments have provided the first evidence that OspA may be an important protein in the T cell response, at least in the response of CB6F1 to the TLS strain.

OspA may have considerable heterogeneity in various strains of the spirochete. Should this heterogeneity be manifest at the level of the primary amino acid sequence and OspA prove to be major T cell antigen in humans, this data might significantly limit the potential for vaccine development.

REFERENCES

1. STEERE, A. C. 1983. The spirochetal etiology of Lyme disease. N. Engl. J. Med. **308:** 733–740.
2. BERGER, B. W. 1986. Treating erythema chronicum migrans of Lyme disease. J. Am. Acad. Dermatol. **15:** 459–463.
3. PACHNER, A. R. & A. C. STEERE. 1985. The triad neurologic manifestations of Lyme disease. Neurology **35:** 47–53.
4. STEERE, A. C., R. T. SCHOEN & E. TAYLOR. 1987. The clinical evolution of Lyme arthritis. Ann. Intern. Med. **107:** 725–731.
5. PACHNER, A. R. & A. ITANO. 1990. *Borrelia burgdorferi* infection of the brain—characterization of the organism and response to antibiotics and immune sera in the mouse model. Neurology. In press.
6. PACHNER, A. R. & F. S. KANTOR. 1984. The relationship of clinical disease to antibody titer, proliferative responses, and neurophysiology in murine experimental autoimmune myasthenia gravis. Clin. Exp. Immunol. **56:** 614.

T Cell Receptor Gene Rearrangements in the Human Response to Myelin Basic Protein

J. R. RICHERT,[a] E. D. ROBINSON,[a] R. MARTIN,[b]
H. F. McFARLAND,[b] AND C. K. HURLEY[c]

Departments of [a]Neurology and Microbiology[c]
Georgetown University Medical Center
Washington, DC 20007
and
[b]Neuroimmunology Branch
Building 10, Room 5B-16
National Institute of Neurological Diseases and Stroke
National Institutes of Health
Bethesda, Maryland 20892

We previously reported the existence of multiple human T cell epitopes on the human myelin basic protein (MBP) molecule.[1,2] This suggested, but did not prove, that multiple T cell receptors (TCRs) were utilized in the human T cell response to MBP. The TCR_β gene rearrangements generated by 17 HLA DRw13-restricted T lymphocyte clones (TLCs), isolated from a subject with multiple sclerosis (MS) and reactive with a synthetic peptide corresponding to residues 152–170 of the MBP molecule, were studied by Southern blot analysis. Studies with *Bgl*II, *Eco*RI, *Bam*HI, *Hind*III, and a human TCR_β constant region probe demonstrated 12 different rearrangement patterns, indicating that multiple T cell populations were generated in the human response to this epitope.

Anchored polymerase chain reaction (PCR) was used to sequence the expressed TCR_α genes utilized by 9 of the TLCs and by 4 MBP-reactive T cell lines (TCLs) generated from 3 additional MS patients and a normal subject. Six of the TLCs and one of the MS TCLs expressed V_α 8.2 and a J_α sequence that has not previously been published (TABLE 1). Three of the TLCs and a second MS TCL expressed V_α 3.1 and a J_α gene segment that is nearly identical to that seen in TABLE 1 (TABLE 2). The J_α sequences differ from one another predominantly at the V-J junction. The TCL that expressed V_α 3.1 was monospecific for a synthetic peptide corresponding to residues 86–105 of the MBP molecule and was restricted by HLA DR2. The remaining two TCLs expressed a variety of V_α and J_α sequences (5 from one and 8 from the other). The latter suggests that multiple T cell populations have survived long-term culture of these lines.

The novel J_α gene segment reported here contains conserved J region sequences that indicate that it is indeed a J region segment. Its association with more than one V region strongly suggests that it is not a laboratory contaminant. These findings have been demonstrated in 2 separate PCRs but must still be confirmed by alternative means. Subsequent studies will be performed to determine if there is any association between this J_α usage and the presence of disease. Other than this finding, the TCR_α and $_\beta$ gene usage in the anti-MBP response appears to be quite heterogeneous. This suggests that sensitization of a large

TABLE 1. TCR$_\alpha$ Sequence from a T Cell Clone Expressing V$_\alpha$ 8.2 and a Previously Undescribed J$_\alpha$ Sequence

V$_\alpha$:
5′   ATGGCAGGCATTCGAGCTTTATTTATGTACTTGTGGCTGCAGCTGGACTGGGTGAGC

AGAGGAGAGAGTGTGGGGCTGCATCTTCCTACCCTGAGTGTCCAGGAGGGTGACAAC

TCTATTATCAACTGTGCTTATTCAAACAGCGCCTCAGACTACTTCATTTGGTACAAG

CAAGAATCTGGAAAAGGTCCTCAATTCATTATAGACATTCGTTCAAATATGGACAAA

AGGCAAGGCCAAAGAGTCACCGTTTTATTGAATAAGACAGTGAAACATCTCTCTCTG

CAAATTGCAGCTACTCAACCTGGAGACTCAGCTGTCTACTTTGTGCA   3′

J$_\alpha$:
5′   GAGAACTACCTCGGAGGAAGCCAAGGAAATCTCATCTTTGGAAAAGGCACTAAACTC

TCTGTGAGAACTACCTCTAAACCA   3′

TABLE 2. TCR$_\alpha$ Sequence from a T Cell Clone Expressing V$_\alpha$ 3.1 and a J$_\alpha$ Sequence Similar to That Shown in TABLE 1, but with a Different Sequence at the V-J Junction[a]

V$_\alpha$:
5'   ATGGAAACTCTCCTGGGAGTGTCTTTGGTGATTCTATGGCTTCAACTGGCTAGGGTG
AACAGTCAACAGGGAGAAGAGGATCCTCAGGCCTTGAGCATCCAGGAGGGTGAAAAT
GCCACCATGAACTGCAGTTACAAAACTAG(C)ATAAACAATTTACAGTGGTATAGAC
AAAATTCAGGTAGAGGCCTTGTCCACCTAATTTTAATACGTTCAAATGAAAGAGAAA
AACACAGTGGAAGATTAAGAGTCACGTTGACACTTCGTTCAAATGAAACCAAGAAA
AGCAGTTCCTTGTTGATCACGGCTTCCCGGGCAGCAGACACTGCTTCTTACTTCTGT
GCT   3'

J$_\alpha$:
5'   (ACGGACAATTAT)GGAGGAAGCC(G)AGGAAATCTCATCTTTGGAAAAGGCACT
AAACTCTCTGTTAAACCA   3'

[a] The (C) in the V$_\alpha$ sequence differs from the published sequence for V$_\alpha$ 3.1, which has (T) at that site, instead. The J$_\alpha$ sequences in parentheses denote sites at which this J$_\alpha$ sequence differs from that shown in TABLE 1.

population of MS patients with a restricted number of TCR peptides is unlikely to fully suppress the human T cell response to MBP.

REFERENCES

1. RICHERT, J. R., E. D. ROBINSON, G. E. DEIBLER, R. E. MARTENSON, L. J. DRAGOVIC & M. W. KIES. 1989. J. Neuroimmunol. **23:** 55–66.
2. MARTIN, R., D. JARAQUEMADA, M. FLERLAGE, J. RICHERT, J. WHITAKER, E. LONG, D. MCFARLIN & H. MCFARLAND. 1990. J. Immunol. **145:** 540–548.

Immunological Alterations during Photopheresis and D-Penicillamine Treatment of Systemic Sclerosis

ROBERT L. RIETSCHEL[a] AND E. SHANNON COOPER

[a]*Department of Dermatology*
and
Blood Bank
Ochsner Clinic
and
Alton Ochsner Medical Foundation
1514 Jefferson Highway
New Orleans, Louisiana 70121

An increased T cell helper/suppressor ratio (CD4+/CD8+), an increase in activation markers (activated CD4+ and CD8+ cells) and a decrease in suppressor inducer cells (Leu 18+Leu 3+ or CD45R+4) have been observed in Swedish systemic sclerosis patients.[1] As part of a multicenter randomized comparison of d-penicillamine therapy with extracorporeal photopheresis treatment, we followed changes in immunologic parameters to assess the impact of the two treatments on the immune system.

Eight females and one male with progressive systemic sclerosis were randomly assigned to receive either d-penicillamine or photopheresis therapy. All had had the disease no longer than four years (affecting 30% of the skin surface), evidence of progression, and no therapy affecting collagen metabolism in the antecedent 3 months. The following lymphocyte subsets were measured by fluorescence-activated cell sorter analysis: T cells (Leu 4); T helper cells (Leu 3a); T suppressor/cytotoxic cells (Leu 2a); T helper inducer cells (Leu 3+, Leu 8−); suppressor inducer cells (Leu 3+Leu 18+); Leu 2+Leu 7+ (a cytotoxic subset); activated Leu 2a cells (Leu 2a+Ta1+); activated Leu 3a cells (Leu 3a+Ta1+); helper/suppressor ratio; and helper inducer/suppressor inducer ratio.

Our findings confirmed the alterations noted in Swedish systemic sclerosis patients, including an increase in activated CD4+ and CD8+ cells and a decrease in suppressor inducer cells (Leu 3+Leu 18+) (TABLE 1). While favorable treatment responses were seen in patients treated with both D-penicillamine and photopheresis, only patients with the most significant skin improvement who were treated with photopheresis showed consistent immunologic alterations in activated T cell subsets. In these two patients, a fall in activated Leu 2a cells accompanied by an increase in activated Leu 3a cells was observed. Results in both treatment groups showed a decline in suppressor/inducer cell populations. A decrease in the suppressor/inducer population has previously been related to the duration of disease, and since this decrease occurred regardless of the benefit of treatment on skin sclerosis, it would appear to be a poor correlate of treatment effects.

TABLE 1. Immunologic Features of Progressive Sytemic Sclerosis

Cell Population	Leu #	CD #	Swedish Study		This Study
			Systemic Sclerosis (Average %)	Control (Average %)	Systemic Sclerosis (Average %)
Helper/inducer	3	4	51	53	49.8
Suppressor/cytotoxic	2	8	21	29	20.1
Activated Leu 3	DR+ 3+ / Ta1+ 3a+	—	5.0	2.0	16.2
Activated Leu 2	DR+ 2+ / Ta1+ 2a+	—	9.0	4.5	10.9
Suppressor inducer	3+ 18+	45R + 4	26	55	15.3
Helper inducer	3+ 8−				42.2
Suppressor T	15 + 2	11b + 8	10	12	2.6
Helper/suppressor ratio	3/2	4/8	2.8	1.9	6.5
Helper inducer/suppressor inducer	3+8−/3+18+				

REFERENCE

1. GUSTAFSSON, R., T. H. TOLTERMAN, L. KLARESKOG *et al.* 1990. Increase in activated T cells and reduction in suppressor inducer T cells in systemic sclerosis. Ann. Rheum. Dis. **49:** 40–45.

DAB$_{486}$IL-2 (IL-2 Toxin) Selectively Inactivates High-Affinity IL-2 Receptor-Bearing Human Peripheral Blood Mononuclear Cells

CORY A. WATERS,[a] CATHERINE E. SNIDER,[a]
KYOGO ITOH,[b] LOUIS POISSON,[a] TERRY B. STROM,[c]
JOHN R. MURPHY,[d] AND JEAN C. NICHOLS[a]

[a]Seragen, Inc.
97 South Street
P.O. Box 9104
Hopkinton, Massachusetts 01748
[b]University of Texas
M.D. Anderson Cancer Center
Houston, Texas 77030
[c]Harvard Medical School
and
Beth Israel Hospital
Boston, Massachusetts 02215
[d]University Hospital
Boston University Medical Center
Boston, Massachusetts 02118

The diphtheria toxin-related IL-2 gene fusion protein, DAB$_{486}$IL-2 (IL-2 toxin), has been shown to be selectively cytotoxic to tumor cells which constitutively express high-affinity IL-2 receptors (IL-2R).[1,2] Because these studies underscore the potential utility of DAB$_{486}$IL-2 as a selective immunosuppressive agent in transplantation and autoimmunity, we further investigated the interaction between the fusion protein and resting or activated normal human peripheral blood mononuclear cells (PBMC).

Equilibrium binding studies were performed in order to demonstrate binding of DAB$_{486}$IL-2 to the high-affinity IL-2R on PBMC activated for 72 h with phytohemagglutinin (PHA). Scatchard analysis of these data revealed an average of 1877 high-affinity sites per cell and a K_d of approximately 748 pM (TABLE 1). rIL-2 interacted with a comparable number of sites per cell, but its K_d for high-affinity binding (28 pM) was nearly 25-fold more affinate.

When 72-h PHA-activated PBMC were exposed to DAB$_{486}$IL-2, potent inhibition of (^{14}C)-leucine incorporation was observed, typically occurring at doses $\leq 1 \times 10^{-10}$ M (FIG. 1). The cytotoxic action of DAB$_{486}$IL-2 was blocked by the addition of monoclonal antibodies to either the p75 or p55 subunits of the IL-2R as well as by rIL-2 itself. In addition, a Schild plot of rIL-2 blocking data was linear with a slope of unity, consistent with the observation that DAB$_{486}$IL-2 and rIL-2 compete for a common cellular receptor. Also of interest in this regard is the fact that the IC$_{50}$ for intoxication was characteristically 10-fold lower than the measured K_d. This suggests that the intoxication process mediated by DAB$_{486}$IL-2 is relatively efficient and may require only a small number of occupied receptor sites

TABLE 1. DAB$_{486}$IL-2 Binding Parameters for High-Affinity IL-2 Receptor-Bearing Cells

Cells	Radioligand	Binding Sites/Cell	K_d (pM)[a]
HUT 102/6TG	rIL-2	19579 ± 3079	37 ± 7
	DAB$_{486}$IL-2	9097 ± 1815	682 ± 94
C91/PL	rIL-2	3874 ± 1274	24 ± 16
	DAB$_{486}$IL-2	4640 ± 203	823 ± 147
PHA-activated human PBMC	rIL-2	1730 ± 470	23 ± 1
	DAB$_{486}$IL-2	1877 ± 189	739 ± 16

[a] Average of K_d measurements for the three cell types above: rIL-2, 28 ± 5 pM; DAB$_{486}$IL-2, 748 ± 41 pM.

in order for sufficient fusion toxin to be endocytosed. Resting PBMC with natural killer cell activity, however, were found to be resistant to DAB$_{486}$IL-2 intoxication (IC$_{50}$ ~ 10^{-7} M).[2]

In order to show that DAB$_{486}$IL-2 mediated inhibition of protein synthesis was not merely due to steric blockade of the IL-2R, we examined the ability of activated PBMC to endocytose (^{125}I)-DAB$_{486}$IL-2. Using trypsin-resistance as an index of internalization, we determined that the $t_{1/2}$ of DAB$_{486}$IL-2 internalization (11 min) was not significantly different from that of rIL-2 itself (~5–10 min). In earlier studies we also showed that the extent to which protein synthesis was impaired by DAB$_{486}$IL-2 in IL-2R-expressing cells correlated with inactivation of elongation factor 2, the intracellular target of diphtheria toxin action.[1] These

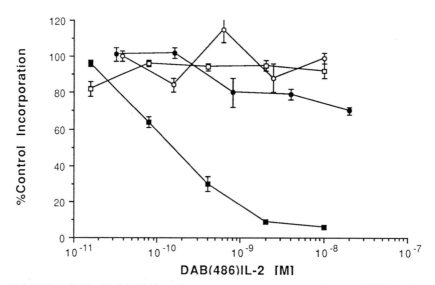

FIGURE 1. DAB$_{486}$IL-2 inhibition of protein synthesis on activated human PBMC is IL-2 receptor-specific. DAB$_{486}$IL-2 was added to 72-h PHA-activated PBMC in the absence (■) or presence of rIL-2 (□), anti-p75 monoclonal antibody (●), or anti-p55 monoclonal antibody (○). Eighteen hours later the cultures were pulsed with (^{14}C)-leucine and the extent of label incorporation determined. Action of the fusion protein was inhibited by all three IL-2 receptor-specific reagents.

observations support the contention that $DAB_{486}IL$-2 mediated inhibition of protein synthesis occurs via a classical toxin-related mechanism.

Because $DAB_{486}IL$-2 has a relatively short serum half-life in humans and primates ($t_{1/2} \sim 10$ min),[3] we investigated both the kinetics with which internalized $DAB_{486}IL$-2 inhibited protein synthesis in activated PBMC and the minimum time the fusion protein must be in contact with the IL-2R. Timed dosing studies revealed that the rate of decrease in protein synthesis essentially obeyed apparent first-order kinetics. At the K_d, half-maximal inhibition of protein synthesis occurred in as little as 4.6 h. Moreover, exposure of activated PBMC to a comparable dose of $DAB_{486}IL$-2 for as little as 15–30 min was sufficient to cause half-maximal inhibition of protein synthesis at the end of an 18-h culture period. Thus, despite its short serum half-life, $DAB_{486}IL$-2 rapidly binds to and intoxicates activated but not resting IL-2R-expressing PBMC, thereby offering a potentially attractive alternative to more broadly immunosuppressive therapies.

REFERENCES

1. BACHA, P., D. P. WILLIAMS, C. WATERS, J. M. WILLIAMS, J. R. MURPHY & T. B. STROM. 1986. Interleukin 2 receptor-targeted cytotoxicity. Interleukin 2 receptor-mediated action of a diphtheria toxin-related interleukin 2 fusion protein. J. Exp. Med. **167:** 612–622.
2. WATERS, C. A., P. A. SCHIMKE, C. E. SNIDER, K. ITOH, K. A. SMITH, J. C. NICHOLS, T. B. STROM & J. R. MURPHY. 1990. Interleukin 2 receptor-targeted cytotoxicity. Receptor binding requirements for entry of a diphtheria toxin-related interleukin 2 fusion protein into cells. Eur. J. Immunol. **20:** 785–791.
3. BACHA, P., S. FORTE, N. KASSAM, J. THOMAS, D. AKIYOSHI, C. WATERS, J. NICHOLS & M. ROSENBLUM. 1990. Pharmacokinetics of the recombinant fusion protein $DAB_{486}IL$-2 in animal models. Cancer Chemother. Pharmacol. **26:** 409–414.

Effect of Prednisolone and Cyclophosphamide on Inhibition of the Response to Alloantigen Induced by Treatment with Photoinactivated Effector T Cells (PET Cells)

YASUHIRO YAMANE, MARITZA PEREZ, LORI JOHN,
AND RICHARD EDELSON

Department of Dermatology
Yale University School of Medicine
333 Ceder Street
P.O. Box 3333
New Haven, Connecticut 06510-8058

Recently using a murine animal model, we showed that inhibition of the *in vivo* (graft rejection and delayed type hypersensitivity (DTH) reaction to alloantigen) and *in vitro* (mixed leucocyte culture and cell-mediated lympholysis) response to alloantigen is induced by immunization of the host with photoinactivated syngeneic splenocytes containing the effector cells of the specific alloantigenic rejection.[1] The hyporesponsiveness to alloantigen is considered to be due to generation of suppressive cell populations capable of inhibiting the response to alloantigen. Herein we investigated the effect of pretreatment with an immunosuppressive agent, prednisolone and an alkylating anticancer drug, cyclophosphamide on the induction of the allogeneic tolerance in this animal model.

Splenocytes from Balb/c(H-2^d) mice undergoing allograft rejection against CBA/J(H-2^k) skin incubated with 100 ng/ml 8-MOP and then exposed to 1 J/cm^2 UVA. After the exposure to UVA, the treated splenocytes containing photoinactivated effector cells (PET cells) of specific graft rejection were intravenously infused into syngeneic recipient mice which were also treated intraperitoneally with either 20 mg/kg prednisolone, 30 mg/kg cyclophosphamide or PBS as control. The injections with PET cells were carried out twice a week for 6 weeks. After 12 infusions with PET cells, the injected Balb/c mice were sacrificed and their splenocytes were adoptively transferred into naive Balb/c mice, in order to exclude a direct effect of the agents on subsequent DTH assay and skin graft survival assay. The data of DTH assay using CBA/J splenocytes as alloantigen showed that the generation of the suppressive cell populations to the alloantigen was reduced by administration of prednisolone (31% suppression) compared with the administration of PBS as control (64% suppression). On the other hand, the administration of cyclophosphamide augmented the induction of the inhibition of the response to the alloantigen (85% suppression) (FIG. 1). In contrast, DTH assay using B10 (H-2^b) splenocytes as irrelevant alloantigen, showed no significant suppression in all groups (FIG. 1), suggesting that the induction and the modulation of the hyporesponsiveness to alloantigen by PET cells and these drugs are alloantigen specific. The results of skin graft survival assay were consistent with those of DTH assay, indicating that the induction of the suppressive cell

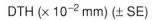

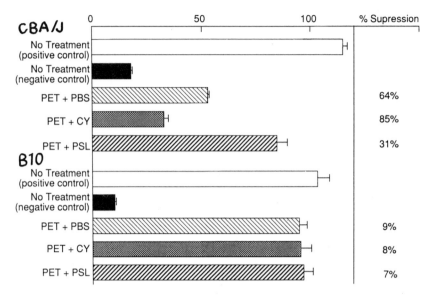

FIGURE 1. Induction of DTH hyporesponsiveness and specificity. Balb/c mice received intravenous infusions of PET cells against CBA/J alloantigen twice a week and intraperitoneal injections of either cyclophosphamide (CY) at 30 mg/kg, prednisolone (PSL) at 20 mg/kg, or PBS as control three times a week. After treatment, the different groups of treated mice were sacrificed and their spleen cells were adoptively transferred into naive Balb/c recipients that were sensitized on the same day with either CBA/J or B10 spleen cells. After 7 days, elicitation was performed and foot pad swelling was measured. Percentage of suppression was calculated from the formula; $100 \times \langle 1\text{-(treated animal-negative control/positive control-negative control)}\rangle$.

TABLE 1. Prolongation of Skin Graft Survival[a]

Group	Donor of Skin	Skin Graft Survival (Days)	Mean Survival Time (± SD)
A) No treatment	CBA/J	8, 8, 9, 8,	8.25 ± 0.50
	B10	9, 9, 9, 9,	9.0 ± 0
B) PET + PBS	CBA/J	16, 14, 14, 15,	14.75 ± 0.96
	B10	9, 10, 9, 10,	9.5 ± 0.58
C) PET + CY	CBA/J	18, 19, 19, 19,	18.75 ± 0.50
	B10	8, 9, 10, 9,	9.0 ± 0.82
D) PET + PSL	CBA/J	9, 9, 10, 10,	9.5 ± 0.58
	B10	8, 9, 10, 8,	8.75 ± 0.96

[a] A one-centimeter-square CBA/J or B10 skin was engrafted onto naive Balb/c recipients of spleen cells from PET-treated mice, pretreated or not with CY or PSL. Grafts were defined as rejected at the time of complete sloughing or when they formed a dry scab.

populations is diminished by prednisolone, on the contrary, is augmented by cyclophosphamide in the alloantigen specific manner (TABLE 1).

These findings indicated that the immunomodulating effects of intravenously administered PET cells can be inhibited by immunosuppressive drugs, such as prednisolone, and actually enhanced by selective alkylating agents such as cyclophosphamide.

REFERENCE

1. PEREZ, M., R. EDELSON, L. LAROCHE & C. BERGER. 1989. J. Invest. Dermatol. **92:** 669–676.

Index of Contributors